P9-DGF-425

*PARZEN • Modern Probability Theory and Its Applications
PILZ • Bayesian Estimation and Experimental Design in Linear Regression Models
PRESS • Bayesian Statistics: Principles, Models, and Applications
PUKELSHEIM • Optimal Experimental Design
PURI and SEN • Nonparametric Methods in General Linear Models
PURI, VILAPLANA, and WERTZ • New Perspectives in Theoretical and Applied Statistics
RAO • Asymptotic Theory of Statistical Inference
RAO • Linear Statistical Inference and Its Applications, *Second Edition*
ROBERTSON, WRIGHT, and DYKSTRA • Order Restricted Statistical Inference
ROGERS and WILLIAMS • Diffusions, Markov Processes, and Martingales, Volume II: Îto Calculus
ROHATGI • An Introduction to Probability Theory and Mathematical Statistics
ROSS • Stochastic Processes
RUBINSTEIN • Simulation and the Monte Carlo Method
RUZSA and SZEKELY • Algebraic Probability Theory
SCHEFFE • The Analysis of Variance
SEBER • Linear Regression Analysis
SEBER • Multivariate Observations
SEBER and WILD • Nonlinear Regression
SERFLING • Approximation Theorems of Mathematical Statistics
SHORACK and WELLNER • Empirical Processes with Applications to Statistics
SMALL and McLEISH • Hilbert Space Methods in Probability and Statistical Inference
STAUDTE and SHEATHER • Robust Estimation and Testing
STOYANOV • Counterexamples in Probability
STYAN • The Collected Papers of T. W. Anderson: 1943–1985
WHITTAKER • Graphical Models in Applied Multivariate Statistics
YANG • The Construction Theory of Denumerable Markov Processes

Applied Probability and Statistics

ABRAHAM and LEDOLTER • Statistical Methods for Forecasting
AGRESTI • Analysis of Ordinal Categorical Data
AGRESTI • Categorical Data Analysis
ANDERSON and LOYNES • The Teaching of Practical Statistics
ANDERSON, AUQUIER, HAUCK, OAKES, VANDAELE, and WEISBERG • Statistical Methods for Comparative Studies
*ARTHANARI and DODGE • Mathematical Programming in Statistics
ASMUSSEN • Applied Probability and Queues
*BAILEY • The Elements of Stochastic Processes with Applications to the Natural Sciences
BARNETT • Interpreting Multivariate Data
BARNETT and LEWIS • Outliers in Statistical Data, *Second Edition*
BARTHOLOMEW, FORBES, and McLEAN • Statistical Techniques for Manpower Planning, *Second Edition*
BATES and WATTS • Nonlinear Regression Analysis and Its Applications
BELSLEY • Conditioning Diagnostics: Collinearity and Weak Data in Regression
BELSLEY, KUH, and WELSCH • Regression Diagnostics: Identifying Influential Data and Sources of Collinearity
BHAT • Elements of Applied Stochastic Processes, *Second Edition*
BHATTACHARYA and WAYMIRE • Stochastic Processes with Applications
BIEMER, GROVES, LYBERG, MATHIOWETZ, and SUDMAN • Measurement Errors in Surveys
BIRKES and DODGE • Alternative Methods of Regression
BLOOMFIELD • Fourier Analysis of Time Series: An Introduction
BOLLEN • Structural Equations with Latent Variables
BOULEAU • Numerical Methods for Stochastic Processes

Continued on back end papers

*Now available in a lower priced paperback edition in the Wiley Classics Library.

BIOSTATISTICS
A Foundation for Analysis
in the Health Sciences

BIOSTATISTICS

A Foundation for Analysis in the Health Sciences

· ·

SIXTH EDITION

Wayne W. Daniel
Georgia State University

John Wiley & Sons, Inc.
New York • Chichester • Brisbane • Toronto • Singapore

Acquisitions Editor   Brad Wiley II
Marketing Manager   Susan Elbe
Production Supervisor   Charlotte Hyland
Designer   Nancy Field
Manufacturing Manager   Susan Stetzer
Illustration   Jaime Perea

This book was set in New Baskerville by Science Typographers and printed and bound by Malloy. The cover was printed by Phoenix Color.

Recognizing the importance of preserving what has been written, it is a policy of John Wiley & Sons, Inc., to have books of enduring value published in the United States printed on acid-free paper, and we exert our best efforts to that end.

Copyright © 1995, by John Wiley & Sons. Inc.

All rights reserved. Published simultaneously in Canada.

Reproduction or translation of any part of
this work beyond that permitted by Sections
107 and 108 of the 1976 United States Copyright
Act without the permission of the copyright
owner is unlawful. Requests for permission
or further information should be addressed to
the Permissions Department, John Wiley & Sons, Inc.

Library of Congress Cataloging in Publication Data:

Daniel, Wayne W., 1929–
    Biostatistics : a foundation for analysis in the health sciences/
Wayne W. Daniel. —6th ed.
      p.   cm.
    Includes bibliographical references and index.
    ISBN 0-471-58852-0 (cloth)
    1. Medical statistics.   2. Statistics.   I. Title
    [DNLM: 1. Biometry.   2. Statistics. WA 950 D184b 1995]
RA409.D35 1995
519.5'02461—dc20
DNLM/DLC
for Library of Congress   94-26060
                                  CIP

Printed in the United States of America

10 9 8 7 6

To my wife, Mary,
and my children, Jean, Carolyn, and John

Preface

• • • • • • • • • • • • • •

This sixth edition of *Biostatistics: A Foundation for Analysis in the Health Sciences* should appeal to the same audience for which the first five editions were written: advanced undergraduate students, beginning graduate students, and health professionals in need of a reference book on statistical methodology.

Like its predecessors, this edition requires few mathematical prerequisites. Only reasonable proficiency in algebra is required for an understanding of the concepts and methods underlying the calculations. The emphasis continues to be on an intuitive understanding of principles rather than an understanding based on mathematical sophistication.

Since the publication of the first edition, the widespread use of microcomputers has had a tremendous impact on the teaching of statistics. It is the rare student who does not now own or have access to a personal computer. Now, more than ever, the statistics instructor can concentrate on teaching concepts and principles and devote less class time to tracking down computational errors made by students. Relieved of the tedium and labor associated with lengthy hand calculations, today's students have more reason than ever before to view their statistics course as an enjoyable experience.

Consequently this edition contains a greater emphasis on computer applications. For most of the statistical techniques covered in this edition, we give the MINITAB commands by which they can be applied. (MINITAB is a registered trademark. Further information may be obtained from MINITAB Data Analysis Software, 3081 Enterprise Drive, State College, PA 16801; telephone: 814/238-3280; telex: 881612.) We also present printouts of the results obtained from the MINITAB calculations. The appendix contains some of the more useful basic MINITAB commands. Included are commands for entering, editing, and sorting data.

We are also, for the first time, including in this edition of *Biostatistics* computer printouts obtained by use of the SAS® software package. We hope that this new feature will be helpful to those students who use SAS® in conjunction with their statistics course.

In response to reviewers and users of previous editions of the text, we have made some major changes in this edition that are designed to make the book more readable, more useful, and more attractive to the student, the professor, and the researcher.

The following are some of the additional specific improvements in the sixth edition of *Biostatistics*:

1. Chapter 1 split. Chapter 1, titled "Organizing and Summarizing Data" in previous editions, has been split into two chapters as follows: Chapter 1 titled "Introduction to Biostatistics" and Chapter 2 titled "Descriptive Statistics." The new Chapter 1 includes the sections on basic concepts and computer usage that were in the old Chapter 1. In addition, the section on measurement and measurement scales, originally in Chapter 11, and the second on simple random sampling formerly in Chapter 4, have been moved to the new Chapter 1. Chapter 2 contains the remainder of the material that has been a part of Chapter 1 in previous editions.

2. Chapter 9 split. Chapter 9, titled "Multiple Regression and Correlation" in previous editions, has been split into two chapters as follows: The section on qualitative independent variables has been moved to a new Chapter 11 titled "Regression Analysis — Some Additional Techniques." To this chapter have been added two new topics covering variable selection procedures and logistic regression. The remaining sections of the old Chapter 9 are now contained in Chapter 10.

3. New Topics. In addition to variable selection procedures and logistic regression, the new topics appearing in this edition of *Biostatistics* include the following:

a. The Type II Error and the Power of a Test (Chapter 7)
b. Determining Sample Size to Control Both Type I and Type II Errors (Chapter 7)
c. The Repeated Measures Design (Chapter 8)
d. The Fisher Exact Test (Chapter 12)
e. Relative Risk (Chapter 12)
f. Odds Ratio (Chapter 12)
g. The Mantel–Haenszel Statistic (Chapter 12)

4. Real Data. In an effort to make the text more relevant to the health sciences student and practitioner, we have made extensive use of real data obtained directly from researchers in the health field and from reports of research findings published in the health sciences literature. More than 250 of the examples and exercises in the text are based on real data.

5. Large Data Sets on Computer Disk. The large data sets that appeared throughout the text in the previous edition are now available only on 3-1/2″ floppy disk and in ASCII file format. Adopters of the text may receive a master copy of the data disk upon contacting:

Brad Wiley II, Editor
College Division
John Wiley & Sons Inc.   *Phone:* 212/850-6027
605 Third Avenue   *Fax:* 212/867-6877
New York, NY 10158-0012   *e-mail:* bwileyii@jwiley.com

The twenty large data sets are designed for analysis by the following techniques: interval estimation (Chapter 6), hypothesis testing (Chapter 7), analysis of variance (Chapter 8), simple linear regression (Chapter 9), multiple regression (Chapter 10), advanced regression analysis (Chapter 11), and chi-square (Chapter 12). Exercises at the end of these chapters instruct the student on how to use the large data sets.

6. Clarity. Many passages and paragraphs within the book have been rewritten in an effort to achieve the highest level of clarity and readability possible. With clarity in mind we have also added new illustrations where it was felt that they would help the reader's understanding of the written material. Many new headings have been added in an effort to highlight important concepts and topics.

7. Design. The sixth edition has been comprehensively redesigned. The new format includes a larger text trim size and typeface as well as bolder chapter titles, section titles, and other pedagogical features of the work. A third of the illustrations have been redrawn. The overall effect should be a more accessible and clearly organized text.

A solutions manual is available to adopters of the text.

For their many helpful suggestions on how to make this edition of *Biostatistics* better, I wish to express my gratitude to the many readers of the previous editions and to the instructors who have used the book in their classrooms. In particular, I thank the following people who made detailed recommendations for this revision:

Howard Kaplan	Towson State University Baltimore, Maryland
K. C. Carriere	University of Manitoba Winnipeg, Manitoba
Michael J. Doviak	Old Dominion University Norfolk, Virginia
Stanley Lemeshow	University of Massachusetts at Amherst Amherst, Massachusetts
Mark S. West	Auburn University Montgomery, Alabama
Dr. Leonard Chiazze, Jr.	Georgetown University School of Medicine Washington, DC
Kevin F. O'Brien	East Carolina University Greenville, North Carolina

I wish to acknowledge the cooperation of Minitab, Inc., for making available to me the latest version of the MINITAB software package for illustrating the use of the microcomputer in statistical analysis.

Special thanks are due to my colleagues at Georgia State University — Professors Geoffrey Churchill and Brian Schott, who wrote computer programs for generating some of the Appendix tables — and Professor Lillian Lin of the Emory University School of Public Health, who read the section on logistic regression and made valuable suggestions for its improvement. I am grateful to the many researchers in the health sciences field who so generously made available to me raw data from their research projects. These data appear in the examples and exercises and are acknowledged individually wherever they appear. I would also like to thank the editors and publishers of the various journals who allowed me to reprint data from their publications for use in many of the examples and exercises.

Despite the help of so many people, I alone accept full responsibility for any deficiencies the book may possess.

Wayne W. Daniel

Contents

• • • • • • • • • • • • • •

BIOSTATISTICS

A Foundation for Analysis
in the Health Sciences

CHAPTER 1

Introduction to Biostatistics

• • • • • • • • • • • • • • • • • • •

CONTENTS

1.1 Introduction

The objectives of this book are twofold: (1) to teach the student to organize and summarize data and (2) to teach the student how to reach decisions about a large body of data by examining only a small part of the data. The concepts and methods necessary for achieving the first objective are presented under the heading of *descriptive statistics*, and the second objective is reached through the study of what is called *inferential statistics*. This chapter discusses descriptive statistics. Chapters 2 through 5 discuss topics that form the foundation of statistical inference, and most of the remainder of the book deals with inferential statistics.

Since this volume is designed for persons preparing for or already pursuing a career in the health field, the illustrative material and exercises reflect the problems and activities that these persons are likely to encounter in the performance of their duties.

1.2
Some Basic Concepts

Like all fields of learning, statistics has its own vocabulary. Some of the words and phrases encountered in the study of statistics will be new to those not previously exposed to the subject. Other terms, though appearing to be familiar, may have specialized meanings that are different from the meanings that we are accustomed to associating with these terms. The following are some terms that we will use extensively in the remainder of this book.

Data   The raw material of statistics is *data*. For our purposes we may define data as *numbers*. The two kinds of numbers that we use in statistics are numbers that result from the taking—in the usual sense of the term—of a *measurement*, and those that result from the process of *counting*. For example, when a nurse weighs a patient or takes a patient's temperature, a measurement, consisting of a number such as 150 pounds or 100 degrees Fahrenheit, is obtained. Quite a different type of number is obtained when a hospital administrator counts the number of patients—perhaps 20—discharged from the hospital on a given day. Each of the three numbers is a *datum*, and the three taken together are data.

Statistics   The meaning of *statistics* is implicit in the previous section. More concretely, however, we may say that *statistics is a field of study concerned with* (1) *the collection, organization, summarization, and analysis of data, and* (2) *the drawing of inferences about a body of data when only a part of the data is observed.*

The person who performs these statistical activities must be prepared to *interpret* and to *communicate* the results to someone else as the situation demands. Simply put, we may say that data are numbers, numbers contain information, and the purpose of statistics is to determine the nature of this information.

Sources of Data   The performance of statistical activities is motivated by the need to answer a question. For example, clinicians may want answers to questions regarding the relative merits of competing treatment procedures. Administrators may want answers to questions regarding such areas of concern as employee morale or facility utilization. When we determine that the appropriate approach to seeking an answer to a question will require the use of statistics, we begin to search for suitable data to serve as the raw material for our investigation. Such data are usually available from one or more of the following sources:

1. *Routinely kept records*   It is difficult to imagine any type of organization that does not keep records of day-to-day transactions of its activities. Hospital medical records, for example, contain immense amounts of information on patients, while hospital accounting records contain a wealth of data on the facility's business activities. When the need for data arises, we should look for them first among routinely kept records.

2. *Surveys* If the data needed to answer a question are not available from routinely kept records, the logical source may be a survey. Suppose, for example, that the administrator of a clinic wishes to obtain information regarding the mode of transportation used by patients to visit the clinic. If admission forms do not contain a question on mode of transportation, we may conduct a survey among patients to obtain this information.

3. *Experiments* Frequently the data needed to answer a question are available only as the result of an experiment. A nurse may wish to know which of several strategies is best for maximizing patient compliance. The nurse might conduct an experiment in which the different strategies of motivating compliance are tried with different patients. Subsequent evaluation of the responses to the different strategies might enable the nurse to decide which is most effective.

4. *External sources* The data needed to answer a question may already exist in the form of published reports, commercially available data banks, or the research literature. In other words, we may find that someone else has already asked the same question, and the answer they obtained may be applicable to our present situation.

Biostatistics The tools of statistics are employed in many fields—business, education, psychology, agriculture, and economics, to mention only a few. When the data being analyzed are derived from the biological sciences and medicine, we use the term *biostatistics* to distinguish this particular application of statistical tools and concepts. This area of application is the concern of this book.

Variable If, as we observe a characteristic, we find that it takes on different values in different persons, places, or things, we label the characteristic a *variable*. We do this for the simple reason that the characteristic is not the same when observed in different possessors of it. Some examples of variables include diastolic blood pressure, heart rate, the heights of adult males, the weights of preschool children, and the ages of patients seen in a dental clinic.

Quantitative Variables A *quantitative variable* is one that can be measured in the usual sense. We can, for example, obtain measurements on the heights of adult males, the weights of preschool children, and the ages of patients seen in a dental clinic. These are examples of *quantitative variables*. Measurements made on quantitative variables convey information regarding amount.

Qualitative Variables Some characteristics are not capable of being measured in the sense that height, weight, and age are measured. Many characteristics can be categorized only, as for example, when an ill person is given a medical diagnosis, a person is designated as belonging to an ethnic group, or a person, place, or object is said to possess or not to possess some characteristic of interest. In such cases measuring consists of categorizing. We refer to variables of this kind as *qualitative variables*. Measurements made on qualitative variables convey information regarding attribute.

Although, in the case of qualitative variables, measurement in the usual sense of the word is not achieved, we can count the number of persons, places, or things belonging to various categories. A hospital administrator, for example, can count the number of patients admitted during a day under each of the various admitting diagnoses. These counts, or *frequencies* as they are called, are the numbers that we manipulate when our analysis involves qualitative variables.

Random Variable   Whenever we determine the height, weight, or age of an individual, the result is frequently referred to as a *value* of the respective variable. When the values obtained arise as a result of chance factors, so that they cannot be exactly predicted in advance, the variable is called a *random variable*. An example of a random variable is adult height. When a child is born, we cannot predict exactly his or her height at maturity. Attained adult height is the result of numerous genetic and environmental factors. Values resulting from measurement procedures are often referred to as *observations* or *measurements*.

Discrete Random Variable   Variables may be characterized further as to whether they are *discrete* or *continuous*. Since mathematically rigorous definitions of discrete and continuous variables are beyond the level of this book, we offer, instead, nonrigorous definitions and give an example of each.

A discrete variable is characterized by gaps or interruptions in the values that it can assume. These gaps or interruptions indicate the absence of values between particular values that the variable can assume. Some examples illustrate the point. The number of daily admissions to a general hospital is a discrete random variable since the number of admissions each day must be represented by a whole number, such as 0, 1, 2, or 3. The number of admissions on a given day cannot be a number such as 1.5, 2.997, or 3.333. The number of decayed, missing, or filled teeth per child in an elementary school is another example of a discrete variable.

Continuous Random Variable   *A continuous random variable does not possess the gaps or interruptions characteristic of a discrete random variable.* A continuous random variable can assume any value within a specified relevant interval of values assumed by the variable. Examples of continuous variables include the various measurements that can be made on individuals such as height, weight, and skull circumference. No matter how close together the observed heights of two people, for example, we can, theoretically, find another person whose height falls somewhere in between.

Because of the limitations of available measuring instruments, however, observations on variables that are inherently continuous are recorded as if they were discrete. Height, for example, is usually recorded to the nearest one-quarter, one-half, or whole inch, whereas, with a perfect measuring device, such a measurement could be made as precise as desired.

Population   The average person thinks of a population as a collection of entities, usually people. A population or collection of entities may, however, consist of animals, machines, planes, or cells. For our purposes, we define a *population of entities as the largest collection of entities for which we have an interest at a particular time*. If we take a measurement of some variable on each of the entities in a population, we generate a population of values of that variable. We may, therefore, define a *population of values as the largest collection of values of a random variable for which we have an interest at a particular time*. If, for example, we are interested in the weights of all the children enrolled in a certain county elementary school system, our population consists of all these weights. If our interest lies only in the weights of first grade students in the system, we have a different population—weights of first grade students enrolled in the school system. Hence, populations are determined or defined by our sphere of interest. Populations may be *finite* or *infinite*. If a population of values consists of a fixed number of these values, the population is said to be *finite*. If, on the other hand, a population consists of an endless succession of values, the population is an *infinite* one.

Sample   A sample may be defined simply as *a part of a population*. Suppose our population consists of the weights of all the elementary school children enrolled in a certain county school system. If we collect for analysis the weights of only a fraction of these children, we have only a part of our population of weights, that is, we have a *sample*.

1.3
Measurement and
Measurement Scales

In the preceding discussion we used the word *measurement* several times in its usual sense, and presumably the reader clearly understood the intended meaning. The word *measurement*, however, may be given a more scientific definition. In fact, there is a whole body of scientific literature devoted to the subject of measurement. Part of this literature is concerned also with the nature of the numbers that result from measurements. Authorities on the subject of measurement speak of measurement scales that result in the categorization of measurements according to their nature. In this section we define measurement and the four resulting measurement scales. A more detailed discussion of the subject is to be found in the writings of Stevens (1, 2).

Measurement   This may be defined as the assignment of numbers to objects or events according to a set of rules. The various measurement scales result from the fact that measurement may be carried out under different sets of rules.

The Nominal Scale   The lowest measurement scale is the *nominal scale*. As the name implies it consists of "naming" observations or classifying them into various mutually exclusive and collectively exhaustive categories. The practice of using numbers to distinguish among the various medical diagnoses constitutes measurement on a nominal scale. Other examples include such dichotomies as male–female, well–sick, under 65 years of age–65 and over, child–adult, and married–not married.

The Ordinal Scale   Whenever observations are not only different from category to category, but can be ranked according to some criterion, they are said to be measured on an ordinal scale. Convalescing patients may be characterized as unimproved, improved, and much improved. Individuals may be classified according to socioeconomic status as low, medium, or high. The intelligence of children may be above average, average, or below average. In each of these examples the members of any one category are all considered equal, but the members of one category are considered lower, worse, or smaller than those in another category, which in turn bears a similar relationship to another category. For example, a much improved patient is in better health than one classified as improved, while a patient who has improved is in better condition than one who has not improved. It is usually impossible to infer that the difference between members of one category and the next adjacent category is equal to the difference between members of that category and the members of the category adjacent to it. The degree of improvement between unimproved and improved is probably not the same as that between improved and much improved. The implication is that if a finer breakdown were made resulting in more categories, these, too, could be ordered in a similar manner. The function of numbers assigned to ordinal data is to order (or rank) the observations from lowest to highest and, hence, the term *ordinal*.

The Interval Scale   The *interval scale* is a more sophisticated scale than the nominal or ordinal in that with this scale it is not only possible to order measurements, but also the distance between any two measurements is known. We know, say, that the difference between a measurement of 20 and a measurement of 30 is equal to the difference between measurements of 30 and 40. The ability to do this implies the use of a unit distance and a zero point, both of which are arbitrary. The selected zero point is not a true zero in that it does not indicate a total absence of the quantity being measured. Perhaps the best example of an interval scale is provided by the way in which temperature is usually measured (degrees Fahrenheit or Celsius). The unit of measurement is the degree and the point of comparison is the arbitrarily chosen "zero degrees," which does not indicate a lack of heat. The interval scale unlike the nominal and ordinal scales is a truly quantitative scale.

The Ratio Scale   The highest level of measurement is the *ratio scale*. This scale is characterized by the fact that equality of ratios as well as equality of intervals may be determined. Fundamental to the ratio scale is a true zero point.

The measurement of such familiar traits as height, weight, and length makes use of the ratio scale.

1.4
The Simple Random Sample

As noted earlier, one of the purposes of this book is to teach the concepts of statistical inference, which we may define as follows:

DEFINITION

Statistical inference is the procedure by which we reach a conclusion about a population on the basis of the information contained in a sample that has been drawn from that population.

There are many kinds of samples that may be drawn from a population. Not every kind of sample, however, can be used as a basis for making valid inferences about a population. In general, in order to make a valid inference about a population, we need a scientific sample from the population. There are also many kinds of scientific samples that may be drawn from a population. The simplest of these is the *simple random sample*. In this section we define a simple random sample and show you how to draw one from a population.

If we use the letter N to designate the size of a finite population and the letter n to designate the size of a sample, we may define a simple random sample as follows.

DEFINITION

If a sample of size n is drawn from a population of size N in such a way that every possible sample of size n has the same chance of being selected, the sample is called a *simple random sample*.

The mechanics of drawing a sample to satisfy the definition of a simple random sample is called *simple random sampling*.

We will demonstrate the procedure of simple random sampling shortly, but first let us consider the problem of whether to sample *with replacement* or *without replacement*. When sampling with replacement is employed, every member of the population is available at each draw. For example, suppose that we are drawing a sample from a population of former hospital patients as part of a study of length of stay. Let us assume that the sampling involves selecting from the shelves in the medical record department a sample of charts of discharged patients. In sampling with replacement we would proceed as follows: select a chart to be in the sample, record the length of stay, and return the chart to the shelf. The chart is back in the "population" and may be drawn again on some subsequent draw, in which case the length of stay will again be recorded. In sampling without replacement, we would not return a drawn chart to the shelf after recording the length of stay, but would lay it aside until the entire sample is drawn. Following this procedure, a given chart could appear in the sample only once. As a rule, in practice, sampling is always done without replacement. The significance and consequences of this will be explained later, but first let us see how one goes about selecting a simple random sample. To ensure true randomness of selection we will need to follow some objective procedure. We certainly will want to avoid using our own judgment to decide which members of the population constitute a random sample. The following example illustrates one method of selecting a simple random sample from a population.

Example 1.4.1

Clasen et al. (A-1) studied the oxidation of sparteine and mephenytoin in a group of subjects living in Greenland. Two populations were represented in their study: inhabitants of East Greenland and West Greenlanders. The investigators were interested in comparing the two groups with respect to the variables of interest. Table 1.4.1 shows the ages of 169 of the subjects from West Greenland. For illustrative purposes, let us consider these subjects to be a population of size $N = 169$. We wish to select a simple random sample of size 10 from this population.

Solution: One way of selecting a simple random sample is to use a table of random numbers like that shown in Appendix II Table A. As the first step we locate a random starting point in the table. This can be done in a number of ways, one of which is to look away from the page while touching it with the point of a pencil. The random starting point is the digit closest to where the pencil touched the page. Let us assume that following this procedure led to a random starting point in Table A at the intersection of row 21 and column 28. The digit at this point is 5. Since we have 169 values to choose from, we can use only the random numbers 1 through 169. It will be convenient to pick three-digit numbers so that the numbers 001 through 169 will be the only eligible numbers. The first three-digit number, beginning at our random starting point, is 532, a number we cannot use. Let us move down past 196, 372, 654, and 928 until we come to 137, a number we can use. The age of the 137th subject from Table 1.4.1 is 42, the first value in our sample. We record the random number and the corresponding age in Table 1.4.2. We record the random number to keep track of the random numbers selected. Since we want to sample without replacement, we do not want to include the same individual's age twice. Proceeding in the manner just described leads us to the remaining nine random numbers and their corresponding ages shown in Table 1.4.2. Notice that when we get to the end of the column we simply move over three digits to 028 and proceed up the column. We could have started at the top with the number 369.

TABLE 1.4.1 Ages of 169 Subjects Who Participated in a Study of Sparteine and Mephenytoin Oxidation

Subject No.	Age	Subject No.	Age	Subject No.	Age
1	27	57	29	113	45
2	27	58	26	114	28
3	42	59	52	115	42
4	23	60	20	116	40
5	37	61	37	117	26
6	47	62	27	118	29
7	30	63	63	119	48
8	27	64	44	120	53
9	47	65	22	121	27
10	41	66	44	122	38
11	19	67	45	123	53
12	52	68	40	124	33
13	48	69	48	125	24
14	48	70	36	126	25
15	32	71	51	127	43
16	35	72	31	128	39
17	22	73	28	129	40
18	23	74	44	130	22
19	37	75	63	131	25
20	33	76	30	132	21
21	26	77	21	133	26
22	22	78	50	134	41
23	48	79	30	135	47
24	43	80	31	136	30
25	34	81	30	137	42
26	28	82	24	138	33
27	23	83	26	139	31
28	61	84	56	140	29
29	24	85	31	141	37
30	29	86	26	142	40
31	32	87	23	143	31
32	38	88	18	144	26
33	62	89	38	145	30
34	25	90	53	146	27
35	34	91	40	147	26
36	46	92	23	148	36
37	24	93	24	149	24
38	45	94	18	150	50
39	26	95	49	151	31
40	29	96	49	152	42
41	48	97	39	153	34
42	34	98	32	154	27
43	41	99	25	155	28
44	53	100	32	156	31
45	30	101	23	157	40
46	27	102	47	158	28
47	22	103	34	159	29
48	27	104	26	160	29
49	38	105	46	161	24
50	26	106	21	162	28
51	27	107	19	163	22
52	30	108	37	164	50
53	32	109	36	165	30
54	43	110	24	166	38
55	29	111	51	167	28
56	24	112	30	168	23
				169	39

SOURCE: Kim Brøsen, M. D. Used with permission.

TABLE 1.4.2 Sample of 10 Ages Drawn from the Ages in Table 1.4.1

Random Number	Sample Subject Number	Age
137	1	42
114	2	28
155	3	28
028	4	61
085	5	31
018	6	23
164	7	50
042	8	34
053	9	32
108	10	37

Thus we have drawn a simple random sample of size 10 from a population of size 169. In future discussion, whenever the term simple random sample is used, it will be understood that the sample has been drawn in this or an equivalent manner.

EXERCISES

1.4.1 Using the table of random numbers, select a new random starting point, and draw another simple random sample of size 10 from the data in Table 1.4.1. Record the ages of the subjects in this new sample. Save your data for future use. What is the variable of interest is this exercise? What measurement scale was used to obtain the measurements?

1.4.2 Select another simple random sample of size 10 from the population represented in Table 1.4.1. Compare the subjects in this sample with those in the sample drawn in Exercise 1.4.1. Are there any subjects who showed up in both samples? How many? Compare the ages of the subjects in the two samples. How many ages in the first sample were duplicated in the second sample?

1.5
Computers and Biostatistical Analysis

The relatively recent widespread use of computers has had a tremendous impact on health sciences research in general and biostatistical analysis in particular. The necessity to perform long and tedious arithmetic computations as part of the statistical analysis of data lives only in the memory of those researchers and practitioners whose careers antedate the so-called computer revolution. Computers can perform more calculations faster and far more accurately than can human technicians. The use of computers makes it possible for investigators to devote more time to the improvement of the quality of raw data and the interpretation of the results.

The current prevalence of microcomputers and the abundance of available statistical software programs have further revolutionized statistical computing. The reader in search of a statistical software package will find the book by Woodward et al. (3) extremely helpful. This book describes approximately 140 packages. Each entry contains detailed facts such as hardware and additional software requirements, ordering and price information, available documentation and telephone support, statistical functions, graphic capabilities, and listings of published reviews. An article by Carpenter et al. (4) also provides help in choosing a statistical software program. The authors propose and define comparative features that are important in the selection of a package. They also describe general characteristics of the hardware and operating-system requirements, documentation, ease of use, and the statistical options that one may expect to find. The article examines and compares 24 packages. An article by Berk (5) focuses on important aspects of microcomputer statistical software such as documentation, control language, data entry, data listing and editing, data manipulation, graphics, statistical procedures, output, customizing, system environment, and support. Berk's primary concern is that a package encourage good statistical practice. A person about to use a computer for the first time will find the article on basic computer concepts by Sadler (6) useful. Reviews of available statistical software packages are a regular feature of *The American Statistician*, a quarterly publication of the American Statistical Association.

Many of the computers currently on the market are equipped with random number generating capabilities. As an alternative to using printed tables of random numbers, investigators may use computers to generate the random numbers they need. Actually, the "random" numbers generated by most computers are in reality *pseudorandom numbers* because they are the result of a deterministic formula. However, as Fishman (7) points out, the numbers appear to serve satisfactorily for many practical purposes.

The usefulness of the computer in the health sciences is not limited to statistical analysis. The reader interested in learning more about the use of computers in biology, medicine, and the other health sciences will find the books by Krasnoff (8), Ledley (9), Lindberg (10), Sterling and Pollack (11), and Taylor (12) helpful.

Current developments in the use of computers in biology, medicine, and related fields are reported in several periodicals devoted to the subject. A few such periodicals are *Computers in Biology and Medicine*, *Computers and Biomedical Research*, *International Journal of Bio-Medical Computing*, *Computer Methods and Programs in Biomedicine*, *Computers and Medicine*, *Computers in Healthcare*, and *Computers in Nursing*.

Computer printouts are used throughout this book to illustrate the use of computers in biostatistical analysis. The MINITAB and SAS® statistical software packages for the personal computer have been used for this purpose. Appendix I at the end of the book contains a list of some basic MINITAB commands for handling data.

1.6
Summary

In this chapter we introduced the reader to the basic concepts of statistics. We defined statistics as an area of study concerned with collecting and describing data and with making statistical inferences. We defined statistical inference as the procedure by which we reach a conclusion about a population on the basis of information contained in a sample drawn from that population. We learned that a basic type of sample that will allow us to make valid inferences is the simple random sample. We learned how to use a table of random numbers to draw a simple random sample from a population.

The reader is provided with the definitions of some basic terms, such as variable and sample, that are used in the study of statistics. We also discussed measurement and defined four measurement scales—nominal, ordinal, interval, and ratio.

Finally we discussed the importance of computers in the performance of the activities involved in statistics.

REVIEW QUESTIONS AND EXERCISES

1. Explain what is meant by descriptive statistics.

2. Explain what is meant by inferential statistics.

3. Define:
   a. Statistics
   b. Biostatistics
   c. Variable
   d. Quantitative variable
   e. Qualitative variable
   f. Random variable
   g. Population
   h. Finite population
   i. Infinite population
   j. Sample
   k. Discrete variable
   l. Continuous variable
   m. Simple random sample.
   n. Sampling with replacement.
   o. Sampling without replacement.

4. Define the word *measurement*.

5. List in order of sophistication and describe the four measurement scales.

6. For each of the following variables indicate whether it is quantitative or qualitative and specify the measurement scale that is employed when taking measurements on each:
   a. Class standing of the members of this class relative to each other.
   b. Admitting diagnosis of patients admitted to a mental health clinic.
   c. Weights of babies born in a hospital during a year.
   d. Gender of babies born in a hospital during a year.
   e. Range of motion of elbow joint of students enrolled in a university health sciences curriculum.
   f. Under-arm temperature of day-old infants born in a hospital.

7. For each of the following situations, answer questions a through e:

    a. What is the sample in the study?

    b. What is the population?

    c. What is the variable of interest?

    d. How many measurements were used in calculating the reported results?

    e. What measurement scale was used?

      Situation A. A study of 300 households in a small southern town revealed that 20 percent had at least one school-age child present.

      Situation B. A study of 250 patients admitted to a hospital during the past year revealed that, on the average, the patients lived 15 miles from the hospital.

REFERENCES

References Cited

1. S. S. Stevens, "On the Theory of Scales of Measurement," *Science*, *103* (1946), 677–680.

2. S. S. Stevens, "Mathematics, Measurement and Psychophysics," in S. S. Stevens (editor), *Handbook of Experimental Psychology*, Wiley, New York, 1951.

3. Wayne A. Woodward, Alan C. Elliott, Henry L. Gray, and Douglas C. Matlock, *Directory of Statistical Microcomputer Software*, *1988 Edition*, Marcel Dekker, New York, 1987.

4. James Carpenter, Dennis Deloria, and David Morganstein, "Statistical Software for Microcomputers," *Byte*, April (1984), 234–264.

5. Kenneth N. Berk, "Effective Microcomputer Statistical Software," *The American Statistician*, *41* (1987), 222–228.

6. Charles Sadler, "A Primer for the Novice: Basic Computer Concepts," *Orthopedic Clinics of North America*, *17* (October 1986), 515–517.

7. George S. Fishman, *Concepts and Methods in Discrete Event Digital Simulation*, Wiley, New York, 1973.

8. Sidney O. Krasnoff, *Computers in Medicine*, Charles C. Thomas, Springfield, Ill., 1967.

9. Robert Steven Ledley, *Use of Computers in Biology and Medicine*, McGraw-Hill, New York, 1965.

10. Donald A. B. Lindberg, *The Computer and Medical Care*, Charles C. Thomas, Springfield, Ill., 1968.

11. Theodor D. Sterling and Seymour V. Pollack, *Computers and the Life Sciences*, Columbia University Press, New York, 1965.

12. Thomas R. Taylor, *The Principles of Medical Computing*, Blackwell Scientific Publications, Oxford, 1967.

Applications Reference

A-1. Knud Clasen, Laila Madsen, Kim Brøsen, Kurt Albøge, Susan Misfeldt, and Lars F. Gram, "Sparteine and Mephenytoin Oxidation: Genetic Polymorphisms in East and West Greenland," *Clinical Pharmacology* & *Therapeutics*, *49* (1991), 624–631.

CHAPTER 2

Descriptive Statistics

● ●

CONTENTS

2.1
Introduction

In Chapter 1 we stated that the taking of a measurement and the process of counting yield numbers that contain information. The objective of the person applying the tools of statistics to these numbers is to determine the nature of this information. This task is made much easier if the numbers are organized and summarized. When measurements of a random variable are taken on the entities of a population or sample, the resulting values are made available to the researcher or statistician as a mass of unordered data. Measurements that have not been organized, summarized, or otherwise manipulated are called *raw data*. Unless the number of observations is extremely small, it will be unlikely that these raw data will impart much information until they have been put in some kind of order.

In this chapter we learn several techniques for organizing and summarizing data so that we may more easily determine what information they contain. The ultimate in summarization of data is the calculation of a single number that in some way conveys important information about the data from which it was calculated. Such single numbers that are used to describe data are called *descriptive measures*. After studying this chapter you will be able to compute several descriptive measures for both populations and samples of data.

2.2
The Ordered Array

A first step in organizing data is the preparation of an *ordered array*. An *ordered array* is a listing of the values of a collection (either population or sample) in order of magnitude from the smallest value to the largest value. If the number of measurements to be ordered is of any appreciable size, the use of a computer to prepare the ordered array is highly desirable.

An ordered array enables one to determine quickly the value of the smallest measurement, the value of the largest measurement, and other facts about the arrayed data that might be needed in a hurry. We illustrate the construction of an ordered array with the data discussed in Example 1.4.1.

Example 2.2.1   Table 1.4.1 contains a list of the ages of subjects who participated in the study of Greenland residents discussed in Example 1.4.1. As can be seen, this unordered table requires considerable searching for us to ascertain such elementary information as the age of the youngest and oldest subjects.

Solution: Table 2.2.1 presents the data of Table 1.4.1 in the form of an ordered array. By referring to Table 2.2.1 we are able to determine quickly the age of the

TABLE 2.2.1 Ordered Array of Ages of Subjects from Table 1.4.1

18	18	19	19	20	21	21	21	22	22	22	22	22
22	23	23	23	23	23	23	23	24	24	24	24	24
24	24	24	24	25	25	25	25	26	26	26	26	26
26	26	26	26	26	26	27	27	27	27	27	27	27
27	27	27	28	28	28	28	28	28	28	29	29	29
29	29	29	29	29	30	30	30	30	30	30	30	30
30	30	31	31	31	31	31	31	31	32	32	32	32
32	33	33	33	34	34	34	34	34	35	36	36	36
37	37	37	37	37	38	38	38	38	38	39	39	39
40	40	40	40	40	40	41	41	41	42	42	42	42
43	43	43	44	44	44	45	45	45	46	46	47	47
47	47	48	48	48	48	48	48	49	49	50	50	50
51	51	52	52	53	53	53	53	56	61	62	63	63

youngest subject (18), and the age of the oldest subject (63). We also readily note that about three-fourths of the subjects are under 40 years of age.

Computer Analysis If additional computations and organization of a data set have to be done by hand, the work may be facilitated by working from an ordered array. If the data are to be analyzed by a computer, it may be undesirable to prepare an ordered array, unless one is needed for reference purposes or for some other use. A computer does not need to first construct an ordered array before constructing frequency distributions and performing other analyses of the data.

If an ordered array is desired, most computer software packages contain routines for its construction. Suppose, for example, that we are using MINITAB and that the ages in Table 1.4.1 exist in Column 1. The command SORT C1 C2 will sort the ages and put them in Column 2 as shown in Table 2.2.1.

2.3
Grouped Data —
The Frequency Distribution

Although a set of observations can be made more comprehensible and meaningful by means of an ordered array, further useful summarization may be achieved by grouping the data. Before the days of computers one of the main objectives in grouping large data sets was to facilitate the calculation of various descriptive measures such as percentages and averages. Because computers can perform these calculations on large data sets without first grouping the data, the main purpose in grouping data now is summarization. One must bear in mind that data contain information and that summarization is a way of making it easier to determine the nature of this information.

To group a set of observations we select a set of contiguous, nonoverlapping intervals such that each value in the set of observations can be placed in one, and only one, of the intervals. These intervals are usually referred to as *class intervals*.

One of the first considerations when data are to be grouped is how many intervals to include. Too few intervals are undesirable because of the resulting loss of information. On the other hand, if too many intervals are used, the objective of summarization will not be met. The best guide to this, as well as to other decisions to be made in grouping data, is your knowledge of the data. It may be that class intervals have been determined by precedent, as in the case of annual tabulations, when the class intervals of previous years are maintained for comparative purposes. A commonly followed rule of thumb states that there should be no fewer than six intervals and no more than 15. If there are fewer than six intervals the data have been summarized too much and the information they contain has been lost. If there are more than 15 intervals the data have not been summarized enough.

Those who wish more specific guidance in the matter of deciding how many class intervals are needed may use a formula given by Sturges (1). This formula gives $k = 1 + 3.322(\log_{10} n)$, where k stands for the number of class intervals and n is the number of values in the data set under consideration. The answer obtained by applying *Sturges' rule* should not be regarded as final, but should be considered as a guide only. The number of class intervals specified by the rule should be increased or decreased for convenience and clear presentation.

Suppose, for example, that we have a sample of 275 observations that we want to group. The logarithm to the base 10 of 275 is 2.4393. Applying Sturges' formula gives $k = 1 + 3.322(2.4393) \simeq 9$. In practice, other considerations might cause us to use 8 or fewer or perhaps 10 or more class intervals.

Another question that must be decided regards the width of the class intervals. Although this is sometimes impossible, class intervals generally should be of the same width. This width may be determined by dividing the range by k, the number of class intervals. Symbolically, the class interval width is given by

$$ w = \frac{R}{k} \tag{2.3.1} $$

where R (the range) is the difference between the smallest and the largest observation in the data set. As a rule this procedure yields a width that is inconvenient for use. Again, we may exercise our good judgment and select a width (usually close to the one given by Equation 2.3.1) that is more convenient.

There are other rules of thumb that are helpful in setting up useful class intervals. When the nature of the data make them appropriate, class interval widths of 5 units, 10 units, and widths that are multiples of 10 tend to make the summarization more comprehensible. When these widths are employed it is generally good practice to have the lower limit of each interval end in a zero or 5. Usually class intervals are ordered from smallest to largest; that is, the first class interval contains the smaller measurements and the last class interval contains the larger measurements. When this is the case, the lower limit of the first class interval should be equal to or smaller than the smallest measurement in the data set, and the upper limit of the last class interval should be equal to or greater than the largest measurement.

Although most microcomputer software packages contain routines for constructing class intervals, they frequently require user input regarding interval widths and the number of intervals desired. Let us use the 169 ages shown in Table 1.4.1 and arrayed in Table 2.2.1 to illustrate the construction of a frequency distribution.

Example 2.3.1   We wish to know how many class intervals to have in the frequency distribution of the data. We also want to know how wide the intervals should be.

Solution: To get an idea as to the number of class intervals to use, we can apply Sturges' rule to obtain

$$k = 1 + 3.322(\log 169)$$

$$= 1 + 3.322(2.227886705)$$

$$\approx 8$$

Now let us divide the range by 8 to get some idea about the class interval width. We have

$$\frac{R}{k} = \frac{63 - 18}{8} = \frac{45}{8} = 5.625$$

It is apparent that a class interval width of 5 or 10 will be more convenient to use, as well as more meaningful to the reader. Suppose we decide on 10. We may now construct our intervals. Since the smallest value in Table 2.2.1 is 18 and the largest value is 63, we may begin our intervals with 10 and end with 69. This gives the following intervals:

10–19
20–29
30–39
40–49
50–59
60–69

We see that there are six of these intervals, two fewer than the number suggested by Sturges' rule.

When we group data manually, determining the number of values falling into each class interval is merely a matter of looking at the ordered array and counting the number of observations falling in the various intervals. When we do this for our example, we have Table 2.2.2.

A table such as Table 2.2.2 is called a *frequency distribution*. This table shows the way in which the values of the variable are distributed among the specified class intervals. By consulting it, we can determine the frequency of occurrence of values within any one of the class intervals shown.

Relative Frequencies It may be useful at times to know the proportion, rather than the number, of values falling within a particular class interval. We obtain this information by dividing the number of values in the particular class interval by the total number of values. If, in our example, we wish to know the

TABLE 2.2.2 Frequency Distribution of Ages of
169 Subjects Shown in Tables 1.4.1 and 2.2.1

Class Interval	Frequency
10–19	4
20–29	66
30–39	47
40–49	36
50–59	12
60–69	4
Total	169

proportion of values between 30 and 39, inclusive, we divide 47 by 169, obtaining
.2781. Thus we say that 47 out of 169, or 47/169ths, or .2781, of the values
are between 30 and 39. Multiplying .2781 by 100 gives us the percentage of values
between 30 and 39. We can say, then, that 27.81 percent of the subjects
are between 30 and 39 years of age. We may refer to the proportion of values
falling within a class interval as the *relative frequency of occurrence* of values in that
interval.

In determining the frequency of values falling within two or more class
intervals, we obtain the sum of the number of values falling within the class
intervals of interest. Similarly, if we want to know the relative frequency of
occurrence of values falling within two or more class intervals, we add the
respective relative frequencies. We may sum, or *cumulate*, the frequencies and
relative frequencies to facilitate obtaining information regarding the frequency or
relative frequency of values within two or more contiguous class intervals. Table
2.2.3 shows the data of Table 2.2.2 along with the *cumulative frequencies,* the *relative
frequencies*, and *cumulative relative frequencies*.

Suppose that we are interested in the relative frequency of values between 30
and 59. We use the cumulative relative frequency column of Table 2.2.3 and
subtract .4142 from .9763, obtaining .5621.

TABLE 2.2.3 Frequency, Cumulative Frequency, Relative Frequency, and Cumulative
Relative Frequency Distributions of the Ages of Subjects Described in Example 1.4.1

Class Interval	Frequency	Cumulative Frequency	Relative Frequency	Cumulative Relative Frequency
10–19	4	4	.0237	.0237
20–29	66	70	.3905	.4142
30–39	47	117	.2781	.6923
40–49	36	153	.2130	.9053
50–59	12	165	.0710	.9763
60–69	4	169	.0237	1.0000
Total	169		1.0000	

The Histogram We may display a frequency distribution (or a relative frequency distribution) graphically in the form of a *histogram*, which is a special type of bar graph. Figure 2.3.1 is the histogram of the ages of the subjects shown in Table 2.2.2.

When we construct a histogram the values of the variable under consideration are represented by the horizontal axis, while the vertical axis has as its scale the frequency (or relative frequency if desired) of occurrence. Above each class interval on the horizontal axis a rectangular bar, or cell, as it is sometimes called, is erected so that the height corresponds to the respective frequency. The cells of a histogram must be joined and, to accomplish this, we must take into account the true boundaries of the class intervals to prevent gaps from occurring between the cells of our graph.

The level of precision observed in reported data that are measured on a continuous scale indicates some order of rounding. The order of rounding reflects either the reporter's personal preference or the limitations of the measuring instrument employed. When a frequency distribution is constructed from the data, the class interval limits usually reflect the degree of precision of the raw data. This has been done in our illustrative example. We know, however, that some of the values falling in the second class interval, for example, when measured precisely, would probably be a little less than 20 and some would be a little greater than 29. Considering the underlying continuity of our variable, and assuming that the data were rounded to the nearest whole number, we find it convenient to think of 19.5

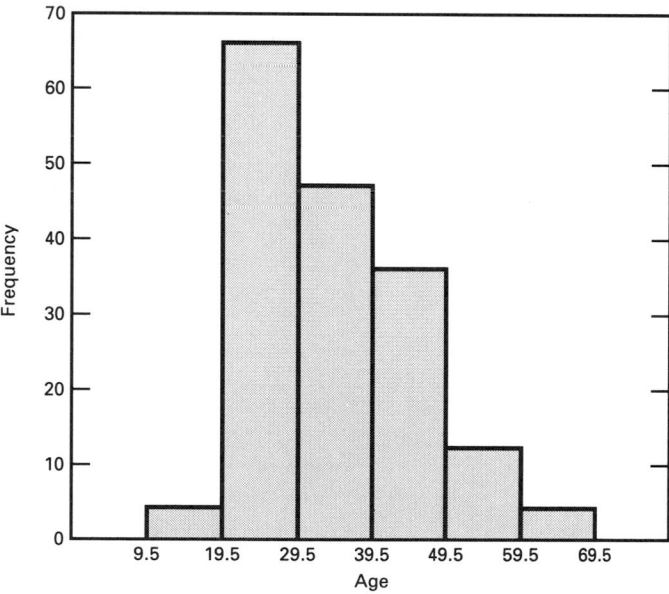

Figure 2.3.1 Histogram of ages of 169 subjects from Table 2.2.2.

TABLE 2.2.4 The Data of Table 2.2.2 Showing True Class Limits

True Class Limits	Frequency
9.5–19.5	4
19.5–29.5	66
29.5–39.5	47
39.5–49.5	36
49.5–59.5	12
59.5–69.5	4
Total	169

and 29.5 as the *true limits* of this second interval. The true limits for each of the class intervals, then, we take to be as shown in Table 2.2.4.

If we draw a graph using these class limits as the base of our rectangles, no gaps will result, and we will have the histogram shown in Figure 2.3.1. Consider the space enclosed by the horizontal axis and the exterior boundary formed by the bars in Figure 2.3.1. We refer to this space as the *area* of the histogram.

Each observation is allotted one unit of this area. Since we have 169 observations, the histogram consists of a total of 169 units. Each cell contains a certain proportion of the total area, depending on the frequency. The second cell, for example, contains 66/169 of the area. This, as we have learned, is the relative frequency of occurrence of values between 19.5 and 29.5. From this we see that subareas of the histogram defined by the cells correspond to the frequencies of occurrence of values between the horizontal scale boundaries of the areas. The ratio of a particular subarea to the total area of the histogram is equal to the relative frequency of occurrence of values between the corresponding points on the horizontal axis.

Computer Analysis   Many computer software packages contain programs for the construction of histograms. One such package is MINITAB. Figure 2.3.2 shows the histogram constructed from the age data in Table 2.2.1 by the MINITAB program. After the data were entered into the computer, the computer was instructed to construct a histogram with a first midpoint of 14.5 and an interval

```
Midpoint    Count
   14.5        4    **
   24.5       66    ********************************
   34.5       47    ***********************
   44.5       36    *****************
   54.5       12    ******
   64.5        4    **
```

Figure 2.3.2   Computer-constructed histogram using the ages from Table 2.2.1 and the MINITAB software package.

width of 10. With the data stored in column 1, the MINITAB commands are as follows:

```
HISTOGRAM C1;
INCREMENT 10;
START AT 14.5.
```

The Frequency Polygon A frequency distribution can be portrayed graphically in yet another way by means of a *frequency polygon*, which is a special kind of line graph. To draw a frequency polygon we first place a dot above the midpoint of each class interval represented on the horizontal axis of a graph like the one shown in Figure 2.3.1. The height of a given dot above the horizontal axis corresponds to the frequency of the relevant class interval. Connecting the dots by straight lines produces the frequency polygon. Figure 2.3.3 is the frequency polygon for the ages data in Table 2.2.1.

Note that the polygon is brought down to the horizontal axis at the ends at points that would be the midpoints if there were an additional cell at each end of the corresponding histogram. This allows for the total area to be enclosed. The total area under the frequency polygon is equal to the area under the histogram. Figure 2.3.4 shows the frequency polygon of Figure 2.3.3 superimposed on the histogram of Figure 2.3.1. This figure allows you to see, for the same set of data, the relationship between the two graphic forms.

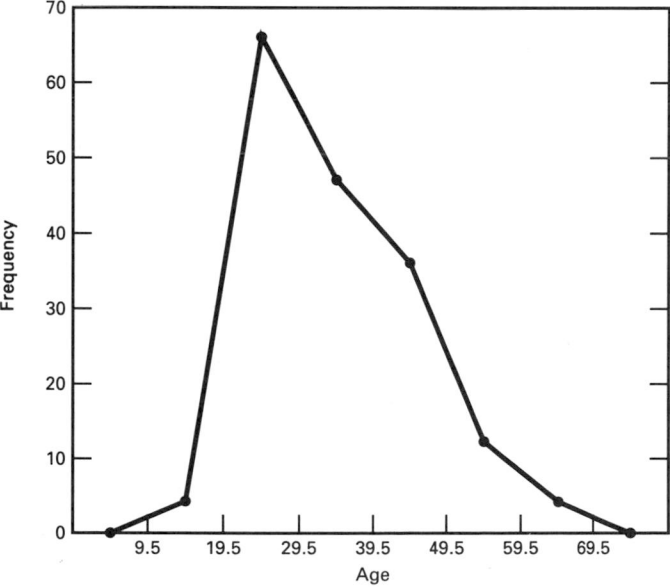

Figure 2.3.3 Frequency polygon for the ages of 169 subjects shown in Table 2.2.1.

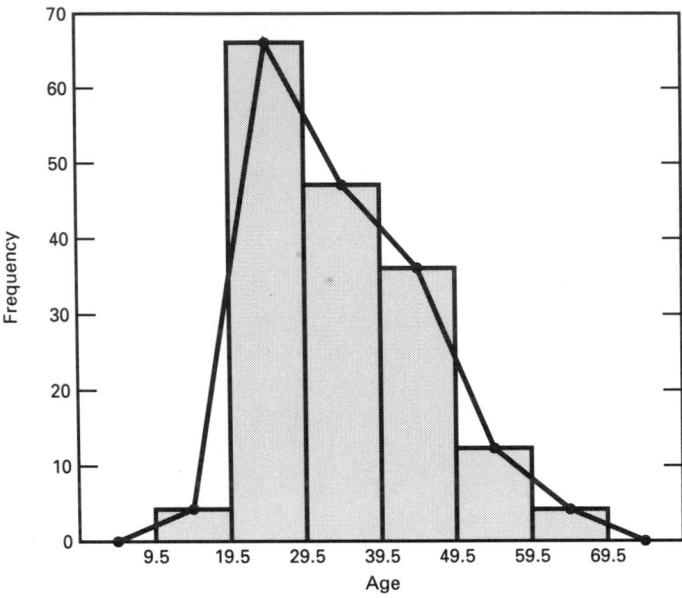

Figure 2.3.4 Histogram and frequency polygon for the ages of 169 subjects shown in Table 2.2.1.

Stem-and-Leaf Displays   Another graphical device that is useful for representing relatively small quantitative data sets is the *stem-and-leaf display*. A stem-and-leaf display bears a strong resemblance to a histogram and serves the same purpose. A properly constructed stem-and-leaf display, like a histogram, provides information regarding the range of the data set, shows the location of the highest concentration of measurements, and reveals the presence or absence of symmetry. An advantage of the stem-and-leaf display over the histogram is the fact that it preserves the information contained in the individual measurements. Such information is lost when measurements are assigned to the class intervals of a histogram. As will become apparent, another advantage of stem-and-leaf displays is the fact that they can be constructed during the tallying process, so the intermediate step of preparing an ordered array is eliminated.

To construct a stem-and-leaf display we partition each measurement into two parts. The first part is called the *stem*, and the second part is called the *leaf*. The stem consists of one or more of the initial digits of the measurement, and the leaf is composed of one or more of the remaining digits. All partitioned numbers are shown together in a single display; the stems form an ordered column with the smallest stem at the top and the largest at the bottom. We include in the stem column all stems within the range of the data even when a measurement with that stem is not in the data set. The rows of the display contain the leaves, ordered and listed to the right of their respective stems. When leaves consist of more than one digit, all digits after the first may be deleted. Decimals when present in the original data are omitted in the stem-and-leaf display. The stems are separated from their leaves by a vertical line. Thus we see that a stem-and-leaf display is also an ordered array of the data.

Stem-and-leaf displays are most effective with relatively small data sets. As a rule they are not suitable for use in annual reports or other communications aimed at the general public. They are primarily of value in helping researchers and decision makers understand the nature of their data. Histograms are more appropriate for externally circulated publications. The following example illustrates the construction of a stem-and-leaf display.

Example 2.3.2

Let us use the age data shown in Table 2.2.1 to construct a stem-and-leaf display.

Solution: Since the measurements are all two-digit numbers, we will have one-digit stems and one-digit leaves. For example, the measurement 18 has a stem of 1 and a leaf of 8. Figure 2.3.5 shows the stem-and-leaf display for the data.

The MINITAB statistical software package may be used to construct stem-and-leaf displays. Figure 2.3.6 shows, for the age data in Table 2.2.1, the stem-and-leaf display constructed by MINITAB.

```
Stem   Leaf

   1 | 8899
   2 | 011122222233333334444444445555666666666667777777777888888899999999
   3 | 00000000000111111122222333444445666777778888899
   4 | 0000001112222333444555667777788888899
   5 | 000112233336
   6 | 1233
```

Figure 2.3.5 Stem-and-leaf display of ages of 169 subjects shown in Table 2.2.1 (stem unit = 10, leaf unit = 1).

```
Stem-and-leaf of c1  N = 169
Leaf unit = 1.0
    4   1  8899
   70   2  011122222233333334444444445555666666666667777777777888888899999999 +
  (47)  3  00000000000111111122222333444445666777778888899
   52   4  0000001112222333444555667777788888899
   16   5  000112233336
    4   6  1233
```

Figure 2.3.6 Stem-and-leaf display prepared by MINITAB from the data on subjects' ages shown in Table 2.2.1.

With the data in column 1, the MINITAB commands are as follows:

```
STEM AND LEAF C1;
INCREMENT 10.
```

The increment subcommand specifies the distance from one stem to the next. The numbers in the leftmost column of Figure 2.3.6 provide information regarding the number of observations (leaves) on a given line and above or the number of observations on a given line and below. For example, the number 70 on the second line shows that there are 70 observations (or leaves) on that line and the one above it. The number 52 on the fourth line from the top tells us that there are 52 observations on that line and all the ones below. The number in parentheses tells us that there are 47 observations on that line. The parentheses mark the line containing the middle observation if the total number of observations is odd or the two middle observations if the total number of observations is even.

The + at the end of the second line in Figure 2.3.6 indicates that the frequency for that line (age group 20 through 29) exceeds the line capacity, and that there is at least one additional leaf that is not shown. In this case, the frequency for the 20–29 age group was 66. The line contains only 65 leaves, so the + indicates that there is one more leaf, a 9, that is not shown.

One way to avoid exceeding the capacity of a line is to have more lines. This is accomplished by making the distance between lines shorter; that is, by decreasing the widths of the class intervals. For the present example, we may use class interval widths of 5, so that the distance between lines is 5. Figure 2.3.7 shows the result when MINITAB is used to produce the stem-and-leaf display.

```
Stem-and-leaf of c1  N = 169
Leaf unit = 1.0
     4      1 8899
    30      2 0111222222333333344444444
    70      2 555566666666666777777777788888889999999
   (30)     3 000000000011111112222233344444
    69      3 5666777788888999
    52      4 0000001112222333444
    33      4 555667777888888899
    16      5 00011223333
     5      5 6
     4      6 1233
```

Figure 2.3.7 Stem-and-leaf display prepared by MINITAB from the data on subjects' ages shown in Table 2.2.1, class interval width = 5.

EXERCISES

2.3.1 In a study of the proliferative activity of breast cancers, Veronese and Gambacorta (A-1) used the Ki-67 monoclonal antibody and immunohistochemical methods. The investigators obtained tumor tissues from 203 patients with breast carcinoma. The patients ranged in age from 26 to 82 years. The following table shows the Ki-67 values (expressed as percents) for these patients.

10.12	10.80	10.54	27.30	8.38
10.15	5.48	23.50	32.60	42.70
19.30	16.40	4.40	26.80	16.60
33.00	11.65	26.30	1.73	35.90
9.63	9.31	7.40	9.35	14.78
21.42	25.11	12.60	17.96	41.12
28.30	19.50	15.92	19.40	7.19
4.65	73.00	17.84	10.90	2.74
21.09	11.95	33.30	4.53	19.40
1.00	27.00	9.03	51.20	6.40
13.72	32.90	9.80	2.43	2.00
8.77	9.40	35.40	51.70	43.50
3.00	4.70	14.00	15.00	3.60
4.09	9.20	6.20	5.00	15.00
17.60	50.00	10.00	20.00	30.00
5.22	5.00	15.00	25.00	10.00
12.70	30.00	10.00	15.00	20.00
7.39	4.00	25.00	20.00	30.00
21.36	49.85	29.70	19.95	5.00
11.36	24.89	29.55	10.00	38.90
8.12	28.85	19.80	4.99	6.00
3.14	5.00	44.20	30.00	9.88
4.33	9.20	4.87	10.00	29.10
5.07	2.00	3.00	2.00	2.96
8.10	4.84	9.79	5.00	9.50
4.23	10.00	19.83	20.00	4.77
13.11	75.00	20.00	5.00	4.55
4.07	14.79	8.99	3.97	30.00
6.07	15.00	40.00	18.79	13.76
45.82	4.32	5.69	1.42	18.57
5.58	12.82	4.50	4.41	1.88
5.00	10.00	4.12	14.24	9.11
9.69	8.37	6.20	2.07	3.12
4.14	2.03	2.69	3.69	5.42
4.59	10.00	6.27	6.37	13.78
27.55	9.83	6.55	8.21	3.42
3.51	9.10	11.20	6.88	7.53
8.58	5.00	29.50	9.60	6.03
14.70	5.60	28.10	5.48	7.00
6.72	3.32	13.52	5.70	17.80
13.10	9.75	7.37		

SOURCE: Silvio M. Veronese, Ph.D. Used with permission.

Use these data to prepare:
a. A frequency distribution.
b. A relative frequency distribution.
c. A cumulative frequency distribution.
d. A cumulative relative frequency distribution.
e. A histogram.
f. A frequency polygon.

2.3.2 Jarjour et al (A-2) conducted a study in which they measured bronchoalveolar lavage (BAL) fluid histamine levels in subjects with allergic rhinitis, subjects with asthma, and normal volunteers. One of the measurements obtained was the total protein (μg/ml) in BAL samples. The following are the results for the 61 samples they analyzed.

76.33	57.73	74.78	100.36	73.50
77.63	88.78	77.40	51.16	62.20
149.49	86.24	57.90	72.10	67.20
54.38	54.07	91.47	62.32	44.73
55.47	95.06	71.50	73.53	57.68
51.70	114.79	61.70	47.23	
78.15	53.07	106.00	35.90	
85.40	72.30	61.10	72.20	
41.98	59.36	63.96	66.60	
69.91	59.20	54.41	59.76	
128.40	67.10	83.82	95.33	
88.17	109.30	79.55		
58.50	82.60	153.56		
84.70	62.80	70.17		
44.40	61.90	55.05		

Source: Nizar N. Jarjour, M.D. Used with permission.

Use these data to prepare:
a. A frequency distribution.
b. A relative frequency distribution.
c. A cumulative frequency distribution.
d. A cumulative relative frequency distribution.
e. A histogram.
f. A frequency polygon.

2.3.3 Ellis et al. (A-3) conducted a study to explore the platelet imipramine binding characteristics in manic patients and to compare the results with equivalent data for healthy controls and depressed patients. As part of the study the investigators obtained maximal receptor binding (B_{max}) values on their subjects. The following are the values for the 57 subjects in the study who had a diagnosis of unipolar depression.

1074	392	286	179
372	475	511	530
473	319	147	446
797	301	476	328

385	556	416	348
769	300	528	773
797	339	419	697
485	488	328	520
334	1114	1220	341
670	761	438	604
510	571	238	420
299	306	867	397
333	80	1657	
303	607	790	
768	1017	479	

SOURCE: Peter E. Ellis. Used with permission.

Use these data to construct:
a. A frequency distribution.
b. A relative frequency distribution.
c. A cumulative frequency distribution.
d. A cumulative relative frequency distribution.
e. A histogram.
f. A frequency polygon.

2.3.4 The objective of a study by Herrman et al. (A-4) was to estimate the prevalence of severe mental disorders in a representative sample of prisoners in three metropolitan prisons in Melbourne, Australia. Three groups of prisoners were identified: those who agreed to be interviewed, those who refused to be interviewed, and those who agreed to serve as replacements for the subjects who initially refused to be interviewed. In addition to assessing the prevalence of mental disorders among the subjects, the investigators obtained data on length of sentence and length of incarceration at the time of the study. The following data are the lengths of minimum sentence (in days) for the subjects who refused to be interviewed.

18	4380	0	360
4955	720	1095	727
2190	730	365	1275
450	455	180	344
3650	0	2340	2555
2920	540	360	545
270	545	180	90
1000	0	2005	60
270	150	717	540
180	1825	3710	90
910	2920	180	660
90	270	2555	365
253	284	4015	3100
450	330	2885	1050
360	0	730	90
1460	1000	3160	450
1095	1460	910	1200

635	360	360	120
1953	0	466	1460
844	120	2920	409
360	1095	240	910
570	330	4745	0
951	540	88	1125
540	730	545	
450		90	
450		1670	
730			

Source: Helen Herrman, M.D. Used with permission.

Use these data to construct:
a. A frequency distribution.
b. A relative frequency distribution.
c. A cumulative frequency distribution.
d. A cumulative relative frequency distribution.
e. A histogram.
f. A frequency polygon.

2.3.5 The following table shows the number of hours 45 hospital patients slept following the administration of a certain anesthetic.

7	10	12	4	8	7	3	8	5
12	11	3	8	1	1	13	10	4
4	5	5	8	7	7	3	2	3
8	13	1	7	17	3	4	5	5
3	1	17	10	4	7	7	11	8

From these data construct:

a. A frequency distribution.   **b.** A relative frequency distribution.
c. A histogram.   **d.** A frequency polygon.

2.3.6 The following are the number of babies born during a year in 60 community hospitals.

30	55	27	45	56	48	45	49	32	57	47	56
37	55	52	34	54	42	32	59	35	46	24	57
32	26	40	28	53	54	29	42	42	54	53	59
39	56	59	58	49	53	30	53	21	34	28	50
52	57	43	46	54	31	22	31	24	24	57	29

From these data construct:

a. A frequency distribution.   **b.** A relative frequency distribution.
c. A frequency polygon.

2.3.7 In a study of physical endurance levels of male college freshmen the following composite endurance scores based on several exercise routines were collected.

254	281	192	260	212	179	225	179	181	149
182	210	235	239	258	166	159	223	186	190
180	188	135	233	220	204	219	211	245	151
198	190	151	157	204	238	205	229	191	200
222	187	134	193	264	312	214	227	190	212
165	194	206	193	218	198	241	149	164	225
265	222	264	249	175	205	252	210	178	159
220	201	203	172	234	198	173	187	189	237
272	195	227	230	168	232	217	249	196	223
232	191	175	236	152	258	155	215	197	210
214	278	252	283	205	184	172	228	193	130
218	213	172	159	203	212	117	197	206	198
169	187	204	180	261	236	217	205	212	218
191	124	199	235	139	231	116	182	243	217
251	206	173	236	215	228	183	204	186	134
188	195	240	163	208					

From these data construct:

a. A frequency distribution.　　**b.** A relative frequency distribution.

c. A frequency polygon.　　**d.** A histogram.

2.3.8 The following are the ages of 30 patients seen in the emergency room of a hospital on a Friday night. Construct a stem-and-leaf display from these data.

35	32	21	43	39	60
36	12	54	45	37	53
45	23	64	10	34	22
36	45	55	44	55	46
22	38	35	56	45	57

2.3.9 The following are the emergency room charges made to a sample of 25 patients at two city hospitals. Construct a stem-and-leaf display for each set of data. What does a comparison of the two displays suggest regarding the two hospitals?

Hospital A

249.10	202.50	222.20	214.40	205.90
214.30	195.10	213.30	225.50	191.40
201.20	239.80	245.70	213.00	238.80
171.10	222.00	212.50	201.70	184.90
248.30	209.70	233.90	229.80	217.90

Hospital B				
199.50	184.00	173.20	186.00	214.10
125.50	143.50	190.40	152.00	165.70
154.70	145.30	154.60	190.30	135.40
167.70	203.40	186.70	155.30	195.90
168.90	166.70	178.60	150.20	212.40

2.3.10   Refer to the ages of Greenland residents discussed in Example 1.4.1 and displayed in Table 1.4.1. Use class interval widths of 5 and construct:

a. A frequency distribution.
b. A relative frequency distribution.
c. A cumulative frequency distribution.
d. A cumulative relative frequency distribution.
e. A histogram.
f. A frequency polygon.

2.4
Descriptive Statistics —
Measures of Central Tendency

Although frequency distributions serve useful purposes, there are many situations that require other types of data summarization. What we need in many instances is the ability to summarize the data by means of a single number called a *descriptive measure*. Descriptive measures may be computed from the data of a sample or the data of a population. To distinguish between them we have the following definitions.

DEFINITIONS

1. A descriptive measure computed from the data of a sample is called a *statistic*.
2. A descriptive measure computed from the data of a population is called a *parameter*.

Several types of descriptive measures can be computed from a set of data. In this chapter, however, we limit discussion to *measures of central tendency* and *measures of dispersion*. We consider measures of central tendency in this section and measures of dispersion in the following one.

In each of the measures of central tendency, of which we discuss three, we have a single value that is considered to be typical of the set of data as a whole. Measures of central tendency convey information regarding the average value of a set of values. As we will see, the word *average* can be defined in different ways.

The three most commonly used measures of central tendency are the *mean*, the *median*, and the *mode*.

Arithmetic Mean The most familiar measure of central tendency is the arithmetic mean. It is the descriptive measure most people have in mind when they speak of the "average." The adjective *arithmetic* distinguishes this mean from other means that can be computed. Since we are not covering these other means in this book, we shall refer to the arithmetic mean simply as the *mean*. The mean is obtained by adding all the values in a population or sample and dividing by the number of values that are added.

Example 2.4.1

We wish to obtain the mean age of the population of 169 subjects represented in Table 1.4.1.

Solution: We proceed as follows:

$$\text{mean age} = \frac{27 + 27 + \cdots + 23 + 39}{169} = \frac{5797}{169} = 34.302$$

The three dots in the numerator represent the values we did not show in order to save space.

General Formula for the Mean It will be convenient if we can generalize the procedure for obtaining the mean and, also, represent the procedure in a more compact notational form. Let us begin by designating the random variable of interest by the capital letter X. In our present illustration we let X represent the random variable, age. Specific values of a random variable will be designated by the lowercase letter x. To distinguish one value from another we attach a subscript to the x and let the subscript refer to the first, the second, the third value, and so on. For example, from Table 1.4.1 we have

$$x_1 = 27, \qquad x_2 = 27, \ldots, \qquad \text{and} \qquad x_{169} = 39$$

In general, a typical value of a random variable will be designated by x_i and the final value, in a finite population of values, by x_N where N is the number of values in the population. Finally, we will use the Greek letter μ to stand for the population mean. We may now write the general formula for a finite population mean as follows:

$$\mu = \frac{\sum\limits_{i=1}^{N} x_i}{N} \tag{2.4.1}$$

The symbol $\sum_{i=1}^{N}$ instructs us to add all values of the variable from the first to the last. This symbol, $\sum$, called the *summation sign*, will be used extensively in this book. When from the context it is obvious which values are to be added, the symbols above and below $\sum$ will be omitted.

The Sample Mean   When we compute the mean for a sample of values, the procedure just outlined is followed with some modifications in notation. We use $\bar{x}$ to designate the sample mean and n to indicate the number of values in the sample. The sample mean then is expressed as

$$\bar{x} = \frac{\sum\limits_{i=1}^{n} x_i}{n} \tag{2.4.2}$$

Example 2.4.2   In Chapter 1 we selected a simple random sample of 10 subjects from the population of subjects represented in Table 1.4.1. Let us now compute the mean age of the 10 subjects in our sample.

Solution: We recall (see Table 1.4.2) that the ages of the 10 subjects in our sample were $x_1 = 42$, $x_2 = 28$, $x_3 = 28$, $x_4 = 61$, $x_5 = 31$, $x_6 = 23$, $x_7 = 50$, $x_8 = 34$, $x_9 = 32$, $x_{10} = 37$. Substitution of our sample data into Equation 2.4.2 gives

$$\bar{x} = \frac{\sum\limits_{i=1}^{n} x_i}{n} = \frac{42 + 28 + \cdots + 37}{10} = \frac{366}{10} = 36.6$$

Properties of the Mean   The arithmetic mean possesses certain properties, some desirable and some not so desirable. These properties include the following.

1. Uniqueness. For a given set of data there is one and only one arithmetic mean.
2. Simplicity. The arithmetic mean is easily understood and easy to compute.
3. Since each and every value in a set of data enters into the computation of the mean, it is affected by each value. Extreme values, therefore, have an influence on the mean and, in some cases, can so distort it that it becomes undesirable as a measure of central tendency.

As an example of how extreme values may affect the mean, consider the following situation. Suppose the five physicians who practice in an area are surveyed to determine their charges for a certain procedure. Assume that they report these charges: $75, $75, $80, $80, and $280. The mean charge for the five physicians is found to be $118, a value that is not very representative of the set of data as a whole. The single atypical value had the effect of inflating the mean.

Median   The median of a finite set of values is that value which divides the set into two equal parts such that the number of values equal to or greater than the median is equal to the number of values equal to or less than the median. If the number of values is odd, the median will be the middle value when all values have been arranged in order of magnitude. When the number of values is even, there is no single middle value. Instead there are two middle values. In this case the median is taken to be the mean of these two middle values, when all values have been arranged in the order of their magnitude. In other words, the median observation of a data set is the $(n + 1)/2$th one when the observations have been ordered. If, for example, we have 11 observations, the median is the $(11 + 1)/2 = $ 6th ordered observation. If we have 12 observations the median is the $(12 + 1)/2 = 6.5$th ordered observation, and is a value halfway between the 6th and 7th ordered observation.

Example 2.4.3

Let us illustrate by finding the median of the data in Table 2.2.1.

Solution:　The values are already ordered so we need only to find the two middle values. The middle value is the $(n + 1)/2 = (169 + 1)/2 = 170/2 = 85$th one. Counting from the smallest up to the 85th value we see that it is 31. Thus the median age of the 169 subjects is 31 years.

Example 2.4.4

We wish to find the median age of the subjects represented in the sample described in Example 2.4.2.

Solution:　Arraying the 10 ages in order of magnitude from smallest to largest gives 23, 28, 28, 31, 32, 34, 37, 42, 50, 61. Since we have an even number of ages, there is no middle value. The two middle values, however, are 32 and 34. The median, then, is $(32 + 34)/2 = 33$.

Properties of the Median　Properties of the median include the following:

1. Uniqueness. As is true with the mean, there is only one median for a given set of data.
2. Simplicity. The median is easy to calculate.
3. It is not as drastically affected by extreme values as is the mean.

The Mode　The mode of a set of values is that value which occurs most frequently. If all the values are different there is no mode; on the other hand, a set of values may have more than one mode.

Example 2.4.5

Find the modal age of the subjects whose ages are given in Table 2.2.1.

Solution:　A count of the ages in Table 2.2.1 reveals that the age 26 occurs most frequently (11 times). The mode for this population of ages is 26.

For an example of a set of values that has more than one mode, let us consider a laboratory with 10 employees whose ages are 20, 21, 20, 20, 34, 22, 24, 27, 27, and

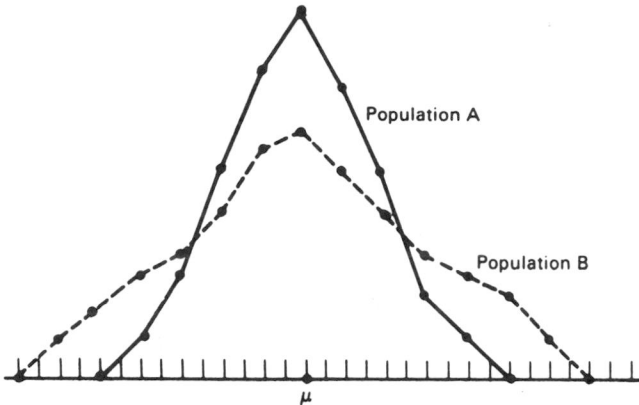

Figure 2.5.1 Two frequency distributions with equal means but different amounts of dispersion.

27. We could say that these data have two modes, 20 and 27. The sample consisting of the values 10, 21, 33, 53, and 54 has no mode since all the values are different.

The mode may be used for describing qualitative data. For example, suppose the patients seen in a mental health clinic during a given year received one of the following diagnoses: mental retardation, organic brain syndrome, psychosis, neurosis, and personality disorder. The diagnosis occurring most frequently in the group of patients would be called the modal diagnosis.

2.5
Descriptive Statistics —
Measures of Dispersion

The *dispersion* of a set of observations refers to the variety that they exhibit. A measure of dispersion conveys information regarding the amount of variabiltiy present in a set of data. If all the values are the same, there is no dispersion; if they are not all the same, dispersion is present in the data. The amount of dispersion may be small, when the values, though different, are close together. Figure 2.5.1 shows the frequency polygons for two populations that have equal means but different amounts of variability. Population B, which is more variable than population A, is more spread out. If the values are widely scattered, the dispersion is greater. Other terms used synonymously with dispersion include *variation*, *spread*, and *scatter*.

The Range   One way to measure the variation in a set of values is to compute the *range*. The range is the difference between the smallest and largest value in a set of observations. If we denote the range by R, the largest value by x_L, and the smallest value by x_S, we compute the range as follows:

$$R = x_L - x_S \qquad (2.5.1)$$

Example 2.5.1

We wish to compute the range of the ages of the sample subjects discussed in Example 2.4.2.

Solution: Since the youngest subject in the sample is 23 years old and the oldest is 61, we compute the range to be

$$R = 61 - 23 = 38$$

The usefulness of the range is limited. The fact that it takes into account only two values causes it to be a poor measure of dispersion. The main advantage in using the range is the simplicity of its computation.

The Variance When the values of a set of observations lie close to their mean, the dispersion is less than when they are scattered over a wide range. Since this is true, it would be intuitively appealing if we could measure dispersion relative to the scatter of the values about their mean. Such a measure is realized in what is known as the *variance*. In computing the variance of a sample of values, for example, we subtract the mean from each of the values, square the resulting differences, and then add up the squared differences. This sum of the squared deviations of the values from their mean is divided by the sample size, minus 1, to obtain the sample variance. Letting s^2 stand for the sample variance, the procedure may be written in notational form as follows:

$$s^2 = \frac{\sum_{i=1}^{n} (x_i - \bar{x})^2}{n - 1} \tag{2.5.2}$$

Example 2.5.2

Let us illustrate by computing the variance of the ages of the subjects discussed in Example 2.4.2.

Solution:

$$s^2 = \frac{(42 - 36.6)^2 + (28 - 36.6)^2 \cdots (37 - 36.6)^2}{9}$$

$$= \frac{1196.399997}{9} = 132.933333$$

Degrees of Freedom The reason for dividing by $n - 1$ rather than n, as we might have expected, is the theoretical consideration referred to as *degrees of freedom*. In computing the variance, we say that we have $n - 1$ *degrees of freedom*. We reason as follows. The sum of the deviations of the values from their mean is equal to zero, as can be shown. If, then, we know the values of $n - 1$ of the deviations from the mean, we know the nth one, since it is automatically determined because of the necessity for all n values to add to zero. From a practical point of view, dividing the squared differences by $n - 1$ rather than n is necessary in order to use the sample variance in the inference procedures discussed later. The concept of degrees of freedom will be discussed again later. Students interested in pursuing the matter further at this time should refer to the article by Walker (2).

Alternative Variance Formula When the number of observations is large, the use of Equation 2.5.2 can be tedious. The following formula may prove to be less troublesome.

$$s^2 = \frac{n \sum\limits_{i=1}^{n} x_i^2 - \left(\sum\limits_{i=1}^{n} x_i \right)^2}{n(n-1)} \tag{2.5.3}$$

When we compute the variance from a finite population of values, the procedures outlined above are followed except that we divide by N rather than $N - 1$. If we let σ^2 stand for the finite population variance, the definitional and computational formulas, respectively, are as follows:

$$\sigma^2 = \frac{\sum\limits_{i=1}^{N} (x_i - \mu)^2}{N} \tag{2.5.4}$$

$$\sigma^2 = \frac{N \sum\limits_{i=1}^{N} x_i^2 - \left(\sum\limits_{i=1}^{N} x_i \right)^2}{N \cdot N} \tag{2.5.5}$$

Standard Deviation The variance represents squared units and, therefore, is not an appropriate measure of dispersion when we wish to express this concept in terms of the original units. To obtain a measure of dispersion in original units, we merely take the square root of the variance. The result is called the *standard deviation*. In general, the standard deviation of a sample is given by

$$s = \sqrt{s^2} = \sqrt{\frac{\sum\limits_{i=1}^{n} (x_i - \bar{x})^2}{n-1}} \tag{2.5.6}$$

The standard deviation of a finite population is obtained by taking the square root of the quantity obtained by Equation 2.5.4.

The Coefficient of Variation   The standard deviation is useful as a measure of variation within a given set of data. When one desires to compare the dispersion in two sets of data, however, comparing the two standard deviations may lead to fallacious results. It may be that the two variables involved are measured in different units. For example, we may wish to know, for a certain population, whether serum cholesterol levels, measured in milligrams per 100 ml, are more variable than body weight, measured in pounds.

Furthermore, although the same unit of measurement is used, the two means may be quite different. If we compare the standard deviation of weights of first grade children with the standard deviation of weights of high school freshmen, we may find that the latter standard deviation is numerically larger than the former, because the weights themselves are larger, not because the dispersion is greater.

What is needed in situations like these is a measure of relative variation rather than absolute variation. Such a measure is found in the *coefficient of variation*, which expresses the standard deviation as a percentage of the mean. The formula is given by

$$\text{C.V.} = \frac{s}{\bar{x}}(100) \qquad\qquad (2.5.7)$$

We see that, since the mean and standard deviations are expressed in the same unit of measurement, the unit of measurement cancels out in computing the coefficient of variation. What we have, then, is a measure that is independent of the unit of measurement.

Example 2.5.3

Suppose two samples of human males yield the following results.

	Sample 1	Sample 2
Age	25 years	11 years
Mean weight	145 pounds	80 pounds
Standard deviation	10 pounds	10 pounds

We wish to know which is more variable, the weights of the 25-year-olds or the weights of the 11-year-olds.

Solution: A comparison of the standard deviations might lead one to conclude that the two samples possess equal variability. If we compute the coefficients of variation, however, we have for the 25-year-olds

$$\text{C.V.} = \frac{10}{145}(100) = 6.9$$

and for the 11-year olds

$$\text{C.V.} = \frac{10}{80}(100) = 12.5$$

If we compare these results we get quite a different impression.

The coefficient of variation is also useful in comparing the results obtained by different persons who are conducting investigations involving the same variable.

N	MEAN	MEDIAN	TRMEAN	STDEV	SEMEAN
10	36.60	33.00	35.25	11.53	3.65

MIN	MAX	Q1	Q3
23.00	61.00	28.00	44.00

Figure 2.5.2 Printout of descriptive measures computed from the sample of ages in Example 2.4.2, MINITAB software package.

Since the coefficient of variation is independent of the scale of measurement, it is a useful statistic for comparing the variability of two or more variables measured on different scales. We could, for example, use the coefficient of variation to compare the variability in weights of one sample of subjects whose weights are expressed in pounds with the variability in weights of another sample of subjects whose weights are expressed in kilograms.

Computer Analysis Computer software packages provide a variety of possibilities in the calculation of descriptive measures. Figure 2.5.2 shows a printout of the descriptive measures available from the MINITAB package. The data consists of the ages from Example 2.4.2. With the data in column 1, the MINITAB command is

```
DESCRIBE C1
```

In the printout Q1 and Q3 are the first and third quartiles, respectively. These measures are described later in this chapter.

TRMEAN stands for *trimmed mean*. The trimmed mean instead of the arithmetic mean is sometimes used as a measure of central tendency. It is computed after some of the extreme values have been discarded. The trimmed mean, therefore, does not possess the disadvantage of being influenced unduly by extreme values as is the case with the arithmetic mean. The term SEMEAN stands for *standard error of the mean*. This measure, as well as the trimmed mean, will be discussed in detail in a later chapter. Figure 2.5.3 shows, for the same data, the SAS® printout obtained by using the PROC MEANS statement.

VARIABLE	N	MEAN	STANDARD DEVIATION	MINIMUM VALUE	MAXIMUM VALUE
AGES	10	36.60000000	11.52967187	23.00000000	61.00000000
STD ERROR OF MEAN		SUM	VARIANCE	C.V.	
3.64600238		366.00000000	132.93333333	31.502	

Figure 2.5.3 Printout of descriptive measures computed from the sample of ages in Example 2.4.2, SAS® software package.

EXERCISES

For each of the data sets in the following exercises compute (a) the mean, (b) the median, (c) the mode, (d) the range, (e) the variance, (f) the standard deviation, and (g) the coefficient of variation. Treat each data set as a sample.

2.5.1 Thirteen patients with severe chronic airflow limitation were the subjects of a study by Fernandez et al. (A-5), who investigated the effectiveness of a treatment to improve gas exchange in such subjects. The following are the body surface areas (m^2) of the patients.

2.10	1.74	1.68	1.83	1.57	1.71	1.73
1.65	1.74	1.57	2.76	1.90	1.77	

SOURCE: Enrique Fernandez, Paltiel Weiner, Ephraim Meltzer, Mary M. Lutz, David B. Badish, and Reuben M. Cherniack, "Sustained Improvement in Gas Exchange After Negative Pressure Ventilation for 8 Hours Per Day on 2 Successive Days in Chronic Airflow Limitation," *American Review of Respiratory Disease, 144* (1991), 390–394.

2.5.2 The results of a study by Dosman et al. (A-6) allowed them to conclude that breathing cold air increases the bronchial reactivity to inhaled histamine in asthmatic patients. The study subjects were seven asthmatic patients aged 19 to 33 years. The baseline forced expiratory values (in liters per minute) for the subjects in their sample were as follows:

3.94	1.47	2.06	2.36	3.74	3.43	3.78

SOURCE: J. A. Dosman, W. C. Hodgson, and D. W. Cockcroft, "Effect of Cold Air on the Bronchial Response to Inhaled Histamine in Patients with Asthma," *American Review of Respiratory Disease, 144* (1991), 45–50.

2.5.3 Seventeen patients admitted to the Aberdeen Teaching Hospitals in Scotland between 1980 and mid-1988 were diagnosed as having pyogenic liver abscess. Nine of the patients died. In an article in the journal *Age and Ageing*, Sridharan et al. (A-7) state that "The high fatality of pyogenic liver abscess seems to be at least in part due to a lack of clinical suspicion." The following are the ages of the subjects in the study:

63	72	62	69	71	84	81	78	61	76	84	67	86
69	64	87	76									

SOURCE: G. V. Sridharan, S. P. Wilkinson, and W. R. Primrose, "Pyogenic Liver Abscess in the Elderly," *Age and Ageing, 19* (1990), 199–203. Used by permission of Oxford University Press.

2.5.4 Arinami et al. (A-8) analyzed the auditory brain-stem responses in a sample of 12 mentally retarded males with the fragile X syndrome. The IQs of the subjects were as follows:

17	22	17	18	17	19	34	26	14	33	21	29

SOURCE: Tadao Arinami, Miki Sato, Susumu Nakajima, and Ikuko Kondo, "Auditory Brain-Stem Responses in the Fragile X Syndrome," *American Journal of Human Genetics, 43* (1988), 46–51. © 1988 by The American Society of Human Genetics. All rights reserved. Published by the University of Chicago.

2.5.5 In an article in the *American Journal of Obstetrics and Gynecology*, Dr. Giancarlo Mari (A-9) discusses his study of arterial blood flow velocity waveforms of the pelvis and lower extremities in normal and growth-retarded fetuses. He states that his preliminary data suggest that "the femoral artery pulsatility index cannot be used as an indicator of adverse fetal outcome, whereas absent or reverse flow of the umbilical artery seems to be better correlated with adverse fetal outcome." The following are the gestational ages (in weeks) of 20 growth-retarded fetuses that he studied:

24	26	27	28	28	28	29	30	30	31	32	32	33
33	34	34	35	35	35	36						

SOURCE: Giancarlo Mari, "Arterial Bood Flow Velocity Waveforms of the Pelvis and Lower Extremities in Normal and Growth-Retarded Fetuses," *American Journal of Obstetrics and Gynecology*, *165* (1991), 143–151.

2.5.6 The objective of a study by Kuhnz et al (A-10) was to analyze certain basic pharmacokinetic parameters in women who were treated with a triphasic oral contraceptive. The weights (in kilograms) of the 10 women who participated in the study were:

62	53	57	55	69	64	60	59	60	60

SOURCE: Wilhelm Kuhnz, Durda Sostarek, Christiane Gansau, Tom Louton, and Marianne Mahler, "Single and Multiple Administration of a New Triphasic Oral Contraceptive to Women: Pharmacokinetics of Ethinyl Estradiol and Free and Total Testosterone Levels in Serum," *American Journal of Obstetrics and Gynecology*, *165* (1991), 596–602.

2.6
Measures of Central Tendency Computed from Grouped Data

After data have been grouped into a frequency distribution it may be desirable to compute some of the descriptive measures, such as the mean and variance. Frequently an investigator does not have access to the raw data in which he or she is interested, but does have a frequency distribution. Data frequently are published in the form of a frequency distribution without an accompanying list of individual values or descriptive measures. Readers interested in a measure of central tendency or a measure of dispersion for these data must compute their own.

When data are grouped the individual observations lose their identity. By looking at a frequency distribution we are able to determine the number of observations falling into the various class intervals, but the actual values cannot be determined. Because of this we must make certain assumptions about the values when we compute a descriptive measure from grouped data. As a consequence of making these assumptions our results are only approximations to the true values.

The Mean Computed from Grouped Data   In calculating the mean from grouped data, we assume that all values falling into a particular class interval are located at the *midpoint* of the interval. The midpoint of a class interval is obtained by computing the mean of the upper and lower limits of the interval. The midpoint of the first class interval of the distribution shown in Table 2.2.2, for example, is equal to $(10 + 19)/2 = 29/2 = 14.5$. The midpoints of successive class intervals may be found by adding the class interval width to the previous midpoint. The midpoint of the second class interval in Table 2.2.2 is equal to $14.5 + 10 = 24.5$.

To find the mean we multiply each midpoint by the corresponding frequency, sum these products, and divide by the sum of the frequencies. If the data represent a sample of observations, the computation of the mean may be shown symbolically as

$$\bar{x} = \frac{\sum\limits_{i=1}^{k} m_i f_i}{\sum\limits_{i=1}^{k} f_i} \tag{2.6.1}$$

where k = the number of class intervals, m_i = the midpoint of the ith class interval, and f_i = the frequency of the ith class interval.

Example 2.6.1   Let us use the frequency distribution of Table 2.2.2 to compute the mean age of the 169 subjects, which we now treat as a sample.

Solution: When we compute the mean from grouped data, it is convenient to prepare a work table such as Table 2.6.1, which has been prepared for the data of Table 2.2.2.

TABLE 2.6.1 Work Table for Computing the Mean Age from the Grouped Data of Table 2.2.2

Class Interval	Class Midpoint m_I	Class Frequency f_I	$m_I f_I$
10–19	14.5	4	58.0
20–29	24.5	66	1617.0
30–39	34.5	47	1621.5
40–49	44.5	36	1602.0
50–59	54.5	12	654.0
60–69	64.5	4	258.0
Total		169	5810.5

We may now compute the mean.

$$\bar{x} = \frac{\sum_{i=1}^{k} m_i f_i}{\sum_{i=1}^{k} f_i} = \frac{5810.5}{169} = 34.48$$

We get an idea of the accuracy of the mean computed from grouped data by noting that, for our sample, the mean computed from the individual observations is 34.302.

The computation of a mean from a population of values grouped into a finite number of classes is performed in exactly the same manner.

The Median — Grouped Data When computing a mean from grouped data, we assume that the values within a class interval are located at the midpoint; however, in computing the median, we assume that they are evenly distributed through the interval.

The first step in computing the median from grouped data is to locate the class interval in which it is located. We do this by finding the interval containing the $n/2$ value.

The median then may be computed by the following formula:

$$\text{median} = L_i + \frac{j}{f_i}(U_i - L_i) \tag{2.6.2}$$

where L_i = the true lower limit of the interval containing the median, U_i = the true upper limit of the interval containing the median, j = the number of observations still lacking to reach the median, after the lower limit of the interval containing the median has been reached, and f_i = the frequency of the interval containing the median.

Example 2.6.2 Again, let us use the frequency distribution of Table 2.2.2 to compute the median age of the 169 subjects.

Solution: The $n/2$ value is $169/2 = 84.5$. Looking at Table 2.2.2 we see that the first two class intervals account for 70 of the observations and that 117 observations are accounted for by the first three class intervals. The median value, therefore, is in the third class interval. It is somewhere between 29.5 and 39.5 if we consider the true class limits. The question now is: How far must we proceed into this interval before reaching the median? Under the assumption that the values are evenly distributed through the interval, it seems reasonable that we should move a distance equal to $(84.5 - 70)/47$ of the total distance of the class interval. After reaching the lower limit of the class interval containing the median we need 14.5 more observations, and there are a total of 47 observations in the interval. The value of the median then is equal to the value of the lower limit of the interval containing the median plus $14.5/47$ of the interval width. For the data of Table 2.2.2 we compute the median to be $29.5 + (14.5/47)(10) = 32.6 \approx 33$.

The median computed from the individual ages is 31. Note that when we locate the median value for grouped data we use $n/2$ rather than $(n + 1)/2$, which we used with ungrouped data.

The Mode — Grouped Data We have defined the mode of a set of values as the value that occurs most frequently. When designating the mode of grouped data, we usually refer to the *modal class* where the modal class is the class interval with the highest frequency. In Table 2.2.2 the modal class would be the second class, 20–29, or 19.5–29.5, using the true class limits. If a single value for the mode of grouped data must be specified, it is taken as the midpoint of the modal class. In the present example this is 24.5. The assumption is made that all values in the interval fall at the midpoint.

Percentiles and Quartiles The mean and median are special cases of a family of parameters known as *location parameters*. These descriptive measures are called location parameters because they can be used to designate certain positions on the horizontal axis when the distribution of a variable is graphed. In that sense the so-called location parameters "locate" the distribution on the horizontal axis. For example, a distribution with a median of 100 is located to the right of a distribution with a median of 50 when the two distributions are graphed. Other location parameters include percentiles and quartiles. We may define a percentile as follows:

DEFINITION

Given a set of n observations $x_1, x_2, \ldots, x_n$, the pth percentile P is the value of X such that p percent or less of the observations are less than P and $(100 - p)$ percent or less of the observations are greater than P.

Subscripts on P serve to distinguish one percentile from another. The 10th percentile, for example, is designated P_{10}, the 70th is designated P_{70}, and so on. The 50th percentile is the median and is designated P_{50}. All percentiles are computed by the method described earlier for computing the median. Usually one calculates percentiles only for large data sets.

For grouped data the location of the kth percentile P_k is given by

$$P_k = \frac{k}{100}n \tag{2.6.3}$$

Example 2.6.3

Let us find the 80th percentile of the ages shown in Table 2.2.2.

Solution: By Equation 2.6.3 we find that $P_{80} = (80/100)(169) = 135.2$. By Equation 2.6.2, then, we compute

$$P_{80} = 39.5 + \frac{(135.2 - 117)}{36}(49.5 - 39.5)$$

$$= 44.56$$

We see that 80 percent of the subjects are younger than 44.56 years.

Percentiles for Ungrouped Data   The 25th percentile is often referred to as the *first quartile* and denoted Q_1. The 50th percentile (the median) is referred to as the second or *middle quartile* and written Q_2, and the 75th percentile is referred to as the *third quartile*, Q_3.

When we wish to find the quartiles of ungrouped data, the following formulas are used:

$$Q_1 = \frac{n+1}{4}\text{th} \qquad \text{ordered observation}$$

$$Q_2 = \frac{2(n+1)}{4} = \frac{n+1}{2}\text{th} \qquad \text{ordered observation}$$

$$Q_3 = \frac{3(n+1)}{4}\text{th} \qquad \text{ordered observation}$$

Box-and-Whisker Plots   A useful visual device for communicating the information contained in a data set is the *box-and-whisker plot*. The construction of a box-and-whisker plot (sometimes called, simply, a *boxplot*) makes use of the quartiles of a data set and may be accomplished by following these five steps:

1. Represent the variable of interest on the horizontal axis.

2. Draw a box in the space above the horizontal axis in such a way that the left end of the box aligns with the first quartile Q_1 and the right end of the box aligns with the third quartile Q_3.

3. Divide the box into two parts by a vertical line that aligns with the median Q_2.

4. Draw a horizontal line called a *whisker* from the left end of the box to a point that aligns with the smallest measurement in the data set.

5. Draw another horizontal line, or whisker, from the right end of the box to a point that aligns with the largest measurement in the data set.

Examination of a box-and-whisker plot for a set of data reveals information regarding the amount of spread, location of concentration, and symmetry of the data.

The following example illustrates the construction of a box-and-whisker plot.

Example 2.6.4

In a medical journal article, Pitts et al. (A-11) state that "Carcinomas with metaplasia and sarcomas arising within the breast are difficult to accurately diagnose and classify because of their varied histologic patterns and rarity." The authors investigated a series of pure sarcomas and carcinomas exhibiting metaplasia in an attempt to further study their biologic characteristics. Table 2.6.2 contains the ordered diameters in centimeters of the neoplasms removed from the breasts of 20 subjects with pure sarcomas.

TABLE 2.6.2 Diameters (cm) of Pure Sarcomas Removed from the Breasts of 20 Women

.5	1.2	2.1	2.5	2.5	3.0	3.8	4.0	4.2	4.5	5.0
5.0	5.0	5.0	6.0	6.5	7.0	8.0	9.5	13.0		

SOURCE: William C. Pitts, Virginia A. Rojas, Michael J. Gaffey, Robert V. Rouse, Jose Esteban, Henry F. Frierson, Richard L. Kempson, and Lawrence M. Weiss, "Carcinomas With Metaplasia and Sarcomas of the Breast," *American Journal of Clinical Pathology, 95* (1991), 623–632.

Solution: The smallest and largest measures are .5 and 13.0, respectively. The first quartile is the $Q_1 = (20 + 1)/4 = 5.25$th measurement, which is $2.5 + (.25)(3.0 - 2.5) = 2.625$. The median is the $Q_2 = (20 + 1)/2 = 10.5$th measurement or $4.5 + (.5)(5.0 - 4.5) = 4.75$, and the third quartile is the $Q_3 = 3(20 + 1)/4 = 15.75$th measurement, which is equal to $6.0 + (.75)(6.5 - 6.0) = 6.375$. The resulting box-and-whisker plot is shown in Figure 2.6.1.

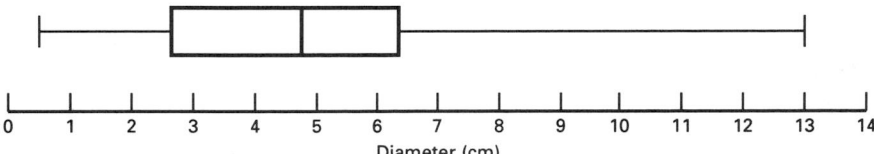

Figure 2.6.1 Box-and-whisker plot for Example 2.6.4.

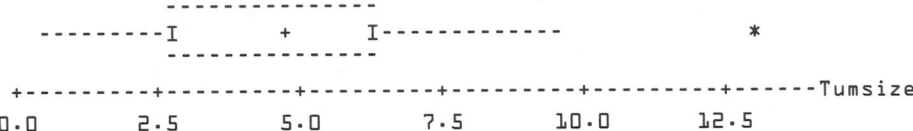

```
                    ---------------
        ---------I     +     I------------                    *
                    ---------------

      +---------+---------+---------+---------+---------+------Tumsize
      0.0       2.5       5.0       7.5      10.0      12.5
```

Figure 2.6.2 Box-and-whisker plot constructed by MINITAB from the data of Table 2.6.2.

Examination of Figure 2.6.1 reveals that 50 percent of the measurements are between about 2.6 and 6.4, the approximate values of the first and third quartiles, respectively. The vertical bar inside the box shows that the median is about 4.75. The longer right-hand whisker indicates that the distribution of diameters is skewed to the right.

Many statistical software packages have the capability of constructing box-and-whisker plots. Figure 2.6.2 shows one constructed by MINITAB from the patient age data of Table 2.2.2. We put the data into column 1 and issue the MINITAB command

```
Boxplot C1
```

The asterisk in Figure 2.6.2 alerts us to the fact that the data set contains an unusually large value, called an *outlier*. It is the melanoma that was 13 cm in diameter. The right whisker in Figure 2.6.2, therefore, stops at 9.5, the largest value not considered to be an outlier.

The SAS® statement PROC UNIVARIATE may be used to obtain a box-and-whisker plot. The statement also produces other descriptive measures and displays, including stem-and-leaf plots, means, variances, and quartiles.

Exploratory Data Analysis Box-and-whisker plots and stem-and-leaf displays are examples of what are known as *exploratory data analysis* techniques. These techniques, made popular as a result of the work of Tukey (3), allow the investigator to examine data in ways that reveal trends and relationships, identify unique features of data sets, and facilitate their description and summarization. Breckenridge (4) uses exploratory data analysis in the study of change in the age pattern of fertility. A book by Du Toit et al. (5) provides an overview of most of the well-known and widely used methods of analyzing and portraying data graphically with emphasis on exploratory techniques.

2.7
The Variance and Standard Deviation — Grouped Data

In calculating the variance and standard deviation from grouped data we assume that all values falling into a particular class interval are located at the midpoint of the interval. This, it will be recalled, is the assumption made in computing the mean and the mode. The variance of a sample, then, is given by

$$s^2 = \frac{\sum_{i=1}^{k} (m_i - \bar{x})^2 f_i}{\sum_{i=1}^{k} f_i - 1} \qquad (2.7.1)$$

where the symbols to the right of the equal sign have the definitions given in Equation 2.6.1.

The following computing formula for the sample variance on occasion may be preferred:

$$s^2 = \frac{n \sum_{i=1}^{k} m_i^2 f_i - \left(\sum_{i=1}^{k} m_i f_i \right)^2}{n(n-1)} \qquad (2.7.2)$$

where

$$n = \sum_{i=1}^{k} f_i$$

The definitional formula for σ^2 is the same as for s^2 except that μ replaces $\bar{x}$ and the denominator is $\sum_{i=1}^{k} f_i$. The computational formula for σ^2 has $N \cdot N$ in the denominator rather than $n(n-1)$.

Example 2.7.1

Let us now illustrate the computation of the variance and standard deviation, by both the definitional and the computational formula, using the data of Table 2.2.2.

Solution: Another work table such as Table 2.7.1 will be useful.

Dividing the total of column 6 by the total of column 3, less 1, we have

$$s^2 = \frac{\sum_{i=1}^{k} (m_i - \bar{x})^2 f_i}{\sum_{i=1}^{k} f_i - 1} = \frac{20197.6336}{168} = 120.224$$

The standard deviation is

$$s = \sqrt{120.224} = 10.9647$$

TABLE 2.7.1 Work Table for Computing the Variance and Standard Deviation from the Data in Table 2.2.2

	Calculations for Equation 2.7.1					Calculations for Equation 2.7.2		
(1) Class Interval	(2) Class Midpoint m_i	(3) Class Frequency f_i	(4) $(m_i - \bar{x})$	(5) $(m_i - \bar{x})^2$	(6) $(m_i - \bar{x})^2 f_i$	(7) m_i^2	(8) $m_i^2 f_i$	(9) $m_i f_i$
10–19	14.5	4	−19.88	395.2144	1,580.8576	210.25	841.00	58.0
20–29	24.5	66	−9.88	97.6144	6,442.5504	600.25	39,616.50	1617.0
30–39	34.5	47	.12	.0144	.6768	1190.25	55,941.75	1621.5
40–49	44.5	36	10.18	102.4144	3,686.9184	1980.25	71,289.00	1602.0
50–59	54.5	12	20.12	404.2144	4,857.7728	2970.25	35,643.00	654.0
60–69	64.5	4	30.12	907.2144	3,628.8576	4160.25	16,641.00	258.0
Total $\bar{x} = 34.48$		169		1907.2864	20,197.6336		219,972.25	5810.5

If we use the computing formula of Equation 2.7.2, we have

$$s^2 = \frac{169(219972.25) - (5810.5)^2}{169(168)} = 120.224$$

For comparative purposes, we note that the standard deviation is 10.328 when computed from the 169 ages and the formula for ungrouped data is used.

EXERCISES

In the following exercises, treat the data sets as samples.

2.7.1 See Exercise 2.3.1. Find:

    a. The mean.   **b.** The median.
    c. The modal class.   **d.** The variance.
    e. The standard deviation.

2.7.2 See Exercise 2.3.2. Find:

    a. The mean.   **b.** The median.
    c. The modal class.   **d.** The variance.
    e. The standard deviation.

2.7.3 See Exercise 2.3.3. Find:

    a. The mean.   **b.** The median.
    c. The modal class.   **d.** The variance.
    e. The standard deviation.

2.7.4 See Exercise 2.3.4. Find:
- **a.** The mean.
- **b.** The median.
- **c.** The modal class.
- **d.** The variance.
- **e.** The standard deviation.

2.7.5 See Exercises 2.3.5. Find:
- **a.** The mean.
- **b.** The median.
- **c.** The variance.
- **d.** The standard deviation.

2.7.6 See Exercise 2.3.6. Find:
- **a.** The mean.
- **b.** The median.
- **c.** The variance.
- **d.** The standard deviation.

2.7.7 See Exercise 2.3.7. Find:
- **a.** The mean.
- **b.** The median.
- **c.** The variance.
- **d.** The standard deviation.

2.7.8 Stein and Uhde (A-12) examined the dynamic status of the hypothalamic–pituitary–thyroid axis in panic disorder by studying the neuroendocrine responses to protirelin in a sample of patients with panic disorder and a sample of normal controls. Among the data collected on the subjects were behavioral ratings as measured by the Zung Anxiety scale (ZAS). The following are the ZAS scores of the 26 subjects who had a diagnosis of panic disorder:

> 53 59 45 36 69 51 51 38 40 41 46 45 53 41 46 45 60 43 41 38 40
> 35 31 38 36 35

> SOURCE: Thomas W. Uhde, M.D. Used with permission.

Construct a box-and-whisker plot for these data.

2.8
Summary

In this chapter various descriptive statistical procedures are explained. These include the organization of data by means of the ordered array, the frequency distribution, the relative frequency distribution, the histogram, and the frequency polygon. The concepts of central tendency and variation are described, along with methods for computing their more common measures: the mean, median, mode, range, variance, and standard deviation. The concepts and methods are presented in a way that makes possible the handling of both grouped and ungrouped data. The reader is introduced to exploratory data analysis through a description of stem-and-leaf displays and box-and-whisker plots.

We emphasize the use of the computer as a tool for calculating descriptive measures and constructing various distributions from large data sets.

REVIEW QUESTIONS AND EXERCISES

1. Define:
   a. Stem-and-leaf display
   b. Box-and-whisker plot
   c. Percentile
   d. Quartile
   e. Location parameter
   f. Exploratory data analysis
   g. Ordered array
   h. Frequency distribution
   i. Relative frequency distribution
   j. Statistic
   k. Parameter
   l. Frequency polygon
   m. True class limits
   n. Histogram

2. Define and compare the characteristics of the mean, the median, and the mode.

3. What are the advantages and limitations of the range as a measure of dispersion?

4. Explain the rationale for using $n - 1$ to compute the sample variance.

5. What is the purpose of the coefficient of variation?

6. What is the purpose of Sturges' rule?

7. What assumptions does one make when computing the mean from grouped data? The median? The variance?

8. Describe from your field of study a population of data where knowledge of the central tendency and dispersion would be useful. Obtain real or realistic synthetic values from this population and compute the mean, median, mode, variance, and standard deviation, using the techniques for ungrouped data.

9. Collect a set of real, or realistic, data from your field of study and construct a frequency distribution, a relative frequency distribution, a histogram, and a frequency polygon.

10. Compute the mean, median, modal class, variance, and standard deviation for the data in Exercise 9, using the techniques for grouped data.

11. Find an article in a journal from your field of study in which some measure of central tendency and dispersion have been computed.

12. Exercise 2.7.8 uses Zung Anxiety Scale (ZAS) scores of 26 subjects with panic disorder who participated in a study conducted by Stein and Uhde (A-12). In their study these investigators also used 22 healthy control subjects (that is, subjects who did not have panic disorder). The following are the ZAS scores of 21 of these healthy controls:

    26 28 34 26 25 26 26 30 34 28 25 26 31 25 25 25 25 28 25 25 25
    SOURCE: Thomas W. Uhde, M.D. Used with permission.

    a. Combine these scores with the scores for the 26 patients with panic disorder and construct a stem-and-leaf plot.
    b. Based on the stem-and-leaf plot, what one word would you use to describe the nature of the data?
    c. Why do you think the stem-and-leaf plot looks the way it does?
    d. For the combined ZAS data, and using formulas for ungrouped data, compute the mean, median, variance, and standard deviation.

13. Refer to Exercise 12. Compute, for the 21 healthy controls alone, the mean, median, variance, and standard deviation.

14. Refer to Exercise 12. Compute the mean, median, variance, and standard deviation for the 26 patients with panic disorder.

15. Which set of ZAS scores are more variable: Those for the combined subjects, those for the healthy controls, or those for the patients with panic disorder? How do you justify your answer?

16. Refer to Exercise 12. Which measure of central tendency do you think is more appropriate to use to describe the ZAS scores, the mean or the median? Why?

17. Swift et al. (A-13) conducted a study concerned with the presence of significant psychiatric illness in heterozygous carriers of the gene for the Wolfram syndrome. According to the investigators, the Wolfram syndrome is an autosomal recessive neurodegenerative syndrome in which 25 percent of the individuals who are homozygous for the condition have severe psychiatric symptoms that lead to suicide attempts or psychiatric hospitalizations. Among the subjects studied were 543 blood relatives of patients with Wolfram syndrome. The following is a frequency distribution of the ages of these blood relatives:

Age	Number
20–29	55
30–39	93
40–49	113
50–59	90
60–69	85
70–79	73
80–89	29
90–99	5
Total	543

SOURCE: Ronnie Gorman Swift, Diane O. Perkins, Charles L. Chase, Debra B. Sadler, and Michael Swift, "Psychiatric Disorders in 36 Families With Wolfram Syndrome," *American Journal of Psychiatry*, *148* (1991), 775–779.

a. For these data construct a relative frequency distribution, a cumulative frequency distribution, and a cumulative relative frequency distribution.

b. Compute the mean, median, variance, and standard deviation. Use formulas for computing sample descriptive measures.

18. A concern that current recommendations on dietary energy requirements may underestimate the total energy needs of young adult men was the motivation for a study by Roberts et al, (A-14). Subjects for the study were 14 young, healthy adult men of normal body weight who were employed full-time in sedentary occupations as students or laboratory technicians. The following are the body mass index values (kg/m^2) for the 14 subjects in the sample:

24.4   30.4   21.4   25.1   21.3   23.8   20.8   22.9   20.9   23.2   21.1
23.0   20.6   26.0

SOURCE: Susan B. Roberts, Melvin B. Heyman, William J. Evans, Paul Fuss, Rita Tsay, and Vernon R. Young, "Dietary Energy Requirements of Young Adult Men, Determined by Using the Doubly Labeled Water Method," *American Journal of Clinical Nutrition*, *54* (1991), 499–505.

    a. Compute the mean, median, variance, standard deviation, and coefficient of variation.

    b. Construct a stem-and-leaf display.

    c. Construct a box-and-whisker plot.

    d. What percentage of the measurements are within one standard deviation of the mean? Within two standard deviations? Three standard deviations?

19. Refer to Exercise 18. The following are the weights (kg) and heights (cm) of the 14 subjects in the sample studied by Roberts et al. (A-14):

    Weight: 83.9 99.0 63.8 71.3 65.3 79.6 70.3 69.2 56.4
               66.2 88.7 59.7 64.6 78.8
    Height: 185 180 173 168 175 183 184 174 164 169 205
               161 177 174

    Source: Susan B. Roberts, Melvin B. Heyman, William J. Evans, Paul Fuss, Rita Tsay, and Vernon R. Young, "Dietary Energy Requirements of Young Adult Men, Determined by Using the Doubly Labeled Water Method," *American Journal of Clinical Nutrition*, *54* (1991), 499–505.

    a. For each variable, compute the mean, median, variance, standard deviation, and coefficient of variation.

    b. For each variable, construct a stem-and-leaf display and a box-and-whisker plot.

    c. Which set of measurements is more variable, weight or height? On what do you base your answer?

20. The following table shows the age distribution of cases of a certain disease reported during a year in a particular state.

Age	Number of Cases
5–14	5
15–24	10
25–34	20
35–44	22
45–54	13
55–64	5
Total	75

Compute the sample mean, median, variance, and standard deviation.

21. Give three synonyms for variation (variability).

22. As part of a research project, investigators obtained the following data on serum lipid peroxide (SLP) levels from laboratory reports of a sample of 10 adult subjects undergoing treatment for diabetes mellitus: 5.85, 6.17, 6.09, 7.70, 3.17, 3.83, 5.17, 4.31, 3.09, 5.24. Compute the mean, median, variance, and standard deviation.

23. The following are the SLP values obtained from a sample of 10 apparently healthy adults: 4.07, 2.71, 3.64, 3.37, 3.84, 3.83, 3.82, 4.21, 4.04, 4.50. For these data compute the mean, the variance, and the standard deviation.

24. The following are the ages of 48 patients admitted to the emergency room of a hospital. Construct a stem-and-leaf display from these data.

32	63	33	57	35	54	38	53	42	51	42	48
43	46	61	53	12	13	16	16	31	30	28	28
25	23	23	22	21	17	13	30	14	29	16	28
17	27	21	24	22	23	61	55	34	42	13	26

25. Researchers compared two methods of collecting blood for coagulation studies. The following are the arterial activated partial thromboplastin time (APTT) values recorded for 30 patients in each of the two groups. Construct a box-and-whisker plot from each set of measurements. Compare the two plots. Do they indicate a difference in the distributions of APTT times for the two methods?

Method 1:

20.7	29.6	34.4	56.6	22.5	29.7
31.2	38.3	28.5	22.8	44.8	41.6
24.9	29.0	30.1	33.9	39.7	45.3
22.9	20.3	28.4	35.5	22.8	54.7
52.4	20.9	46.1	35.0	46.1	22.1

Method 2:

23.9	23.2	56.2	30.2	27.2	21.8
53.7	31.6	24.6	49.8	22.6	48.9
23.1	34.6	41.3	34.1	26.7	20.1
38.9	24.2	21.1	40.7	39.8	21.4
41.3	23.7	35.7	29.2	27.4	23.2

26. Express in words the following properties of the sample mean:

a. $\sum(x - \bar{x})^2 = $ a minimum

b. $n\bar{x} = \sum x$

c. $\sum(x - \bar{x}) = 0$

27. Your statistics instructor tells you on the first day of class that there will be five tests during the term. From the scores on these tests for each student he will compute a measure of central tendency that will serve as the student's final course grade. Before taking the first test you must choose whether you want your final grade to be the mean or the median of the five test scores. Which would you choose? Why?

28. Consider the following possible class intervals for use in constructing a frequency distribution of serum cholesterol levels of subjects who participated in a mass screening:

a. 50–74	**b.** 50–74	**c.** 50–75
75–99	75–99	75–100
100–149	100–124	100–125
150–174	125–149	125–150
175–199	150–174	150–175
200–249	175–199	175–200
250–274	200–224	200–225
etc.	225–249	225–250
	etc.	etc.

Which set of class intervals do you think is most appropriate for the purpose? Why? State specifically for each one why you think the other two are less desirable.

29. On a statistics test students were asked to construct a frequency distribution of the blood creatine levels (Units/liter) for a sample of 300 healthy subjects. The mean was 95 and the standard deviation was 40. The following class interval widths were used by the students:

a. 1   **b.** 5
c. 10   **d.** 15
e. 20   **f.** 25

Comment on the appropriateness of these choices of widths.

30. Give a health sciences related example of a population of measurements for which the mean would be a better measure of central tendency than the median.

31. Give a health sciences related example of a population of measurements for which the median would be a better measure of central tendency than the mean.

32. Indicate for the following variables which you think would be a better measure of central tendency, the mean, the median, or mode and justify your choice:

a. Annual incomes of licensed practical nurses in the Southeast.

b. Diagnoses of patients seen in the emergency department of a large city hospital.

c. Weights of high-school male basketball players.

REFERENCES

References Cited

1. H. A. Sturges, "The Choice of a Class Interval," *Journal of the American Statistical Association*, *21* (1926), 65–66.
2. Helen M. Walker, "Degrees of Freedom," *The Journal of Educational Psychology*, *31* (1040), 253–269.
3. John W. Tukey, *Exploratory Data Analysis*, Addison-Wesley, Reading, Mass., 1977.
4. Mary B. Breckenridge, *Age, Time, and Fertility: Applications of Exploratory Data Analysis*, Academic Press, New York, 1983.
5. S. H. C. Du Toit, A. G. W. Steyn, and R. H. Stumpf, *Graphical Exploratory Data Analysis*, Springer-Verlag, New York, 1986.

Other References, Books

1. Harvey J. Brightman, *Statistics in Plain English*, South-Western, Cincinnati, 1986.
2. Wilfred J. Dixon and Frank J. Massey, Jr., *Introduction to Statistical Analysis*, Fourth Edition, McGraw-Hill, New York, 1985.
3. Bernard G. Greenberg, "Biostatistics," in Hugh Rodman Leavell and E. Gurney Clark, *Preventive Medicine*, McGraw-Hill, New York, 1965.
4. George W. Snedecor and William G. Cochran, *Statistical Methods*, Seventh Edition, The Iowa State University Press, Ames, 1980.
5. Robert G. D. Steel and James H. Torrie, *Principles and Procedures of Statistics: A Biometrical Approach*, Second Edition, McGraw-Hill, New York, 1980.

Other References, Journal Articles

1. I. Altmann and A. Ciocco, "Introduction to Occupational Health Statistics I," *Journal of Occupational Medicine, 6* (1964), 297–301.

2. W. F. Bodmer, "Understanding Statistics," *Journal of the Royal Statistical Society-A, 148* (1985), 69–81.

3. Darrell L. Butler and William Neudecker, "A Comparison of Inexpensive Statistical Packages for Microcomputers Running MS-DOS," *Behavior Research Methods, Instruments, & Computers, 21* (1989), 113–120.

4. Editorial, "Limitations of Computers in Medicine," *Canadian Medical Association Journal, 104* (1971), 234–235.

5. A. R. Feinstein, "Clinical Biostatistics I, A New Name and Some Other Changes of the Guard," *Clinical Pharmacology and Therapeutics,* (1970), 135–138.

6. Alva R. Feinstein, "Clinical Biostatistics VI, Statistical Malpractice—and the Responsibility of a Consultant," *Clinical Pharmacology and Therapeutics, 11* (1970), 898–914.

7. Lyon Hyams, "The Practical Psychology of Biostatistical Consultation," *Biometrics, 27* (1971), 201–211.

8. Johannes Ipsen, "Statistical Hurdles in the Medical Career," *American Statistician, 19* (June 1965), 22–24.

9. D. W. Marquardt, "The Importance of Statisticians," *Journal of the American Statistical Association, 82* (1987), 1–7.

10. Richard K. Means, "Interpreting Statistics: An Art," *Nursing Outlook, 13* (May 1965), 34–37.

11. Carol M. Newton, "Biostatistical Computing," *Federation Proceeding, Federation of American Societies for Experimental Biology, 33* (1974), 2317–2319.

12. E. S. Pearson, "Studies in the History of Probability and Statistics. XIV. Some Incidents in the Early History of Biometry and Statistics, 1890–94," *Biometrika, 52* (1965), 3–18.

13. Robert I. Rollwagen, "Statistical Methodology in Medicine," *Canadian Medical Association Journal, 112* (1975), 677.

14. D. S. Salsburg, "The Religion of Statistics as Practiced in Medical Journals," *The American Statistician, 39* (1985), 220–223.

15. Harold M. Schoolman, "Statistics in Medical Research," *The New England Journal of Medicine, 280* (1969), 218–219.

16. Stanley Schor and Irving Karten, "Statistical Evaluation of Medical Journal Manuscripts," *Journal of the American Medical Association, 195* (1966), 1123–1128.

17. H. C. Selvin and A. Stuart, "Data—Dredging Procedures in Surgery Analysis," *American Statistician, 20* (June 1966), 20–22.

18. Robert L. Stearman, "Statistical Concepts in Microbiology," *Bacteriological Reviews, 19* (1955), 160–215.

19. Harry E. Ungerleider and Courtland C. Smith, "Use and Abuse of Statistics," *Geriatrics, 22* (Feb. 1967), 112–120.

20. James P. Zimmerman, "Statistical Data and Their Use," *Physical Therapy, 49* (1969), 301–302.

Applications References

A-1. Silvio M. Veronese and Marcello Gambacorta, "Detection of Ki-67 Proliferation Rate in Breast Cancer," *American Journal of Clinical Pathology, 95* (1991), 30–34.

A-2. Nizar N. Jarjour, William J. Calhoun, Lawrence B. Schwartz, and William W. Busse, "Elevated Bronchoalveolar Lavage Fluid Histamine Levels in Allergic Asthmatics Are Associated with Increased Airway Obstruction," *American Review of Respiratory Disease, 144* (1991), 83–87.

A-3. Peter M. Ellis, Graham W. Mellsop, Ruth Beeston, and Russell R. Cooke, "Platelet Tritiated Imipramine Binding in Patients Suffering from Mania," *Journal of Affective Disorders, 22* (1991), 105–110.

A-4. Helen Herrman, Patrick McGorry, Jennifer Mills, and Bruce Singh, "Hidden Severe Psychiatric Morbidity in Sentenced Prisoners: An Australian Study," *American Journal of Psychiatry*, *148* (1991), 236–239.

A-5. Enrique Fernandez, Paltiel Weiner, Ephraim Meltzer, Mary M. Lutz, David B. Badish, and Reuben M. Cherniack, "Sustained Improvement in Gas Exchange After Negative Pressure Ventilation for 8 Hours Per Day on 2 Successive Days in Chronic Airflow Limitation," *American Review of Respiratory Disease*, *144* (1991), 390–394.

A-6. J. A. Dosman, W. C. Hodgson, and D. W. Cockcroft, "Effect of Cold Air on the Bronchial Response to Inhaled Histamine in Patients with Asthma," *American Review of Respiratory Disease*, *144* (1991), 45–50.

A-7. G. V. Sridharan, S. P. Wilkinson, and W. R. Primrose, "Pyogenic Liver Abscess in the Elderly," *Age and Ageing*, *19* (1990), 199–203.

A-8. Tadao Arinami, Miki Sato, Susumu Nakajima, and Ikuko Kondo, "Auditory Brain-Stem Responses in the Fragile X Syndrome," *American Journal of Human Genetics*, *43* (1988), 46–51.

A-9. Giancarlo Mari, "Arterial Blood Flow Velocity Waveforms of the Pelvis and Lower Extremities in Normal and Growth-Retarded Fetuses," *American Journal of Obstetrics and Gynecology*, *165* (1991), 143–151.

A-10. Welhelm Kuhnz, Durda Sostarek, Christiane Gansau, Tom Louton, and Marianne Mahler, "Single and Multiple Administration of a New Triphasic Oral Contraceptive to Women: Pharmacokinetics of Ethinyl Estradiol and Free and Total Testosterone Levels in Serum," *American Journal of Obstetrics and Gynecology*, *165* (1991), 596–602.

A-11. William C. Pitts, Virginia A. Rojas, Michael J. Gaffey, Robert V. Rouse, Jose Esteban, Henry F. Frierson, Richard L. Kempson, and Lawrence M. Weiss, "Carcinomas With Metaplasia and Sarcomas of the Breast," *American Journal of Clinical Pathology*, *95* (1991), 623–632.

A-12. Murray B. Stein and Thomas W. Uhde, "Endocrine, Cardiovascular, and Behavioral Effects of Intravenous Protirelin in Patients With Panic Disorder," *Archives of General Psychiatry*, *48* (1991), 148–156.

A-13. Ronnie Gorman Swift, Diane O. Perkins, Charles L. Chase, Debra B. Sadler, and Michael Swift, "Psychiatric Disorders in 36 Families With Wolfram Syndrome," *American Journal of Psychiatry*, *148* (1991), 775–779.

A-14. Susan B. Roberts, Melvin B. Heyman, William J. Evans, Pauls Fuss, Rita Tsay, and Vernon R. Young, "Dietary Energy Requirements of Young Adult Men, Determined by Using the Doubly Labeled Water Method," *American Journal of Clinical Nutrition*, *54* (1991), 499–505.

CHAPTER 3

Some Basic Probability Concepts

• •

CONTENTS

3.1
Introduction

The theory of probability provides the foundation for statistical inference. However, this theory, which is a branch of mathematics, is not the main concern of this book, and, consequently, only its fundamental concepts are discussed here. Students who desire to pursue this subject should refer to the books on probability by Bates (1), Dixon (2), Mosteller et al. (3), Earl et al. (4), Berman (5), Hausner (6), and Mullins and Rosen (7). They will also find helpful the books on mathematical statistics by Freund and Walpole (8), Hogg and Craig (9), and Mood et al. (10). For those interested in the history of probability, the books by Todhunter (11) and David (12) are recommended. From the latter, for example, we learn that the first mathematician to calculate a theoretical probability correctly was Girolamo Cardano, an Italian who lived from 1501 to 1576. The objectives of this chapter are to help students gain some mathematical ability in the area of probability and to assist them in developing an understanding of the more important concepts.

Progress along these lines will contribute immensely to their success in understanding the statistical inference procedures presented later in this book.

The concept of probability is not foreign to health workers and is frequently encountered in everyday communication. For example, we may hear a physician say that a patient has a 50–50 chance of surviving a certain operation. Another physician may say that she is 95 percent certain that a patient has a particular disease. A public health nurse may say that nine times out of ten a certain client will break an appointment. As these examples suggest, most people express probabilities in terms of percentages. In dealing with probabilities mathematically it is more convenient to express probabilities as fractions. (Percentages result from multiplying the fractions by 100.) Thus we measure the probability of the occurrence of some event by a number between zero and one. The more likely the event, the closer the number is to one; and the more unlikely the event, the closer the number is to zero. An event that cannot occur has a probability of zero, and an event that is certain to occur has a probability of one.

3.2
Two Views of Probability —
Objective and Subjective

Until fairly recently, probability was thought of by statisticians and mathematicians only as an *objective* phenomenon derived from objective processes.

The concept of *objective probability* may be categorized further under the headings of (1) *classical*, or *a priori*, *probability* and (2) the *relative frequency*, or *a posteriori*, concept of probability.

Classical Probability   The classical treatment of probability dates back to the 17th century and the work of two mathematicians, Pascal and Fermat (11, 12). Much of this theory developed out of attempts to solve problems related to games of chance, such as those involving the rolling of dice. Examples from games of chance illustrate very well the principles involved in classical probability. For example, if a fair six-sided die is rolled, the probability that a 1 will be observed is equal to 1/6 and is the same for the other five faces. If a card is picked at random from a well-shuffled deck of ordinary playing cards, the probability of picking a heart is 13/52. Probabilities such as these are calculated by the processes of abstract reasoning. It is not necessary to roll a die or draw a card to compute these probabilities. In the rolling of the die we say that each of the six sides is *equally likely* to be observed if there is no reason to favor any one of the six sides. Similarly, if there is no reason to favor the drawing of a particular card from a deck of cards we say that each of the 52 cards is equally likely to be drawn. We may define probability in the classical sense as follows.

DEFINITION

If an event can occur in N mutually exclusive and equally likely ways, and if m of these possess a characteristic, E, the probability of the occurrence of E is equal to m/N.

If we read $P(E)$ as "the probability of E," we may express this definition as

$$P(E) = \frac{m}{N} \qquad (3.2.1)$$

Relative Frequency Probability The relative frequency approach to probability depends on the repeatability of some process and the ability to count the number of repetitions, as well as the number of times that some event of interest occurs. In this context we may define the probability of observing some characteristic, E, of an event as follows.

DEFINITION

If some process is repeated a large number of times n, and if some resulting event with the characteristic E occurs m times, the relative frequency of occurrence of E, m/n, will be approximately equal to the probability of E.

To express this definition in compact form we write

$$P(E) = \frac{m}{n} \qquad (3.2.2)$$

We must keep in mind, however, that strictly speaking, m/n is only an estimate of $P(E)$.

Subjective Probability In the early 1950s, L. J. Savage (13) gave considerable impetus to what is called the "personalistic" or subjective concept of probability. This view holds that probability measures the confidence that a particular individual has in the truth of a particular proposition. This concept does not rely on the repeatability of any process. In fact, by applying this concept of probability, one may evaluate the probability of an event that can only happen once, for example, the probability that a cure for cancer will be discovered within the next 10 years.

Although the subjective view of probability has enjoyed increased attention over the years, it has not been fully accepted by statisticians who have traditional orientations.

3.3
Elementary Properties of Probability

In 1933 the axiomatic approach to probability was formalized by the Russian mathematician A. N. Kolmogorov (14). The basis of this approach is embodied in three properties from which a whole system of probability theory is constructed through the use of mathematical logic. The three properties are as follows.

1. Given some process (or experiment) with n mutually exclusive outcomes (called events), $E_1, E_2, \ldots, E_n$, the probability of any event E_i is assigned a nonnegative number. That is,

$$P(E_i) \geq 0 \tag{3.3.1}$$

In other words, all events must have a probability greater than or equal to zero, a reasonable requirement in view of the difficulty of conceiving of negative probability. A key concept in the statement of this property is the concept of *mutually exclusive* outcomes. Two events are said to be mutually exclusive if they cannot occur simultaneously.

2. The sum of the probabilities of all mutually exclusive outcomes is equal to 1.

$$P(E_1) + P(E_2) + \cdots + P(E_n) = 1 \tag{3.3.2}$$

This is the property of *exhaustiveness* and refers to the fact that the observer of a probabilistic process must allow for all possible events, and when all are taken together, their total probability is 1. The requirement that the events be mutually exclusive is specifying that the events $E_1, E_2, \ldots, E_n$ do not overlap.

3. Consider any two mutually exclusive events, E_i and E_j. The probability of the occurrence of either E_i or E_j is equal to the sum of their individual probabilities.

$$P(E_i \text{ or } E_j) = P(E_i) + P(E_j) \tag{3.3.3}$$

Suppose the two events were not mutually exclusive; that is, suppose they could occur at the same time. In attempting to compute the probability of the occurrence of either E_i or E_j the problem of overlapping would be discovered, and the procedure could become quite complicated.

3.4
Calculating the Probability of an Event

We now make use of the concepts and techniques of the previous sections in calculating the probabilities of specific events. Additional ideas will be introduced as needed.

Example 3.4.1

In an article in *The American Journal of Drug and Alcohol Abuse*, Erickson and Murray (A-1) state that women have been identified as a group at particular risk for cocaine addiction and that it has been suggested that their problems with cocaine are greater than those of men. Based on their review of the scientific literature and their analysis of the results of an original research study, the authors argue that there is no evidence that women's cocaine use exceeds that of men, that women's rates of use are growing faster than men's, or that female cocaine users experience more problems than male cocaine users. The subjects in the study by Erickson and Murray consisted of a sample of 75 men and 36 women. The authors state that the subjects are a fairly representative sample of "typical" adult users who were neither in treatment nor in jail. Table 3.4.1 shows the lifetime frequency of cocaine use and the gender of these subjects. Suppose we pick a person at random from this sample. What is the probability that this person will be a male?

TABLE 3.4.1 Frequency of Cocaine Use by Gender Among Adult Cocaine Users

Lifetime Frequency of Cocaine Use	Male (M)	Female (F)	Total
1–19 times (A)	32	7	39
20–99 times (B)	18	20	38
100 + times (C)	25	9	34
Total	75	36	111

SOURCE: Reprinted from Patricia G. Erickson and Glenn F. Murray, "Sex Differences in Cocaine Use and Experiences: A Double Standard?" *American Journal of Drug and Alcohol Abuse*, 15 (1989), 135–152, by courtesy of Marcel Dekker, Inc.

Solution: We assume that male and female are mutually exclusive categories and that the likelihood of selecting any one person is equal to the likelihood of selecting any other person. We define the desired probability as the number of subjects with the characteristic of interest (male) divided by the total number of subjects. We may write the result in probability notation as follows:

$$P(M) = \text{Number of males/Total number of subjects}$$

$$= 75/111 = .6757$$

Conditional Probability   On occasion, the set of "all possible outcomes" may constitute a subset of the total group. In other words, the size of the group of interest may be reduced by conditions not applicable to the total group. When probabilities are calculated with a subset of the total group as the denominator, the result is a *conditional probability*.

The probability computed in Example 3.4.1, for example, may be thought of as an unconditional probability, since the size of the total group served as the denominator. No conditions were imposed to restrict the size of the denominator. We may also think of this probability as a *marginal probability* since one of the marginal totals was used as the numerator.

We may illustrate the concept of conditional probability by referring again to Table 3.4.1.

Example 3.4.2   Suppose we pick a subject at random from the 111 subjects and find that he is a male (M). What is the probability that this male will be one who has used cocaine 100 times or more during his lifetime (C)?

Solution: The total number of subjects is no longer of interest, since, with the selection of a male, the females are eliminated. We may define the desired probability, then, as follows: Given that the selected subject is a male (M), what is the probability that the subject has used cocaine 100 times or more (C) during his lifetime? This is a conditional probability and is written as $P(C|M)$ in which the vertical line is read "given". The 75 males become the denominator of this conditional probability, and 25, the number of males who have used cocaine 100 times or more during their lifetime, becomes the numerator. Our desired probability, then, is

$$P(C|M) = 25/75 = .33$$

Joint Probability   Sometimes we want to find the probability that a subject picked at random from a group of subjects possesses two characteristics at the same time. Such a probability is referred to as a *joint probability*. We illustrate the calculation of a joint probability with the following example.

Example 3.4.3   Let us refer again to Table 3.4.1. What is the probability that a person picked at random from the 111 subjects will be a male (M) *and* be a person who has used cocaine 100 times or more during his lifetime (C)?

Solution: The probability we are seeking may be written in symbolic notation as $P(M \cap C)$ in which the symbol $\cap$ is read either as "intersection" or "and." The statement $M \cap C$ indicates the joint occurrence of conditions M and C. The number of subjects satisfying both of the desired conditions is found in Table 3.4.1 at the intersection of the column labeled M and the row labeled C and is seen to be 25. Since the selection will be made from the total set of subjects, the denominator is 111. Thus, we may write the joint probability as

$$P(M \cap C) = 25/111 = .2252$$

The Multiplication Rule A probability may be computed from other probabilities. For example, a joint probability may be computed as the product of an appropriate marginal probability and an appropriate conditional probability. This relationship is known as the *multiplication rule* of probability. We illustrate with the following example.

Example 3.4.4

We wish to compute the joint probability of male (M) and a lifetime frequency of cocaine use of 100 times or more (C) from a knowledge of an appropriate marginal probability and an appropriate conditional probability.

Solution: The probability we seek is $P(M \cap C)$. We have already computed a marginal probability, $P(M) = 75/111 = .6757$, and a conditional probability, $P(C|M) = 25/75 = .3333$. It so happens that these are appropriate marginal and conditional probabilities for computing the desired joint probability. We may now compute $P(M \cap C) = P(M)P(C|M) = (.6757)(.3333) = .2252$. This, we note, is, as expected, the same result we obtained earlier for $P(M \cap C)$.

We may state the multiplication rule in general terms as follows:
For any two events A and B,

$$P(A \cap B) = P(B)P(A|B), \qquad \text{if } P(B) \neq 0 \qquad (3.4.1)$$

For the same two events A and B, the multiplication rule may also be written as $P(A \cap B) = P(A)P(B|A)$, if $P(A) \neq 0$.

We see that through algebraic manipulation the multiplication rule as stated in Equation 3.4.1 may be used to find any one of the three probabilities in its statement if the other two are known. We may, for example, find the conditional probability $P(A|B)$ by dividing $P(A \cap B)$ by $P(B)$. This relationship allows us to formally define conditional probability as follows.

DEFINITION

The *conditional probability* of A given B is equal to the probability of $A \cap B$ divided by the probability of B, provided the probability of B is not zero.

That is,

$$P(A|B) = \frac{P(A \cap B)}{P(B)}, \qquad P(B) \neq 0 \qquad (3.4.2)$$

We illustrate the use of the multiplication rule to compute a conditional probability with the following example.

Example 3.4.5

We wish to use Equation 3.4.2 and the data in Table 3.4.1 to find the conditional probability, $P(C|M)$.

Solution: According to Equation 3.4.2

$$P(C|M) = P(C \cap M)/P(M)$$

Earlier we found $P(C \cap M) = P(M \cap C) = 25/111 = .2252$. We have also determined that $P(M) = 75/111 = .6757$. Using these results we are able to compute $P(C|M) = .2252/.6757 = .3333$ which, as expected, is the same result we obtained by using the frequencies directly from Table 3.4.1.

The Addition Rule   The third property of probability given previously states that the probability of the occurrence of either one or the other of two mutually exclusive events is equal to the sum of their individual probabilities. Suppose, for example, that we pick a person at random from the 111 represented in Table 3.4.1. What is the probability that this person will be a male (M) or a female (F)? We state this probability in symbols as $P(M \cup F)$ where the symbol $\cup$ is read either as "union" or "or." Since the two genders are mutually exclusive, $P(M \cup F) = P(M) + P(F) = (75/111) + (36/111) = .6757 + .3243 = 1$.

What if two events are not mutually exclusive? This case is covered by what is known as the *addition rule*, which may be stated as follows.

DEFINITION

Given two events A and B, the probability that event A, or event B, or both occur is equal to the probability that event A occurs, plus the probability that event B occurs, minus the probability that the events occur simultaneously.

The addition rule may be written

$$P(A \cup B) = P(A) + P(B) - P(A \cap B) \tag{3.4.3}$$

Let us illustrate the use of the addition rule by means of an example.

Example 3.4.6

If we select a person at random from the 111 subjects represented in Table 3.4.1, what is the probability that this person will be a male (M) or will have used cocaine 100 times or more during his lifetime (C) or both?

Solution: The probability we seek is $P(M \cup C)$. By the addition rule as expressed by Equation 3.4.3, this probability may be written as $P(M \cup C) = P(M) + P(C) - P(M \cap C)$. We have already found that $P(M) = 75/111 = .6757$ and $P(M \cap C) = 25/111 = .2252$. From the information in Table 3.4.1 we calculate $P(C) = 34/111 = .3063$. Substituting these results into the equation for $P(M \cup C)$ we have $P(M \cup C) = .6757 + .3063 - .2252 = .7568$

Note that the 25 subjects who are *both* male *and* have used cocaine 100 times or more are included in the 75 who are male as well as in the 34 who have used cocaine 100 times or more. Since, in computing the probability, these 25 have been added into the numerator twice, they have to be subtracted out once to overcome the effect of duplication, or overlapping.

Independent Events Suppose that, in Equation 3.4.1, we are told that event B has occurred, but that this fact has no effect on the probability of A. That is, suppose that the probability of event A is the same regardless of whether or not B occurs. In this situation, $P(A|B) = P(A)$. In such cases we say that A and B are *independent events*. The multiplication rule for two independent events, then, may be written as

$$P(A \cap B) = P(B)P(A); \quad P(A) \neq 0, \quad P(B) \neq 0 \qquad (3.4.4)$$

Thus, we see that if two events are independent, the probability of their joint occurrence is equal to the product of the probabilities of their individual occurrences.

Note that when two events with nonzero probabilities are independent, each of the following statements is true:

$$P(A|B) = P(A), \quad P(B|A) = P(B), \quad P(A \cap B) = P(A)P(B)$$

Two events are not independent unless all these statements are true.

Let us illustrate the concept of independence by means of the following example.

Example 3.4.7

In a certain high school class, consisting of 60 girls and 40 boys, it is observed that 24 girls and 16 boys wear eyeglasses. If a student is picked at random from this class, the probability that the student wears eyeglasses, $P(E)$, is 40/100, or .4.

a. What is the probability that a student picked at random wears eyeglasses, given that the student is a boy?

Solution: By using the formula for computing a conditional probability we find this to be

$$P(E|B) = \frac{P(E \cap B)}{P(B)} = \frac{16/100}{40/100} = .4$$

Thus the additional information that a student is a boy does not alter the probability that the student wears eyeglasses, and $P(E) = P(E|B)$. We say that the events being a boy and wearing eyeglasses for this group are independent. We may also show that the event of wearing eyeglasses, E, and *not* being a boy, $\bar{B}$, are also independent as follows:

$$P(E|\bar{B}) = \frac{P(E \cap \bar{B})}{P(\bar{B})} = \frac{24/100}{60/100} = \frac{24}{60} = .4$$

b. What is the probability of the joint occurrence of the events of wearing eyeglasses and being a boy?

Solution: Using the rule given in Equation 3.4.1, we have

$$P(E \cap B) = P(B)P(E|B)$$

but, since we have shown that events E and B are independent we may replace $P(E|B)$ by $P(E)$ to obtain, by Equation 3.4.4

$$P(E \cap B) = P(B)P(E)$$

$$= \left(\frac{40}{100}\right)\left(\frac{40}{100}\right)$$

$$= .16$$

Complementary Events   Earlier, using the data in Table 3.4.1, we computed the probability that a person picked at random from the 111 subjects will be a male as $P(M) = 75/111 = .6757$. We found the probability of a female to be $P(F) = 36/111 = .3243$. The sum of these two probabilities we found to be equal to 1. This is true because the events being male and being female are *complementary events*. In general, we may make the following statement about complementary events. The probability of an event A is equal to 1 minus the probability of its complement, which is written $\bar{A}$, and

$$P(\bar{A}) = 1 - P(A) \tag{3.4.5}$$

This follows from the third property of probability since the event, A, and its complement, $\bar{A}$, are mutually exclusive.

**Example
3.4.8**   Suppose that of 1200 admissions to a general hospital during a certain period of time, 750 are private admissions. If we designate these as set A, then $\bar{A}$ is equal to

1200 minus 750, or 450. We may compute

$$P(A) = 750/1200 = .625$$

and

$$P(\overline{A}) = 450/1200 = .375$$

and see that

$$P(\overline{A}) = 1 - P(A)$$

$$.375 = 1 - .625$$

$$.375 = .375$$

Marginal Probability Earlier we used the term *marginal probability* to refer to a probability in which the numerator of the probability is a marginal total from a table such as Table 3.4.1. For example, when we compute the probability that a person picked at random from the 111 persons represented in Table 3.4.1 is a male, the numerator of the probability is the total number of males, 75. Thus $P(M) = 75/111 = .6757$. We may define marginal probability more generally as follows.

DEFINITION

Given some variable that can be broken down into m categories designated by $A_1, A_2, \ldots, A_i, \ldots, A_m$ and another jointly occurring variable that is broken down into n categories designated by $B_1, B_2, \ldots, B_j, \ldots, B_n$, the *marginal probability* of A_i, $P(A_i)$, is equal to the sum of the joint probabilities of A_i with all the categories of B. That is,

$$P(A_i) = \sum P(A_i \cap B_j), \qquad \text{for all values of } j \qquad (3.4.6)$$

The following example illustrates the use of Equation 3.4.6 in the calculation of a marginal probability.

Example 3.4.9

We wish to use Equation 3.4.6 and the data in Table 3.4.1 to compute the marginal probability $P(M)$.

Solution: The variable gender is broken down into two categories, male (M) and female (F). The variable frequency of cocaine use is broken down into three categories, 1–19 times (A), 20–99 times (B), and 100+ times (C). The category male occurs jointly with all three categories of the variable frequency of cocaine use. The three joint probabilities that may be computed are $P(M \cap A) = 32/111 = .2883$, $P(M \cap B) = 18/111 = .1622$, and $P(M \cap C) = 25/111 = .2252$. We obtain the marginal probability $P(M)$ by adding these three joint probabilities as follows:

$$P(M) = P(M \cap A) + P(M \cap B) + P(M \cap C)$$

$$= .2883 + .1622 + .2252$$

$$= .6757$$

The result, as expected, is the same as the one obtained by using the marginal total for male as the numerator and the total number of subjects as the denominator.

EXERCISES

3.4.1 In a study of the influence of social and political violence on the risk of pregnancy complications, Zapata et al. (A-2) collected extensive information on a sample of 161 pregnant women between the ages of 19 and 40 years who were enrolled for prenatal care in six health centers in Santiago, Chile. The following table shows the sample subjects cross-classified according to education level and number of pregnancy complications:

Education (years)	Number of Pregnancy Complications		
	≥ 2	0–1	Total
1–3	22	53	75
4–8	9	23	32
9–10	10	27	37
≥ 11	5	12	17
Total	46	115	161

SOURCE: B. Cecilia Zapata, Annabella Rebolledo, Eduardo Atalah, Beth Newman, and Mary-Clair King, "The Influence of Social and Political Violence on the Risk of Pregnancy Complications," *American Journal of Public Health*, *82* (1992), 685–690. © 1992 American Public Health Association.

a. Suppose we pick a woman at random from this group. What is the probability that this woman will be one with two or more pregnancy complications?
b. What do we call the probability calculated in part a?
c. Show how to calculate the probability asked for in part a by two additional methods.
d. If we pick a woman at random, what is the probability that she will be one with two or more pregnancy complications and have four to eight years of education?

    e. What do we call the probability calculated in part d?

    f. Suppose we pick a woman at random and find that she has zero or one pregnancy complication. What is the probability that she has 11 years or more of education?

    g. What do we call the probability calculated in part f?

    h. Suppose we pick a woman at random. What is the probability that she is one with two or more pregnancy complications or has less than four years of education or both?

    i. What do we call the method by which you obtained the probability in part h?

3.4.2 In an article in the *Canadian Journal of Public Health*, Hammoud and Grindstaff (A-3) state that it is estimated that approximately 15 percent of the adult Canadian population is physically disabled to some degree. The authors reviewed a national sample of Canadian adults to determine the characteristics of the physically disabled, compared to a random sample of able-bodied in the same age groups. The following table shows the sample subjects cross-classified according to disability status and occupation:

	Disability Status		
Occupation	**Disabled**	**Able-bodied**	**Total**
Management	333	451	784
Clerical	260	281	541
Services	320	316	636
Primary	68	62	130
Manufacturing	297	317	614
Total	1278	1427	2705

SOURCE: Ali M. Hammoud and Carl F. Grindstaff, "Sociodemographic Characteristics of the Physically Disabled in Canada," *Canadian Journal of Public Health*, *83* (1992), 57–60.

    a. How many marginal probabilities can be calculated from these data? State each in probability notation and do the calculations.

    b. How many joint probabilities can be calculated? State each in probability notation and do the calculations.

    c. How many conditional probabilities can be calculated? State each in probability notation and do the calculations.

    d. Use the multiplication rule to find the probability that a person picked at random is able-bodied and is employed in a clerical occupation.

    e. What do we call the probability calculated in part d?

    f. Use the multiplication rule to find the probability that a person picked at random is disabled, given that he/she is employed in manufacturing.

    g. What do we call the probability calculated in part f?

    h. Use the concept of complementary events to find the probability that a person picked at random is employed in management.

3.4.3 Refer to the data in Exercise 3.4.2. State the following probabilities in words:

    a. $P(\text{Clerical} \cap \text{Able-bodied})$

    b. $P(\text{Clerical} \cup \text{Able-bodied})$

    c. $P(\text{Clerical} | \text{Able-bodied})$

    d. $P(\text{Clerical})$

3.4.4 Sninsky et al. (A-4) conducted a study to evaluate the efficacy and safety of a pH-sensitive, polymer-coated oral preparation of mesalamine in patients with mildly to moderately active ulcerative colitis. The following table shows the results of treatment at the end of six weeks by treatment received:

Outcome	Treatment Group		
	Placebo	Mesalamine, 1.6 g / d	Mesalamine, 2.4 g / d
In remission	2	6	6
Improved	8	13	15
Maintained	12	11	14
Worsened	22	14	8

SOURCE: Reproduced with permission from Charles A. Sninsky, David H. Cort, Fergus Shanahan, Bernard J. Powers, John T. Sessions, Ronald E. Pruitt, Walter H. Jacobs, Simon K. Lo, Stephan R. Targan, James J. Cerda, Daniel E. Gremillion, William J. Snape, John Sabel, Horacio Jinich, James M. Swinehart, and Michael P. DeMicco, "Oral Mesalamine (Asacol) for Mildly to Moderately Active Ulcerative Colitis," *Annals of Internal Medicine*, *115* (1991), 350–355.

  a. What is the probability that a randomly selected patient will be in remission at the end of six weeks?
  b. What is the probability that a patient placed on placebo will be in remission at the end of six weeks?
  c. What is the probability that a randomly selected patient will be in remission and one who received the placebo?
  d. What is the probability that a patient selected at random will be one who received a dose of 2.4 g/d or was listed as improved or both?

3.4.5 If the probability of left-handedness in a certain group of people is .05, what is the probability of right-handedness (assuming no ambidexterity)?

3.4.6 The probability is .6 that a patient selected at random from the current residents of a certain hospital will be a male. The probability that the patient will be a male who is in for surgery is .2. A patient randomly selected from current residents is found to be a male; what is the probability that the patient is in the hospital for surgery?

3.4.7 In a certain population of hospital patients the probability is .35 that a randomly selected patient will have heart disease. The probability is .86 that a patient with heart disease is a smoker. What is the probability that a patient randomly selected from the population will be a smoker *and* have heart disease?

3.5
Summary

In this chapter some of the basic ideas and concepts of probability were presented. The objective has been to provide enough of a "feel" for the subject so that the probabilistic aspects of statistical inference can be more readily understood and appreciated when this topic is presented later.

We defined probability as a number between 0 and 1 that measures the likelihood of the occurrence of some event. We distinguished between subjective probability and objective probability. Objective probability can be categorized further as either classical or relative frequency probability. After stating the three properties of probability, we defined and illustrated the calculation of the following kinds of probabilities: marginal, joint, and conditional. We also learned how to apply the addition and multiplication rules to find certain probabilities. Finally we learned the meaning of independent, mutually exclusive, and complementary events.

REVIEW QUESTIONS AND EXERCISES

1. Define the following:

a. Probability

b. Objective probability

c. Subjective probability

d. Classical probability

e. The relative frequency concept of probability

f. Mutually exclusive events

g. Independence

h. Marginal probability

i. Joint probability

j. Conditional probability

k. The addition rule

l. The multiplication rule

m. Complementary events

2. Name and explain the three properties of probability.

3. Des Jarlais et al. (A-5) examined the failure to maintain AIDS risk reduction in a study of intravenous drug users from New York City. The following table shows the study subjects cross-classified according to risk reduction status and number of sexual partners in an average month:

Number of Sexual Partners / Month	Risk Reduction Status			
	None	**Not Maintained**	**Maintained**	**Total**
None	20	17	43	80
1	37	45	95	177
> 1	20	54	67	141
Total	77	116	205	398

SOURCE: Reprinted from Don C. Des Jarlais, Abu Abdul-Quader, and Susan Tross, "The Next Problem: Maintenance of AIDS Risk Reduction Among Intravenous Drug Users," *The International Journal of the Addictions, 26* (1991), 1279–1292, by courtesy of Marcel Dekker, Inc.

a. We select a subject at random. What is the probability that he/she did not initiate any risk reduction?

b. We select a subject at random and find that he/she had more than one sexual partner. What is the probability that he/she maintained risk reduction?

c. We select a subject at random. What is the probability that he/she had no sexual partners and did not maintain risk reduction?

d. We select a subject at random. What is the probability that he/she had one sexual partner or initiated no risk reduction?

4. The purpose of a study by Gehan et al. (A-6) was to define the optimum dose of lignocaine required to reduce pain on injection of propofol. According to these researchers, propofol is a rapidly acting intravenous agent used for induction of anesthesia. Despite its many advantages, however, pain induced by its injection limits its use. Other studies have shown that intravenous lignocaine given before or with propofol reduced the frequency of pain. Subjects used in the study by Gehan et al. (A-6) were 310 patients undergoing anesthesia. Patients were allocated to four categories according to lignocaine dosage. Group A received no lignocaine, while Groups B, C, and D received .1, .2, and .4 mg kg^{-1}, respectively mixed with propofol. The degree of pain experienced by patients was scored from 0 to 3, with patients experiencing no pain receiving a score of 0. The following table shows the patients cross-classified by dose level group and pain score:

Pain Score	Group				
	A	**B**	**C**	**D**	**Total**
0	49	73	58	62	242
1	16	7	7	8	38
2	8	5	6	6	25
3	4	1	0	0	5
Total	77	86	71	76	310

SOURCE: G. Gehan, P. Karoubi, F. Quinet, A. Leroy, C. Rathat, and J. L. Pourriat, "Optimal Dose of Lignocaine for Preventing Pain on Injection of Propofol," *British Journal of Anaesthesia*, *66* (1991), 324–326.

a. Find the following probabilities and explain their meaning:
   1. $P(0 \cap D)$
   2. $P(B \cup 2)$
   3. $P(3 | A)$
   4. $P(C)$

b. Explain why each of the following equations is or is not a true statement:
   1. $P(0 \cap D) = P(D \cap 0)$
   2. $P(2 \cup C) = P(C \cup 2)$
   3. $P(A) = P(A \cap 0) + P(A \cap 1) + P(A \cap 2) + P(A \cap 3)$
   4. $P(B \cup 2) = P(B) + P(2)$
   5. $P(D | 0) = P(D)$
   6. $P(C \cap 1) = P(C)P(1)$
   7. $P(A \cap B) = 0$
   8. $P(2 \cap D) = P(D)P(2 | D)$
   9. $P(B \cap 0) = P(B)P(B | 0)$

5. One hundred married women were asked to specify which type of birth control method they preferred. The following table shows the 100 responses cross-classified by educational level of the respondent.

Birth Control Method	Educational Level			
	High School (A)	College (B)	Graduate School (C)	Total
S	15	8	7	30
T	3	7	20	30
V	5	5	15	25
W	10	3	2	15
Total	33	23	44	100

Specify the number of members of each of the following sets:

a. S **b.** $V \cup C$ **c.** A **d.** $\overline{W}$

e. U **f.** $\overline{B}$ **g.** $T \cap B$ **h.** $\overline{(T \cap C)}$

6. A certain county health department has received 25 applications for an opening that exists for a public health nurse. Of these applicants ten are over 30 and fifteen are under 30. Seventeen hold bachelor's degrees only, and eight have master's degrees. Of those under 30, six have master's degrees. If a selection from among these 25 applicants is made at random, what is the probability that a person over 30 *or* a person with a master's degree will be selected?

7. The following table shows 1000 nursing school applicants classified according to scores made on a college entrance examination and the quality of the high school from which they graduated, as rated by a group of educators.

Score	Quality of High Schools			
	Poor (P)	Average (A)	Superior (S)	Total
Low (L)	105	60	55	220
Medium (M)	70	175	145	390
High (H)	25	65	300	390
Total	200	300	500	1000

a. Calculate the probability that an applicant picked at random from this group:
   1. Made a low score on the examination.
   2. Graduated from a superior high school.
   3. Made a low score on the examination and graduated from a superior high school.
   4. Made a low score on the examination given that he or she graduated from a superior high school.
   5. Made a high score or graduated from a superior high school.

b. Calculate the following probabilities:

   1. $P(A)$ **2.** $P(H)$ **3.** $P(M)$

   4. $P(A|H)$ **5.** $P(M \cap P)$ **6.** $P(H|S)$

8. If the probability that a public health nurse will find a client at home is .7, what is the probability (assuming independence) that on two home visits made in a day both clients will be home?

9. The following table shows the outcome of 500 interviews completed during a survey to study the opinions of residents of a certain city about legalized abortion. The data are also classified by the area of the city in which the questionnaire was attempted.

Area of City	Outcome			Total
	For (F)	Against (Q)	Undecided (R)	
A	100	20	5	125
B	115	5	5	125
D	50	60	15	125
E	35	50	40	125
Total	300	135	65	500

a. If a questionnaire is selected at random from the 500, what is the probability that:
  1. The respondent was for legalized abortion?
  2. The respondent was against legalized abortion?
  3. The respondent was undecided?
  4. The respondent lived in area A? B? D? E?
  5. The respondent was for legalized abortion, given that he/she resided in area B?
  6. The respondent was undecided or resided in area D?
b. Calculate the following probabilities:
  1. $P(A \cap R)$ 2. $P(Q \cup D)$ 3. $P(\overline{D})$
  4. $P(Q|D)$ 5. $P(B|R)$ 6. $P(F)$

10. In a certain population the probability that a randomly selected subject will have been exposed to a certain allergen and experience a reaction to the allergen is .60. The probability is .8 that a subject exposed to the allergen will experience an allergic reaction. If a subject is selected at random from this population, what is the probability that he/she will have been exposed to the allergen?

11. Suppose that 3 percent of the people in a population of adults have attempted suicide. It is also known that 20 percent of the population are living below the poverty level. If these two events are independent, what is the probability that a person selected at random from the population will have attempted suicide *and* be living below the poverty level?

12. In a certain population of women 4 percent have had breast cancer, 20 percent are smokers, and 3 percent are smokers and have had breast cancer. A woman is selected at random from the population. What is the probability that she has had breast cancer or smokes or both?

13. The probability that a person selected at random from a population will exhibit the classic symptom of a certain disease is .2, and the probability that a person selected at random has the disease is .23. The probability that a person who has the symptom also has the disease is .18. A person selected at random from the population does not have the symptom; what is the probability that the person has the disease?

14. For a certain population we define the following events for mother's age at time of giving birth: A = under 20 years; B = 20–24 years; C = 25–29 years; D = 30–44 years. Are the events A, B, C, and D pairwise mutually exclusive?

15. Refer to Exercise 14. State in words the event $E = (A \cup B)$.

16. Refer to Exercise 14. State in words the event $F = (B \cup C)$.

17. Refer to Exercise 14. Comment on the event $G = (A \cap B)$.

18. For a certain population we define the following events with respect to plasma lipoprotein levels (mg/dl): $A = (10–15)$; $B - (\geq 30)$; $C - (\leq 20)$. Are the events A and B mutually exclusive? A and C? B and C? Explain your answer to each question.

19. Refer to Exercise 18. State in words the meaning of the following events:
a. $A \cup B$ **b.** $A \cap B$ **c.** $A \cap C$ **d.** $A \cup C$

20. Refer to Exercise 18. State in words the meaning of the following events:
a. $\bar{A}$ **b.** $\bar{B}$ **c.** $\bar{C}$

REFERENCES

References Cited

1. Grace E. Bates, *Probability*, Addison-Wesley, Reading, Mass., 1965.

2. John R. Dixon, *A Programmed Introduction to Probability*, Wiley, New York, 1964.

3. Frederick Mosteller, Robert E. K. Rourke, and George T. Thomas, Jr., *Probability With Statistical Applications*, Second Edition, Addison-Wesley, Reading, Mass., 1970.

4. Boyd Earl, William Moore, and Wendell I. Smith, *Introduction to Probability*, McGraw-Hill, New York, 1963.

5. Simeon M. Berman, *The Elements of Probability*, Addison-Wesley, Reading, Mass., 1969.

6. Melvin Hausner, *Elementary Probability Theory*, Harper & Row, New York, 1971.

7. E. R. Mullins, Jr., and David Rosen, *Concepts of Probability*, Bogden and Quigley, New York, 1972.

8. John E. Freund and Ronald E. Walpole, *Mathematical Statistics*, Fourth Edition, Prentice-Hall, Englewood Cliffs, N.J., 1987.

9. Robert V. Hogg and Allen T. Craig, *Introduction to Mathematical Statistics*, Fourth Edition, Macmillan, New York, 1978.

10. Alexander M. Mood, Franklin A. Graybill, and Duane C. Boes, *Introduction to the Theory of Statistics*, Third Edition, McGraw-Hill, New York, 1974.

11. I. Todhunter, *A History of the Mathematical Theory of Probability*, G. E. Stechert, New York, 1931.

12. F. N. David, *Games, Gods and Gambling*, Hafner, New York, 1962.

13. L. J. Savage, *Foundations of Statistics*, Second Revised Edition, Dover, New York, 1972.

14. A. N. Kolmogorov, *Foundations of the Theory of Probability*, Chelsea, New York, 1964. (Original German edition published in 1933.)

Applications References

A-1. Patricia G. Erickson and Glenn F. Murray, "Sex Differences in Cocaine Use and Experiences: A Double Standard?" *American Journal of Drug and Alcohol Abuse*, *15* (1989), 135–152, Marcel Dekker, Inc., New York.

A-2. B. Cecilia Zapata, Annabella Rebolledo, Eduardo Atalah, Beth Newman, and Mary-Clair King, "The Influence of Social and Political Violence on the Risk of Pregnancy Complications," *American Journal of Public Health*, *82* (1992), 685–690.

A-3. Ali M. Hammoud and Carl F. Grindstaff, "Sociodemographic Characteristics of the Physically Disabled in Canada," *Canadian Journal of Public Health*, *83* (1992), 57–60.

A-4. Charles A. Sninsky, David H. Cort, Fergus Shanahan, Bernard J. Powers, John T. Sessions, Ronald E. Pruitt, Walter H. Jacobs, Simon K. Lo, Stephan R. Targan, James J. Cerda, Daniel E. Gremillion, William J. Snape, John Sabel, Horacio Jinich, James M. Swinehart, and Michael P. DeMicco, "Oral Mesalamine (Asacol) for Mildly to Moderately Active Ulcerative Colitis," *Annals of Internal Medicine*, *115* (1991), 350–355.

A-5. Don C. Des Jarlais, Abu Abdul-Quader, and Susan Tross, "The Next Problem: Maintenance of AIDS Risk Reduction Among Intravenous Drug Users," *The International Journal of the Addictions*, *26* (1991), 1279–1292, Marcel Dekker, Inc., New York.

A-6. G. Gehan, P. Karoubi, F. Quinet, A. Leroy, C. Rathat, and J. L. Pourriat, "Optimal Dose of Lignocaine for Preventing Pain on Injection of Propofol," *British Journal of Anaesthesia*, *66* (1991), 324–326.

CHAPTER 4

Probability Distributions

· ·

CONTENTS

4.1
Introduction

In the preceding chapter we introduced the basic concepts of probability as well as methods for calculating the probability of an event. We build on these concepts in the present chapter and explore ways of calculating the probability of an event under somewhat more complex conditions.

4.2
Probability Distributions of Discrete Variables

Let us begin our discussion of probability distributions by considering the probability distribution of a discrete variable, which we shall define as follows:

79

DEFINITION

The *probability distribution* of a discrete random variable is a table, graph, formula, or other device used to specify all possible values of a discrete random variable along with their respective probabilities.

Example 4.2.1

In an article in the *American Journal of Obstetrics and Gynecology*, Buitendijk and Bracken (A-1) state that during the previous 25 years there had been an increasing awareness of the potentially harmful effects of drugs and chemicals on the developing fetus. The authors assessed the use of medication in a population of women who were delivered of infants at a large Eastern hospital between 1980 and 1982, and studied the association of medication use with various maternal characteristics such as alcohol, tobacco, and illegal drug use. Their findings suggest that women who engage in risk-taking behavior during pregnancy are also more likely to use medications while pregnant. Table 4.2.1 shows the prevalence of prescription and nonprescription drug use in pregnancy among the study subjects.

We wish to construct the probability distribution of the discrete variable X = number of prescription and nonprescription drugs used by the study subjects.

Solution: The values of X are $x_1 = 0$, $x_2 = 1, \ldots, x_{11} = 10$, and $x_{12} = 12$. We compute the probabilities for these values by dividing their respective frequencies

TABLE 4.2.1 Prevalence of Prescription and Nonprescription Drug Use in Pregnancy Among Women Delivered of Infants at a Large Eastern Hospital

Number of Drugs	Frequency
0	1425
1	1351
2	793
3	348
4	156
5	58
6	28
7	15
8	6
9	3
10	1
12	1
Total	4185

SOURCE: Simone Buitendijk and Michael B. Bracken, "Medication in Early Pregnancy: Prevalence of Use and Relationship to Maternal Characteristics," *American Journal of Obstetrics and Gynecology, 165* (1991), 33–40.

TABLE 4.2.2 Probability Distribution of Number of Prescription and Nonprescription Drugs Used During Pregnancy Among the Subjects Described in Example 4.2.1

Number of Drugs (x)	$P(X = x)$
0	.3405
1	.3228
2	.1895
3	.0832
4	.0373
5	.0139
6	.0067
7	.0036
8	.0014
9	.0007
10	.0002
12	.0002
Total	1.0000

by the total, 4185. Thus, for example, $P(X = x_1) = 1425/4185 = .3405$. We display the results in Table 4.2.2, which is the desired probability distribution.

Alternatively, we can present this probability distribution in the form of a graph, as in Figure 4.2.1. In Figure 4.2.1 the length of each vertical bar indicates the probability for the corresponding value of x.

It will be observed in Table 4.2.2 that the values of $P(X = x)$ are all positive, they are all less than 1, and their sum is equal to 1. These are not phenomena peculiar to this particular example, but are characteristics of all probability distributions of discrete variables. We may then give the following two essential properties of a probability distribution of a discrete variable:

$$(1) \quad 0 \le P(X = x) \le 1$$

$$(2) \quad \sum P(X = x) = 1$$

The reader will also note that each of the probabilities in Table 4.2.2 is the *relative frequency of occurrence* of the corresponding value of X.

With its probability distribution available to us, we can make probability statements regarding the random variable X. We illustrate with some examples.

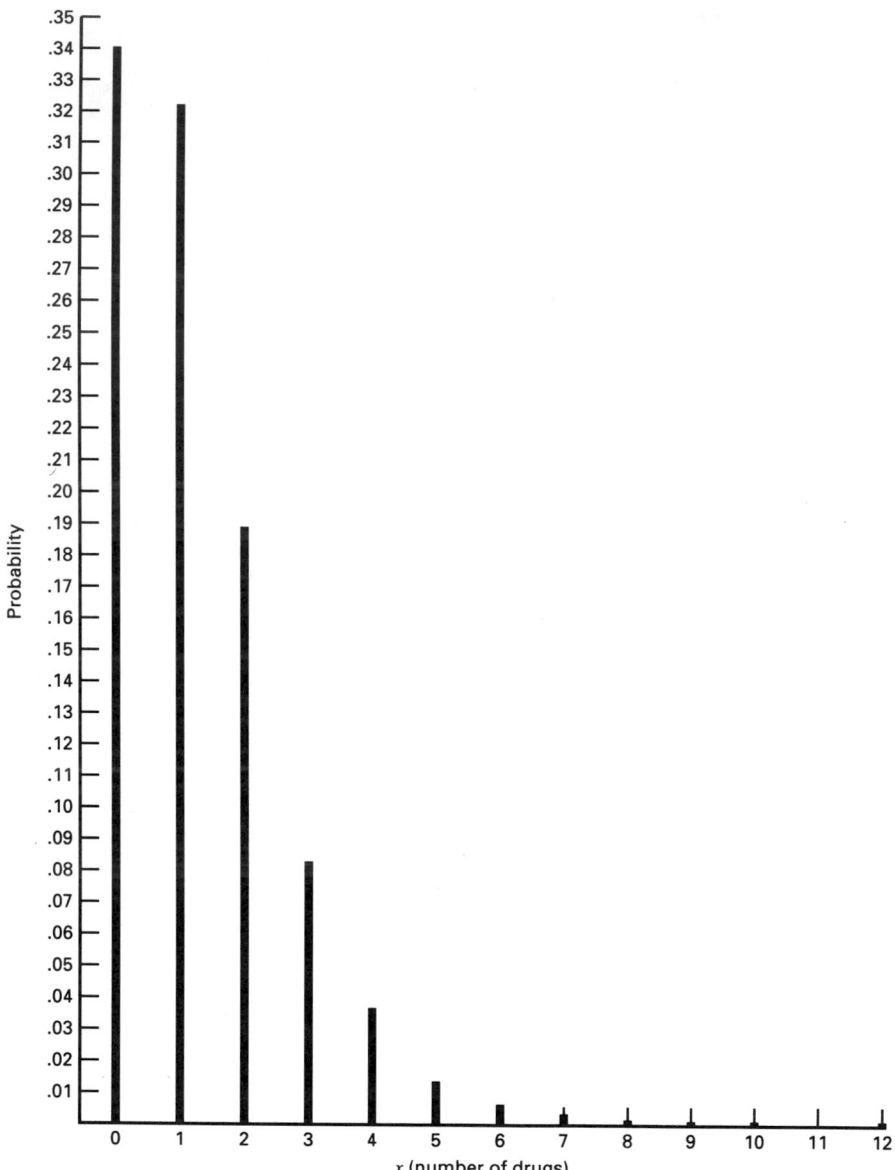

Figure 4.2.1   Graphical representation of the probability distribution shown in Table 4.2.1.

Example 4.2.2   What is the probability that a randomly selected woman will be one who used three prescription and nonprescription drugs?

Solution: We may write the desired probability as $P(X = 3)$. We see in Table 4.2.2 that the answer is .0832.

Example 4.2.3

What is the probability that a randomly selected woman used either one or two drugs?

Solution: To answer this question, we use the addition rule for mutually exclusive events. Using probability notation and the results in Table 4.2.2, we write the answer as $P(1 \cup 2) = P(1) + P(2) = .3228 + .1895 = .5123$.

Cumulative Distributions Sometimes it will be more convenient to work with the *cumulative probability distribution* of a random variable. The cumulative probability distribution for the discrete variable whose probability distribution is given in Table 4.2.2 may be obtained by successively adding the probabilities, $P(X = x)$, given in the last column. The cumulative probability for x_i is written as $F(x) = P(X \leq x_i)$. It gives the probability that X is less than or equal to a specified value, x_i.

The resulting cumulative probability distribution is shown in Table 4.2.3 The graph of the cumulative probability distribution is shown in Figure 4.2.2. The graph of a cumulative probability distribution is called an *ogive*. In Figure 4.2.2 the graph of $F(x)$ consists solely of the horizontal lines. The vertical lines only give the graph a connected appearance. The length of each vertical line represents the same probability as that of the corresponding line in Figure 4.2.1. For example, the length of the vertical line at $X = 3$ in Figure 4.2.2 represents the same probability as the length of the line erected at $X = 3$ in Figure 4.2.1, or .0832 on the vertical scale.

By consulting the cumulative probability distribution we may answer quickly questions like those in the following examples.

TABLE 4.2.3 Cumulative Probability Distribution of Number of Prescription and Nonprescription Drugs Used During Pregnancy Among the Subjects Described in Example 4.2.1

Number of Drugs (x)	Cumulative Frequency $P(X \leq 2)$
0	.3405
1	.6633
2	.8528
3	.9360
4	.9733
5	.9872
6	.9939
7	.9975
8	.9989
9	.9996
10	.9998
12	1.0000

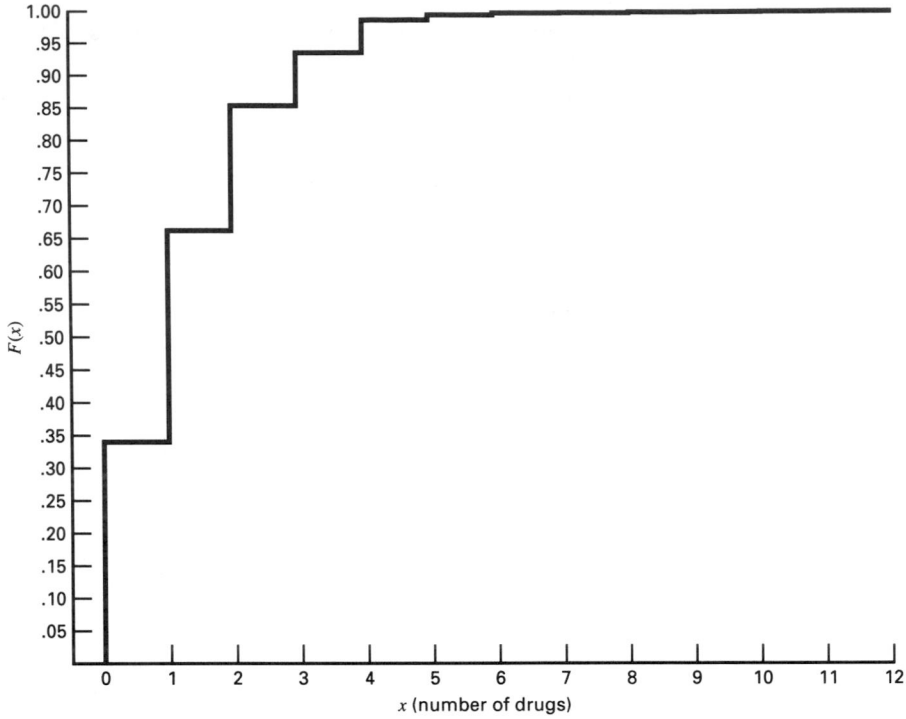

Figure 4.2.2 Cumulative probability distribution of number of prescription and nonprescription drugs used during pregnancy among the subjects described in Example 4.2.1.

Example 4.2.4   What is the probability that a woman picked at random will be one who used two or fewer drugs?

Solution: The probability we seek may be found directly in Table 4.2.3 by reading the cumulative probability opposite $x = 2$, and we see that it is .8528. That is, $P(x \leq 2) = .8528$. We also may find the answer by inspecting Figure 4.2.2 and determining the height of the graph (as measured on the vertical axis) above the value $x = 2$.

Example 4.2.5   What is the probability that a randomly selected woman will be one who used fewer than two drugs?

Solution: Since a woman who used fewer than two drugs used either one or no drugs, the answer is the cumulative probability for 1. That is, $P(x < 2) = P(x \leq 1) = .6633$.

Example 4.2.6

What is the probability that a randomly selected woman used five or more drugs?

Solution: To find the answer we make use of the concept of complementary probabilities. The set of women who used five or more drugs is the complement of the set of women who used fewer than five (that is, four or fewer) drugs. The sum of the two probabilities associated with these sets is equal to 1. We write this relationship in probability notation as $P(x \geq 5) + P(x \leq 4) = 1$. Therefore, $P(x \geq 5) = 1 - P(x \leq 4) = 1 - .9733 = .0267$.

Example 4.2.7

What is the probability that a randomly selected woman is one who used between three and five drugs, inclusive?

Solution: $P(x \leq 5) = .9872$ is the probability that a woman used between zero and five drugs, inclusive. To get the probability of between three and five drugs, we subtract from .9872, the probability of two or fewer. Using probability notation we write the answer as $P(3 \leq x \leq 5) = P(x \leq 5) - P(x \leq 2) = .9872 - .8528 = .1344$.

The probability distribution given in Table 4.2.1 was developed out of actual experience, so to find another variable following this distribution would be coincidental. The probability distributions of many variables of interest, however, can be determined or assumed on the basis of theoretical considerations. In the following sections, we study in detail three of these theoretical probability distributions, the *binomial*, the *Poisson*, and the *normal*.

4.3
The Binomial Distribution

The *binomial distribution* is one of the most widely encountered probability distributions in applied statistics. The distribution is derived from a process known as a *Bernoulli trial*, named in honor of the Swiss mathematician James Bernoulli (1654–1705), who made significant contributions in the field of probability, including, in particular, the binomial distribution. When a process or experiment, called a trial, can result in only one of two mutually exclusive outcomes, such as dead or alive, sick or well, male or female, the trial is called a Bernoulli trial.

The Bernoulli Process   A sequence of Bernoulli trials forms a *Bernoulli process* under the following conditions.

1. Each trial results in one of two possible, mutually exclusive, outcomes. One of the possible outcomes is denoted (arbitrarily) as a success, and the other is denoted a failure.

2. The probability of a success, denoted by p, remains constant from trial to trial. The probability of a failure, $1 - p$, is denoted by q.

3. The trials are independent; that is, the outcome of any particular trial is not affected by the outcome of any other trial.

Example 4.3.1

We are interested in being able to compute the probability of x successes in n Bernoulli trials. For example, suppose that in a certain population 52 percent of all recorded births are males. We interpret this to mean that the probability of a recorded male birth is .52. If we randomly select five birth records from this population, what is the probability that exactly three of the records will be for male births?

Solution: Let us designate the occurrence of a record for a male birth as a "success," and hasten to add that this is an arbitrary designation for purposes of clarity and convenience and does not reflect an opinion regarding the relative merits of male versus female births. The occurrence of a birth record for a male will be designated a success, since we are looking for birth records of males. If we are looking for birth records of females, these would be designated successes, and birth records of males would be designated failures.

It will also be convenient to assign the number 1 to a success (record for a male birth) and the number 0 to a failure (record of a female birth).

The process that eventually results in a birth record we consider to be a Bernoulli process.

Suppose the five birth records selected resulted in this sequence of sexes:

$$\text{MFMMF}$$

In coded form we would write this as

$$10110$$

Since the probability of a success is denoted by p and the probability of a failure is denoted by q, the probability of the above sequence of outcomes is found by means of the multiplication rule to be

$$P(1, 0, 1, 1, 0) = pqppq = q^2p^3$$

The multiplication rule is appropriate for computing this probability since we are seeking the probability of a male, and a female, and a male, and a male, and a female, in that order or, in other words, the joint probability of the five events. For simplicity, commas, rather than intersection notation, have been used to separate the outcomes of the events in the probability statement.

The resulting probability is that of obtaining the specific sequence of outcomes in the order shown. We are not, however, interested in the order of occurrence of records for male and female births but, instead, as has been stated already, the probability of the occurrence of exactly three records of male births out of five randomly selected records. Instead of occurring in the sequence shown above (call it sequence number 1), three successes and two failures could occur in any one of the following additional sequences as well:

Number	Sequence
2	11100
3	10011
4	11010
5	11001
6	10101
7	01110
8	00111
9	01011
10	01101

Each of these sequences has the same probability of occurring, and this probability is equal to $q^2 p^3$, the probability computed for the first sequence mentioned.

When we draw a single sample of size five from the population specified, we obtain only one sequence of successes and failures. The question now becomes, what is the probability of getting sequence number 1 or sequence number 2 . . . or sequence number 10? From the addition rule we know that this probability is equal to the sum of the individual probabilities. In the present example we need to sum the 10 $q^2 p^3$'s or, equivalently, multiply $q^2 p^3$ by 10. We may now answer our original question: What is the probability, in a random sample of size 5, drawn from the specified population, of observing three successes (record of a male birth) and two failures (record of a female birth)? Since in the population, $p = .52$, $q = (1 - p) = (1 - .52) = .48$, the answer to the question is

$$10(.48)^2(.52)^3 = 10(.2304)(.140608) = .32$$

Large Sample Procedure   We can easily anticipate that, as the size of the sample increases, listing the number of sequences becomes more and more difficult and tedious. What is needed is an easy method of counting the number of sequences. Such a method is provided by means of a counting formula that allows us to determine quickly how many subsets of objects can be formed when we use in the subsets different numbers of the objects that make up the set from which the objects are selected. When the order of the objects in a subset is immaterial, the subset is called a combination of objects. If a set consists of n objects, and we wish to form a subset of x objects from these n objects, without regard to the order of the objects in the subset, the result is called a *combination*. For emphasis, we define a combination as follows when the combination is formed by taking x objects from a set of n objects.

DEFINITION

A combination of n objects taken x at a time is an unordered subset of x of the n objects.

The number of combinations of n objects that can be formed by taking x of them at a time is given by

$$_nC_x = \frac{n!}{x!(n-x)!} \qquad (4.3.1)$$

where $x!$, read x factorial, is the product of all the whole numbers from x down to 1. That is, $x! = x(x-1)(x-2)\ldots(1)$. We note that, by definition, $0! = 1$.

Let us return to our example in which we have a sample of $n = 5$ birth records, and we are interested in finding the probability that three of them will be for male births.

The number of sequences in our example is found by Equation 4.3.1 to be

$$_5C_2 = \frac{5 \cdot 4 \cdot 3 \cdot 2 \cdot 1}{2 \cdot 1 \cdot 3 \cdot 2 \cdot 1} = 120/12 = 10$$

In our example we may let $x = 3$, the number of successes, so that $n - x = 2$, the number of failures. We then may write the probability of obtaining exactly x successes in n trials as

$$f(x) = {_nC_x}q^{n-x}p^x = {_nC_x}p^xq^{n-x} \qquad \text{for } x = 0, 1, 2, \ldots, n$$

$$= 0, \text{ elsewhere} \qquad (4.3.2)$$

This expression is called the binomial distribution. In Equation 4.3.2 $f(x) = P(X = x)$ where X is the random variable, number of successes in n trials. We use $f(x)$ rather than $P(X = x)$ because of its compactness and because of its almost universal use.

We may present the binomial distribution in tabular form as in Table 4.3.1.

We establish the fact that Equation 4.3.2 is a probability distribution by showing that

1. $f(x) \geq 0$ for all real values of x. This follows from the fact that n and p are both nonnegative and, hence, $_nC_x$, p^x, and $(1-p)^{n-x}$ are all nonnegative and, therefore, their product is greater than or equal to zero.

2. $\Sigma f(x) = 1$. This is seen to be true if we recognize that $\Sigma {_nC_x}q^{n-x}p^x$ is equal to $[(1-p) + p]^n = 1^n = 1$, the familiar binomial expansion. If the binomial $(q + p)^n$ is expanded we have

$$(q+p)^n = q^n + nq^{n-1}p^1 + \frac{n(n-1)}{2}q^{n-2}p^2 + \cdots + nq^1p^{n-1} + p^n$$

If we compare the terms in the expansion, term for term, with the $f(x)$ in

TABLE 4.3.1 The Binomial Distribution

Number of Successes, x	Probability, $f(x)$
0	$_nC_0 q^{n-0}p^0$
1	$_nC_1 q^{n-1}p^1$
2	$_nC_2 q^{n-2}p^2$
$\vdots$	$\vdots$
x	$_nC_x q^{n-x}p^x$
$\vdots$	$\vdots$
n	$_nC_n q^{n-n}p^n$
Total	1

Table 4.3.1 we see that they are, term for term, equivalent, since

$$f(0) = {_nC_0} q^{n-0}p^0 = q^n$$

$$f(1) = {_nC_1} q^{n-1}p^1 = nq^{n-1}p^1$$

$$f(2) = {_nC_2} q^{n-2}p^2 = \frac{n(n-1)}{2} q^{n-2}p^2$$

$$\vdots \qquad \vdots \qquad \vdots$$

$$f(n) = {_nC_n} q^{n-n}p^n = p^n$$

Example 4.3.2

As another example of the use of the binomial distribution, suppose that it is known that 30 percent of a certain population are immune to some disease. If a random sample of size 10 is selected from this population, what is the probability that it will contain exactly four immune persons?

Solution: We take the probability of an immune person to be .3. Using Equation 4.3.1 we find

$$f(4) = {_{10}C_4}(.7)^6(.3)^4$$

$$= \frac{10!}{4!6!}(.117649)(.0081)$$

$$= .2001$$

Binomial Table The calculation of a probability using Equation 4.3.1 can be a tedious undertaking if the sample size is large. Fortunately, probabilities for different values of n, p, and x have been tabulated, so that we need only to consult an appropriate table to obtain the desired probability. Table B of Appendix II is one of many such tables available. It gives the probability that x is less than or equal to some specified value. That is, the table gives the cumulative probabilities from $x = 0$ up through some specified value.

Let us illustrate the use of the table by using Example 4.3.2 where it was desired to find the probability that $x = 4$ when $n = 10$ and $p = .3$. Drawing on our knowledge of cumulative probability distributions from the previous section, we know that $P(x = 4)$ may be found by subtracting $P(X \leq 3)$ from $P(X \leq 4)$. If in Table B we locate $p = .3$ for $n = 10$, we find that $P(X \leq 4) = .8497$ and $P(X \leq 3) = .6496$. Subtracting the latter from the former gives $.8497 - .6496 = .2001$, which agrees with our hand calculation.

Frequently we are interested in determining probabilities, not for specific values of X, but for intervals such as the probability that X is between, say, 5 and 10. Let us illustrate with an example.

**Example
4.3.3**

Suppose it is known that in a certain population 10 percent of the population is color blind. If a random sample of 25 people is drawn from this population, use Table B in Appendix II to find the probability that:

a. Five or fewer will be color blind.

Solution: This probability is an entry in the table. No addition or subtraction is necessary. $P(X \leq 5) = .9666$.

b. Six or more will be color blind.

Solution: This set is the complement of the set specified in part a; therefore,

$$P(X \geq 6) = 1 - P(X \leq 5) = 1 - .9666 = .0334$$

c. Between six and nine inclusive will be color blind.

Solution: We find this by subtracting the probability that X is less than or equal to 5 from the probability that X is less than or equal to 9. That is,

$$P(6 \leq X \leq 9) = P(X \leq 9) - P(X \leq 5) = .9999 - .9666 = .0333$$

d. Two, three, or four will be color blind.

Solution: This is the probability that X is between 2 and 4 inclusive.

$$P(2 \leq X \leq 4) = P(X \leq 4) - P(X \leq 1) = .9020 - .2712 = .6308$$

Using Table B When $p > .5$ Table B does not give probabilities for values of p greater than .5. We may obtain probabilities from Table B, however, by restating the problem in terms of the probability of a failure, $1 - p$, rather than in terms of the probability of a success, p. As part of the restatement, we must also think in terms of the number of failures, $n - x$, rather than the number of successes, x. We may summarize this idea as follows:

$$P(X = x \mid n, p > .50) = P(X = n - x \mid n, 1 - p) \qquad (4.3.3)$$

In words, Equation 4.3.3 says, "The probability that X is equal to some specified value given the sample size and a probability of success greater than .5 is equal to the probability that X is equal to $n - x$ given the sample size and the probability of a failure of $1 - p$." For purposes of using the binomial table we treat the probability of a failure as though it were the probability of a success. When p is greater than .5, we may obtain cumulative probabilities from Table B by using the following relationship:

$$P(X \leq x|n, p > .5) = P(X \geq n - x|n, 1 - p) \qquad (4.3.4)$$

Finally, to use Table B to find the probability that X is greater than or equal to some x when $p > .5$, we use the following relationship:

$$P(X \geq x|n, p > .5) = P(X \leq n - x|n, 1 - p) \qquad (4.3.5)$$

Example 4.3.4

In a certain community, on a given evening, someone is at home in 85 percent of the households. A health research team conducting a telephone survey selects a random sample of 12 households. Use Table B to find the probability that:

a. The team will find someone at home in exactly 7 households.

Solution: We restate the problem as follows: What is the probability that the team conducting the survey gets no answer from exactly 5 calls out of 12, if no one is at home in 15 percent of the households? We find the answer as follows:

$$P(X = 5|n = 12, p = .15) = P(X \leq 5) - P(X \leq 4)$$
$$= .9954 - .9761 = .0193$$

b. The team will find someone at home in 5 or fewer households.

Solution: The probability we want is

$$P(X \leq 5|n = 12, p = .85) = P(X \geq 12 - 5|n = 12, p = .15)$$
$$= P(X \geq 7|n = 12, p = .15)$$
$$= 1 - P(X \leq 6|n = 12, p = .15)$$
$$= 1 - .9993 = .0007$$

c. The team will find someone at home in 8 or more households.

Solution: The probability we desire is

$$P(X \geq 8|n = 12, p = .85) = P(X \leq 4|n = 12, p = .15) = .9761$$

Figure 4.3.1 provides a visual representation of the solution to the three parts of Example 4.3.4.

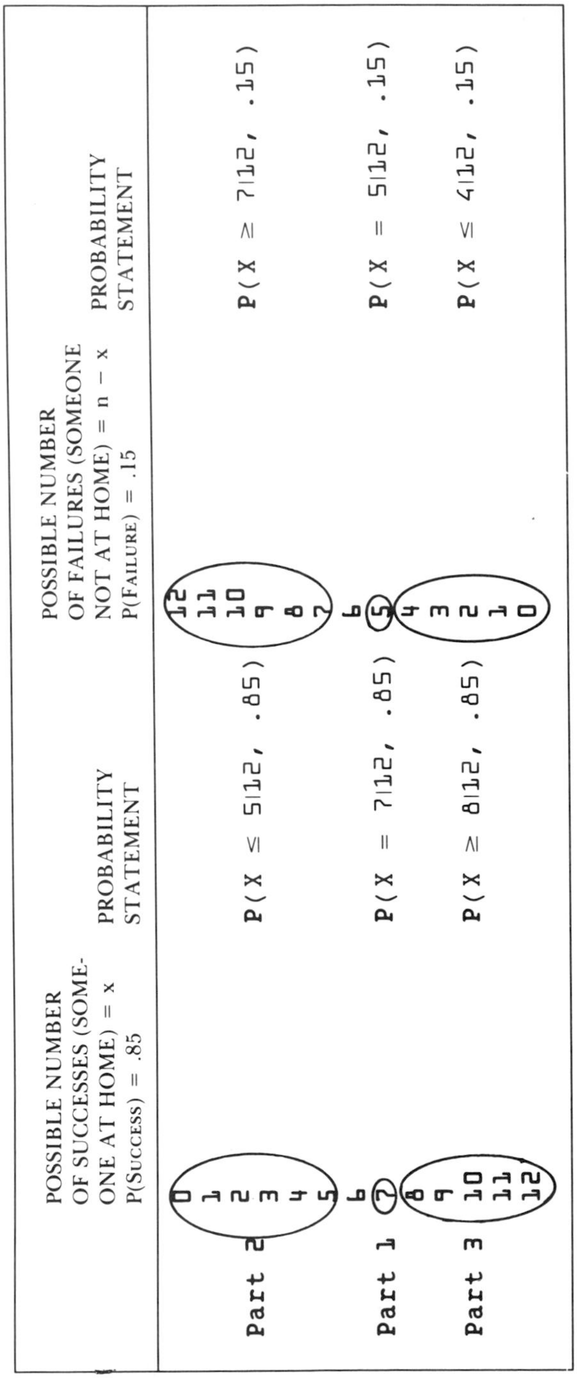

POSSIBLE NUMBER OF SUCCESSES (SOMEONE AT HOME) = x $P(\text{Success}) = .85$	PROBABILITY STATEMENT	POSSIBLE NUMBER OF FAILURES (SOMEONE NOT AT HOME) = n − x $P(\text{Failure}) = .15$	PROBABILITY STATEMENT
Part 2 (0 1 2 3 4 5) 6 (7) (8 9 10 11 12)	$P(X \leq 5 \mid 12, .85)$	(12 11 10 9 8 7) 6 (5) (4 3 2 1 0)	$P(X \geq 7 \mid 12, .15)$
Part 1	$P(X = 7 \mid 12, .85)$		$P(X = 5 \mid 12, .15)$
Part 3	$P(X \geq 8 \mid 12, .85)$		$P(X \leq 4 \mid 12, .15)$

Figure 4.3.1 Schematic representation of solutions to Example 4.3.4 (the relevant number of successes and failures in each case are circled).

The Binomial Parameters The binomial distribution has two parameters, n and p. They are parameters in the sense that they are sufficient to specify a binomial distribution. The binomial distribution is really a family of distributions with each possible value of n and p designating a different member of the family. The mean and variance of the binomial distribution are $\mu = np$ and $\sigma^2 = np(1 - p)$, respectively.

Strictly speaking, the binomial distribution is applicable in situations where sampling is from an infinite population or from a finite population with replacement. Since in actual practice samples are usually drawn without replacement from finite populations, the question naturally arises as to the appropriateness of the binomial distribution under these circumstances. Whether or not the binomial is appropriate depends on how drastic is the effect of these conditions on the constancy of p from trial to trial. It is generally agreed that when n is small relative to N, the binomial model is appropriate. Some writers say that n is small relative to N if N is at least 10 times as large as n.

EXERCISES

In each of the following exercises, assume that N is sufficiently large relative to n that the binomial distribution may be used to find the desired probabilities.

4.3.1 Based on their analysis of data collected by the National Center for Health Statistics, Najjar and Rowland (A-2) report that 25.7 percent of U. S. adults are overweight. If we select a simple random sample of 20 U. S. adults, find the probability that the number of overweight people in the sample will be (round the percentage to 26 for computation purposes):

a. Exactly three.　　**b.** Three or more.
c. Fewer than three.　　**d.** Between three and seven, inclusive.

4.3.2 Refer to Exercise 4.3.1. How many overweight adults would you expect to find in a sample of 20?

4.3.3 Refer to Exercise 4.3.1. Suppose we select a simple random sample of five adults. Use Equation 4.3.2 to find the probability that the number of overweight people in the sample will be:

a. Zero.　　　　　　　　　　　　　　**b.** More than one.
c. Between one and three, inclusive.　　**d.** Two or fewer.
e. Five.

4.3.4 A National Center for Health Statistics report based on 1985 data states that 30 percent of American adults smoke (A-3). Consider a simple random sample of 15 adults selected at that time. Find the probability that the number of smokers in the sample would be:

a. Three.　　　　　　　　　　　　　**b.** Less than five.
c. Between five and nine, inclusive.　　**d.** More than five, but less than 10.
e. Six or more.

4.3.5 Refer to Exercise 4.3.4. Find the mean and variance of the number of smokers in samples of size 15.

4.3.6   Refer to Exercise 4.3.4. Suppose we were to take a simple random sample of 25 adults today and find that two are smokers. Would these results cause you to suspect that the percentage of adults who smoke has decreased since 1985? Why or why not?

4.3.7   The probability that a person suffering from migraine headache will obtain relief with a particular drug is .9. Three randomly selected sufferers from migraine headache are given the drug. Find the probability that the number obtaining relief will be:

    a. Exactly zero.   **b**. Exactly one.

    c. More than one.   **d**. Two or fewer.

    e. Two or three.   **f**. Exactly three.

4.3.8.   In a survey of nursing students pursuing a master's degree, 75 percent stated that they expect to be promoted to a higher position within one month after receiving their degree. If this percentage holds for the entire population, find, for a sample of 15, the probability that the number expecting a promotion within a month after receiving their degree is:

    a. Six   **b**. At least seven

    c. No more than five   **d**. Between six and nine, inclusive

4.4
The Poisson Distribution

The next discrete distribution that we consider is the *Poisson distribution*, named for the French mathematician Simeon Denis Poisson (1781–1840), who is generally credited for publishing its derivation in 1837 (1, 2). This distribution has been used extensively, as a probability model in biology and medicine. Haight (2) presents a fairly extensive catalog of such applications in Chapter 7 of his book.

If x is the number of occurrences of some random event in an interval of time or space (or some volume of matter), the probability that x will occur is given by

$$f(x) = \frac{e^{-\lambda}\lambda^x}{x!}, \qquad x = 0, 1, 2, \ldots \qquad (4.4.1)$$

The Greek letter λ (lambda) is called the parameter of the distribution and is the average number of occurrences of the random event in the interval (or volume). The symbol e is the constant (to four decimals) 2.7183.

It can be shown that $f(x) \geq 0$ for every x and that $\sum_x f(x) = 1$, so that the distribution satisfies the requirements for a probability distribution.

The Poisson Process   We have seen that the binomial distribution results from a set of assumptions about an underlying process yielding a set of numerical observations. Such, also, is the case with the Poisson distribution. The following statements describe what is known as the *Poisson process*.

1. The occurrences of the events are independent. The occurrence of an event in an interval[1] of space or time has no effect on the probability of a second occurrence of the event in the same, or any other, interval.

2. Theoretically, an infinite number of occurrences of the event must be possible in the interval.

3. The probability of the single occurrence of the event in a given interval is proportional to the length of the interval.

4. In any infinitesimally small portion of the interval, the probability of more than one occurrence of the event is negligible.

An interesting feature of the Poisson distribution is the fact that the mean and variance are equal.

When to Use the Poisson Model   The Poisson distribution is employed as a model when counts are made of events or entities that are distributed at random in space or time. One may suspect that a certain process obeys the Poisson law, and under this assumption probabilities of the occurrence of events or entities within some unit of space or time may be calculated. For example, under the assumption that the distribution of some parasite among individual host members follows the Poisson law, one may, with knowledge of the parameter λ, calculate the probability that a randomly selected individual host will yield x number of parasites. In a later chapter we will learn how to decide whether the assumption that a specified process obeys the Poisson law is plausible.

To illustrate the use of the Poisson distribution for computing probabilities, let us consider the following examples.

Example 4.4.1   In a study of suicides, Gibbons et al. (A-4) found that the monthly distribution of adolescent suicides in Cook County, Illinois, between 1977 and 1987 closely followed a Poisson distribution with parameter $\lambda = 2.75$. Find the probability that a randomly selected month will be one in which three adolescent suicides occurred.

Solution: By Equation 4.4.1, we find the answer to be

$$P(X = 3) = \frac{e^{-2.75}2.75^3}{3!} = \frac{(.063928)(20.796875)}{6} = .221584$$

Example 4.4.2   Refer to Example 4.4.1. Assume that future adolescent suicides in the studied population will follow a Poisson distribution. What is the probability that a randomly selected future month will be one in which either three or four suicides will occur?

[1]For simplicity, the Poisson is discussed in terms of intervals, but other units, such as a volume of matter, are implied.

Solution: Since the two events are mutually exclusive, we use the addition rule to obtain

$$P(X = 3) + P(X = 4) = .221584 + \frac{e^{-2.75}2.75^4}{4!}$$

$$= .221584 + .152338 = .373922$$

In the foregoing examples the probabilities were evaluated directly from the equation. We may, however, use Appendix II Table C, which gives cumulative probabilities for various values of λ and X.

Example 4.4.3 In the study of a certain aquatic organism, a large number of samples were taken from a pond, and the number of organisms in each sample was counted. The average number of organisms per sample was found to be two. Assuming that the number of organisms follows a Poisson distribution, find the probability that the next sample taken will contain one or fewer organisms.

Solution: In Table C we see that when $\lambda = 2$, the probability that $X \leq 1$ is .406. That is, $P(X \leq 1|2) = .406$.

Example 4.4.4 Refer to Example 4.4.3. Find the probability that the next sample taken will contain exactly three organisms.

Solution:

$$P(X = 3|2) = P(X \leq 3) - P(X \leq 2) = .857 - .677 = .180$$

Example 4.4.5 Refer to Example 4.4.3. Find the probability that the next sample taken will contain more than five organisms.

Solution: Since the set of more than five organisms does not include five, we are asking for the probability that six or more organisms will be observed. This is obtained by subtracting the probability of observing five or fewer from 1. That is,

$$P(X > 5|2) = 1 - P(X \leq 5) = 1 - .983 = .017$$

EXERCISES

4.4.1 Suppose it is known that in a certain area of a large city the average number of rats per quarter block is five. Assuming that the number of rats follows a Poisson distribution, find the probability that in a randomly selected quarter block:

a. There are exactly five rats.

b. There are more than five rats.

c. There are fewer than five rats.

d. There are between five and seven rats, inclusive.

4.4.2 Suppose that over a period of several years the average number of deaths from a certain noncontagious disease has been 10. If the number of deaths from this disease follows the Poisson distribution, what is the probability that during the current year:

a. Exactly seven people will die from the disease?

b. Ten or more people will die from the disease?

c. There will be no deaths from the disease?

4.4.3 If the mean number of serious accidents per year in a large factory (where the number of employees remains constant) is five, find the probability that in the current year there will be:

a. Exactly seven accidents. **b.** Ten or more accidents.

c. No accidents. **d.** Fewer than five accidents.

4.4.4 In a study of the effectiveness of an insecticide against a certain insect, a large area of land was sprayed. Later the area was examined for live insects by randomly selecting squares and counting the number of live insects per square. Past experience has shown the average number of live insects per square after spraying to be .5. If the number of live insects per square follows a Poisson distribution, what is the probability that a selected square will contain:

a. Exactly one live insect? **b.** No live insects?

c. Exactly four live insects? **d.** One or more live insects?

4.4.5 In a certain population an average of 13 new cases of esophageal cancer are diagnosed each year. If the annual incidence of esophageal cancer follows a Poisson distribution, find the probability that in a given year the number of newly diagnosed cases of esophageal cancer will be:

a. Exactly 10. **b.** At least 8.

c. No more than 12. **d.** Between 9 and 15, inclusive.

e. Fewer than 7.

4.5
Continuous Probability Distributions

The probability distributions considered thus far, the binomial and the Poisson, are distributions of discrete variables. Let us now consider distributions of continuous random variables. In Chapter 1 we stated that a continuous variable is one that can assume any value within a specified interval of values assumed by the variable. Consequently, between any two values assumed by a continuous variable, there exist an infinite number of values.

To help us understand the nature of the distribution of a continuous random variable, let us consider the data presented in Table 1.4.1 and Figure 2.3.1. In the table we have 169 values of the random variable, age. The histogram of Figure 2.3.1 was constructed by locating specified points on a line representing the measurement of interest and erecting a series of rectangles, whose widths were the distances between two specified points on the line, and whose heights represented the number of values of the variable falling between the two specified points. The intervals defined by any two consecutive specified points we called class intervals. As was noted in Chapter 2, subareas of the histogram correspond to the frequencies of occurrence of values of the variable between the horizontal scale boundaries of these subareas. This provides a way whereby the relative frequency of occurrence of values between any two specified points can be calculated: merely determine the proportion of the histogram's total area falling between the specified points. This can be done more conveniently by consulting the relative frequency or cumulative relative frequency columns of Table 2.2.3.

Imagine now the situation where the number of values of our random variable is very large and the width of our class intervals is made very small. The resulting histogram could look like that shown in Figure 4.5.1.

If we were to connect the midpoints of the cells of the histogram in Figure 4.5.1 to form a frequency polygon, clearly we would have a much smoother figure than the frequency polygon of Figure 2.2.3.

In general, as the number of observations, n, approaches infinity, and the width of the class intervals approaches zero, the frequency polygon approaches a smooth curve such as is shown in Figure 4.5.2. Such smooth curves are used to represent graphically the distributions of continuous random variables. This has some important consequences when we deal with probability distributions. First, the total area under the curve is equal to one, as was true with the histogram, and the relative

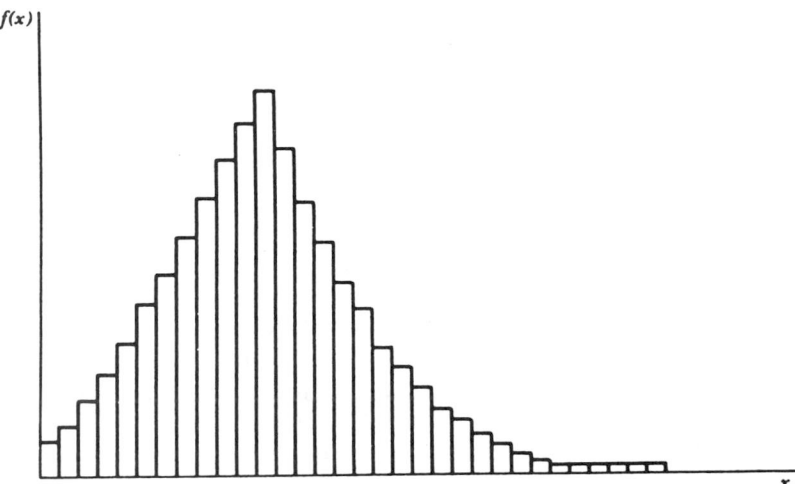

Figure 4.5.1 A histogram resulting from a large number of values and small class intervals.

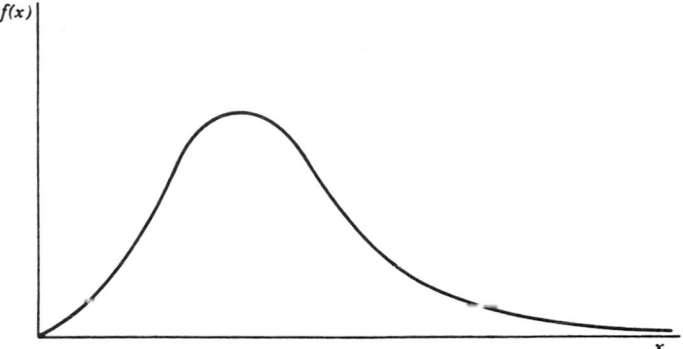

Figure 4.5.2 Graphical representation of a continuous distribution.

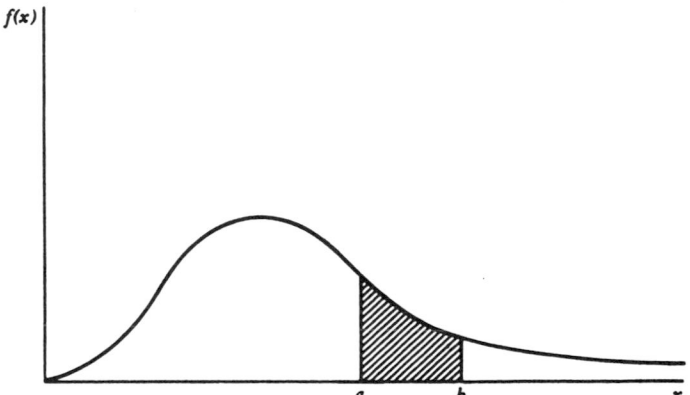

Figure 4.5.3 Graph of a continuous distribution showing area between *a* and *b*.

frequency of occurrence of values between any two points on the *x*-axis is equal to the total area bounded by the curve, the *x*-axis, and perpendicular lines erected at the two points on the *x*-axis. See Figure 4.5.3. The probability of *any specific value* of the random variable is *zero*. This seems logical, since a specific value is represented by a point on the *x*-axis and the area above a point is zero.

Finding Area Under a Smooth Curve   With a histogram, as we have seen, subareas of interest can be found by adding areas represented by the cells. We have no cells in the case of a smooth curve, so we must seek an alternate method of finding subareas. Such a method is provided by integral calculus. To find the area under a smooth curve between any two points *a* and *b*, the *density function* is integrated from *a* to *b*. A *density function* is a formula used to represent the distribution of a continuous random variable. Integration is the limiting case of summation, but we will not perform any integrations, since the mathematics involved are beyond the scope of this book. As we will see later, for all the continuous distributions we will consider, there will be an easier way to find areas under their curves.

Although the definition of a probability distribution for a continuous random variable has been implied in the foregoing discussion, by way of summary, we present it in a more compact form as follows.

DEFINITION

A nonnegative function $f(x)$ is called a *probability distribution* (sometimes called a probability density function) of the continuous random variable X if the total area bounded by its curve and the x-axis is equal to 1 and if the subarea under the curve bounded by the curve, the x-axis, and perpendiculars erected at any two points a and b gives the probability that X is between the points a and b.

4.6
The Normal Distribution

We come now to the most important distribution in all of statistics—the *normal distribution*. The formula for this distribution was first published by Abraham De Moivre (1667–1754) on November 12, 1733 (3). Many other mathematicians figure prominently in the history of the normal distribution, including Carl Friedrich Gauss (1777–1855). The distribution is frequently called the *Gaussian distribution* in recognition of his contributions.

The normal density is given by

$$f(x) = \frac{1}{\sqrt{2\pi}\,\sigma} e^{-(x-\mu)^2/2\sigma^2}, \qquad -\infty < x < \infty \qquad (4.6.1)$$

In Equation 4.6.1, π and e are the familiar constants, 3.14159 and 2.71828, respectively, which are frequently encountered in mathematics. The two parameters of the distribution are μ, the mean, and σ, the standard deviation. For our purposes we may think of μ and σ of a normal distribution, respectively, as measures of central tendency and dispersion as discussed in Chapter 2. Since, however, a normally distributed random variable is continuous and takes on values between $-\infty$ and $+\infty$, its mean and standard deviation may be more rigorously defined; but such definitions cannot be given without using calculus. The graph of the normal distribution produces the familiar bell-shaped curve shown in Figure 4.6.1.

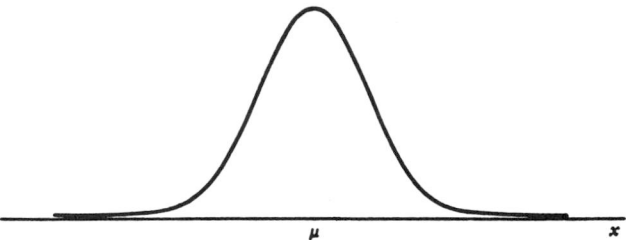

Figure 4.6.1 Graph of a normal distribution.

Characteristics of the Normal Distribution The following are some important characteristics of the normal distribution.

1. It is symmetrical about its mean, μ. As is shown in Figure 4.6.1, the curve on either side of μ is a mirror image of the other side.

2. The mean, the median, and the mode are all equal.

3. The total area under the curve above the x-axis is one square unit. This characteristic follows from the fact that the normal distribution is a probability distribution. Because of the symmetry already mentioned, 50 percent of the area is to the right of a perpendicular erected at the mean, and 50 percent is to the left.

4. If we erect perpendiculars a distance of 1 standard deviation from the mean in both directions, the area enclosed by these perpendiculars, the x-axis, and the curve will be approximately 68 percent of the total area. If we extend these lateral boundaries a distance of 2 standard deviations on either side of the mean, approximately 95 percent of the area will be enclosed, and extending them a distance of 3 standard deviations will cause approximately 99.7 percent of the total area to be enclosed. These approximate areas are illustrated in Figure 4.6.2.

5. The normal distribution is completely determined by the parameters μ and σ. In other words, a different normal distribution is specified for each different value of μ and σ. Different values of μ shift the graph of the distribution along the x-axis as is shown in Figure 4.6.3. Different values of σ determine the degree of flatness or peakedness of the graph of the distribution as is shown in Figure 4.6.4.

The Standard Normal Distribution The last-mentioned characteristic of the normal distribution implies that the normal distribution is really a family of distributions in which one member is distinguished from another on the basis of the values of μ and σ. The most important member of this family is the *standard normal distribution* or *unit normal distribution*, as it is sometimes called, because it has a mean of 0 and a standard deviation of 1. It may be obtained from Equation 4.6.1 by creating a random variable $z = (x - \mu)/\sigma$. The equation for the standard

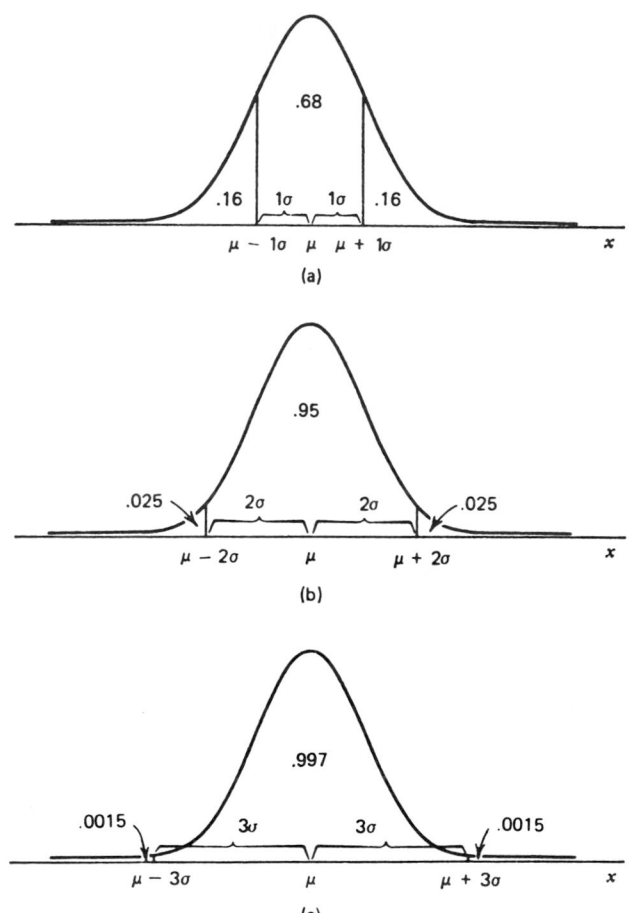

Figure 4.6.2 Subdivision of the area under the normal curve (areas are approximate).

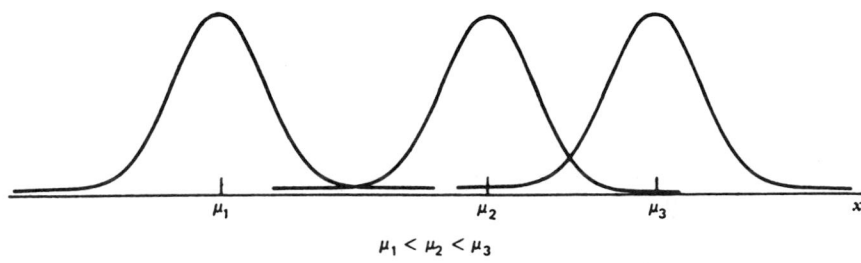

Figure 4.6.3 Three normal distributions with different means but the same amount of variability.

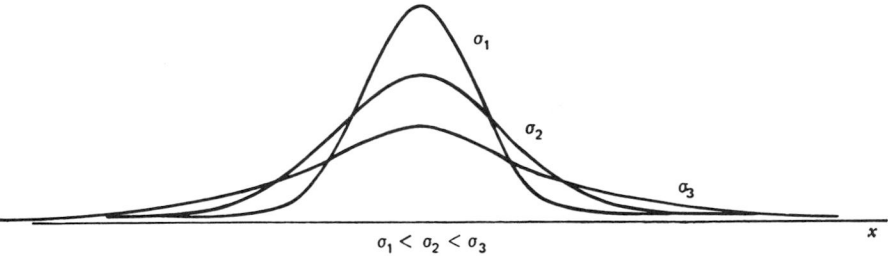

Figure 4.6.4 Three normal distributions with different standard deviations but the same mean.

normal distribution is written

$$f(z) = \frac{1}{\sqrt{2\pi}}e^{-z^2/2}, \qquad -\infty < z < \infty \qquad (4.6.2)$$

The graph of the standard normal distribution is shown in Figure 4.6.5.

To find the probability that z takes on a value between any two points on the z-axis, say z_0 and z_1, we must find the area bounded by perpendiculars erected at these points, the curve, and the horizontal axis. As we mentioned previously, areas under the curve of a continuous distribution are found by integrating the function between two values of the variable. In the case of the standard normal, then, to find the area between z_0 and z_1, we need to evaluate the following integral:

$$\int_{z_0}^{z_1} \frac{1}{\sqrt{2\pi}}e^{-z^2/2}\,dz$$

Fortunately, we do not have to concern ourselves with the mathematics, since there

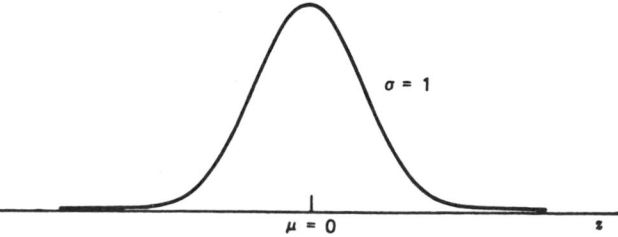

Figure 4.6.5 The standard normal distribution.

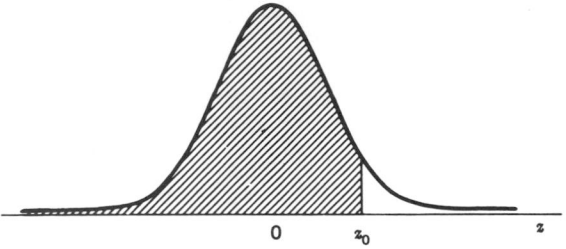

Figure 4.6.6 Area given by Appendix II Table D.

are tables available that provide the results of all such integrations in which we might be interested. Table D of Appendix II is an example of these tables. In the body of Table D are found the areas under the curve between $-\infty$ and the values of z shown in the left-most column of the table. The shaded area of Figure 4.6.6 represents the area listed in the table as being between $-\infty$ and z_0 where z_0 is the specified value of z.

We now illustrate the use of Table D by several examples.

Example 4.6.1

Given the standard normal distribution, find the area under the curve, above the z-axis between $z = -\infty$ and $z = 2$.

Solution: It will be helpful to draw a picture of the standard normal distribution and shade the desired area, as in Figure 4.6.7. If we locate $z = 2$ in Table D and read the corresponding entry in the body of the table, we find the desired area to be .9772. We may interpret this area in several ways. We may interpret it as the probability that a z picked at random from the population of z's will have a value between $-\infty$ and 2. We may also interpret it as the relative frequency of

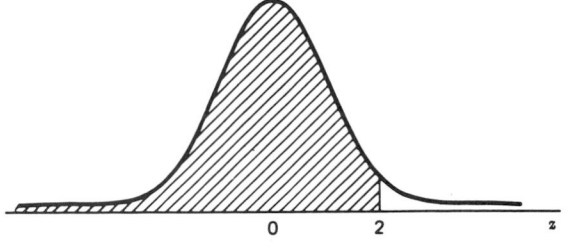

Figure 4.6.7 The standard normal distribution showing area between $z = -\infty$ and $z = 2$.

occurrence (or proportion) of values of z between $-\infty$ and 2, or we may say that 97.72 percent of the z's have a value between $-\infty$ and 2.

Example 4.6.2

What is the probability that a z picked at random from the population of z's will have a value between -2.55 and $+2.55$?

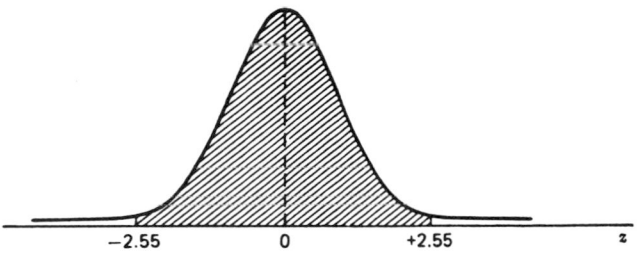

Figure 4.6.8 Standard normal curve showing $P(-2.55 < z < 2.55)$.

Solution: Figure 4.6.8 shows the area desired. Table D gives us the area between $-\infty$ and 2.55, which is found by locating 2.5 in the left-most column of the table and then moving across until we come to the entry in the column headed by .05. We find this area to be .9946. If we look at the picture we draw, we see that this is more area than is desired. We need to subtract from .9946 the area to the left of -2.55. Reference to Table D shows that the area to the left of -2.55 is .0054. Thus the desired probability is

$$P(-2.55 < z < 2.55) = .9946 - .0054 = .9892.$$

Suppose we had been asked to find the probability that z is between -2.55 and 2.55 inclusive. The desired probability is expressed as $P(-2.55 \leq z \leq 2.55)$. Since, as we noted in Section 4.5, $P(z = z_0) = 0$, $P(-2.55 \leq z \leq 2.55) = P(-2.55 < z < 2.55) = .9892$.

Example 4.6.3

What proportion of z values are between -2.74 and 1.53?

Solution: Figure 4.6.9 shows the area desired. We find in Table D that the area between $-\infty$ and 1.53 is .9370, and the area between $-\infty$ and -2.74 is .0031. To obtain the desired probability we subtract .0031 from .9370. That is,

$$P(-2.74 \leq z \leq 1.53) = .9370 - .0031 = .9339$$

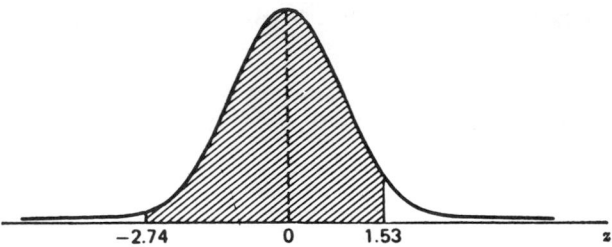

Figure 4.6.9 Standard normal curve showing proportion of z values between $z = -2.74$ and $z = 1.53$.

Example 4.6.4

Given the standard normal distribution, find $P(z \geq 2.71)$.

Solution: The area desired is shown in Figure 4.6.10. We obtain the area to the right of $z = 2.71$ by subtracting the area between $-\infty$ and 2.71 from 1. Thus,

$$P(z \geq 2.71) = 1 - P(z \leq 2.71)$$

$$= 1 - .9966$$

$$= .0034$$

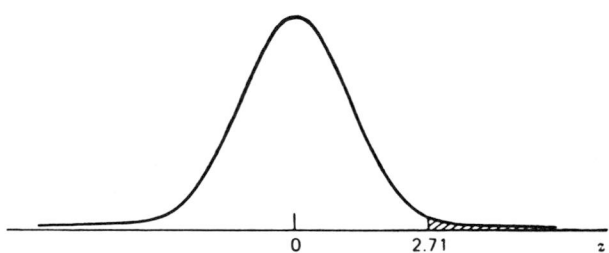

Figure 4.6.10 Standard normal distribution showing $P(z \geq 2.71)$.

Example 4.6.5

Given the standard normal distribution, find $P(.84 \leq z \leq 2.45)$.

Solution: The area we are looking for is shown in Figure 4.6.11. We first obtain the area between $-\infty$ and 2.45 and from that subtract the area between $-\infty$ and

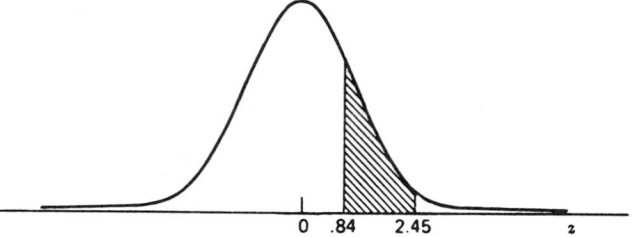

Figure 4.6.11   Standard normal curve showing $P(.84 \leq z \leq 2.45)$.

.84. In other words,

$$P(.84 \leq z \leq 2.45) = P(z \leq 2.45) - P(z \leq .84)$$

$$= .9929 - .7995$$

$$= .1934$$

EXERCISES

Given the standard normal distribution find:

4.6.1   The area under the curve between $z = 0$ and $z = 1.43$.

4.6.2   The probability that a z picked at random will have a value between $z = -2.87$ and $z = 2.64$.

4.6.3 $P(z \geq .55)$.   **4.6.4** $P(z \geq -.55)$.

4.6.5 $P(z < -2.33)$.   **4.6.6** $P(z < 2.33)$.

4.6.7 $P(-1.96 \leq z \leq 1.96)$.   **4.6.8** $P(-2.58 \leq z \leq 2.58)$.

4.6.9 $P(-1.65 \leq z \leq 1.65)$.   **4.6.10** $P(z = .74)$.

Given the following probabilities, find z_1:

4.6.11 $P(z \leq z_1) = .0055$ **4.6.12** $P(-2.67 \leq z \leq z_1) = .9718$

4.6.13 $P(z > z_1) = .0384$ **4.6.14** $P(z_1 \leq z \leq 2.98) = .1117$

4.6.15 $P(-z_1 \leq z \leq z_1) = .8132$

4.7
Normal Distribution Applications

Although its importance in the field of statistics is indisputable, one should realize that the normal distribution is not a law that is adhered to by all measurable characteristics occurring in nature. It is true, however, that many of these characteristics are approximately normally distributed. Consequently, even though no variable encountered in practice is precisely normally distributed, the normal distribution can be used to model the distribution of many variables that are of interest. Using the normal distribution as a model allows us to make useful probability statements about some variables much more conveniently than would be the case if some more complicated model had to be used.

Human stature and human intelligence are frequently cited as examples of variables that are approximately normally distributed. On the other hand, Elveback et al. (4) and Nelson et al. (5) have pointed out that many distributions relevant to the health field cannot be described adequately by a normal distribution. Whenever it is known that a random variable is approximately normally distributed or when, in the absence of complete knowledge, it is considered reasonable to make this assumption, the statistician is aided tremendously in his or her efforts to solve practical problems relative to this variable.

There are several other reasons why the normal distribution is so important in statistics, and these will be considered in due time. For now, let us see how we may answer simple probability questions about random variables when we know, or are willing to assume, that they are, at least, approximately normally distributed.

Example 4.7.1   As part of a study of Alzheimer's disease, Dusheiko (A-5) reported data that are compatible with the hypothesis that brain weights of victims of the disease are normally distributed. From the reported data, we may compute a mean of 1076.80 grams and a standard deviation of 105.76 grams. If we assume that these results are applicable to all victims of Alzheimer's disease, find the probability that a randomly selected victim of the disease will have a brain that weighs less than 800 grams.

Solution: First let us draw a picture of the distribution and shade the area corresponding to the probability of interest. This has been done in Figure 4.7.1.

If our distribution were the standard normal distribution with a mean of 0 and a standard deviation of 1, we could make use of Table D and find the probability with little effort. Fortunately, it is possible for any normal distribution to be

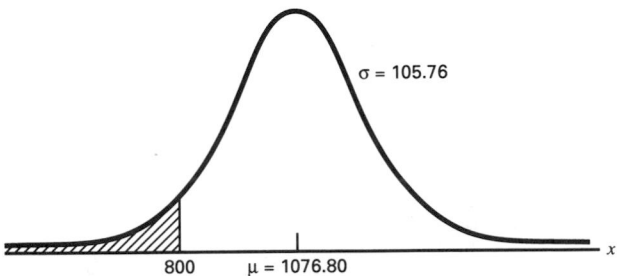

Figure 4.7.1 Normal distribution to approximate distribution of brain weights of patients with Alzheimer's disease (mean and standard deviation estimated).

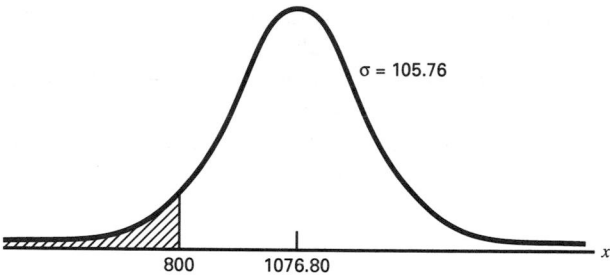

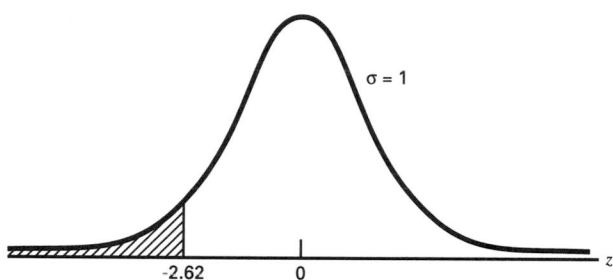

Figure 4.7.2 Normal distribution of brain weights (x) and the standard normal distribution (z).

transformed easily to the standard normal. What we do is transform all values of X to corresponding values of z. This means that the mean of X must become 0, the mean of z. In Figure 4.7.2 both distributions are shown. We must determine what value of z, say z_0, corresponds to an x of 800. This is done by the following formula:

$$z = \frac{x - \mu}{\sigma} \qquad (4.7.1)$$

which transforms any value of x in any normal distribution to the corresponding value of z in the standard normal distribution. For the present example we have

$$z = \frac{800 - 1076.80}{105.76} = -2.62$$

The value of z_0 we seek, then, is -2.62.

Let us examine these relationships more closely. It is seen that the distance from the mean, 1076.80, to the x-value of interest, 800, is $800 - 1076.80 = -276.80$, which is a distance of 2.62 standard deviations. When we transform brain weight values to z values, the distance of the z value of interest from its mean, 0, is equal to the distance of the corresponding x value from its mean, 1076.80, in standard deviation units. We have seen that this latter distance is 2.62 standard deviations. In the z distribution a standard deviation is equal to 1, and consequently the point on the z scale located a distance of 2.62 standard deviations below 0 is $z = -2.62$, the result obtained by employing the formula. By consulting Table D, we find that the area to the left of $z = -2.62$ is .0044. We may summarize this discussion as follows:

$$P(x < 800) = P\left(z < \frac{800 - 1076.80}{105.76}\right) = P(z < -2.62) = .0044$$

To answer the original question, we say that the probability is .0044 that a randomly selected patient will have a brain weight of less than 800 grams.

Example 4.7.2   Suppose it is known that the heights of a certain population of individuals are approximately normally distributed with a mean of 70 inches and a standard deviation of 3 inches. What is the probability that a person picked at random from this group will be between 65 and 74 inches tall?

Solution: In Figure 4.7.3 are shown the distribution of heights and the z distribution to which we transform the original values to determine the desired probabilities. We find the z value corresponding to an x of 65 by

$$z = \frac{65 - 70}{3} = -1.67$$

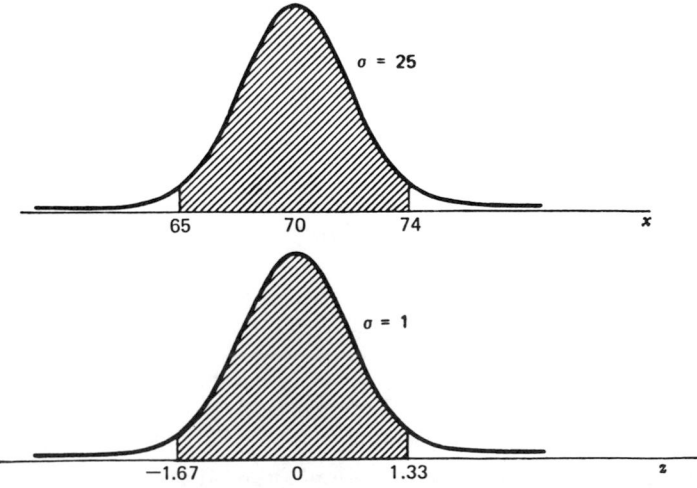

Figure 4.7.3 Distribution of heights (x) and the corresponding standard normal distribution (z).

Similarly, for $x = 74$ we have

$$z = \frac{74 - 70}{3} = 1.33$$

From Table D we find the area between $-\infty$ and -1.67 to be .0475 and the area between $-\infty$ and 1.33 to be .9082. The area desired is the difference between these, $.9082 - .0475 = .8607$. To summarize

$$P(65 \leq x \leq 74) = P\left(\frac{65 - 70}{3} \leq z \leq \frac{74 - 70}{3}\right)$$

$$= P(-1.67 \leq z \leq 1.33)$$

$$= P(-\infty \leq z \leq 1.33) - P(-\infty \leq z \leq -1.67)$$

$$= .9082 - .0475$$

$$= .8607$$

The probability asked for in our original question, then, is .8607.

Example 4.7.3

In a population of 10,000 of the people described in Example 4.7.2, how many would you expect to be 6 feet 5 inches tall or taller?

Solution: We first find the probability that one person selected at random from the population would be 6 feet 5 inches tall or taller. That is,

$$P(x > 77) = P\left(z > \frac{77 - 70}{3}\right) = P(z > 2.33) = 1 - .9901 = .0099$$

Out of 10,000 people we would expect $10,000(.0099) = 99$ to be 6 feet 5 inches (77 inches) tall or taller.

EXERCISES

4.7.1 Suppose the ages at time of onset of a certain disease are approximately normally distributed with a mean of 11.5 years and a standard deviation of 3 years. A child has just come down with the disease. What is the probability that the child is:

a. Between the ages of $8\frac{1}{2}$ and $14\frac{1}{2}$ years?

b. Over 10 years of age?

c. Under 12?

4.7.2 In the study of fingerprints an important quantitative characteristic is the total ridge count for the 10 fingers of an individual. Suppose that the total ridge counts of individuals in a certain population are approximately normally distributed with a mean of 140 and a standard deviation of 50. Find the probability that an individual picked at random from this population will have a ridge count:

a. Of 200 or more.

b. Less than 100.

c. Between 100 and 200.

d. Between 200 and 250.

e. In a population of 10,000 people how many would you expect to have a ridge count of 200 or more?

4.7.3 If the capacities of the cranial cavities of a certain population are approximately normally distributed with a mean of 1400 cc and a standard deviation of 125, find the probability that a person randomly picked from this population will have a cranial cavity capacity:

a. Greater than 1450 cc.   **b.** Less than 1350 cc.

c. Between 1300 cc and 1500 cc.

4.7.4 Suppose the average length of stay in a chronic disease hospital of a certain type of patient is 60 days with a standard deviation of 15. If it is reasonable to assume an approximately normal distribution of lengths of stay, find the probability that a randomly selected patient from this group will have a length of stay:

a. Greater than 50 days.   **b.** Less than 30 days.

c. Between 30 and 60 days.   **d.** Greater than 90 days.

4.7.5 If the total cholesterol values for a certain population are approximately normally distributed with a mean of 200 mg/100 ml and a standard deviation of 20 mg/100 ml, find the probability that an individual picked at random from this population will have a cholesterol value:

a. Between 180 and 200 mg/100 ml.   **b.** Greater than 225 mg/100 ml.

c. Less than 150 mg/100 ml.   **d.** Between 190 and 210 mg/100 ml.

4.7.6 Given a normally distributed population with a mean of 75 and a variance of 625, find:

a. $P(50 \leq x \leq 100)$.   **b.** $P(x > 90)$.

c. $P(x < 60)$.   **d.** $P(x \geq 85)$.

e. $P(30 \leq x \leq 110)$.

4.7.7 The weights of a certain population of young adult females are approximately normally distributed with a mean of 132 pounds and a standard deviation of 15. Find the probability that a subject selected at random from this population will weigh:

a. More than 155 pounds.   **b.** 100 pounds or less.

c. Between 105 and 145 pounds.

4.8
Summary

In the present chapter the concepts of probability described in the preceding chapter are further developed. The concepts of discrete and continuous random variables and their probability distributions are discussed. In particular, two discrete probability distributions, the binomial and the Poisson, and one continuous probability distribution, the normal, are examined in considerable detail. We have seen how these theoretical distributions allow us to make probability statements about certain random variables that are of interest to the health professional.

REVIEW QUESTIONS AND EXERCISES

1. What is a discrete random variable? Give three examples that are of interest to the health professional.

2. What is a continuous random variable? Give three examples of interest to the health professional.

3. Define the probability distribution of a discrete random variable.

4. Define the probability distribution of a continuous random variable.

5. What is a cumulative probability distribution?

6. What is a Bernoulli trial?

7. Describe the binomial distribution.

8. Give an example of a random variable that you think follows a binomial distribution.

9. Describe the Poisson distribution.

10. Give an example of a random variable that you think is distributed according to the Poisson law.

11. Describe the normal distribution.

12. Describe the standard normal distribution and tell how it is used in statistics.

13. Give an example of a random variable that you think is, at least approximately, normally distributed.

14. Using the data of your answer to question 13, demonstrate the use of the standard normal distribution in answering probability questions related to the variable selected.

15. The usual method for teaching a particular self-care skill to retarded persons is effective in 50 percent of the cases. A new method is tried with 10 persons. If the new method is no better than the standard, what is the probability that seven or more will learn the skill?

16. Personnel records of a large hospital show that 10 percent of housekeeping and maintenance employees quit within one year after being hired. If 10 new employees have just been hired:

   a. What is the probability that exactly half of them will still be working after one year?

   b. What is the probability that all will be working after one year?

   c. What is the probability that 3 of the 10 will quit before the year is up?

17. In a certain developing country, 30 percent of the children are undernourished. In a random sample of 25 children from this area, what is the probability that the number of undernourished will be:

   a. Exactly 10?   **b.** Less than five?

   c. Five or more?   **d.** Between three and five inclusive?

   e. Less than seven, but more than four?

18. On the average, two students per hour report for treatment to the first-aid room of a large elementary school.

   a. What is the probability that during a given hour three students come to the first-aid room for treatment?

   b. What is the probability that during a given hour two or fewer students will report to the first-aid room?

   c. What is the probability that between three and five students, inclusive, will report to the first-aid room during a given hour?

19. On the average, five smokers pass a certain street corner every 10 minutes. What is the probability that during a given 10-minute period the number of smokers passing will be:

   a. Six or fewer?   **b.** Seven or more?

   c. Exactly eight?

20. In a certain metropolitan area there is an average of one suicide per month. What is the probability that during a given month the number of suicides will be:

   a. Greater than one?   **b.** Less than one?

   c. Greater than three?

21. The IQs of individuals admitted to a state school for the mentally retarded are approximately normally distributed with a mean of 60 and a standard deviation of 10.

   a. Find the proportion of individuals with IQs greater than 75.

   b. What is the probability that an individual picked at random will have an IQ between 55 and 75?

   c. Find $P(50 \leq X \leq 70)$.

22. A nurse supervisor has found that staff nurses, on the average, complete a certain task in 10 minutes. If the times required to complete the task are approximately normally distributed with a standard deviation of 3 minutes, find:

   a. The proportion of nurses completing the task in less than 4 minutes.

   b. The proportion of nurses requiring more than 5 minutes to complete the task.

   c. The probability that a nurse who has just been assigned the task will complete it within 3 minutes.

23. Scores made on a certain aptitude test by nursing students are approximately normally distributed with a mean of 500 and a variance of 10,000.

   a. What proportion of those taking the test score below 200?

   b. A person is about to take the test; what is the probability that he or she will make a score of 650 or more?

   c. What proportion of scores fall between 350 and 675?

24. Given a binomial variable with a mean of 20 and a variance of 16, find n and p.

25. Suppose a variable X is normally distributed with a standard deviation of 10. Given that .0985 of the values of X are greater than 70, what is the mean value of X?

26. Given the normally distributed random variable X, find the numerical value of k such that $P(\mu - k\sigma \leq X \leq \mu + k\sigma) = .754$.

27. Given the normally distributed random variable X with mean 100 and standard deviation 15, find the numerical value of k such that:

   a. $P(X \leq k) = .0094$

   b. $P(X \geq k) = .1093$

   c. $P(100 \leq X \leq k) = .4778$

   d. $P(k' \leq X \leq k) = .9660$, where k' and k are equidistant from μ.

28. Given the normally distributed random variable X with $\sigma = 10$ and $P(X \leq 40) = .0080$, find μ.

29. Given the normally distributed random variable X with $\sigma = 15$ and $P(X \leq 50) = .9904$, find μ.

30. Given the normally distributed random variable X with $\sigma = 5$ and $P(X \geq 25) = .0526$, find μ.

31. Given the normally distributed random variable X with $\mu = 25$ and $P(X \leq 10) = .0778$, find σ.

32. Given the normally distributed random variable X with $\mu = 30$ and $P(X \leq 50) = .9772$, find σ.

33. Explain why each of the following measurements is or is not the result of a Bernoulli trial:

   a. The gender of a newborn child.

   b. The classification of a hospital patient's condition as stable, critical, fair, good, or poor.

   c. The weight in grams of a newborn child.

34. Explain why each of the following measurements is or is not the result of a Bernoulli trial:

   a. The number of surgical procedures performed in a hospital in a week.

   b. A Hospital patient's temperature in degrees Celsius.

   c. A hospital patient's vital signs recorded as normal or not normal.

35. Explain why each of the following distributions is or is not a probability distribution.

a.
x	$P(X = x)$
0	0.15
1	0.25
2	0.10
3	0.25
4	0.30

b.
x	$P(X = x)$
0	0.15
1	0.20
2	0.30
3	0.10

c.
x	$P(X = x)$
0	0.15
1	−0.20
2	0.30
3	0.20
4	0.15

d.
x	$P(X = x)$
− 1	0.15
0	0.30
1	0.20
2	0.15
3	0.10
4	0.10

REFERENCES

References Cited

1. Norman L. Johnson and Samuel Kotz, *Discrete Distributions*, Houghton-Mifflin, Boston, 1969.

2. Frank A. Haight, *Handbook of the Poisson Distribution*, Wiley, New York, 1967.

3. Helen M. Walker, *Studies in the History of Statistical Method*, Williams & Wilkins, Baltimore, 1931.

4. Lila R. Elveback, Claude L. Gulliver, and F. Raymond Deating, Jr., "Health, Normality and the Ghost of Gauss," *The Journal of the American Medical Association*, *211* (1970), 69–75.

5. Jerald C. Nelson, Elizabeth Haynes, Rodney Willard, and Jan Kuzma, "The Distribution of Euthyroid Serum Protein-Bound Iodine Levels," *The Journal of the American Medical Association*, *216* (1971), 1639–1641.

Other References

1. Sam Duker, "The Poisson Distribution in Educational Research," *Journal of Experimental Education*, *23* (1955), 265–269.

2. M. S. Lafleur, P. R. Hinrchsen, P. C. Landry, and R. B. Moore, "The Poisson Distribution: An Experimental Approach to Teaching Statistics," *Physics Teacher*, *10* (1972), 314–321.

Applications References

A-1. Simone Buitendijk and Michael B. Bracken, "Medication in Early Pregnancy: Prevalence of Use and Relationship to Maternal Characteristics," *American Journal of Obstetrics and Gynecology*, *165* (1991), 33–40.

A-2. National Center for Health Statistics, M. F. Najjar and M. Rowland, Anthropometric Reference Data and Prevalence of Overweight, United States, 1976–80, *Vital and Health Statistics*, Series 11, No. 238. DHHS Pub. No. (PHS) 87–1688, Public Health Service. Washington, U.S. Government Printing Office, Oct. 1987.

A-3. National Center for Health Statistics, O. T. Thornberry, R. W. Wilson, and P. M. Golden, "Health Promotion Data for the 1990 Objectives, Estimates from the National Health Interview Survey of Health Promotion and Disease Prevention, United States, 1985," *Advance Data From Vital and Health Statistics*, No. 126. DHHS Pub. No. (PHS) 86–1250, Public Health Service, Hyattsville, Md., Sept. 19, 1986.

A-4. Robert D. Gibbons, David C. Clark, and Jan Fawcett, "A Statistical Method for Evaluating Suicide Clusters and Implementing Cluster Surveillance," *American Journal of Epidemiology*, *132* (Supplement No. 1, July 1990), S183–S191.

A-5. S. D. Dusheiko, "Some Questions Concerning the Pathological Anatomy of Alzheimer's Disease," *Soviet Neurological Psychiatry*, *7* (Summer 1974), 56–64. Published by International Arts and Sciences Press, White Plains, N.Y.

CHAPTER 5

Some Important Sampling Distributions

CONTENTS

5.1 Introduction

Before we examine the subject matter of this chapter, let us review the high points of what we have covered thus far. Chapter 1 introduces some basic and useful statistical vocabulary and discusses the basic concepts of data collection. In Chapter 2 the organization and summarization of data are emphasized. It is here that we encounter the concepts of central tendency and dispersion and learn how to compute their descriptive measures. In Chapter 3 we are introduced to the fundamental ideas of probability, and in Chapter 4 we consider the concept of a probability distribution. These concepts are fundamental to an understanding of statistical inference, the topic that comprises the major portion of this book.

The present chapter serves as a bridge between the preceding material, which is essentially descriptive in nature, and most of the remaining topics, which have been selected from the area of statistical inference.

5.2
Sampling Distributions

The topic of this chapter is *sampling distributions*. The importance of a clear understanding of sampling distributions cannot be overemphasized, as this concept is the very key to the understanding of statistical inference. Probability distributions serve two purposes: (1) They allow us to answer probability questions about sample statistics, and (2) they provide the necessary theory for making statistical inference procedures valid. In this chapter we use sampling distributions to answer probability questions about sample statistics. In the chapters that follow we will see how sampling distributions make statistical inferences valid.

We begin with the following definition.

DEFINITION

The distribution of all possible values that can be assumed by some statistic, computed from samples of the same size randomly drawn from the same population, is called the *sampling distribution* of that statistic.

Sampling Distributions: Construction   Sampling distributions may be constructed empirically when sampling from a discrete, finite population. To construct a sampling distribution we proceed as follows:

1. From a finite population of size N, randomly draw all possible samples of size n.

2. Compute the statistic of interest for each sample.

3. List in one column the different distinct observed values of the statistic, and in another column list the corresponding frequency of occurrence of each distinct observed value of the statistic.

The actual construction of a sampling distribution is a formidable undertaking if the population is of any appreciable size and is an impossible task if the population is infinite. In such cases, sampling distributions may be approximated by taking a large number of samples of a given size.

Sampling Distributions: Important Characteristics   We usually are interested in knowing three things about a given sampling distribution: its *mean*, its *variance*, and its *functional form* (how it looks when graphed).

We can recognize the difficulty of constructing a sampling distribution according to the steps given above when the population is large. We also run into a problem when considering the construction of a sampling distribution when the population is infinite. The best we can do experimentally in this case is to approximate the sampling distribution of a statistic.

Both these problems may be obviated by means of mathematics. Although the procedures involved are not compatible with the mathematical level of this text, sampling distributions can be derived mathematically. The interested reader can consult one of many mathematical statistics textbooks, for example, Larsen and Marx (1) or Rice (2).

In the sections that follow some of the more frequently encountered sampling distributions are discussed.

5.3
Distribution of the Sample Mean

An important sampling distribution is the distribution of the sample mean. Let us see how we might construct the sampling distribution by following the steps outlined in the previous section.

Example 5.3.1

Suppose we have a population of size $N = 5$, consisting of the ages of five children who are outpatients in a community mental health center. The ages are as follows: $x_1 = 6$, $x_2 = 8$, $x_3 = 10$, $x_4 = 12$, and $x_5 = 14$. The mean, μ, of this population is equal to $\Sigma x_i / N = 10$ and the variance

$$\sigma^2 = \frac{\Sigma(x_i - \mu)^2}{N} = \frac{40}{5} = 8$$

Let us compute another measure of dispersion and designate it by capital S as follows:

$$S^2 = \frac{\Sigma(x_i - \mu)^2}{N - 1} = \frac{40}{4} = 10$$

We will refer to this quantity again in the next chapter. We wish to construct the sampling distribution of the sample mean, $\bar{x}$, based on samples of size $n = 2$ drawn from this population.

Solution: Let us draw all possible samples of size $n = 2$ from this population. These samples, along with their means, are shown in Table 5.3.1.

We see in this example that when sampling is with replacement, there are 25 possible samples. In general, when sampling is with replacement, the number of possible samples is equal to N^n.

TABLE 5.3.1 All Possible Samples of Size $n = 2$ From a Population of Size $N = 5$. Samples Above or Below the Principal Diagonal Result When Sampling is Without Replacement. Sample Means are in Parentheses

| | | Second Draw | | | | |
		6	8	10	12	14
	6	6, 6 (6)	6, 8 (7)	6, 10 (8)	6, 12 (9)	6, 14 (10)
	8	8, 6 (7)	8, 8 (8)	8, 10 (9)	8, 12 (10)	8, 14 (11)
First draw	10	10, 6 (8)	10, 8 (9)	10, 10 (10)	10, 12 (11)	10, 14 (12)
	12	12, 6 (9)	12, 8 (10)	12, 10 (11)	12, 12 (12)	12, 14 (13)
	14	14, 6 (10)	14, 8 (11)	14, 10 (12)	14, 12 (13)	14, 14 (14)

We may construct the sampling distribution of $\bar{x}$ by listing the different values of $\bar{x}$ in one column and their frequency of occurrence in another, as in Table 5.3.2.

We see that the data of Table 5.3.2 satisfy the requirements for a probability distribution. The individual probabilities are all greater than 0, and their sum is equal to 1.

It was stated earlier that we are usually interested in the functional form of a sampling distribution, its mean, and its variance. We now consider these characteristics for the sampling distribution of the sample mean, $\bar{x}$.

Sampling Distribution of $\bar{x}$: Functional Form   Let us look at the distribution of $\bar{x}$ plotted as a histogram, along with the distribution of the population, both

TABLE 5.3.2 Sampling Distribution of $\bar{x}$ Computed From Samples in Table 5.3.1

$\bar{x}$	Frequency	Relative Frequency
6	1	1/25
7	2	2/25
8	3	3/25
9	4	4/25
10	5	5/25
11	4	4/25
12	3	3/25
13	2	2/25
14	1	1/25
Total	25	25/25

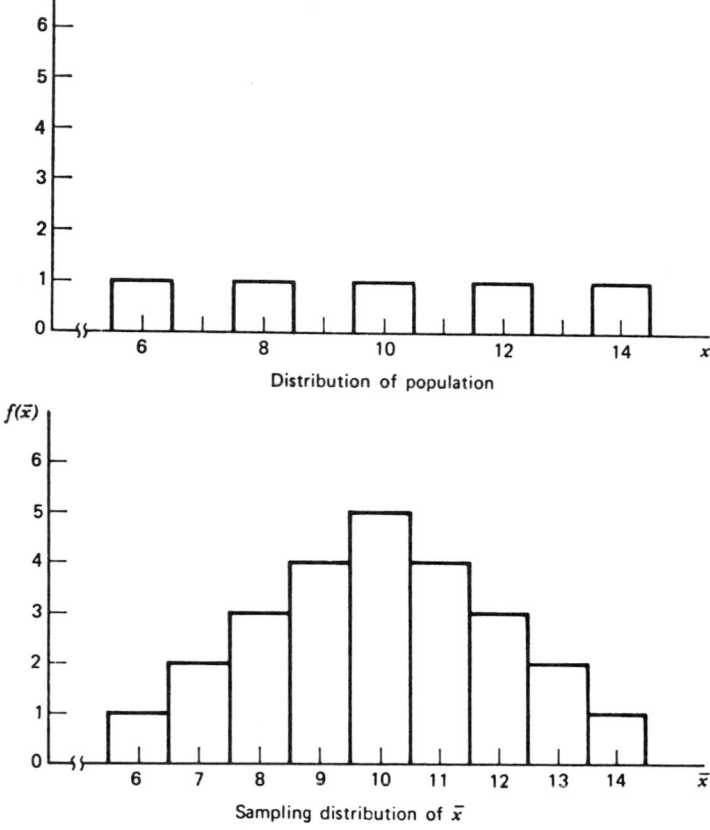

Figure 5.3.1 Distribution of population and sampling distribution of $\bar{x}$.

of which are shown in Figure 5.3.1. We note the radical difference in appearance between the histogram of the population and the histogram of the sampling distribution of $\bar{x}$. Whereas the former is uniformly distributed, the latter gradually rises to a peak and then drops off with perfect symmetry.

Sampling Distribution of $\bar{x}$: Mean   Now let us compute the mean, which we will call $\mu_{\bar{x}}$, of our sampling distribution. To do this we add the 25 sample means and divide by 25. Thus

$$\mu_{\bar{x}} = \frac{\Sigma \bar{x}_i}{N^n} = \frac{6 + 7 + 7 + 8 + \cdots + 14}{25} = \frac{250}{25} = 10$$

We note with interest that the mean of the sampling distribution of $\bar{x}$ has the same value as the mean of the original population.

Sampling Distribution of $\bar{x}$: Variance   Finally, we may compute the variance of $\bar{x}$, which we call $\sigma_{\bar{x}}^2$, as follows:

$$\sigma_{\bar{x}}^2 = \frac{\Sigma(\bar{x}_i - \mu_{\bar{x}})^2}{N^n}$$

$$= \frac{(6-10)^2 + (7-10)^2 + (7-10)^2 + \cdots + (14-10)^2}{25}$$

$$= \frac{100}{25} = 4$$

We note that the variance of the sampling distribution is not equal to the population variance. It is of interest to observe, however, that the variance of the sampling distribution is equal to the population variance divided by the size of the sample used to obtain the sampling distribution. That is,

$$\sigma_{\bar{x}}^2 = \frac{\sigma^2}{n} = \frac{8}{2} = 4$$

The square root of the variance of the sampling distribution, $\sqrt{\sigma_{\bar{x}}^2} = \sigma/\sqrt{n}$, is called the *standard error of the mean* or, simply, the *standard error*.

These results are not coincidences but are examples of the characteristics of sampling distributions in general, when sampling is with replacement or when sampling is from an infinite population. To generalize, we distinguish between two situations: sampling from a normally distributed population and sampling from a nonnormally distributed population.

Sampling Distribution of $\bar{x}$: Sampling From Normally Distributed Populations   When sampling is from a normally distributed population, the distribution of the sample mean will possess the following properties:

1. The distribution of $\bar{x}$ will be normal.
2. The mean, $\mu_{\bar{x}}$, of the distribution of $\bar{x}$ will be equal to the mean of the population from which the samples were drawn.
3. The variance, $\sigma_{\bar{x}}^2$, of the distribution of $\bar{x}$ will be equal to the variance of the population divided by the sample size.

Sampling from Nonnormally Distributed Populations   For the case where sampling is from a nonnormally distributed population, we refer to an important mathematical theorem known as the *central limit theorem*. The importance of this theorem in statistical inference may be summarized in the following statement.

The Central Limit Theorem

Given a population of any nonnormal functional form with a mean μ and finite variance σ^2, the sampling distribution of $\bar{x}$, computed from samples of size n from this population, will have mean μ and variance σ^2/n and will be approximately normally distributed when the sample size is large.

Note that the central limit theorem allows us to sample from nonnormally distributed populations with a guarantee of approximately the same results as would be obtained if the populations were normally distributed provided that we take a large sample.

The importance of this will become evident later when we learn that a normally distributed sampling distribution is a powerful tool in statistical inference. In the case of the sample mean, we are assured of at least an approximately normally distributed sampling distribution under three conditions: (1) when sampling is from a normally distributed population; (2) when sampling is from a nonnormally distributed population and our sample is large; and (3) when sampling is from a population whose functional form is unknown to us as long as our sample size is large.

The logical question that arises at this point is: How large does the sample have to be in order for the central limit theorem to apply? There is no one answer, since the size of the sample needed depends on the extent of nonnormality present in the population. One rule of thumb states that, in most practical situations, a sample of size 30 is satisfactory. In general, the approximation to normality of the sampling distribution of $\bar{x}$ becomes better and better as the sample size increases.

Sampling without Replacement   The foregoing results have been given on the assumption that sampling is either with replacement or that the samples are drawn from infinite populations. In general, we do not sample with replacement, and in most practical situations it is necessary to sample from a finite population; hence, we need to become familiar with the behavior of the sampling distribution of the sample mean under these conditions. Before making any general statements, let us again look at the data in Table 5.3.1. The sample means that result when sampling is without replacement are those above the principal diagonal, which are the same as those below the principal diagonal, if we ignore the order in which the observations were drawn. We see that there are 10 possible samples. In general, when drawing samples of size n from a finite population of size N without replacement, and ignoring the order in which the sample values are drawn, the number of possible samples is given by the combination of N things taken n at a time. In our present example we have

$$_NC_n = \frac{N!}{n!(N-n)!} = \frac{5!}{2!3!} = \frac{5 \cdot 4 \cdot 3!}{2!3!} = 10 \text{ possible samples}$$

The mean of the 10 sample means is

$$\mu_{\bar{x}} = \frac{\Sigma \bar{x}_i}{{}_N C_n} = \frac{7 + 8 + 9 + \cdots + 13}{10} = \frac{100}{10} = 10$$

We see that once again the mean of the sampling distribution is equal to the population mean.

The variance of this sampling distribution is found to be

$$\sigma_{\bar{x}}^2 = \frac{\Sigma(\bar{x}_i - \mu_{\bar{x}})^2}{{}_N C_n} = \frac{30}{10} = 3$$

and we note that this time the variance of the sampling distribution is not equal to the population variance divided by the sample size, since $\sigma_{\bar{x}}^2 = 3 \neq 8/2 = 4$. There is, however, an interesting relationship that we discover by multiplying σ^2/n by $(N - n)/(N - 1)$. That is,

$$\frac{\sigma^2}{n} \cdot \frac{N - n}{N - 1} = \frac{8}{2} \cdot \frac{5 - 2}{4} = 3$$

This result tells us that if we multiply the variance of the sampling distribution that would be obtained if sampling were with replacement, by the factor $(N - n)/(N - 1)$, we obtain the value of the variance of the sampling distribution that results when sampling is without replacement. We may generalize these results with the following statement.

When sampling is without replacement from a finite population, the sampling distribution of $\bar{x}$ will have mean μ and variance

$$\frac{\sigma^2}{n} \cdot \frac{N - n}{N - 1}$$

If the sample size is large, the central limit theorem applies and the sampling distribution of $\bar{x}$ will be approximately normally distributed.

The Finite Population Correction   The factor $(N - n)/(N - 1)$ is called the finite population correction and can be ignored when the sample size is small in comparison with the population size. When the population is much larger than the sample, the difference between σ^2/n and $(\sigma^2/n)[(N - n)/(N - 1)]$ will be negligible. Suppose a population contains 10,000 observations and a sample from this population consists of 25 observations; the finite population correction would be equal to $(10{,}000 - 25)/(9999) = .9976$. To multiply .9976 times σ^2/n is almost equivalent to multiplying by 1. Most practicing statisticians do not use the finite population correction unless the sample contains more than 5 percent of the observations in the population. That is, the finite population correction is usually ignored when $n/N \leq .05$.

The Sampling Distribution of $\bar{x}$—A Summary   Let us summarize the characteristics of the sampling distribution of $\bar{x}$ under two conditions.

1. When sampling is from a normally distributed population with a known population variance:
   a. $\mu_{\bar{x}} = \mu$
   b. $\sigma_{\bar{x}} = \sigma/\sqrt{n}$
   c. The sampling distribution of $\bar{x}$ is normal.

2. Sampling is from a nonnormally distributed population with a known population variance:
   a. $\mu_{\bar{x}} = \mu$
   b. $\sigma_{\bar{x}} = \sigma/\sqrt{n}$ when $n/N \leq .05$
   $$\sigma_{\bar{x}} = (\sigma/\sqrt{n})\sqrt{\frac{N-n}{N-1}}$$
   c. The sampling distribution of $\bar{x}$ is approximately normal.

Applications   As we will see in succeeding chapters, a knowledge and understanding of sampling distributions will be necessary for understanding the concepts of statistical inference. The simplest application of our knowledge of the sampling distribution of the sample mean is in computing the probability of obtaining a sample with a mean of some specified magnitude. Let us illustrate with some examples.

Example 5.3.2   Suppose it is known that in a certain large human population cranial length is approximately normally distributed with a mean of 185.6 mm and a standard deviation of 12.7 mm. What is the probability that a random sample of size 10 from this population will have a mean greater than 190?

Solution: We know that the single sample under consideration is one of all possible samples of size 10 that can be drawn from the population, so that the mean that it yields is one of the $\bar{x}$'s constituting the sampling distribution of $\bar{x}$ that, theoretically, could be derived from this population.

When we say that the population is approximately normally distributed, we assume that the sampling distribution of $\bar{x}$ will be, for all practical purposes, normally distributed. We also know that the mean and standard deviation of the sampling distribution are equal to 185.6 and $\sqrt{(12.7)^2/10} = 12.7/\sqrt{10} = 4.0161$, respectively. We assume that the population is large relative to the sample so that the finite population correction can be ignored.

We learned in Chapter 4 that whenever we have a random variable that is normally distributed, we may very easily transform it to the standard normal distribution. Our random variable now is $\bar{x}$, the mean of its distribution is $\mu_{\bar{x}}$, and its standard deviation is $\sigma_{\bar{x}} = \sigma / \sqrt{n}$. By appropriately modifying the formula given previously, we arrive at the following formula for transforming the normal distribution of $\bar{x}$ to the standard normal distribution.

$$z = \frac{\bar{x} - \mu_{\bar{x}}}{\sigma / \sqrt{n}} \tag{5.3.1}$$

The probability that answers our question is represented by the area to the right of $\bar{x} = 190$ under the curve of the sampling distribution. This area is equal to the area

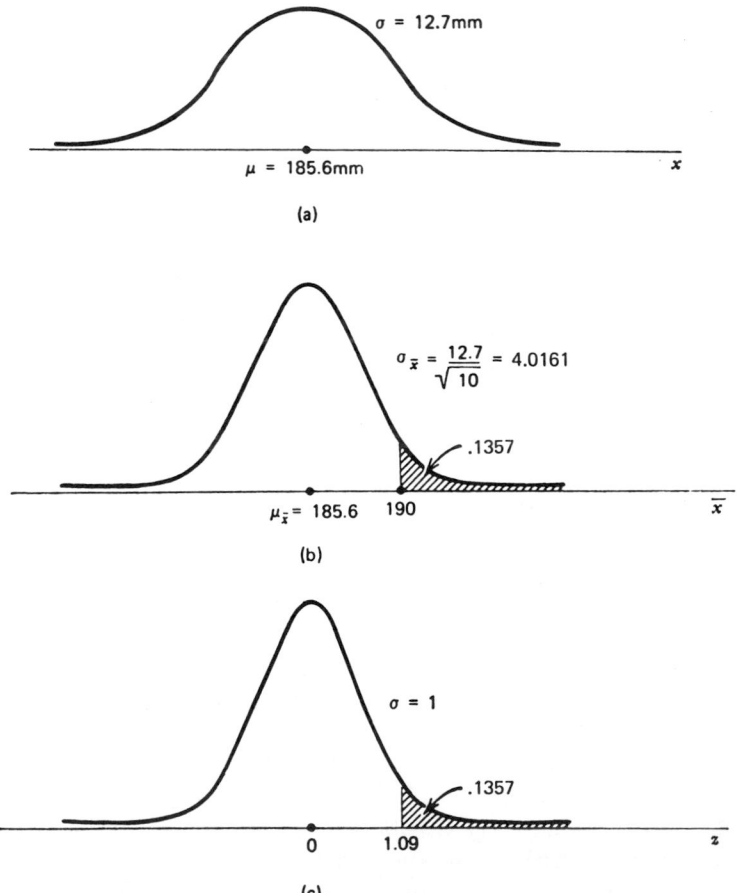

Figure 5.3.2 Population distribution, sampling distribution, and standard normal distribution, Example 5.3.2: (a) population distribution; (b) sampling distribution of $\bar{x}$ for samples of size 10; (c) standard normal distribution.

to the right of

$$z = \frac{190 - 185.6}{4.0161} = \frac{4.4}{4.0161} = 1.10$$

By consulting the standard normal table we find that the area to the right of 1.10 is .1357; hence, we say that the probability is .1357 that a sample of size 10 will have a mean greater than 190.

Figure 5.3.2 shows the relationship between the original population, the sampling distribution of $\bar{x}$, and the standard normal distribution.

Example 5.3.3

If the mean and standard deviation of serum iron values for healthy men are 120 and 15 micrograms per 100 ml, respectively, what is the probability that a random sample of 50 normal men will yield a mean between 115 and 125 micrograms per 100 ml?

Solution: The functional form of the population of serum iron values is not specified, but since we have a sample size greater than 30, we make use of the central limit theorem and transform the resulting approximately normal sampling distribution of $\bar{x}$ (which has a mean of 120 and a standard deviation of $15/\sqrt{50} = 2.1213$) to the standard normal. The probability we seek is

$$P(115 \le \bar{x} \le 125) = P\left(\frac{115 - 120}{2.12} \le z \le \frac{125 - 120}{2.12} \right)$$

$$= P(-2.36 \le z \le 2.36)$$

$$= .9909 - .0091$$

$$- .9818$$

EXERCISES

5.3.1 The National Health and Nutrition Examination Survey of 1976–80 (A-1) found that the mean serum cholesterol level for U. S. males aged 20–74 years was 211. The standard deviation was approximately 90. Consider the sampling distribution of the sample mean based on samples of size 50 drawn from this population of males. What is the mean of the sampling distribution? The standard error?

5.3.2 The study cited in Exercise 5.3.1 reported a serum cholesterol level of 180 for men aged 20–24 years. The standard deviation was approximately 43. If a simple random sample of size 60 is drawn from this population, find the probability that the sample mean serum cholesterol level will be:

a. Between 170 and 195.   **b**. Below 175.

c. Greater than 190.

5.3.3   If the uric acid values in normal adult males are approximately normally distributed with a mean and standard deviation of 5.7 and 1 mg percent respectively, find the probability that a sample of size 9 will yield a mean:

  a. Greater than 6.   **b.** Between 5 and 6.

  c. Less than 5.2.

5.3.4   For a certain large segment of the population, for a particular year, suppose the mean number of days of disability is 5.4 with a standard deviation of 2.8 days. Find the probability that a random sample of size 49 from this population will have a mean:

  a. Greater than 6 days.   **b.** Between 4 and 6 days.

  c. Between $4\frac{1}{2}$ and $5\frac{1}{2}$ days.

5.3.5   Given a normally distributed population with a mean of 100 and a standard deviation of 20, find the following probabilities based on a sample of size 16:

  a. $P(\bar{x} \geq 100)$.   **b.** $P(96 \leq \bar{x} \leq 108)$.

  c. $P(\bar{x} \leq 110)$.

5.3.6   Given: $\mu = 50$, $\sigma = 16$, $n = 64$, find:

  a. $P(45 \leq \bar{x} \leq 55)$.   **b.** $P(\bar{x} > 53)$.

  c. $P(\bar{x} < 47)$.   **d.** $P(49 \leq \bar{x} \leq 56)$.

5.3.7   Suppose a population consists of the following values: $1, 3, 5, 7, 9$. Construct the sampling distribution of $\bar{x}$ based on samples of size two selected without replacement. Find the mean and variance of the sampling distribution.

5.3.8   Use the data of Example 5.3.1 to construct the sampling distribution of $\bar{x}$ based on samples of size three selected without replacement. Find the mean and variance of the sampling distribution.

5.3.9   For a population of 17-year-old boys, the mean subscapular skinfold thickness (in millimeters) is 9.7 and the standard deviation is 6.0. For a simple random sample of size 40 drawn from this population find the probability that the sample mean will be:

  a. Greater than 11.   **b.** Less than or equal to 7.5.

  c. Between 7 and 10.5.

5.4
Distribution of the Difference Between Two Sample Means

Frequently the interest in an investigation is focused on two populations. Specifically, an investigator may wish to know something about the difference between two population means. In one investigation, for example, a researcher may wish to know if it is reasonable to conclude that two population means are different. In another situation, the researcher may desire knowledge about the magnitude of the difference between two population means. A medical research team, for example, may want to know whether or not the mean serum cholesterol level is higher in a population of sedentary office workers than in a population of laborers. If the researchers are able to conclude that the population means are different, they may wish to know by how much they differ. A knowledge of the sampling distribution of the difference between two means is useful in investigations of this type.

Sampling from Normally Distributed Populations The following example illustrates the construction of and the characteristics of the sampling distribution of the difference between sample means when sampling is from two normally distributed distributions.

Example 5.4.1

Suppose we have two populations of individuals—one population (population 1) has experienced some condition thought to be associated with mental retardation, and the other population (population 2) has not experienced the condition. The distribution of intelligence scores in each of the two populations is believed to be approximately normally distributed with a standard deviation of 20.

Suppose, further, that we take a sample of 15 individuals from each population and compute for each sample the mean intelligence score with the following results: $\bar{x}_1 = 92$ and $\bar{x}_2 = 105$. If there is no difference between the two populations, with respect to their true mean intelligence scores, what is the probability of observing a difference this large or larger ($\bar{x}_1 - \bar{x}_2$) between sample means?

Solution: To answer this question we need to know the nature of the sampling distribution of the relevant statistic, the *difference between two sample means*, $\bar{x}_1 - \bar{x}_2$. Notice that we seek a probability associated with the difference between two sample means rather than a single mean.

Sampling Distribution of $\bar{x}_1 - \bar{x}_2$—Construction Although, in practice, we would not attempt to construct the desired sampling distribution, we can conceptualize the manner in which it could be done when sampling is from finite populations. We would begin by selecting from population 1 all possible samples of size 15 and computing the mean for each sample. We know that there would be $_{N_1}C_{n_1}$ such samples where N_1 is the group size and $n_1 = 15$. Similarly, we would select all possible samples of size 15 from population 2 and compute the mean for each of these samples. We would then take all possible pairs of sample means, one from population 1 and one from population 2, and take the difference. Table 5.4.1 shows the results of following this procedure. Note that the 1's and 2's in the last line of this table are not exponents, but indicators of population 1 and 2, respectively.

Sampling Distribution of $\bar{x}_1 - \bar{x}_2$—Characteristics It is the distribution of the differences between sample means that we seek. If we plotted the sample differences against their frequency of occurrence, we would obtain a normal distribution with a mean equal to $\mu_1 - \mu_2$, the difference between the two

TABLE 5.4.1 Working Table for Constructing The Distribution of the Difference Between Two Sample Means

Samples From Population 1	Samples From Population 2	Sample Means Population 1	Sample Means Population 2	All Possible Differences Between Means
n_{11}	n_{12}	$\bar{x}_{11}$	$\bar{x}_{12}$	$\bar{x}_{11} - \bar{x}_{12}$
n_{21}	n_{22}	$\bar{x}_{21}$	$\bar{x}_{22}$	$\bar{x}_{11} - \bar{x}_{22}$
n_{31}	n_{32}	$\bar{x}_{31}$	$\bar{x}_{32}$	$\bar{x}_{11} - \bar{x}_{32}$
⋮	⋮	⋮	⋮	⋮
$n_{N_1 c_{n_1}}1$	$n_{N_2 c_{n_2}}2$	$\bar{x}_{N_1 c_{n_1}}1$	$\bar{x}_{N_2 c_{n_2}}2$	$\bar{x}_{N_1 c_{n_1}}1 - \bar{x}_{N_2 c_{n_2}}2$

population means, and a variance equal to $(\sigma_1^2/n_1) + (\sigma_2^2/n_2)$. That is, the standard error of the difference between sample means would be equal to $\sqrt{(\sigma_1^2/n_1) + (\sigma_2^2/n_2)}$.

For our present example we would have a normal distribution with a mean of 0 (if there is no difference between the two population means) and a variance of $[(20)^2/15] + [(20)^2/15] = 53.3333$. The graph of the sampling distribution is shown in Figure 5.4.1.

Converting to z We know that the normal distribution described in Example 5.4.1 can be transformed to the standard normal distribution by means of a modification of a previously learned formula. The new formula is as follows:

$$z = \frac{(\bar{x}_1 - \bar{x}_2) - (\mu_1 - \mu_2)}{\sqrt{\dfrac{\sigma_1^2}{n_1} + \dfrac{\sigma_2^2}{n_2}}} \tag{5.4.1}$$

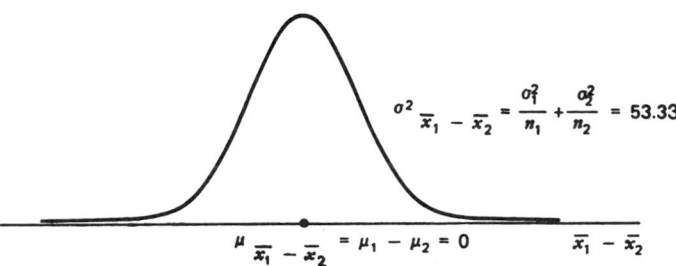

$$\sigma^2_{\bar{x}_1 - \bar{x}_2} = \frac{\sigma_1^2}{n_1} + \frac{\sigma_2^2}{n_2} = 53.33$$

$$\mu_{\bar{x}_1 - \bar{x}_2} = \mu_1 - \mu_2 = 0 \qquad \bar{x}_1 - \bar{x}_2$$

Figure 5.4.1 Graph of the sampling distribution of $\bar{x}_1 - \bar{x}_2$ when there is no difference between population means, Example 5.4.1.

The area under the curve of $\bar{x}_1 - \bar{x}_2$ corresponding to the probability we seek is the area to the left of $\bar{x}_1 - \bar{x}_2 = 92 - 105 = -13$. The z value corresponding to -13, assuming there is no difference between population means, is

$$z = \frac{-13 - 0}{\sqrt{\dfrac{(20)^2}{15} + \dfrac{(20)^2}{15}}} = \frac{-13}{\sqrt{53.3}} = \frac{-13}{7.3} = -1.78$$

By consulting Table D, we find that the area under the standard normal curve to the left of -1.78 is equal to .0375. In answer to our original question, we say that if there is no difference between population means, the probability of obtaining a difference between sample means as large as or larger than 13 is .0375.

Sampling from Normal Populations The procedure we have just followed is valid even when the sample sizes, n_1 and n_2, are different and when the population variances, σ_1^2 and σ_2^2 have different values. The theoretical results on which this procedure is based may be summarized as follows.

Given two normally distributed populations with means, μ_1 and μ_2, and variances, σ_1^2 and σ_2^2, respectively, the sampling distribution of the difference, $\bar{x}_1 - \bar{x}_2$, between the means of independent samples of size n_1 and n_2 drawn from these populations is normally distributed with mean $\mu_1 - \mu_2$ and variance $(\sigma_1^2/n_1) + (\sigma_2^2/n_2)$.

Sampling from Nonnormal Populations Many times a researcher is faced with one or the other of the following problems: the necessity of (1) sampling from nonnormally distributed populations, or (2) sampling from populations whose functional forms are not known. A solution to these problems is to take large samples, since when the sample sizes are large the central limit theorem applies and the distribution of the difference between two sample means is at least approximately normally distributed with a mean equal to $\mu_1 - \mu_2$ and a variance of $(\sigma_1^2/n_1) + (\sigma_2^2/n_2)$. To find probabilities associated with specific values of the statistic, then, our procedure would be the same as that given when sampling is from normally distributed populations.

Example 5.4.2

Suppose it has been established that for a certain type of client the average length of a home visit by a public health nurse is 45 minutes with a standard deviation of 15 minutes, and that for a second type of client the average home visit is 30 minutes long with a standard deviation of 20 minutes. If a nurse randomly visits 35 clients from the first and 40 from the second population, what is the probability that the average length of home visit will differ between the two groups by 20 or more minutes?

Solution: No mention is made of the functional form of the two populations, so let us assume that this characteristic is unknown, or that the populations are not normally distributed. Since the sample sizes are large (greater than 30) in both cases, we draw on the results of the central limit theorem to answer the question posed. We know that the difference between sample means is at least approximately normally distributed with the following mean and variance:

$$\mu_{\bar{x}_1 - \bar{x}_2} = \mu_1 - \mu_2 = 45 - 30 = 15$$

$$\sigma^2_{\bar{x}_1 - \bar{x}_2} = \frac{\sigma_1^2}{n_1} + \frac{\sigma_2^2}{n_2} = \frac{(15)^2}{35} + \frac{(20)^2}{40} = 16.4286$$

The area under the curve of $\bar{x}_1 - \bar{x}_2$ that we seek is that area to the right of 20. The corresponding value of z in the standard normal is

$$z = \frac{(\bar{x}_1 - \bar{x}_2) - (\mu_1 - \mu_2)}{\sqrt{\dfrac{\sigma_1^2}{n_1} + \dfrac{\sigma_2^2}{n_2}}} = \frac{20 - 15}{\sqrt{16.4286}} = \frac{5}{4.0532} = 1.23$$

In Table D we find that the area to the right of $z = 1.23$ is $1 - .8907 = .1093$. We say, then, that the probability of the nurse's random visits resulting in a difference between the two means as great as or greater than 20 minutes is .1093. The curve of $\bar{x}_1 - \bar{x}_2$ and the corresponding standard normal curve are shown in Figure 5.4.2.

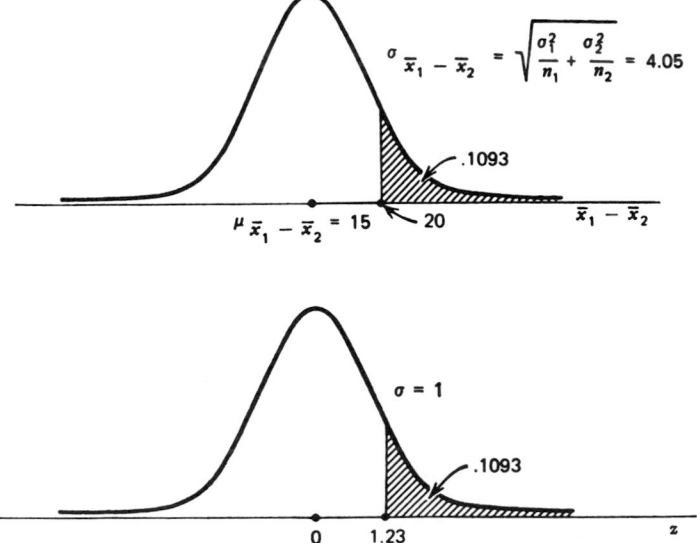

Figure 5.4.2 Sampling distribution of $\bar{x}_1 - \bar{x}_2$ and the corresponding standard normal distribution, home visit example.

EXERCISES

5.4.1 The reference cited in Exercises 5.3.1 and 5.3.2 gives the following data on serum cholesterol levels in U.S. males:

Group	Age	Mean	Standard Deviation
A	20–24	180	43
B	25–34	199	49

Suppose we select a simple random sample of size 50 independently from each population. What is the probability that the difference between sample means $(\bar{x}_B - \bar{x}_A)$ will be more than 25?

5.4.2 In a study of annual family expenditures for general health care, two populations were surveyed with the following results:

$$\text{Population 1: } n_1 = 40, \bar{x}_1 = \$346$$

$$\text{Population 2: } n_2 = 35, \bar{x}_2 = \$300$$

If it is known that the population variances are $\sigma_1^2 = 2800$ and $\sigma_2^2 = 3250$, what is the probability of obtaining sample results $(\bar{x}_1 - \bar{x}_2)$ as large as those shown if there is no difference in the means of the two populations?

5.4.3 Given two normally distributed populations with equal means and variances of $\sigma_1^2 = 100$ and $\sigma_2^2 = 80$, what is the probability that samples of size $n_1 = 25$ and $n_2 = 16$ will yield a value of $\bar{x}_1 - \bar{x}_2$ greater than or equal to 8?

5.4.4 Given two normally distributed populations with equal means and variances of $\sigma_1^2 = 240$ and $\sigma_2^2 = 350$, what is the probability that samples of size $n_1 = 40$ and $n_2 = 35$ will yield a value of $\bar{x}_1 - \bar{x}_2$ as large as or larger than 12?

5.4.5 For a population of 17-year-old boys and 17-year-old girls the means and standard deviations, respectively, of their subscapular skinfold thickness values are as follows: boys, 9.7 and 6.0; girls, 15.6 and 9.5. Simple random samples of 40 boys and 35 girls are selected from the populations. What is the probability that the difference between sample means $(\bar{x}_{girls} - \bar{x}_{boys})$ will be greater than 10?

5.5
Distribution of the Sample Proportion

In the previous sections we have dealt with the sampling distributions of statistics computed from measured variables. We are frequently interested, however, in the sampling distribution of statistics, such as a sample proportion, that result from counts or frequency data.

Example 5.5.1 Suppose we know that in a certain human population .08 are color blind. If we designate a population proportion by *p*, we can say that in this example *p* = .08. If we randomly select 150 individuals from this population, what is the probability that the proportion in the sample who are color blind will be as great as .15?

Solution: To answer this question we need to know the properties of the sampling distribution of the sample proportion. We will designate the sample proportion by the symbol $\hat{p}$.

You will recognize the similarity between this example and those presented in Section 4.3, which dealt with the binomial distribution. The variable color blindness is a *dichotomous variable*, since an individual can be classified into one or the other of two mutually exclusive categories, color blind or not color blind. In Section 4.3, we were given similar information and were asked to find the number with the characteristic of interest, whereas here we are seeking the proportion in the sample possessing the characteristic of interest. We could with a sufficiently large table of binomial probabilities, such as Table B, determine the probability associated with the number corresponding to the proportion of interest. As we will see, this will not be necessary, since there is available an alternative procedure, when sample sizes are large, that is generally more convenient.

Sampling Distribution of $\hat{p}$ — Construction   The sampling distribution of a sample proportion would be constructed experimentally in exactly the same manner as was suggested in the case of the arithmetic mean and the difference between two means. From the population, which we assume to be finite, we would take all possible samples of a given size and for each sample compute the sample proportion, $\hat{p}$. We would then prepare a frequency distribution of $\hat{p}$ by listing the different distinct values of $\hat{p}$ along with their frequencies of occurrence. This frequency distribution (as well as the corresponding relative frequency distribution) would constitute the sampling distribution of $\hat{p}$.

Sampling Distribution of $\hat{p}$ — Characteristics   When the sample size is large, the distribution of sample proportions is approximately normally distributed by virtue of the central limit theorem. The mean of the distribution, $\mu_{\hat{p}}$, that is, the average of all the possible sample proportions, will be equal to the true population proportion p, and the variance of the distribution $\sigma_{\hat{p}}^2$ will be equal to $p(1 - p)/n$. To answer probability questions about p, then, we use the following formula:

$$z = \frac{\hat{p} - p}{\sqrt{\dfrac{p(1 - p)}{n}}} \tag{5.5.1}$$

The question that now arises is: How large does the sample size have to be for the use of the normal approximation to be valid? A widely used criterion is that both np and $n(1 - p)$ must be greater than 5, and we will abide by that rule in this text.

We are now in a position to answer the question regarding color blindness in the sample of 150 individuals from a population in which .08 are color-blind. Since both np and $n(1 - p)$ are greater than 5 ($150 \times .08 = 12$ and $150 \times .92 = 138$), we can say that, in this case, $\hat{p}$ is approximately normally distributed with a mean $\mu_{\hat{p}} = p = .08$ and $\sigma_{\hat{p}}^2 = p(1 - p)/n = (.08)(.92)/150 = .00049$. The probability we seek is the area under the curve of $\hat{p}$ that is to the right of .15. This area is equal to the area under the standard normal curve to the right of

$$z = \frac{\hat{p} - p}{\sqrt{\dfrac{p(1 - p)}{n}}} = \frac{.15 - .08}{\sqrt{.00049}} = \frac{.07}{.0222} = 3.15$$

The transformation to the standard normal distribution has been accomplished in the usual manner: z is found by dividing the standard error into the difference between a value of the statistic and its mean. Using Table D we find that the area to the right of $z = 3.15$ is $1 - .9992 = .0008$. We may say, then, that the probability of observing $\hat{p} \geq .15$ in a random sample of size $n = 150$ from a population in which $p = .08$ is .0008. If we should, in fact, draw such a sample most people would consider it a rare event.

Correction for Continuity The normal approximation may be improved by the *correction for continuity*, a device that makes an adjustment for the fact that a discrete distribution is being approximated by a continuous distribution. Suppose we let $x = n\hat{p}$, the number in the sample with the characteristic of interest when the proportion is $\hat{p}$. To apply the correction for continuity we compute

$$z_c = \frac{\dfrac{x + .5}{n} - p}{\sqrt{pq/n}}, \qquad \text{for } x < np \tag{5.5.2}$$

or

$$z_c = \frac{\dfrac{x - .5}{n} - p}{\sqrt{pq/n}}, \qquad \text{for } x > np \tag{5.5.3}$$

where $q = 1 - p$. The correction for continuity will not make a great deal of difference when n is large. In the above example $n\hat{p} = 150(.15) = 22.5$, and

$$z_c = \frac{\dfrac{22.5 - .5}{150} - .08}{\sqrt{.00049}} = 3.01$$

and $P(\hat{p} \geq .15) = 1 - .9987 = .0013$, a result not greatly different from that obtained without the correction for continuity.

Example 5.5.2   Suppose it is known that in a certain population of women, 90 percent entering their third trimester of pregnancy have had some prenatal care. If a random sample of size 200 is drawn from this population, what is the probability that the sample proportion who have had some prenatal care will be less than .85?

Solution: We can assume that the sampling distribution of $\hat{p}$ is approximately normally distributed with $\mu_{\hat{p}} = .90$ and $\sigma_{\hat{p}}^2 = (.1)(.9)/200 = .00045$. We compute

$$z = \frac{.85 - .90}{\sqrt{.00045}} = \frac{-.05}{.0212} = -2.36$$

The area to the left of -2.36 under the standard normal curve is .0091. Therefore, $P(\hat{p} \le .85) = P(z \le -2.36) = .0091$.

EXERCISES

5.5.1   A Survey by the National Center for Health Statistics (A-2) found that 33.2 percent of women 40 years of age and over had undergone a breast physical examination (BPE) within the previous year. If we select a simple random sample of size 200 from this population, what is the probability that the sample proportion of women who have had a BPE within the previous year will be between .28 and .37?

5.5.2   In the mid-seventies, according to a report by the National Center for Health Statistics (A-3), 19.4 percent of the adult U.S. male population was obese. What is the probability that in a simple random sample of size 150 from this population fewer than 15 percent will be obese?

5.5.3   In a survey conducted in 1990 by the National Center for Health Statistics (A-4), 19 percent of respondents 18 years of age and over stated that they had not heard of the AIDS virus HIV. What is the probability that in a sample of size 175 from this population 25 percent or more will not have heard of the AIDS virus HIV?

5.5.4   The standard drug used to treat a certain disease is known to prove effective within three days in 75 percent of the cases in which it is used. In evaluating the effectiveness of a new drug in treating the same disease, it was given to 150 persons suffering from the disease. At the end of three days 97 persons had recovered. If the new drug is equally as effective as the standard, what is the probability of observing this small a proportion recovering?

5.5.5   Given a population in which $p = .6$ and a random sample from this population of size 100, find:

    a $P(\hat{p} \ge .65)$.   **b.** $P(\hat{p} \le .58)$.
    c. $P(.56 \le \hat{p} \le .63)$.

5.5.6   It is known that 35 percent of the members of a certain population suffer from one or more chronic diseases. What is the probability that in a sample of 200 subjects drawn at random from this population 80 or more will have at least one chronic disease?

5.6
Distribution of the Difference Between
Two Sample Proportions

Often there are two population proportions in which we are interested and we desire to assess the probability associated with a difference in proportions computed from samples drawn from each of these populations. The relevant sampling distribution is the distribution of the difference between the two sample proportions.

Sampling Distribution of $\hat{p}_1 - \hat{p}_2$ — Characteristics   The characteristics of this sampling distribution may be summarized as follows:

If independent random samples of size n_1 and n_2 are drawn from two populations of dichotomous variables where the proportion of observations with the characteristic of interest in the two populations are p_1 and p_2, respectively, the distribution of the difference between sample proportions, $\hat{p}_1 - \hat{p}_2$, is approximately normal with mean

$$\mu_{\hat{p}_1 - \hat{p}_2} = p_1 - p_2$$

and variance

$$\sigma^2_{\hat{p}_1 - \hat{p}_2} = \frac{p_1(1 - p_1)}{n_1} + \frac{p_2(1 - p_2)}{n_2}$$

when n_1 and n_2 are large.

We consider n_1 and n_2 sufficiently large when $n_1 p_1$, $n_2 p_2$, $n_1(1 - p_1)$, and $n_2(1 - p_2)$ are all greater than 5.

Sampling Distribution of $\hat{p}_1 - \hat{p}_2$ — Construction   To physically construct the sampling distribution of the difference between two sample proportions, we would proceed in the manner described in Section 5.4 for constructing the sampling distribution of the difference between two means.

Given two sufficiently small populations, one would draw, from population 1, all possible simple random samples of size n_1 and compute, from each set of sample data, the sample proportion $\hat{p}_1$. From population 2, one would draw independently all possible simple random samples of size n_2 and compute, for each set of sample data, the sample proportion $\hat{p}_2$. One would compute the differences between all possible pairs of sample proportions, where one number of each pair was a value of $\hat{p}_1$ and the other a value of $\hat{p}_2$. The sampling distribution of the difference between sample proportions, then, would consist of all such distinct differences, accompanied by their frequencies (or relative frequencies) of occurrence. For large finite or infinite populations one could approximate the sampling distribution of the difference between sample proportions by drawing a large number of independent simple random samples and proceeding in the manner just described.

To answer probability questions about the difference between two sample proportions, then, we use the following formula:

$$z = \frac{(\hat{p}_1 - \hat{p}_2) - (p_1 - p_2)}{\sqrt{\dfrac{p_1(1 - p_1)}{n_1} + \dfrac{p_2(1 - p_2)}{n_2}}} \tag{5.6.1}$$

Example 5.6.1

Suppose that the proportion of moderate to heavy users of illegal drugs in population 1 is .50 while in population 2 the proportion is .33. What is the probability that samples of size 100 drawn from each of the populations will yield a value of $\hat{p}_1 - \hat{p}_2$ as large as .30?

Solution: We assume that the sampling distribution of $\hat{p}_1 - \hat{p}_2$ is approximately normal with mean

$$\mu_{\hat{p}_1 - \hat{p}_2} = .50 - .33 = .17$$

and variance

$$\sigma^2_{\hat{p}_1 - \hat{p}_2} = \frac{(.33)(.67)}{100} + \frac{(.5)(.5)}{100}$$

$$= .004711$$

The area corresponding to the probability we seek is the area under the curve of $\hat{p}_1 - \hat{p}_2$ to the right of .30. Transforming to the standard normal distribution gives

$$z = \frac{(\hat{p}_1 - \hat{p}_2) - (p_1 - p_2)}{\sqrt{\dfrac{p_1(1 - p_1)}{n_1} + \dfrac{p_2(1 - p_2)}{n_2}}} = \frac{.30 - .17}{\sqrt{.004711}} = 1.89$$

Consulting Table D, we find that the area under the standard normal curve that lies to the right of $z = 1.89$ is $1 - .9706 = .0294$. The probability of observing a difference as large as .30 is, then, .0294.

Example 5.6.2

In a certain population of teenagers it is known that 10 percent of the boys are obese. If the same proportion of girls in the population are obese, what is the probability that a random sample of 250 boys and 200 girls will yield a value of $\hat{p}_1 - \hat{p}_2 \geq .06$?

Solution: We assume that the sampling distribution of $\hat{p}_1 - \hat{p}_2$ is approximately normal. If the proportion of obese individuals is the same in the two populations, the mean of the distribution will be 0 and the variance will be

$$\sigma^2_{\hat{p}_1 - \hat{p}_2} = \frac{p_1(1 - p_1)}{n_1} + \frac{p_2(1 - p_2)}{n_2} = \frac{(.1)(.9)}{250} + \frac{(.1)(.9)}{200}$$

$$= .00081$$

The area of interest under the curve of $\hat{p}_1 - \hat{p}_2$ is that to the right of .06. The corresponding z value is

$$z = \frac{.06 - 0}{\sqrt{.00081}} = 2.11$$

Consulting Table D, we find that the area to the right of $z = 2.11$ is $1 - .9826 = .0174$.

___

EXERCISES

5.6.1 In a certain population of retarded children, it is known that the proportion who are hyperactive is .40. A random sample of size 120 was drawn from this population, and a random sample of size 100 was drawn from another population of retarded children. If the proportion of hyperactive children is the same in both populations, what is the probability that the sample would yield a difference, $\hat{p}_1 - \hat{p}_2$, of .16 or more?

5.6.2 In a certain area of a large city it is hypothesized that 40 percent of the houses are in a dilapidated condition. A random sample of 75 houses from this section and 90 houses from another section yielded a difference, $\hat{p}_1 - \hat{p}_2$, of .09. If there is no difference between the two areas in the proportion of dilapidated houses, what is the probability of observing a difference this large or larger?

5.6.3 A survey conducted by the National Center for Health Statistics (A-5) revealed that 14 percent of males and 23.8 percent of females between the ages of 20 and 74 years deviated from their desirable weight by 20 percent or more. Suppose we select a simple random sample of size 120 males and an independent simple random sample of size 130 females. What is the probability that the difference between sample proportions, $\hat{p}_F - \hat{p}_M$, will be between .04 and .20?

5.7
Summary

This chapter is concerned with sampling distributions. The concept of a sampling distribution is introduced and the following important sampling distributions are covered:

1. The distribution of a single sample mean.
2. The distribution of the difference between two sample means.
3. The distribution of a sample proportion.
4. The distribution of the difference between two sample proportions.

We emphasize the importance of this material and urge readers to make sure that they understand it before proceeding to the next chapter.

REVIEW QUESTIONS AND EXERCISES

1. What is a sampling distribution?

2. Explain how a sampling distribution may be constructed from a finite population.

3. Describe the sampling distribution of the sample mean when sampling is with replacement from a normally distributed population.

4. Explain the central limit theorem.

5. How does the sampling distribution of the sample mean, when sampling is without replacement, differ from the sampling distribution obtained when sampling is with replacement?

6. Describe the sampling distribution of the difference between two sample means.

7. Describe the sampling distribution of the sample proportion when large samples are drawn.

8. Describe the sampling distribution of the difference between two sample means when large samples are drawn.

9. Explain the procedure you would follow in constructing the sampling distribution of the difference between sample proportions based on large samples from finite populations.

10. Suppose it is known that the response time of healthy subjects to a particular stimulus is a normally distributed random variable with a mean of 15 seconds and a variance of 16. What is the probability that a random sample of 16 subjects will have a mean response time of 12 seconds or more?

11. A certain firm has 2000 employees. During a recent year, the mean amount per employee spent on personal medical expenses was $31.50, and the standard deviation was $6.00. What is the probability that a simple random sample of 36 employees will yield a mean between $30 and $33?

12. Suppose it is known that in a certain population of drug addicts the mean duration of abuse is 5 years and the standard deviation is 3 years. What is the probability that a random sample of 36 subjects from this population will yield a mean duration of abuse between 4 and 6 years?

13. Suppose the mean daily protein intake for a certain population is 125 grams, while for another population the mean is 100 grams. If daily protein intake values in the two populations are normally distributed with a standard deviation of 15 grams, what is the probability that random and independent samples of size 25 from each population will yield a difference between sample means of 12 or less?

14. Suppose that two drugs, purported to reduce the response time to a certain stimulus, are under study by a drug manufacturer. The researcher is willing to assume that response times, following administration of the two drugs, are normally distributed with equal variances of 60. As part of the evaluation of the two drugs, drug A is to be administered to 15 subjects and drug B is to be administered to 12 subjects. The researcher would like to know between what two values the central 95 percent of all differences between sample means would lie if the drugs were equally effective and the experiment were repeated a large number of times using these sample sizes.

15. Suppose it is known that the serum albumin concentration in a certain population of individuals is normally distributed with a mean of 4.2 g/100 ml and a standard deviation of .5. A random sample of nine of these individuals placed on a daily dosage of a certain oral steroid yielded a mean serum albumin concentration value of 3.8 g/100 ml. Does it appear likely from these results that the oral steroid reduces the level of serum albumin?

16. A survey conducted in a large metropolitan area revealed that among high school students, 35 percent have, at one time or another, smoked marijuana. If, in a random sample of 150 of these students, only 40 admit to having ever smoked marijuana, what would you conclude?

17. A 1989 survey by the National Center for Health Statistics (A-6) revealed that 7.1 percent of the patients discharged from short-stay hospitals in the United States were between the ages of 20 and 24 years, inclusive. If we select a simple random sample of size 150 from the relevant population, what is the probability that the proportion of patients between the ages of 20 and 24 will be between .05 and .10?

18. A psychiatric social worker believes that in both community A and community B the proportion of adolescents suffering from some emotional or mental problem is .20. In a sample of 150 adolescents from community A, 15 had an emotional or mental problem. In a sample of 100 from community B, the number was 16. If the social worker's belief is correct, what is the probability of observing a difference as great as was observed between these two samples?

19. A report by the National Center for Health Statistics (A-7) shows that in the United States 5.7 percent of males and 7.3 percent of females between the ages of 20 and 74 years have diabetes. Suppose we take a simple random sample of 100 males and an independent simple random sample of 150 females from the relevant populations. What is the probability that the difference between sample proportions with diabetes, $\hat{p}_F - \hat{p}_M$, will be more than .05?

20. How many simple random samples (without replacement) of size 5 can be selected from a population of size 10?

21. It is known that 27 percent of the members of a certain adult population have never smoked. Consider the sampling distribution of the sample proportion based on simple random samples of size 110 drawn from this population. What is the functional form of the sampling distribution?

22. Refer to Exercise 21. Compute the mean and variance of the sampling distribution.

23. Refer to Exercise 21. What is the probability that a single simple random sample of size 110 drawn from this population will yield a sample proportion smaller than .18?

24. In a population of subjects who died from lung cancer following exposure to asbestos it was found that the mean number of years elapsing between exposure and death was 25. The standard deviation was 7 years. Consider the sampling distribution of sample means based on samples of size 35 drawn from this population. What will be the shape of the sampling distribution?

25. Refer to Exercise 24. What will be the mean and variance of the sampling distribution?

26. Refer to Exercise 24. What is the probability that a single simple random sample of size 35 drawn from this population will yield a mean between 22 and 29?

27. For each of the following populations of measurements, state whether the sampling distribution of the sample mean is normally distributed, approximately normally distributed, or not approximately normally distributed when computed from samples of size (A) 10, (B) 50, and (B) 200.
   a. The logarithm of metabolic ratios. The population is normally distributed.
   b. Resting vagal tone in healthy adults. The population is normally distributed.
   c. Insulin action in obese subjects. The population is not normally distributed.

28. For each of the following sampling situations indicate whether the sampling distribution of the sample proportion can be approximated by a normal distribution and explain why or why not.
   a. $p = .50, n = 8$ **b.** $p = .40, n = 30$
   c. $p = .10, n = 30$ **d.** $p = .01, n = 1,000$
   e. $p = .90, n = 100$ **f.** $p = .05, n = 150$

REFERENCES

References Cited

1. Richard J. Larsen and Morris L. Marx, *An Introduction to Mathematical Statistics and Its Applications*, Prentice-Hall, Englewood Cliffs, N.J., 1981.
2. John A. Rice, *Mathematical Statistics and Data Analysis*, Wadsworth & Brooks/Cole Advanced Books & Software, Pacific Grove, Calif., 1988.

Applications References

A-1. National Center for Health Statistics, R. Fulwood, W. Kalsbeek, B. Rifkind, et al., "Total serum cholesterol levels of adults 20–74 years of age: United States, 1976–80," *Vital and Health Statistics*, Series 11, No. 236. DHHS Pub. No. (PHS) 86–1686, Public Health Service, Washington, D.C., U.S. Government Printing Office, May 1986.
A-2. D. A. Dawson and G. B. Thompson, "Breast cancer risk factors and screening: United States, 1987," National Center for Health Statistics, *Vital and Health Statistics*, 10(172), 1989.

A-3. National Center for Health Statistics, S. Abraham, "Obese and Overweight Adults in the United States," *Vital and Health Statistics*. Series 11, No. 230, DHHS Pub. No. 83–1680, Public Health Service, Washington, D.C., U.S. Government Printing Office, Jan. 1983.

A-4. A. M. Hardy, "AIDS Knowledge and Attitudes for October–December 1990"; Provisional data from the National Health Interview Survey. Advance data from vital and health statistics; No. 204, Hyattsville, Md., National Center for Health Statistics, 1991.

A-5. National Center for Health Statistics. Advance data from vital and health statistics: Nos. 51–60. National Center for Health Statistics. *Vital and Health Statistics*, *16*(6), 1991.

A-6. E. J. Graves and L. J. Kozak "National Hospital Discharge Survey: Annual Summary, 1989." National Center for Health Statistics *Vital and Health Statistics*, *13*(109), 1992.

A-7. National Center for Health Statistics, W. C. Hadden and M. I. Harris, "Prevalence of Diagnosed Diabetes, Undiagnosed Diabetes, and Impaired Glucose Tolerance in Adults 20–74 Years of Age, United States, 1976–80," *Vital and Health Statistics*, Series 11, No. 237, DHHS Pub. No. (PHS) 87–1687, Public Health Service, Washington, D.C., U.S. Government Printing Office, Feb. 1987.

CHAPTER 6

Estimation

· · · · · · · · · · · · · · · · ·

CONTENTS

6.1 Introduction

We come now to a consideration of *estimation*, the first of the two general areas of statistical inference. The second general area, *hypothesis testing*, is examined in the next chapter.

We learned in Chapter 1 that inferential statistics is defined as follows.

DEFINITION

Statistical inference is the procedure by which we reach a conclusion about a population on the basis of the information contained in a sample drawn from that population.

The process of estimation entails calculating, from the data of a sample, some statistic that is offered as an approximation of the corresponding parameter of the population from which the sample was drawn.

The rationale behind estimation in the health sciences field rests on the assumption that workers in this field have an interest in the parameters, such as means and proportions, of various populations. If this is the case, there are two good reasons why one must rely on estimating procedures to obtain information regarding these parameters. First, many populations of interest, although finite, are so large that a 100 percent examination would be prohibitive from the standpoint of cost. Second, populations that are infinite are incapable of complete examination.

Suppose the administrator of a large hospital is interested in the mean age of patients admitted to his hospital during a given year. He may consider it too expensive to go through the records of all patients admitted during that particular year and, consequently, elects to examine a sample of the records from which he can compute an estimate of the mean age of patients admitted that year.

A physician in general practice may be interested in knowing what proportion of a certain type of individual, treated with a particular drug, suffers undesirable side effects. No doubt, her concept of the population consists of all those persons who ever have been or ever will be treated with this drug. Deferring a conclusion until the entire population has been observed could have an adverse effect on her practice.

These two examples have implied an interest in estimating, respectively, a population mean and a population proportion. Other parameters, the estimation of which we will cover in this chapter, are the difference between two means, the difference between two proportions, the population variance, and the ratio of two variances.

We will find that for each of the parameters we discuss, we can compute two types of estimate: a point estimate and an interval estimate.

DEFINITION

A *point estimate* is a single numerical value used to estimate the corresponding population parameter.

DEFINITION

An *interval estimate* consists of two numerical values defining a range of values that, with a specified degree of confidence, we feel includes the parameter being estimated.

These concepts will be elaborated on in the succeeding sections.

Choosing an Appropriate Estimator Note that a single computed value has been referred to as an *estimate*. The rule that tells us how to compute this value, or estimate, is referred to as an *estimator*. Estimators are usually presented as formulas. For example,

$$\bar{x} = \frac{\sum x_i}{n}$$

is an estimator of the population mean, μ. The single numerical value that results from evaluating this formula is called an estimate of the parameter μ.

In many cases, a parameter may be estimated by more than one estimator. For example, we could use the sample median to estimate the population mean. How then do we decide which estimator to use for estimating a given parameter? The decision is based on criteria that reflect the "goodness" of particular estimators. When measured against these criteria, some estimators are better than others. One of these criteria is the property of *unbiasedness*.

DEFINITION

An estimator, say T, of the parameter θ is said to be an *unbiased estimator* of θ if $E(T) = \theta$.

$E(T)$ is read, "the expected value of T." For a finite population, $E(T)$ is obtained by taking the average value of T computed from all possible samples of a given size that may be drawn from the population. That is, $E(T) = \mu_T$. For an infinite population, $E(T)$ is defined in terms of calculus.

In the previous chapter we have seen that the sample mean, the sample proportion, the difference between two sample means, and the difference between two sample proportions are each unbiased estimates of their corresponding parameters. This property was implied when the parameters were said to be the means of the respective sampling distributions. For example, since the mean of the sampling distribution of $\bar{x}$ is equal to μ, we know that $\bar{x}$ is an unbiased estimator of μ. The other criteria of good estimators will not be discussed in this book. The interested reader will find them covered in detail by Freund and Walpole (1) and Mood et al. (2), among others. A much less mathematically rigorous treatment may be found in Yamane (3).

Sampled Populations and Target Populations   The health researcher who uses statistical inference procedures must be aware of the difference between two kinds of population—the *sampled population* and the *target population*.

DEFINITION

The sampled population is the population from which one actually draws a sample.

DEFINITION

The target population is the population about which one wishes to make an inference.

These two populations may or may not be the same. Statistical inference procedures allow one to make inferences about sampled populations (provided proper sampling methods have been employed). Only when the target population and the sampled population are the same is it possible for one to use statistical inference procedures to reach conclusions about the target population. If the sampled population and the target population are different, the researcher can reach conclusions about the target population only on the basis of nonstatistical considerations.

Suppose, for example, that a researcher wishes to assess the effectiveness of some method for treating rheumatoid arthritis. The target population consists of all patients suffering from the disease. It is not practical to draw a sample from this population. The researcher may, however, select a sample from all rheumatoid arthritis patients seen in some specific clinic. These patients constitute the sampled population, and, if proper sampling methods are used, inferences about this sampled population may be drawn on the basis of the information in the sample. If the researcher wishes to make inferences about all rheumatoid arthritis sufferers, he or she must rely on nonstatistical means to do so. Perhaps the researcher knows that the sampled population is similar, with respect to all important characteristics, to the target population. That is, the researcher may know that the age, sex, severity of illness, duration of illness, and so on are similar in both populations. And on the strength of this knowledge, the researcher may be willing to extrapolate his or her findings to the target population.

In many situations the sampled population and the target population are identical, and, when this is the case, inferences about the target population are straightforward. The researcher should, however, be aware that this is not always the case and not fall into the trap of drawing unwarranted inferences about a population that is different from the one that is sampled.

Random and Nonrandom Samples   In the examples and exercises of this book, we assume that the data available for analysis have come from random samples. The strict validity of the statistical procedures discussed depends on this assumption. In many instances in real-world applications it is impossible or impractical to use truly random samples. In animal experiments, for example, researchers usually use whatever animals are available from suppliers or their own breeding stock. If the researchers had to depend on randomly selected material, very little research of this type would be conducted. Again, nonstatistical considerations must play a part in the generalization process. Researchers may contend that the samples actually used are equivalent to simple random samples, since there is no reason to believe that the material actually used is not representative of the population about which inferences are desired.

In many health research projects, samples of convenience, rather than random samples, are employed. Researchers may have to rely on volunteer subjects or on readily available subjects such as students in their classes. Again, generalizations must be made on the basis of nonstatistical considerations. The consequences of such generalizations, however, may be useful or they may range from misleading to disastrous.

In some situations it is possible to introduce randomization into an experiment even though available subjects are not randomly selected from some well-defined population. In comparing two treatments, for example, each subject may be randomly assigned to one or the other of the treatments. Inferences in such cases apply to the treatments and not the subjects, and hence the inferences are valid.

6.2
Confidence Interval for a Population Mean

Suppose researchers wish to estimate the mean of some normally distributed population. They draw a random sample of size n from the population, and compute $\bar{x}$, which they use as a point estimate of μ. Although this estimator of μ possesses all the qualities of a good estimator, we know that because of the vagaries of sampling, $\bar{x}$ cannot be expected to be equal to μ.

It would be much more meaningful, therefore, to estimate μ by an interval that somehow communicates information regarding the probable magnitude of μ.

Sampling Distributions and Estimation To obtain an interval estimate, we must draw on our knowledge of sampling distributions. In the present case, since we are concerned with the sample mean as an estimator of a population mean, we must recall what we know about the sampling distribution of the sample mean.

In the previous chapter we learned that if sampling is from a normally distributed population, the sampling distribution of the sample mean will be normally distributed with a mean, $\mu_{\bar{x}}$, equal to the population mean μ, and a variance $\sigma_{\bar{x}}^2$, equal to σ^2/n. We could plot the sampling distribution if we only knew where to locate it on the $\bar{x}$-axis. From our knowledge of normal distributions, in general, we know even more about the distribution of $\bar{x}$ in this case. We know, for example, that regardless of where it is located, approximately 95 percent of the possible values of $\bar{x}$ constituting the distribution are within 2 standard deviations of the mean. The two points that are 2 standard deviations from the mean are $\mu - 2\sigma_{\bar{x}}$ and $\mu + 2\sigma_{\bar{x}}$, so that the interval $\mu \pm 2\sigma_{\bar{x}}$ will contain approximately 95 percent of the possible values of $\bar{x}$. We know that μ and, hence, $\mu_{\bar{x}}$ are unknown, but we may arbitrarily place the sampling distribution of $\bar{x}$ on the $\bar{x}$-axis.

Since we do not know the value of μ, not a great deal is accomplished by the expression $\mu \pm 2\sigma_{\bar{x}}$. We do, however, have a point estimate of μ, which is $\bar{x}$. Would it be useful to construct an interval about this point estimate of μ? The answer is, yes. Suppose we constructed intervals about every possible value of $\bar{x}$ computed from all possible samples of size n from the population of interest. We would have a large number of intervals of the form $\bar{x} \pm 2\sigma_{\bar{x}}$ with widths all equal to the width of the interval about the unknown μ. Approximately 95 percent of these intervals would have centers falling within the $\pm 2\sigma_{\bar{x}}$ interval about μ. Each of the intervals whose centers fall within $2\sigma_{\bar{x}}$ of μ would contain μ. These concepts are illustrated

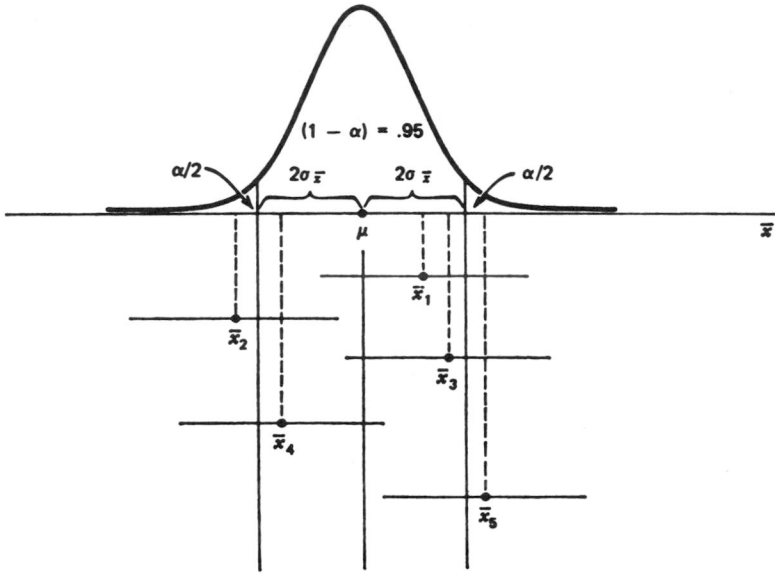

Figure 6.2.1 The 95 percent confidence intervals for μ.

in Figure 6.2.1. In Figure 6.2.1 we see that $x_1, x_3,$ and x_4 all fall within the $2\sigma_{\bar{x}}$ interval about μ, and, consequently, the $2\sigma_{\bar{x}}$ intervals about these sample means include the value of μ. The sample means $\bar{x}_2$ and $\bar{x}_5$ do not fall within the $2\sigma_{\bar{x}}$ interval about μ, and the $2\sigma_{\bar{x}}$ intervals about them do not include μ.

Example 6.2.1

Suppose a researcher, interested in obtaining an estimate of the average level of some enzyme in a certain human population, takes a sample of 10 individuals, determines the level of the enzyme in each, and computes a sample mean of $\bar{x} = 22$. Suppose further it is known that the variable of interest is approximately normally distributed with a variance of 45. We wish to estimate μ.

Solution: An approximate 95 percent confidence interval for μ is given by

$$\bar{x} \pm 2\sigma_{\bar{x}}$$

$$22 \pm 2\sqrt{\tfrac{45}{10}}$$

$$22 \pm 2(2.1213)$$

$$17.76, 26.24$$

Interval Estimate Components Let us examine the composition of the interval estimate constructed in Example 6.2.1. It contains in its center the point estimate of μ. The 2 we recognize as a value from the standard normal distribution that tells us within how many standard errors lie approximately 95 percent of the possible values of $\bar{x}$. This value of z is referred to as the *reliability coefficient*. The last component, $\sigma_{\bar{x}}$, is the standard error, or standard deviation of the sampling distribution of $\bar{x}$. In general, then, an interval estimate may be expressed as follows:

$$\text{estimator} \pm (\text{reliability coefficient}) \times (\text{standard error}) \qquad (6.2.1)$$

In particular, when sampling is from a normal distribution with known variance, an interval estimate for μ may be expressed as

$$\bar{x} \pm z_{(1-\alpha/2)}\sigma_{\bar{x}} \qquad (6.2.2)$$

Interpreting Confidence Intervals How do we interpret the interval given by Expression 6.2.2? In the present example, where the reliability coefficient is equal to 2, we say that in repeated sampling approximately 95 percent of the intervals constructed by Expression 6.2.2 will include the population mean. This interpretation is based on the probability of occurrence of different values of $\bar{x}$. We may generalize this interpretation if we designate the total area under the curve of $\bar{x}$ that is outside the interval $\mu \pm 2\sigma_{\bar{x}}$ as α and the area within the interval as $1 - \alpha$ and give the following *probabilistic interpretation* of Expression 6.2.2.

Probabilistic Interpretation *In repeated sampling, from a normally distributed population with a known standard deviation, $100(1 - \alpha)$ percent of all intervals of the form $\bar{x} \pm z_{(1-\alpha/2)}\sigma_{\bar{x}}$ will in the long run include the population mean, μ.*

The quantity $1 - \alpha$, in this case .95, is called the *confidence coefficient* (or confidence level), and the interval $\bar{x} \pm z_{(1-\alpha/2)}\sigma_{\bar{x}}$ is called a *confidence interval* for μ. When $(1 - \alpha) = .95$, the interval is called the 95 percent confidence interval for μ. In the present example we say that we are 95 percent confident that the population mean is between 17.76 and 26.24. This is called the *practical interpretation* of Expression 6.2.2. In general, it may be expressed as follows.

Practical Interpretation *When sampling is from a normally distributed population with known standard deviation, we are $100(1 - \alpha)$ percent confident that the single computed interval, $\bar{x} \pm z_{(1-\alpha/2)}\sigma_{\bar{x}}$, contains the population mean, μ.*

In the example given here we might prefer, rather than 2, the more exact value of z, 1.96, corresponding to a confidence coefficient of .95. Researchers may use any confidence coefficient they wish; the most frequently used values are .90, .95, and .99, which have associated reliability factors, respectively, of 1.645, 1.96, and 2.58.

Precision The quantity obtained by multiplying the reliability factor by the standard error of the mean is called the *precision* of the estimate. This quantity is also called the *margin of error*.

Example 6.2.2

A physical therapist wished to estimate, with 99 percent confidence, the mean maximal strength of a particular muscle in a certain group of individuals. He is willing to assume that strength scores are approximately normally distributed with a variance of 144. A sample of 15 subjects who participated in the experiment yielded a mean of 84.3.

Solution: The z value corresponding to a confidence coefficient of .99 is found in Table D to be 2.58. This is our reliability coefficient. The standard error is $\sigma_{\bar{x}} = 12/\sqrt{15} = 3.0984$. Our 99 percent confidence interval for μ, then, is

$$84.3 \pm 2.58(3.0984)$$

$$84.3 \pm 8.0$$

$$76.3, 92.3$$

We say we are 99 percent confident that the population mean is between 76.3 and 92.3 since, in repeated sampling, 99 percent of all intervals that could be constructed in the manner just described would include the population mean.

Situations in which the variable of interest is approximately normally distributed with a known variance are so rare as to be almost nonexistent. The purpose of the preceding examples, which assumed that these ideal conditions existed, was to establish the theoretical background for constructing confidence intervals for population means. In most practical situations either the variables are not approximately normally distributed or the population variances are not known or both. Example 6.2.3 and Section 6.3 explain the procedures that are available for use in the less than ideal, but more common, situations.

Sampling from Nonnormal Populations   As noted, it will not always be possible or prudent to assume that the population of interest is normally distributed. Thanks to the central limit theorem, this will not deter us if we are able to select a large enough sample. We have learned that for large samples, the sampling distribution of $\bar{x}$ is approximately normally distributed regardless of how the parent population is distributed.

Example 6.2.3

Punctuality of patients in keeping appointments is of interest to a research team. In a study of patient flow through the offices of general practitioners, it was found that a sample of 35 patients were 17.2 minutes late for appointments, on the average. Previous research had shown the standard deviation to be about 8 minutes. The population distribution was felt to be nonnormal. What is the 90 percent confidence interval for μ, the true mean amount of time late for appointments?

Solution: Since the sample size is fairly large (greater than 30), and since the population standard deviation is known, we draw on the central limit theorem and assume the sampling distribution of $\bar{x}$ to be approximately normally distributed. From Table D we find the reliability coefficient corresponding to a confidence coefficient of .90 to be about 1.645, if we interpolate. The standard error is $\sigma_{\bar{x}} = 8/\sqrt{35} = 1.3522$, so that our 90 percent confidence interval for μ is

$$17.2 \pm 1.645(1.3522)$$

$$17.2 \pm 2.2$$

$$15.0, 19.4$$

Frequently, when the sample is large enough for the application of the central limit theorem the population variance is unknown. In that case we use the sample variance as a replacement for the unknown population variance in the formula for constructing a confidence interval for the population mean.

Computer Analysis When confidence intervals are desired, a great deal of time can be saved if one uses a computer, which can be programmed to construct intervals from raw data.

Example 6.2.4

The following are the activity values (micromoles per minute per gram of tissue) of a certain enzyme measured in normal gastric tissue of 35 patients with gastric carcinoma.

.360	1.189	.614	.788	.273	2.464	.571
1.827	.537	.374	.449	.262	.448	.971
.372	.898	.411	.348	1.925	.550	.622
.610	.319	.406	.413	.767	.385	.674
.521	.603	.533	.662	1.177	.307	1.499

We wish to use the MINITAB computer software package to construct a 95 percent confidence interval for the population mean. Suppose we know that the population variance is .36. It is not necessary to assume that the sampled population of values is normally distributed since the sample size is sufficiently large for application of the central limit theorem.

Solution: We enter the data into column 1 and issue the following MINITAB command:

```
ZINTERVAL 95 .6 C1
```

This command tells the computer that the reliability factor is z, that a 95 percent confidence interval is desired, that the population standard deviation is .6, and that the data are in column 1. We obtain the following printout.

```
THE  ASSUMED  SIGMA = 0.600
N    MEAN    STDEV    SE MEAN    95.0 PERCENT  C.I.
35   0.718   0.511    0.101      (   0.519,    0.917)
```

The printout tells us that the sample mean is .718, the sample standard deviation is .511, and the standard error of the mean, $\sigma / \sqrt{n}$, is $.6 / \sqrt{35} = .101$.

We are 95 percent confident that the population mean is somewhere between .519 and .917.

Confidence intervals may be obtained through the use of many other software packages. Users of SAS®, for example, may wish to use the output from PROC MEANS or PROC UNIVARIATE to construct confidence intervals.

Alternative Estimates of Central Tendency   As noted previously, the mean is sensitive to extreme values—those values that deviate appreciably from most of the measurements in a data set. They are sometimes referred to as *outliers*. We also noted earlier that the median, because it is not so sensitive to extreme measurements, is sometimes preferred over the mean as a measure of central tendency when outliers are present. For the same reason we may prefer to use the sample median as an estimator of the population median when we wish to make an inference about the central tendency of a population. Not only may we use the sample median as a point estimate of the population median, we also may construct a confidence interval for the population median. The formula is not given here, but may be found in the book by Rice (4).

Trimmed Mean   Estimators that are insensitive to outliers are called *robust estimators*. Another robust measure and estimator of central tendency is the *trimmed mean*. For a set of sample data containing n measurements we calculate the 100α percent trimmed mean as follows:

1. Order the measurements.
2. Discard the smallest 100α percent and the largest 100α percent of the measurements. The recommended value of α is something between .1 and .2.
3. Compute the arithmetic mean of the remaining measurements.

Note that the median may be regarded as a 50 percent trimmed mean. The formula for the confidence interval based on the trimmed mean is not given here. The interested reader is referred to the book by Rice (4). Recall that the trimmed mean for a set of data is one of the descriptive measures calculated by MINITAB in response to the DESCRIBE command.

EXERCISES

6.2.1 We wish to estimate the average number of heartbeats per minute for a certain population. The average number of heartbeats per minute for a sample of 49 subjects was found to be 90. If it is reasonable to assume that these 49 patients constitute a random sample, and that the population is normally distributed with a standard deviation of 10, find:

  a. The 90 percent confidence interval for μ.
  b. The 95 percent confidence interval for μ.
  c. The 99 percent confidence interval for μ.

6.2.2 We wish to estimate the mean serum indirect bilirubin level of 4-day-old infants. The mean for a sample of 16 infants was found to be 5.98 mg/100 cc. Assuming bilirubin levels in 4-day-old infants are approximately normally distributed with a standard deviation of 3.5 mg/100 cc find:

  a. The 90 percent confidence interval for μ.
  b. The 95 percent confidence interval for μ.
  c. The 99 percent confidence interval for μ.

6.2.3 In a length of hospitalization study conducted by several cooperating hospitals, a random sample of 64 peptic ulcer patients was drawn from a list of all peptic ulcer patients ever admitted to the participating hospitals and the length of hospitalization per admission was determined for each. The mean length of hospitalization was found to be 8.25 days. If the population standard deviation is known to be 3 days, find:

  a. The 90 percent confidence interval for μ.
  b. The 95 percent confidence interval for μ.
  c. The 99 percent confidence interval for μ.

6.2.4 A sample of 100 apparently normal adult males, 25 years old, had a mean systolic blood pressure of 125. If it is believed that the population standard deviation is 15, find:

  a. The 90 percent confidence interval for μ.
  b. The 95 percent confidence interval for μ.

6.2.5 Some studies of Alzheimer's disease (AD) have shown an increase in $^{14}CO_2$ production in patients with the disease. In one such study the following $^{14}CO_2$ values were obtained from 16 neocortical biopsy samples from AD patients.

1009,	1280,	1180,	1255,	1547,	2352,	1956,	1080,
1776,	1767,	1680,	2050,	1452,	2857,	3100,	1621

Assume that the population of such values is normally distributed with a standard deviation of 350 and construct a 95 percent confidence interval for the population mean.

6.3
The *t* Distribution

In Section 6.2 a procedure was outlined for constructing a confidence interval for a population mean. The procedure requires a knowledge of the variance of the population from which the sample is drawn. It may seem somewhat strange that one can have knowledge of the population variance and not know the value of the population mean. Indeed, it is the usual case, in situations such as have been presented, that the population variance, as well as the population mean, is unknown. This condition presents a problem with respect to constructing confidence intervals. Although, for example, the statistic

$$z = \frac{\bar{x} - \mu}{\sigma/\sqrt{n}}$$

is normally distributed when the population is normally distributed, and is at least approximately normally distributed when n is large, regardless of the functional form of the population, we cannot make use of this fact because σ is unknown. However, all is not lost, and the most logical solution to the problem is the one followed. We use the sample standard deviation

$$s = \sqrt{\sum(x_i - \bar{x})^2 / (n - 1)}$$

to replace σ. When the sample size is large, say greater than 30, our faith in s as an approximation of σ is usually substantial, and we may feel justified in using normal distribution theory to construct a confidence interval for the population mean. In that event, we proceed as instructed in Section 6.2.

It is when we have small samples that it becomes mandatory for us to find an alternative procedure for constructing confidence intervals.

As a result of the work of Gosset (5), writing under the pseudonym of "Student," an alternative, known as *Student's t distribution*, usually shortened to *t distribution*, is available to us.

The quantity

$$t = \frac{\bar{x} - \mu}{s/\sqrt{n}}$$

follows this distribution.

Properties of the *t* Distribution   The *t* distribution has the following properties.

1. It has a mean of 0.
2. It is symmetrical about the mean.

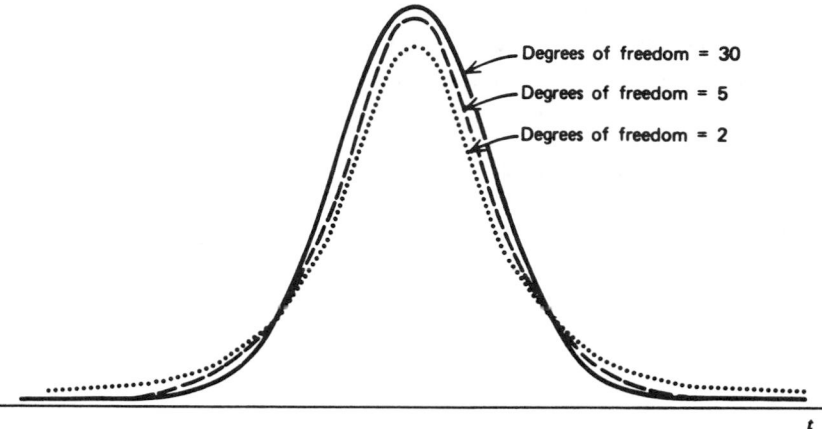

Figure 6.3.1 The *t* distribution for different degrees-of-freedom values.

3. In general, it has a variance greater than 1, but the variance approaches 1 as the sample size becomes large. For $df > 2$, the variance of the *t* distribution is $df/(df - 2)$, where df is the degrees of freedom. Alternatively, since here $df = n - 1$ for $n > 3$, we may write the variance of the *t* distribution as $(n - 1)/(n - 3)$.

4. The variable *t* ranges from $-\infty$ to $+\infty$.

5. The *t* distribution is really a family of distributions, since there is a different distribution for each sample value of $n - 1$, the divisor used in computing s^2. We recall that $n - 1$ is referred to as degrees of freedom. Figure 6.3.1 shows *t* distributions corresponding to several degrees-of-freedom values.

6. Compared to the normal distribution the *t* distribution is less peaked in the center and has higher tails. Figure 6.3.2 compares the *t* distribution with the normal.

7. The *t* distribution approaches the normal distribution as $n - 1$ approaches infinity.

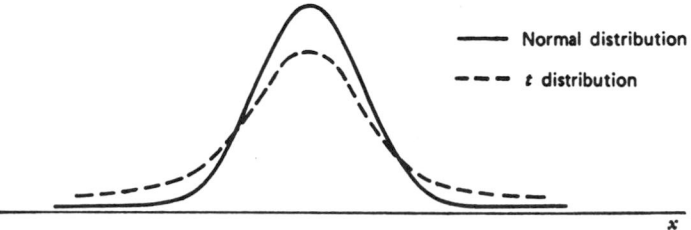

Figure 6.3.2 Comparison of normal distribution and *t* distribution.

The t distribution, like the standard normal, has been extensively tabulated. One such table is given as Table E in Appendix II. As we will see, we must take both the confidence coefficient and degrees of freedom into account when using the table of the t distribution.

Confidence Intervals Using *t* The general procedure for constructing confidence intervals is not affected by our having to use the t distribution rather than the standard normal distribution. We still make use of the relationship expressed by

$$\text{estimator} \pm (\text{reliability coefficient}) \times (\text{standard error})$$

What is different is the source of the reliability coefficient. It is now obtained from the table of the t distribution rather than from the table of the standard normal distribution. To be more specific, *when sampling is from a normal distribution whose standard deviation, σ, is unknown, the $100(1 - \alpha)$ percent confidence interval for the population mean, μ, is given by*

$$\bar{x} \pm t_{(1-\alpha/2)}\frac{s}{\sqrt{n}} \qquad (6.3.1)$$

Notice that a requirement for valid use of the t distribution is that the sample must be drawn from a normal distribution. Experience has shown, however, that moderate departures from this requirement can be tolerated. As a consequence, the t distribution is used even when it is known that the parent population deviates somewhat from normality. Most researchers require that an assumption of, at least, a mound-shaped population distribution be tenable.

Example 6.3.1   Maureen McCauley conducted a study to evaluate the effect of on-the-job body mechanics instruction on the work performance of newly employed young workers (A-1). She used two randomly selected groups of subjects, an experimental group and a control group. The experimental group received one hour of back school training provided by an occupational therapist. The control group did not receive this training. A criterion-referenced Body Mechanics Evaluation Checklist was used to evaluate each worker's lifting, lowering, pulling, and transferring of objects in the work environment. A correctly performed task received a score of 1. The 15 control subjects made a mean score of 11.53 on the evaluation with a standard deviation of 3.681. We assume that these 15 controls behave as a random sample from a population of similar subjects. We wish to use these sample data to estimate the mean score for the population.

Solution: We may use the sample mean, 11.53 as a point estimate of the population mean but, since the population standard deviation is unknown, we must assume the population of values to be at least approximately normally distributed before constructing a confidence interval for μ. Let us assume that such an assumption is reasonable and that a 95 percent confidence interval is desired. We have our estimator, $\bar{x}$, and our standard error is $s/\sqrt{n} = 3.681/\sqrt{15} = .9504$. We need now to find the reliability coefficient, the value of t associated with a confidence coefficient of .95 and $n - 1 = 14$ degrees of freedom. Since a 95 percent

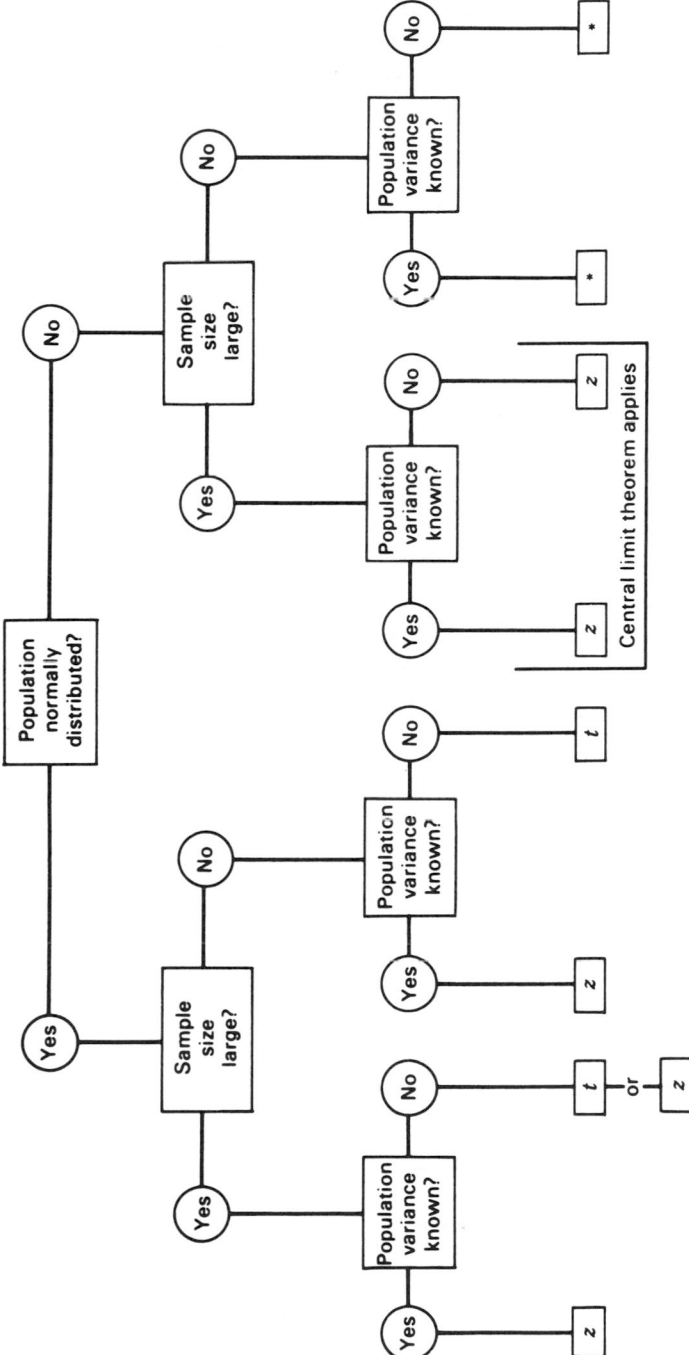

Figure 6.3.3 Flowchart for use in deciding between z and t when making inferences about population means. (*Use a nonparametric procedure. See Chapter 13.)

confidence interval leaves .05 of the area under the curve of t to be equally divided between the two tails, we need the value of t to the right of which lies .025 of the area. We locate in Table E the column headed $t_{.975}$. This is the value of t to the left of which lies .975 of the area under the curve. The area to the right of this value is equal to the desired .025. We now locate the number 14 in the degrees-of-freedom column. The value at the intersection of the row labeled 14 and the column labeled $t_{.975}$ is the t we seek. This value of t, which is our reliability coefficient, is found to be 2.1448. We now construct our 95 percent confidence interval as follows:

$$11.53 \pm 2.1448(.9504)$$

$$11.53 \pm 2.04$$

$$9.49, 13.57$$

This interval may be interpreted from both the probabilistic and practical points of view. We say we are 95 percent confident that the true population mean, μ, is somewhere between 9.49 and 13.57 because, in repeated sampling, 95 percent of intervals constructed in like manner will include μ.

Deciding Between z and t   When we construct a confidence interval for a population mean, we must decide whether to use a value of z or a value of t as the reliability factor. To make an appropriate choice we must consider sample size, whether the sampled population is normally distributed, and whether the population variance is known. Figure 6.3.3 provides a flowchart that one can use to decide quickly whether the reliability factor should be z or t.

Computer Analysis   If you wish to have MINITAB construct a confidence interval for a population mean when the t statistic is the appropriate reliability factor, the command begins with the word TINTERVAL. The remainder of the command is the same as for the ZINTERVAL command minus the sigma designation.

EXERCISES

6.3.1   Use the t distribution to find the reliability factor for a confidence interval based on the following confidence coefficients and sample sizes:

	a	*b*	*c*	*d*
Confidence coefficient	.95	.99	.90	.95
Sample size	15	24	8	30

6.3.2   In an investigation of the flow and volume dependence of the total respiratory system in a group of mechanically ventilated patients with chronic obstructive pulmonary disease, Tantucci et al. (A-2) collected the following baseline values on constant inspiratory flow (L/s): .90, .97, 1.03, 1.10, 1.04, 1.00. Assume that the six subjects constitute a simple random sample from a normally distributed population of similar subjects.

a. What is the point estimate of the population mean?

b. What is the standard deviation of the sample?

c. What is the estimated standard error of the sample mean?

d. Construct a 95 percent confidence interval for the population mean constant inspiratory flow.

e. What is the precision of the estimate?

f. State the probabilistic interpretation of the confidence interval you constructed.

g. State the practical interpretation of the confidence interval you constructed.

6.3.3 Lloyd and Mailloux (A-3) reported the following data on the pituitary gland weight in a sample of four Wistar Furth Rats:

mean = 9.0 mg, standard error of the mean = .3

SOURCE: Ricardo V. Lloyd and Joe Mailloux, "Analysis of S-100 Protein Positive Folliculo-Stellate Cells in Rat Pituitary Tissues," *American Journal of Pathology, 133* (1988), 338–346.

a. What was the sample standard deviation?

b. Construct a 95 percent confidence interval for the mean pituitary weight of a population of similar rats.

c. What assumptions are necessary for the validity of the confidence interval you constructed?

6.3.4 In a study of preeclampsia, Kaminski and Rechberger (A-4) found the mean systolic blood pressure of 10 healthy, nonpregnant women to be 119 with a standard deviation of 2.1.

a. What is the estimated standard error of the mean?

b. Construct the 99 percent confidence interval for the mean of the population from which the 10 subjects may be presumed to be a random sample.

c. What is the precision of the estimate?

d. What assumptions are necessary for the validity of the confidence interval you constructed?

6.3.5 A sample of 16 ten-year-old girls gave a mean weight of 71.5 and a standard deviation of 12 pounds, respectively. Assuming normality, find the 90, 95, and 99 percent confidence intervals for μ.

6.3.6 A simple random sample of 16 apparently healthy subjects yielded the following values of urine excreted arsenic (milligrams per day).

Subject	Value	Subject	Value
1	.007	9	.012
2	.030	10	.006
3	.025	11	.010
4	.008	12	.032
5	.030	13	.006
6	.038	14	.009
7	.007	15	.014
8	.005	16	.011

Construct a 95 percent confidence interval for the population mean.

6.4
Confidence Interval for the Difference Between Two Population Means

Sometimes there arise cases in which we are interested in estimating the difference between two population means. From each of the populations an independent random sample is drawn and, from the data of each, the sample means $\bar{x}_1$ and $\bar{x}_2$, respectively, are computed. We learned in the previous chapter that the estimator $\bar{x}_1 - \bar{x}_2$ yields an unbiased estimate of $\mu_1 - \mu_2$, the difference between the population means. The variance of the estimator is $(\sigma_1^2/n_1) + (\sigma_2^2/n_2)$. We also know from Chapter 5 that, depending on the conditions, the sampling distribution of $\bar{x}_1 - \bar{x}_2$ may be, at least, approximately normally distributed, so that in many cases we make use of the theory relevant to normal distributions to compute a confidence interval for $\mu_1 - \mu_2$. When the population variances are known, the $100(1 - \alpha)$ percent confidence interval for $\mu_1 - \mu_2$ is given by

$$(\bar{x}_1 - \bar{x}_2) \pm z_{1-\alpha/2} \sqrt{\frac{\sigma_1^2}{n_1} + \frac{\sigma_2^2}{n_2}} \qquad (6.4.1)$$

Let us illustrate, for the case where sampling is from normal distributions.

Example 6.4.1

A research team is interested in the difference between serum uric acid levels in patients with and without Down's syndrome. In a large hospital for the treatment of the mentally retarded, a sample of 12 individuals with Down's syndrome yielded a mean of $\bar{x}_1 = 4.5$ mg/100 ml. In a general hospital a sample of 15 normal individuals of the same age and sex were found to have a mean value of $\bar{x}_2 = 3.4$. If it is reasonable to assume that the two populations of values are normally distributed with variances equal to 1 and 1.5, find the 95 percent confidence interval for $\mu_1 - \mu_2$.

Solution: For a point estimate of $\mu_1 - \mu_2$, we use $\bar{x}_1 - \bar{x}_2 = 4.5 - 3.4 = 1.1$. The reliability coefficient corresponding to .95 is found in Table D to be 1.96. The standard error is

$$\sigma_{\bar{x}_1-\bar{x}_2} = \sqrt{\frac{\sigma_1^2}{n_1} + \frac{\sigma_2^2}{n_2}} = \sqrt{\frac{1}{12} + \frac{1.5}{15}} = .4282$$

The 95 percent confidence interval, then, is

$$1.1 \pm 1.96(.4282)$$

$$1.1 \pm .84$$

$$.26, 1.94$$

We say that we are 95 percent confident that the true difference, $\mu_1 - \mu_2$, is somewhere between .26 and 1.94, because, in repeated sampling, 95 percent of the intervals constructed in this manner would include the difference between the true means.

Sampling from Nonnormal Populations   The construction of a confidence interval for the difference between two population means when sampling is from nonnormal populations proceeds in the same manner as in Example 6.4.1 if the sample sizes n_1 and n_2 are large. Again, this is a result of the central limit theorem. If the population variances are unknown, we use the sample variances to estimate them.

Example 6.4.2

Motivated by an awareness of the existence of a body of controversial literature suggesting that stress, anxiety, and depression are harmful to the immune system, Gorman et al. (A-5) conducted a study in which the subjects were homosexual men, some of whom were HIV positive and some of whom were HIV negative. Data were collected on a wide variety of medical, immunological, psychiatric, and neurological measures, one of which was the number of CD4 + cells in the blood. The mean number of CD4 + cells for the 112 men with HIV infection was 401.8 with a standard deviation of 226.4. For the 75 men without HIV infection the mean and standard deviation were 828.2 and 274.9, respectively. We wish to construct a 99 percent confidence interval for the difference between population means.

Solution: No information is given regarding the shape of the distribution of CD4 + cells. Since our sample sizes are large, however, the central limit theorem assures us that the sampling distribution of the difference between sample means will be approximately normally distributed even if the distribution of the variable in the populations is not normally distributed. We may use this fact as justification for using the z statistic as the reliability factor in the construction of our confidence interval. Also, since the population standard deviations are not given, we will use the sample standard deviations to estimate them. The point estimate for the difference between population means is the difference between sample means, $828.2 - 401.8 = 426.4$. In Table D we find the reliability factor to be 2.58. The estimated standard error is

$$s_{\bar{x}_1 - \bar{x}_2} = \sqrt{\frac{274.9^2}{75} + \frac{226.4^2}{112}} = 38.2786$$

By Equation 6.4.1, our 99 percent confidence interval for the difference between population means is

$$426.4 \pm 2.58(38.2786)$$

$$327.6, 525.2$$

We are 99 percent confident that the mean number of CD4 + cells in HIV-positive males differs from the mean for HIV-negative males by somewhere between 327.6 and 525.2.

The *t* Distribution and the Difference Between Means   When population variances are unknown, and we wish to estimate the difference between two population means with a confidence interval, we can use the *t* distribution as a source of the reliability factor if certain assumptions are met. We must know, or be willing to assume, that the two sampled populations are normally distributed. With regard to the population variances, we distinguish between two situations: (1) the situation in which the population variances are equal and (2) the situation in which they are not equal. Let us consider each situation separately.

Population Variances Equal   If the assumption of equal population variances is justified, the two sample variances that we compute from our two independent samples may be considered as estimates of the same quantity, the common variance. It seems logical then that we should somehow capitalize on this in our analysis. We do just that and obtain a *pooled estimate* of the common variance. This pooled estimate is obtained by computing the weighted average of the two sample variances. Each sample variance is weighted by its degrees of freedom. If the sample sizes are equal, this weighted average is the arithmetic mean of the two sample variances. If the two sample sizes are unequal, the weighted average takes advantage of the additional information provided by the larger sample. The pooled estimate is given by the formula:

$$s_p^2 = \frac{(n_1 - 1)s_1^2 + (n_2 - 1)s_2^2}{n_1 + n_2 - 2} \tag{6.4.2}$$

The standard error of the estimate, then, is given by

$$s_{\bar{x}_1 - \bar{x}_2} = \sqrt{\frac{s_p^2}{n_1} + \frac{s_p^2}{n_2}} \tag{6.4.3}$$

and the $100(1 - \alpha)$ percent confidence interval for $\mu_1 - \mu_2$ is given by

$$(\bar{x}_1 - \bar{x}_2) \pm t_{(1 - \alpha/2)}\sqrt{\frac{s_p^2}{n_1} + \frac{s_p^2}{n_2}} \tag{6.4.4}$$

The number of degrees of freedom used in determining the value of *t* to use in constructing the interval is $n_1 + n_2 - 2$, the denominator of Equation 6.4.2. We interpret this interval in the usual manner.

Example 6.4.3

The purpose of a study by Stone et al. (A-6) was to determine the effects of long-term exercise intervention on corporate executives enrolled in a supervised fitness program. Data were collected on 13 subjects (the exercise group) who voluntarily entered a supervised exercise program and remained active for an average of 13 years and 17 subjects (the sedentary group) who elected not to join the fitness program. Among the data collected on the subjects was maximum number of sit-ups completed in 30 seconds. The exercise group had a mean and standard deviation for this variable of 21.0 and 4.9, respectively. The mean and standard deviation for the sedentary group were 12.1 and 5.6, respectively. We assume that the two populations of overall muscle condition measures are approximately normally distributed and that the two population variances are equal. We wish to construct a 95 percent confidence interval for the difference between the means of the populations represented by these two samples.

Solution: First, we use Equation 6.4.2 to compute the pooled estimate of the common population variance.

$$s_p^2 = \frac{(13-1)(4.9^2) + (17-1)(5.6^2)}{13 + 17 - 2} = 28.21$$

When we enter Table E with $13 + 17 - 2 = 28$ degrees of freedom and a desired confidence level of .95, we find that the reliability factor is 2.0484. By Expression 6.4.4 we compute the 95 percent confidence interval for the difference between population means as follows:

$$(21.0 - 12.1) \pm 2.0484\sqrt{\frac{28.21}{13} + \frac{28.21}{17}}$$

$$8.9 \pm 4.0085$$

$$4.9, 12.9$$

We are 95 percent confident that the difference between population means is somewhere between 4.9 and 12.9. We can say this because we know that if we were to repeat the study many, many times, and compute confidence intervals in the same way, about 95 percent of the intervals would include the difference between the population means.

Population Variances Not Equal   When one is unable to ascertain that the variances of two populations of interest are equal, even though the two populations may be assumed to be normally distributed, it is not proper to use the t distribution as just outlined in constructing confidence intervals.

A solution to the problem of unequal variances was proposed by Behrens (6) and later was verified and generalized by Fisher (7, 8). Solutions have also been proposed by Neyman (9), Scheffé (10, 11), and Welch (12, 13). The problem is discussed in detail by Aspin (14), Trickett et al. (15), and Cochran (16). Cochran's approach is also found in Snedecor and Cochran (17).

The problem revolves around the fact that the quantity

$$\frac{(\bar{x}_1 - \bar{x}_2) - (\mu_1 - \mu_2)}{\sqrt{\dfrac{s_1^2}{n_1} + \dfrac{s_2^2}{n_2}}}$$

does not follow a t distribution with $n_1 + n_2 - 2$ degrees of freedom when the population variances are not equal. Consequently, the t distribution cannot be used in the usual way to obtain the reliability factor for the confidence interval for the difference between the means of two populations that have unequal variances. The solution proposed by Cochran consists of computing the reliability factor, $t'_{1-\alpha/2}$, by the following formula:

$$t'_{1-\alpha/2} = \frac{w_1 t_1 + w_2 t_2}{w_1 + w_2} \tag{6.4.5}$$

where $w_1 = s_1^2/n_1$, $w_2 = s_2^2/n_2$, $t_1 = t_{1-\alpha/2}$ for $n_1 - 1$ degrees of freedom, and $t_2 = t_{1-\alpha/2}$ for $n_2 - 1$ degrees of freedom. An approximate $100(1 - \alpha)$ percent confidence interval for $\mu_1 - \mu_2$ is given by

$$(\bar{x}_1 - \bar{x}_2) \pm t'_{(1-\alpha/2)}\sqrt{\frac{s_1^2}{n_1} + \frac{s_2^2}{n_2}} \tag{6.4.6}$$

Example 6.4.4

In the study by Stone et al. (A-6) described in Example 6.4.3, the investigators also reported the following information on a measure of overall muscle condition scores made by the subjects:

Sample	n	Mean	Standard Deviation
Exercise group	13	4.5	.3
Sedentary group	17	3.7	1.0

We assume that the two populations of overall muscle condition scores are approximately normally distributed. We are unwilling to assume, however, that the two population variances are equal. We wish to construct a 95 percent confidence interval for the difference between the mean overall muscle condition scores of the two populations represented by the samples.

Solution: We will use t' as found by Equation 6.4.5 for the reliability factor. Reference to Table E shows that with 12 degrees of freedom and $1 - .05/2 = .975$,

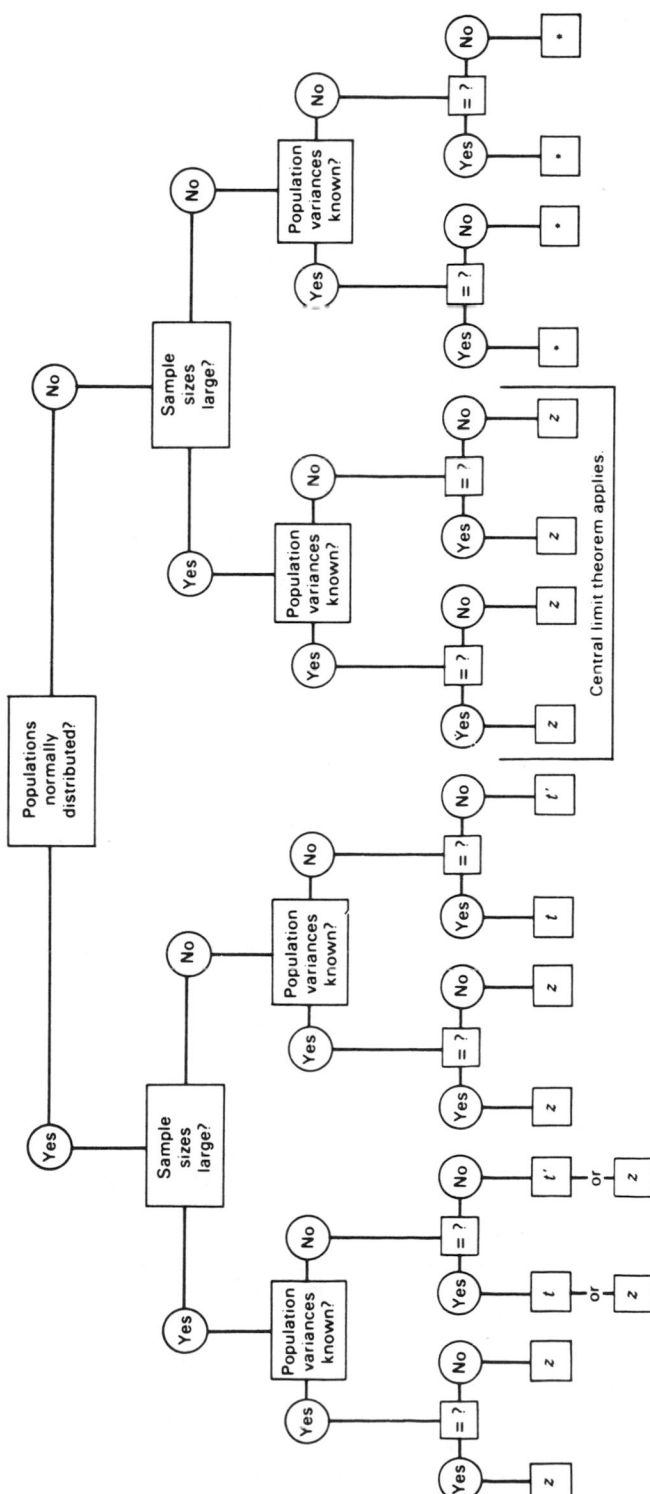

Figure 6.4.1 Flowchart for use in deciding whether the reliability factor should be z, t, or t' when making inferences about the between two population means. (*Use a nonparametric procedure. See Chapter 13.)

$t_1 = 2.1788$. Similarly, with 16 degrees of freedom and $1 - .05/2 = .975$, $t_2 = 2.1199$. We now compute

$$t' = \frac{(.3^2/13)(2.1788) + (1.0^2/17)(2.1199)}{(.3^2/13) + (1.0^2/17)} = \frac{.139784}{.065747}$$

$$= 2.1261$$

By Expression 6.4.6 we now construct the 95 percent confidence interval for the difference between the two population means.

$$(4.5 - 3.7) \pm 2.1261\sqrt{\frac{.3^2}{13} + \frac{1.0^2}{17}}$$

$$.8 \pm 2.1261(.25641101)$$

$$.25, 1.34$$

When constructing a confidence interval for the difference between two population means one may use Figure 6.4.1 to decide quickly whether the reliability factor should be z, t, or t'.

EXERCISES

6.4.1 The objective of an experiment by Buckner et al. (A-7) was to study the effect of pancuronium-induced muscle relaxation on circulating plasma volume. Subjects were newborn infants weighing more than 1700 grams who required respiratory assistance within 24 hours of birth and met other clinical criteria. Five infants paralyzed with pancuronium and seven nonparalyzed infants yielded the following statistics on the second of three measurements of plasma volume (ml) made during mechanical ventilation:

Subject Group	Sample Mean	Sample Standard Deviation
Paralyzed	48.0	8.1
Nonparalyzed	56.7	8.1

The second measurement for the paralyzed group occurred 12 to 24 hours after the first dose of pancuronium. For the nonparalyzed group, measurements were made 12 to 24 hours after commencing mechanical ventilation. State all necessary assumptions and construct the following:
a. The 90 percent confidence interval for $\mu_1 - \mu_2$.
b. The 95 percent confidence interval for $\mu_1 - \mu_2$.
c. The 99 percent confidence interval for $\mu_1 - \mu_2$.

6.4.2 Zucker and Archer (A-8) state that N-NITROSOBIS (2-oxopropyl)amine (BOP) and related β-oxidized nitrosamines produce a high incidence of pancreatic ductular tumors in the Syrian golden hamster. They studied the effect on body weight, plasma glucose, insulin, and plasma glutamate-oxaloacetate transaminase (GOT) levels of exposure of hamsters *in vivo* to BOP. The investigators reported the following results for 8 treated and 12 untreated animals:

Variable	Untreated	Treated
Plasma glucose (mg/dl)	101 ± 5	74 ± 6

SOURCE: Peter F. Zucker and Michael C. Archer, "Alterations in Pancreatic Islet Function Produced by Carcinogenic Nitrosamines in the Syrian Hamster," *American Journal of Pathology*, *133* (1988), 573–577

The data are the sample mean $\pm$ the estimated standard error of the sample mean. State all necessary assumptions and construct the following:

a. The 90 percent confidence interval for $\mu_1 - \mu_2$.
b. The 95 percent confidence interval for $\mu_1 - \mu_2$.
c. The 99 percent confidence interval for $\mu_1 - \mu_2$.

6.4.3 The objectives of a study by Davics et al. (A-9) were to evaluate (1) the effectiveness of the "Time to Quit" self-help smoking cessation program when used on a one-to-one basis in the home and (2) the feasibility of teaching smoking cessation techniques to baccalaureate nursing students. Senior nursing students enrolled in two University of Ottawa research methodology courses were invited to participate in the project. A smoking cessation multiple choice quiz was administered to 120 student nurses who participated and 42 nonparticipating student nurses before and after the study. Differences between pre- and post-study scores were calculated and the following statistics were computed from the differences:

Group	Mean	Standard Deviation
Participants (*A*)	21.4444	15.392
Nonparticipants (*B*)	3.3333	14.595

State all necessary assumptions, and construct the following:

a. The 90 percent confidence interval for $\mu_A - \mu_B$.
b. The 95 percent confidence interval for $\mu_A - \mu_B$.
c. The 99 percent confidence interval for $\mu_A - \mu_B$.

6.4.4 Dr. Ali A. Khraibi (A-10), of the Mayo Clinic and Foundation, conducted a series of experiments to evaluate the natriuretic and diuretic responses of Okamoto spontaneously hypertensive rats (SHR) and Wistar-Kyoto rats (WKY) to direct increases in renal interstitial hydrostatic pressure (RIHP). Direct renal interstitial volume expansion (DRIVE), via a chronically implanted polyethylene matrix in the kidney, was used to increase RIHP. Among the data collected during the study were the following measurements on urinary sodium excretion ($U_{\text{Na}}\dot{V}$) during the DRIVE period.

Group	$U_{\text{Na}}\dot{V}$, (μeq / min)
SHR	6.32, 5.72, 7.96, 4.83, 5.27
2WKY	4.20, 4.69, 4.82, 1.08, 2.10

SOURCE: Dr. Ali A. Khraibi. Used with permission.

State all necessary assumptions and construct a 95 percent confidence interval for the difference between the two population means.

6.4.5 A study by Osberg and Di Scala (A-11) focused on the effectiveness of seat belts in reducing injuries among survivors aged 4 to 14 who were admitted to hospitals. The study contrasted outcomes for 123 belted versus 290 unrestrained children among those involved in motor vehicle crashes who required hospitalization. The study report contained the following statistics on number of ICU days:

Group	Mean	Estimated Standard Error
Belted	.83	.16
No restraint	1.39	.18

State all necessary assumptions, and construct a 95 percent confidence interval for the difference between population means.

6.4.6 Transverse diameter measurements on the hearts of adult males and females gave the following results:

Group	Sample Size	$\bar{x}$ (cm)	s (cm)
Males	12	13.21	1.05
Females	9	11.00	1.01

Assuming normally distributed populations with equal variances, construct the 90, 95, and 99 percent confidence intervals for $\mu_1 - \mu_2$.

6.4.7 Twenty-four experimental animals with vitamin D deficiency were divided equally into two groups. Group 1 received treatment consisting of a diet that provided vitamin D. The second group was not treated. At the end of the experimental period, serum calcium determinations were made with the following results:

Treated group: $\bar{x} = 11.1 \text{ mg}/100 \text{ ml}, s = 1.5$

Untreated group: $\bar{x} = 7.8 \text{ mg}/100 \text{ ml}, s = 2.0$

Assuming normally distributed populations with equal variances, construct the 90, 95, and 99 percent confidence intervals for the difference between population means.

6.4.8 Two groups of children were given visual acuity tests. Group 1 was composed of 11 children who receive their health care from private physicians. The mean score for this group was 26 with a standard deviation of 5. The second group, consisting of 14 children who receive their health care from the health department, had an average score of 21 with a standard deviation of 6. Assuming normally distributed populations with equal variances find the 90, 95, and 99 percent confidence intervals for $\mu_1 - \mu_2$.

6.4.9 The average length of stay of a sample of 20 patients discharged from a general hospital was 7 days with a standard deviation of 2 days. A sample of 24 patients discharged from a chronic disease hospital has an average length of stay of 36 days with a standard deviation of 10 days. Assuming normally distributed populations with unequal variances, find the 95 percent confidence interval for the difference between population means.

6.4.10 In a study of factors thought to be responsible for the adverse effects of smoking on human reproduction, cadmium level determinations (nanograms per gram) were made on placenta tissue of a sample of 14 mothers who were smokers and an independent random sample of 18 nonsmoking mothers. The results were as follows:

Nonsmokers:	10.0, 8.4, 12.8, 25.0, 11.8, 9.8, 12.5, 15.4, 23.5, 9.4, 25.1, 19.5, 25.5, 9.8, 7.5, 11.8, 12.2, 15.0
Smokers:	30.0, 30.1, 15.0, 24.1, 30.5, 17.8, 16.8, 14.8, 13.4, 28.5, 17.5, 14.4, 12.5, 20.4

Construct a 95 percent confidence interval for the difference between population means. Does it appear likely that the mean cadmium level is higher among smokers than nonsmokers? Why do you reach this conclusion?

6.5
Confidence Interval for a Population Proportion

Many questions of interest to the health worker relate to population proportions. What proportion of patients who receive a particular type of treatment recover? What proportion of some population has a certain disease? What proportion of a population are immune to a certain disease?

To estimate a population proportion we proceed in the same manner as when estimating a population mean. A sample is drawn from the population of interest, and the sample proportion, $\hat{p}$, is computed. This sample proportion is used as the point estimator of the population proportion. A confidence interval is obtained by the general formula:

$$\text{estimator} \pm (\text{reliability coefficient}) \times (\text{standard error})$$

In the previous chapter we saw that when both np and $n(1 - p)$ are greater than 5, we may consider the sampling distribution of $\hat{p}$ to be quite close to the normal distribution. When this condition is met, our reliability coefficient is some value of z from the standard normal distribution. The standard error, we have seen, is equal to $\sigma_{\hat{p}} = \sqrt{p(1 - p)/n}$. Since p, the parameter we are trying to estimate, is unknown, we must use $\hat{p}$ as an estimate. Thus we estimate $\sigma_{\hat{p}}$ by $\sqrt{\hat{p}(1 - \hat{p})/n}$, and our $100(1 - \alpha)$ percent confidence interval for p is given by

$$\hat{p} \pm z_{(1-\alpha/2)}\sqrt{\hat{p}(1 - \hat{p})/n} \qquad (6.5.1)$$

We give this interval both the probabilistic and practical interpretations.

Example 6.5.1   Mathers et al. (A-12) found that in a sample of 591 admitted to a psychiatric hospital, 204 admitted to using cannabis at least once in their lifetime. We wish to construct a 95 percent confidence interval for the proportion of lifetime cannabis users in the sampled population of psychiatric hospital admissions.

Solution: The best point estimate of the population proportion is $\hat{p} = 204/591 = .3452$. The size of the sample and our estimate of p are of sufficient magnitude to justify use of the standard normal distribution in constructing a confidence interval. The reliability coefficient corresponding to a confidence level of .95 is 1.96 and our estimate of the standard error $\sigma_{\hat{p}}$ is $\sqrt{\hat{p}(1-\hat{p})/n} = \sqrt{(.3452)(.6548)/591} = .01956$. The 95 percent confidence interval for p, based on these data, is

$$.3452 \pm 1.96(.01956)$$

$$.3452 \pm .0383$$

$$.3069, .3835$$

We say we are 95 percent confident that the population proportion p is between .3069 and .3835 since, in repeated sampling, about 95 percent of the intervals constructed in the manner of the present single interval would include the true p. On the basis of these results we would expect, with 95 percent confidence, to find somewhere between 30.69 percent and 38.35 percent of psychiatric hospital admissions to have a history of cannabis use.

EXERCISES

6.5.1   In a study of childhood abuse in psychiatric patients, Brown and Anderson (A-13) found 166 in a sample of 947 patients reported histories of physical and/or sexual abuse. Construct a 90 percent confidence interval for the population proportion.

6.5.2   Catania et al. (A-14) obtained data regarding sexual behavior from a sample of unmarried men and women between the ages of 20 and 44 residing in geographic areas characterized by high rates of sexually transmitted diseases and admission to drug programs. Fifty percent of 1229 respondents reported that they never used a condom. Construct a 95 percent confidence interval for the population proportion never using a condom.

6.5.3   Rothberg and Lits (A-15) studied the effect on birth weight of maternal stress during pregnancy. Subjects were 86 white mothers with a history of stress who had no known medical or obstetric risk factors for reduced birth weight. The investigators found that 12.8 percent of the mothers in the study gave birth to babies satisfying the criterion for low birth weight. Construct a 99 percent confidence interval for the population proportion.

6.5.4 In a simple random sample of 125 unemployed male high school dropouts between the ages of 16 and 21, inclusive, 88 stated that they were regular consumers of alcoholic beverages. Construct a 95 percent confidence interval for the population proportion.

6.6
Confidence Interval for the Difference Between Two Population Proportions

The magnitude of the difference between two population proportions is often of interest. We may want to compare, for example, men and women, two age groups, two socioeconomic groups, or two diagnostic groups with respect to the proportion possessing some characteristic of interest. An unbiased point estimator of the difference between two population proportions is provided by the difference between sample proportions, $\hat{p}_1 - \hat{p}_2$. Since, as we have seen, n_1 and n_2 are large and the population proportions are not too close to 0 or 1, the central limit theorem applies and normal distribution theory may be employed to obtain confidence intervals. The standard error of the estimate usually must be estimated by

$$\hat{\sigma}_{\hat{p}_1 - \hat{p}_2} = \sqrt{\frac{\hat{p}_1(1 - \hat{p}_1)}{n_1} + \frac{\hat{p}_2(1 - \hat{p}_2)}{n_2}}$$

since, as a rule, the population proportions are unknown. A $100(1 - \alpha)$ percent confidence interval for $p_1 - p_2$ is given by

$$\left(\hat{p}_1 - \hat{p}_2\right) \pm z_{(1-\alpha/2)}\sqrt{\frac{\hat{p}_1(1 - \hat{p}_1)}{n_1} + \frac{\hat{p}_2(1 - \hat{p}_2)}{n_2}} \qquad (6.6.1)$$

We may interpret this interval from both the probabilistic and practical points of view.

Example 6.6.1

Borst et al. (A-16) investigated the relation of ego development, age, gender, and diagnosis to suicidality among adolescent psychiatric inpatients. Their sample consisted of 96 boys and 123 girls between the ages of 12 and 16 years selected from admissions to a child and adolescent unit of a private psychiatric hospital. Suicide attempts were reported by 18 of the boys and 60 of the girls. Let us assume that the girls behave like a simple random sample from a population of similar girls and that the boys likewise may be considered a simple random sample from a population of similar boys. For these two populations, we wish to construct a 99 percent confidence interval for the difference between the proportions of suicide attempters.

Solution: The sample proportions for the girls and boys are, respectively, $\hat{p}_G = 60/123 = .4878$ and $\hat{p}_B = 18/96 = .1875$. The difference between sample proportions is $\hat{p}_G - \hat{p}_B = .4878 - .1875 = .3003$. The estimated standard error of the difference between sample proportions is

$$s_{p_G - p_B} = \sqrt{\frac{(.4878)(.5122)}{123} + \frac{(.1875)(.8125)}{96}}$$

$$= .0602$$

The reliability factor from Table D is 2.58, so that our confidence interval, by Expression 6.6.1, is

$$.3003 \pm 2.58(.0602)$$

$$.1450, .4556$$

We are 99 percent confident that for the sampled populations, the proportion of suicide attempts among girls exceeds the proportion of suicide attempts among boys by somewhere between .1450 and .4556.

EXERCISES

6.6.1 Hartgers et al. (A-17), of the Department of Public Health and Environment in Amsterdam, conducted a study in which the subjects were injecting drug users (IDUs). In a sample of 194 long-term regular methadone (LTM) users, 145 were males. In a sample of 189 IDUs who were not LTM users, 113 were males. State the necessary assumptions about the samples and the represented populations and construct a 95 percent confidence interval for the difference between the proportions of males in the two populations.

6.6.2 Research by Lane et al. (A-18) assessed differences in breast cancer screening practices between samples of predominantly low-income women aged 50 to 75 using county-funded health centers and women in the same age group residing in the towns where the health centers are located. Of the 404 respondents selected from the community at large, 59.2 percent agreed with the following statement about breast cancer: "Women live longer if the cancer is found early." Among the 795 in the sample of health center users, 44.9 percent agreed with the statement. State the assumptions that you think are appropriate and construct a 99 percent confidence interval for the difference between the two relevant population proportions.

6.6.3 Williams et al. (A-19) surveyed a sample of 67 physicians and 133 nurses with chemical-dependent significant others. The purpose of the study was to evaluate the effect on physicians and nurses of being closely involved with one or more chemical-dependent persons. Fifty-two of the physicians and 89 of the nurses said that living with a chemical-dependent person adversely affected their work. State all assumptions that you think are necessary and construct a 95 percent confidence interval for the difference between the proportions in the two populations whose work we would expect to be adversely affected by living with a chemical-dependent person.

6.6.4 Aronow and Kronzon (A-20) identified coronary risk factors among men and women in a long-term health care facility. Of the 215 subjects who were black, 58 had diabetes mellitus. Of the 1140 white subjects, 217 had diabetes mellitus. Construct a 90 percent confidence interval for the difference between the two population proportions. What are the relevant populations? What assumptions are necessary to validate your inferential procedure?

6.7
Determination of Sample Size
for Estimating Means

The question of how large a sample to take arises early in the planning of any survey or experiment. This is an important question that should not be treated lightly. To take a larger sample than is needed to achieve the desired results is wasteful of resources, whereas very small samples often lead to results that are of no practical use. Let us consider, then, how one may go about determining the size sample that is needed in a given situation. In this section, we present a method for determining the sample size required for estimating a population mean, and in the next section we apply this method to the case of sample size determination when the parameter to be estimated is a population proportion. By straightforward extensions of these methods, sample sizes required for more complicated situations can be determined.

Objectives   The objectives in interval estimation are to obtain narrow intervals with high reliability. If we look at the components of a confidence interval, we see that the width of the interval is determined by the magnitude of the quantity

$$(\text{reliability coefficient}) \times (\text{standard error})$$

since the total width of the interval is twice this amount. We have learned that this quantity is usually called the precision of the estimate or the margin of error. For a given standard error, increasing reliability means a larger reliability coefficient. But a larger reliability coefficient for a fixed standard error makes for a wider interval.

On the other hand, if we fix the reliability coefficient, the only way to reduce the width of the interval is to reduce the standard error. Since the standard error is equal to $\sigma / \sqrt{n}$, and since σ is a constant, the only way to obtain a small standard error is to take a large sample. How large a sample? That depends on the size of σ, the population standard deviation, the desired degree of reliability, and the desired interval width.

Let us suppose we want an interval that extends d units on either side of the estimator. We can write

$$d = (\text{reliability coefficient}) \times (\text{standard error}) \qquad (6.7.1)$$

If sampling is to be with replacement, from an infinite population, or from a population that is sufficiently large to warrant our ignoring the finite population correction, Equation 6.7.1 becomes

$$d = z\frac{\sigma}{\sqrt{n}} \tag{6.7.2}$$

which, when solved for n, gives

$$n = \frac{z^2\sigma^2}{d^2} \tag{6.7.3}$$

When sampling is without replacement from a small finite population, the finite population correction is required and Equation 6.7.1 becomes

$$d = z\frac{\sigma}{\sqrt{n}}\sqrt{\frac{N-n}{N-1}} \tag{6.7.4}$$

which, when solved for n, gives

$$n = \frac{Nz^2\sigma^2}{d^2(N-1) + z^2\sigma^2} \tag{6.7.5}$$

If the finite population correction can be ignored, Equation 6.7.5 reduces to Equation 6.7.3.

Estimating σ^2   The formulas for sample size require a knowledge of σ^2 but, as has been pointed out, the population variance is, as a rule, unknown. As a result, σ^2 has to be estimated. The most frequently used sources of estimates for σ^2 are the following:

1. A *pilot* or preliminary sample may be drawn from the population and the variance computed from this sample may be used as an estimate of σ^2. Observations used in the pilot sample may be counted as part of the final sample, so that n (the computed sample size) $- n_1$ (the pilot sample size) $= n_2$ (the number of observations needed to satisfy the total sample size requirement).

2. Estimates of σ^2 may be available from previous or similar studies.

3. If it is thought that the population from which the sample is to be drawn is approximately normally distributed, one may use the fact that the range is approximately equal to 6 standard deviations and compute $\sigma \approx R/6$. This method requires some knowledge of the smallest and largest value of the variable in the population.

Example 6.7.1

A health department nutritionist, wishing to conduct a survey among a population of teenage girls to determine their average daily protein intake (measured in grams), is seeking the advice of a biostatistician relative to the size sample that should be taken.

What procedure does the biostatistician follow in providing assistance to the nutritionist? Before the statistician can be of help to the nutritionist, the latter must provide three items of information: the desired width of the confidence interval, the level of confidence desired, and the magnitude of the population variance.

Solution: Let us assume that the nutritionist would like an interval about 10 grams wide; that is, the estimate should be within about 5 grams of the population mean in either direction. In other words, a margin of error of 5 grams is desired. Let us also assume that a confidence coefficient of .95 is decided on and that, from past experience, the nutritionist feels that the population standard deviation is probably about 20 grams. The statistician now has the necessary information to compute the sample size: $z = 1.96$, $\sigma = 20$, and $d = 5$. Let us assume that the population of interest is large so that the statistician may ignore the finite population correction and use Equation 6.7.3. On making proper substitutions, the value of n is found to be

$$n = \frac{(1.96)^2 (20)^2}{(5)^2}$$

$$= 61.47$$

The nutritionist is advised to take a sample of size 62. When calculating a sample size by Equation 6.7.3 or Equation 6.7.5, we round up to the next largest whole number if the calculations yield a number that is not itself an integer.

EXERCISES

6.7.1 A hospital administrator wishes to estimate the mean weight of babies born in her hospital. How large a sample of birth records should be taken if she wants a 99 percent confidence interval that is 1 pound wide? Assume that a reasonable estimate of σ is 1 pound. What size sample is required if the confidence coefficient is lowered to .95?

6.7.2 The director of the rabies control section in a city health department wishes to draw a sample from the department's records of dog bites reported during the past year in order to estimate the mean age of persons bitten. He wants a 95 percent confidence interval, he will be satisfied to let $d = 2.5$, and from previous studies he estimates the population standard deviation to be about 15 years. How large a sample should be drawn?

6.7.3 A physician would like to know the mean fasting blood glucose value (milligrams per 100 ml) of patients seen in a diabetes clinic over the past 10 years. Determine the number of records the physician should examine in order to obtain a 90 percent confidence interval for μ if the desired width of the interval is 6 units and a pilot sample yields a variance of 60.

6.7.4 For multiple sclerosis patients we wish to estimate the mean age at which the disease was first diagnosed. We want a 95 percent confidence interval that is 10 years wide. If the population variance is 90, how large should our sample be?

6.8
Determination of Sample Size for Estimating Proportions

The method of sample size determination when a population proportion is to be estimated is essentially the same as that described for estimating a population mean. We make use of the fact that one-half the desired interval, d, may be set equal to the product of the reliability coefficient and the standard error.

Assuming random sampling and conditions warranting approximate normality of the distribution of $\hat{p}$ leads to the following formula for n when sampling is with replacement, when sampling is from an infinite population, or when the sampled population is large enough to make the use of the finite population correction unnecessary:

$$n = \frac{z^2 pq}{d^2} \tag{6.8.1}$$

where $q = 1 - p$.

If the finite population correction cannot be disregarded, the proper formula for n is

$$n = \frac{Nz^2 pq}{d^2(N - 1) + z^2 pq} \tag{6.8.2}$$

When N is large in comparison to n (that is, $n/N \leq .05$) the finite population correction may be ignored, and Equation 6.8.2 reduces to Equation 6.8.1.

Estimating p As we see, both formulas require a knowledge of p, the proportion in the population possessing the characteristic of interest. Since this is the parameter we are trying to estimate, it, obviously, will be unknown. One solution to this problem is to take a pilot sample and compute an estimate to be used in place of p in the formula for n. Sometimes an investigator will have some notion of an upper bound for p that can be used in the formula. For example, if it is desired to estimate the proportion of some population who have a certain condition, we may feel that the true proportion cannot be greater than, say, .30.

We then substitute .30 for p in the formula for n. If it is impossible to come up with a better estimate, one may set p equal to .5 and solve for n. Since $p = .5$ in the formula yields the maximum value of n, this procedure will give a large enough sample for the desired reliability and interval width. It may, however, be larger than needed and result in a more expensive sample than if a better estimate of p had been available. This procedure should be used only if one is unable to come up with a better estimate of p.

Example 6.8.1

A survey is being planned to determine what proportion of families in a certain area are medically indigent. It is believed that the proportion cannot be greater than .35. A 95 percent confidence interval is desired with $d = .05$. What size sample of families should be selected?

Solution: If the finite population correction can be ignored, we have

$$n = \frac{(1.96)^2(.35)(.65)}{(.05)^2} = 349.6$$

The necessary sample size, then, is 350.

EXERCISES

6.8.1 An epidemiologist wishes to know what proportion of adults living in a large metropolitan area have subtype ay hepatitis B virus. Determine the size sample that would be required to estimate the true proportion to within .03 with 95 percent confidence. In a similar metropolitan area the proportion of adults with the characteristic is reported to be .20. If data from another metropolitan area were not available and a pilot sample could not be drawn, what size sample would be required?

6.8.2 A survey is planned to determine what proportion of the high school students in a metropolitan school system have regularly smoked marijuana. If no estimate of p is available from previous studies, a pilot sample cannot be drawn, a confidence coefficient of .95 is desired, and $d = .04$ is to be used, determine the appropriate sample size. What size sample would be required if 99 percent confidence were desired?

6.8.3 A hospital administrator wishes to know what proportion of discharged patients are unhappy with the care received during hospitalization. How large a sample should be drawn if we let $d = .05$, the confidence coefficient is .95, and no other information is available? How large should the sample be if p is approximated by .25?

6.8.4 A health planning agency wishes to know, for a certain geographic region, what proportion of patients admitted to hospitals for the treatment of trauma are discharged dead. A 95 percent confidence interval is desired, the width of the interval must be .06, and the population proportion, from other evidence, is estimated to be .20. How large a sample is needed?

6.9
Confidence Interval for the Variance
of a Normally Distributed Population

Point Estimation of the Population Variance   In previous sections it has been suggested that when a population variance is unknown, the sample variance may be used as an estimator. You may have wondered about the quality of this estimator. We have discussed only one criterion of goodness—unbiasedness—so let us see if the sample variance is an unbiased estimator of the population variance. To be unbiased, the average value of the sample variance over all possible samples must be equal to the population variance. That is, the expression $E(s^2) = \sigma^2$ must hold. To see if this condition holds for a particular situation, let us refer to the example of constructing a sampling distribution given in Section 5.3. In Table 5.3.1 we have all possible samples of size 2 from the population consisting of the values 6, 8, 10, 12, and 14. It will be recalled that two measures of dispersion for this population were computed as follows:

$$\sigma^2 = \frac{\sum (x_i - \mu)^2}{N} = 8 \quad \text{and} \quad S^2 = \frac{\sum (x_i - \mu)^2}{N - 1} = 10$$

If we compute the sample variance $s^2 = \sum(x_i - \bar{x})^2/(n - 1)$ for each of the possible samples shown in Table 5.3.1, we obtain the sample variances shown in Table 6.9.1.

Sampling with Replacement   If sampling is with replacement, the expected value of s^2 is obtained by taking the mean of all sample variances in Table 6.9.1. When we do this, we have

$$E(s^2) = \frac{\sum s_i^2}{N^n} = \frac{0 + 2 + \cdots + 2 + 0}{25} = \frac{200}{25} = 8$$

and we see, for example, that when sampling is with replacement $E(s^2) = \sigma^2$, where $s^2 = \sum(x_i - \bar{x})^2/(n - 1)$ and $\sigma^2 = \sum(x_i - \mu)^2/N$.

TABLE 6.9.1 Variances Computed From Samples Shown in Table 5.3.1

		\multicolumn{5}{c}{Second Draw}				
		6	**8**	**10**	**12**	**14**
	6	0	2	8	18	32
	8	2	0	2	8	18
First draw	10	8	2	0	2	8
	12	18	8	2	0	2
	14	32	18	8	2	0

Sampling Without Replacement If we consider the case where sampling is without replacement, the expected value of s^2 is obtained by taking the mean of all variances above (or below) the principal diagonal. That is,

$$E(s^2) = \frac{\sum s_i^2}{_N C_n} = \frac{2 + 8 + \cdots + 2}{10} = \frac{100}{10} = 10$$

which, we see, is not equal to σ^2, but is equal to $S^2 = \sum(x_i - \mu)^2/(N - 1)$.

These results are examples of general principles, as it can be shown that, in general,

$$E(s^2) = \sigma^2 \text{ when sampling is with replacement}$$

$$E(s^2) = S^2 \text{ when sampling is without replacement}$$

When N is large, $N - 1$ and N will be approximately equal and, consequently, σ^2 and S^2 will be approximately equal.

These results justify our use of $s^2 = \sum(x_i - \bar{x})^2/(n - 1)$ when computing the sample variance. In passing, let us note that although s^2 is an unbiased estimator of σ^2, s is not an unbiased estimator of σ. The bias, however, diminishes rapidly as n increases. Those interested in pursuing this point further are referred to the articles by Cureton (18), and Gurland and Tripathi (19).

Interval Estimation of a Population Variance With a point estimate available to us, it is logical to inquire about the construction of a confidence interval for a population variance. Whether we are successful in constructing a confidence interval for σ^2 will depend on our ability to find an appropriate sampling distribution.

The Chi-Square Distribution Confidence intervals for σ^2 are usually based on the sampling distribution of $(n - 1)s^2/\sigma^2$. If samples of size n are drawn from a normally distributed population, this quantity has a distribution known as the *chi-square distribution* with $n - 1$ degrees of freedom. As we will say more about this distribution in a later chapter, we only say here that it is the distribution that the quantity $(n - 1)s^2/\sigma^2$ follows and that it is useful in finding confidence intervals for σ^2 when the assumption that the population is normally distributed holds true.

In Figure 6.9.1 are shown some chi-square distributions for several values of degrees of freedom. Percentiles of the chi-square distribution, designated by the Greek letter χ^2, are given in Table F. The column headings give the values of χ^2 to the left of which lies a proportion of the total area under the curve equal to the subscript of χ^2. The row labels are the degrees of freedom.

To obtain a $100(1 - \alpha)$ percent confidence interval for σ^2, we first obtain the $100(1 - \alpha)$ percent confidence interval for $(n - 1)s^2/\sigma^2$. To do this, we select the values of χ^2 from Table F in such a way that $\alpha/2$ is to the left of the smaller value and $\alpha/2$ is to the right of the larger value. In other words, the two values of χ^2 are selected in such a way that α is divided equally between the two tails of the

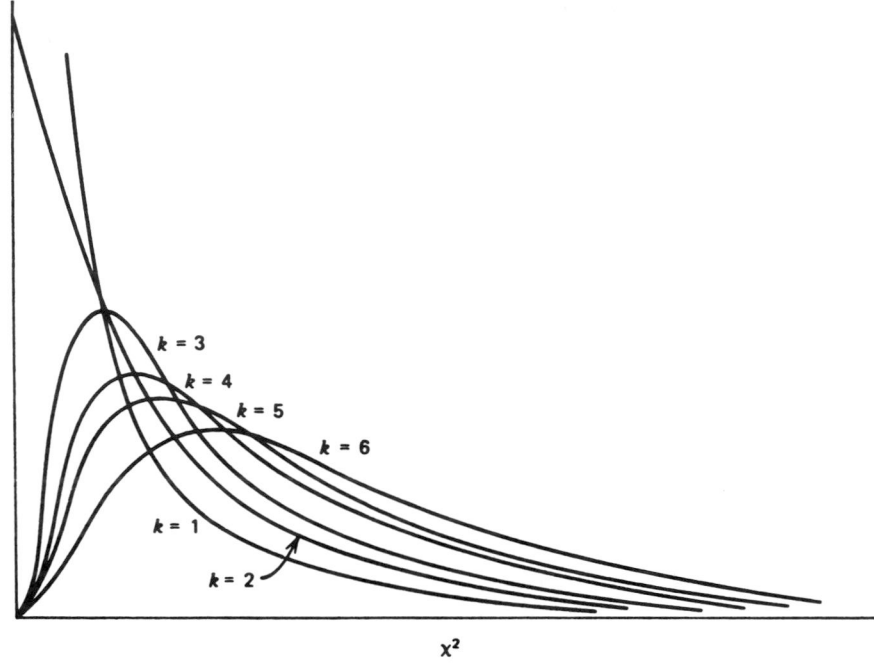

Figure 6.9.1 Chi-square distributions for several values of degrees of freedom k. (*Source:* Paul G. Hoel and Raymond J. Jessen, *Basic Statistics for Business and Economics*, Wiley, 1971. Used by permission.)

distribution. We may designate these two values of χ^2 as $\chi^2_{\alpha/2}$ and $\chi^2_{1-(\alpha/2)}$, respectively. The $100(1 - \alpha)$ percent confidence interval for $(n - 1)s^2/\sigma^2$, then, is given by

$$\chi^2_{\alpha/2} < \frac{(n - 1)s^2}{\sigma^2} < \chi^2_{1-(\alpha/2)}$$

We now manipulate this expression in such a way that we obtain an expression with σ^2 alone as the middle term. First, let us divide each term by $(n - 1)s^2$ to get

$$\frac{\chi^2_{\alpha/2}}{(n - 1)s^2} < \frac{1}{\sigma^2} < \frac{\chi^2_{1-(\alpha/2)}}{(n - 1)s^2}$$

If we take the reciprocal of this expression we have

$$\frac{(n - 1)s^2}{\chi^2_{\alpha/2}} > \sigma^2 > \frac{(n - 1)s^2}{\chi^2_{1-(\alpha/2)}}$$

Note that the direction of the inequalities changed when we took the reciprocals. If we reverse the order of the terms we have

$$\frac{(n-1)s^2}{\chi^2_{1-(\alpha/2)}} < \sigma^2 < \frac{(n-1)s^2}{\chi^2_{\alpha/2}} \tag{6.9.1}$$

which is the $100(1-\alpha)$ percent confidence interval for σ^2. If we take the square root of each term in Expression 6.9.1, we have the following $100(1-\alpha)$ percent confidence interval for σ, the population standard deviation:

$$\sqrt{\frac{(n-1)s^2}{\chi^2_{1-(\alpha/2)}}} < \sigma < \sqrt{\frac{(n-1)s^2}{\chi^2_{\alpha/2}}} \tag{6.9.2}$$

Example 6.9.1

In a study of the effect of diet on low-density lipoprotein cholesterol, Rassias et al. (A-21) used as subjects 12 mildly hypercholesterolemic men and women. The plasma cholesterol levels (mmol/l) of the subjects were as follows: 6.0, 6.4, 7.0, 5.8, 6.0, 5.8, 5.9, 6.7, 6.1, 6.5, 6.3, 5.8. Let us assume that these 12 subjects behave as a simple random sample of subjects from a normally distributed population of similar subjects. We wish to estimate, from the data of this sample, the variance of the plasma cholesterol levels in the population with a 95 percent confidence interval.

Solution: The sample yielded a value of $s^2 = .391868$. The degrees of freedom are $n - 1 = 11$. The appropriate values of χ^2 from Table F are $\chi^2_{1-(\alpha/2)} = 21.920$ and $\chi^2_{\alpha/2} = 3.1816$. Our 95 percent confidence interval for σ^2 is

$$\frac{11(.391868)}{21.920} < \sigma^2 < \frac{11(.391868)}{3.1816}$$

$$.196649087 < \sigma^2 < 1.35483656$$

The 95 percent confidence interval for σ is

$$.4434 < \sigma < 1.1640$$

We say we are 95 percent confident that the parameters being estimated are within the specified limits, because we know that in the long run, in repeated sampling, 95 percent of intervals constructed as illustrated would include the respective parameters.

Some Precautions   Although this method of constructing confidence intervals for σ^2 is widely used, it is not without its drawbacks. First, the assumption of the normality of the population from which the sample is drawn is crucial, and results may be misleading if the assumption is ignored.

Another difficulty with these intervals results from the fact that the estimator is not in the center of the confidence interval, as is the case with the confidence interval for μ. This is because the chi-square distribution, unlike the normal, is not symmetric. The practical implication of this is that the method for the construction of confidence intervals for σ^2, which has just been described, does not yield the shortest possible confidence intervals. Tate and Klett (20) give tables that may be used to overcome this difficulty.

EXERCISES

6.9.1 The objectives of a study by Kennedy and Bhambhani (A-22) were to use physiological measurements to determine the test–retest reliability of the Baltimore Therapeutic Equipment Work Simulator during three simulated tasks performed at light, medium, and heavy work intensities, and to examine the criterion validity of these tasks by comparing them to real tasks performed in a controlled laboratory setting. Subjects were 30 healthy men between the ages of 18 and 35. The investigators reported a standard deviation of .57 for the variable peak oxygen consumption (l/min) during one of the procedures. Describe the population about which data from this sample may be used to make inferences. Construct a 95 percent confidence interval for the population variance for the oxygen consumption variable.

6.9.2 Kubic et al. (A-23) evaluated the hematologic parameters of 11 patients with documented *Bordetella pertussis* infection. The subjects consisted of 11 infected children aged one month to 4.5 years. The white blood cell (WBC) counts ($\times 10^9$/l) for the subjects were 20.2, 15.4, 8.4, 29.8, 40.9, 19.7, 49.5, 12.1, 32.0, 72.9, 13.5. (*Source*: Virginia L. Kubic, Paul T. Kubic, and Richard D. Brunning, "The Morphologic and Immunophenotypic Assessment of the Lymphocytosis Accompanying *Bordetella pertussis* Infection," *American Journal of Clinical Pathology*, *95* (1991), 809–815.) Describe the population about which these data might be used to make inferences. Construct a 90 percent confidence interval for the variance of the WBC counts for this population.

6.9.3 Forced vital capacity determinations were made on 20 healthy adult males. The sample variance was 1,000,000. Construct 90 percent confidence intervals for σ^2 and σ.

6.9.4 In a study of myocardial transit times, appearance transit times were obtained on a sample of 30 patients with coronary artery disease. The sample variance was found to be 1.03. Construct 99 percent confidence intervals for σ^2 and σ.

6.9.5 A sample of 25 physically and mentally healthy males participated in a sleep experiment in which the percentage of each participant's total sleeping time spent in a certain stage of sleep was recorded. The variance computed from the sample data was 2.25. Construct 95 percent confidence intervals for σ^2 and σ.

6.9.6 Hemoglobin determinations were made on 16 animals exposed to a harmful chemical. The following observations were recorded: 15.6, 14.8, 14.4, 16.6, 13.8, 14.0, 17.3,

17.4, 18.6, 16.2, 14.7, 15.7, 16.4, 13.9, 14.8, 17.5. Construct 95 percent confidence intervals for σ^2 and σ.

6.9.7 Twenty air samples taken at the same site over a period of 6 months showed the following amounts of suspended particulate matter (micrograms per cubic meter of air).

68	22	36	32
42	24	28	38
30	44	28	27
28	43	45	50
79	74	57	21

Consider these measurements to be a random sample from a population of normally distributed measurements, and construct a 95 percent confidence interval for the population variance.

6.10
Confidence Interval for the Ratio of the Variances of Two Normally Distributed Populations

It is frequently of interest to compare two variances, and one way to do this is to form their ratio, σ_1^2/σ_2^2. If two variances are equal, their ratio will be equal to 1. We usually will not know the variances of populations of interest, and, consequently, any comparisons we make will have to be based on sample variances. In other words, we may wish to estimate the ratio of two population variances. Again, since this is a form of inference, we must rely on some sampling distribution, and this time the distribution of $(s_1^2/\sigma_1^2)/(s_2^2/\sigma_2^2)$ is utilized provided certain assumptions are met. The assumptions are that s_1^2 and s_2^2 are computed from independent samples of size n_1 and n_2, respectively, drawn from two normally distributed populations. We use s_1^2 to designate the larger of the two sample variances.

The F Distribution If the assumptions are met $(s_1^2/\sigma_1^2)/(s_2^2/\sigma_2^2)$ follows a distribution known as the F *distribution*. We defer a more complete discussion of this distribution until a later chapter, but note that this distribution depends on two-degrees-of-freedom values, one corresponding to the value of $n_1 - 1$ used in computing s_1^2 and the other corresponding to the value of $n_2 - 1$ used in computing s_2^2. These are usually referred to as the *numerator degrees of freedom* and the *denominator degrees of freedom*. Figure 6.10.1 shows some F distributions for several numerator and denominator degrees-of-freedom combinations. Table G contains, for specified combinations of degrees of freedom and values of α, F values to the right of which lies $\alpha/2$ of the area under the curve of F.

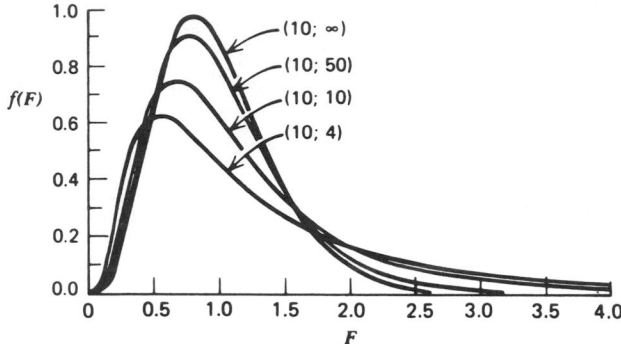

Figure 6.10.1   The F distribution for various degrees of freedom. (From *Documenta Geigy, Scientific Tables*, Seventh Edition, 1970. Courtesy of Ciba-Geigy Limited, Basel, Switzerland.)

A Confidence Interval for σ_1^2/σ_2^2   To find the $100(1-\alpha)$ percent confidence interval for σ_1^2/σ_2^2, we begin with the expression

$$F_{\alpha/2} < \frac{s_1^2/\sigma_1^2}{s_2^2/\sigma_2^2} < F_{1-(\alpha/2)}$$

where $F_{\alpha/2}$ and $F_{1-(\alpha/2)}$ are the values from the F table to the left and right of which, respectively, lies $\alpha/2$ of the area under the curve. The middle term of this expression may be rewritten so that the entire expression is

$$F_{\alpha/2} < \frac{s_1^2}{s_2^2} \cdot \frac{\sigma_2^2}{\sigma_1^2} < F_{1-(\alpha/2)}$$

If we divide through by s_1^2/s_2^2, we have

$$\frac{F_{\alpha/2}}{s_1^2/s_2^2} < \frac{\sigma_2^2}{\sigma_1^2} < \frac{F_{1-(\alpha/2)}}{s_1^2/s_2^2}$$

Taking the reciprocals of the three terms gives

$$\frac{s_1^2/s_2^2}{F_{\alpha/2}} > \frac{\sigma_1^2}{\sigma_2^2} > \frac{s_1^2/s_2^2}{F_{1-(\alpha/2)}}$$

and if we reverse the order we have the following $100(1-\alpha)$ percent confidence interval for σ_1^2/σ_2^2:

$$\frac{s_1^2/s_2^2}{F_{1-(\alpha/2)}} < \frac{\sigma_1^2}{\sigma_2^2} < \frac{s_1^2/s_2^2}{F_{\alpha/2}} \tag{6.10.1}$$

**Example
6.10.1**

Goldberg et al. (A-24) conducted a study to determine if an acute dose of dextroamphetamine might have positive effects on affect and cognition in schizophrenic patients maintained on a regimen of haloperidol. Among the variables measured was the change in patients' tension–anxiety states. For $n_2 = 4$ patients who responded to amphetamine, the standard deviation for this measurement was 3.4. For $n_1 = 11$ patients who did not respond, the standard deviation was 5.8. Let us assume that these patients constitute independent simple random samples from populations of similar patients. Let us also assume that change scores in tension–anxiety state is a normally distributed variable in both populations. We wish to construct a 95 percent confidence interval for the ratio of the variances of these two populations.

Solution: We have the following information:

$$n_1 = 11 \qquad n_2 = 4$$

$$s_1^2 = (5.8)^2 = 33.64 \qquad s_2^2 = (3.4)^2 = 11.56$$

$$df_1 = \text{numerator degrees of freedom} = 10$$

$$df_2 = \text{denominator degrees of freedom} = 3$$

$$\alpha = .05$$

$$F_{.025} = .20704 \qquad F_{.975} = 14.42$$

We are now ready to obtain our 95 percent confidence interval for σ_1^2/σ_2^2 by substituting appropriate values into Expression 6.10.1:

$$\frac{33.64/11.56}{14.42} < \frac{\sigma_1^2}{\sigma_2^2} < \frac{33.64/11.56}{.20704}$$

$$.2018 < \frac{\sigma_1^2}{\sigma_2^2} < 14.0554$$

We give this interval the appropriate probabilistic and practical interpretations.

Finding $F_{1-(\alpha/2)}$ and $F_{\alpha/2}$ At this point we must make a cumbersome, but unavoidable, digression and explain how the values $F_{.975} = 14.42$ and $F_{.025} = .20704$ were obtained. The value of $F_{.975}$ at the intersection of the column headed $df_1 = 10$ and the row labeled $df_2 = 3$ is 14.42. If we had a more extensive table of the F distribution, finding $F_{.025}$ would be no trouble; we would simply find $F_{.025}$ as we found $F_{.975}$. We would take the value at the intersection of the column headed 10 and the row headed 3. To include every possible percentile of F would make for a very lengthy table. Fortunately, however, there exists a relationship that enables us to compute the lower percentile values from our limited table. The relationship is as follows:

$$F_{1-\alpha, df_1, df_2} = \frac{1}{F_{\alpha, df_2, df_1}} \qquad (6.10.2)$$

We proceed as follows.

Interchange the numerator and denominator degrees of freedom and locate the appropriate value of F. For the problem at hand we locate 4.83, which is at the intersection of the column headed 3 and the row labeled 10. We now take the reciprocal of this value, $1/4.83 = .20704$. In summary, the lower confidence limit (LCL) and upper confidence limit (UCL) for σ_1^2/σ_2^2 are as follows:

$$\text{LCL} = \frac{s_1^2}{s_2^2} \frac{1}{F_{\alpha/2, df_1, df_2}} \qquad (6.10.3)$$

$$\text{UCL} = \frac{s_1^2}{s_2^2} \frac{1}{1/F_{1-(\alpha/2), df_1, df_2}} \qquad (6.10.4)$$

Alternative procedures for making inferences about the equality of two variances when the sampled populations are not normally distributed may be found in the book by Daniel (21).

EXERCISES

6.10.1 The objective of a study by Hahn et al. (A-25) was to determine whether breath-alcohol testing was a reliable method to monitor irrigant absorption during prostatectomy in patients suffering from chronic obstructive pulmonary disease (COPD). Subjects were $n_1 = 7$ patients suffering from severe COPD and $n_2 = 7$ control patients with essentially normal pulmonary function. One of the variables measured was weight (kg). The weights of the control subjects were 74, 82, 94, 90, 98, 97, and 84. The weights of the COPD subjects were 81, 58, 93, 58, 51, 96, and 67. Let us assume that these samples constitute independent simple random samples from two populations of similar patients—those with severe COPD and those with essentially normal pulmonary function. Assume also that the weights of the subjects in these populations are normally distributed. Construct a 95 percent confidence interval for the ratio of the two population variances.

6.10.2 The objective of a study by Southwick et al. (A-26) was to better characterize the affective component of posttraumatic stress disorder (PTSD). The subjects were male psychiatric inpatients at a Veterans Administration medical center. Twenty-eight of the subjects met the criteria for PTSD and were veterans of the Vietnam conflict. The remaining 17 suffered from major depressive disorder. The 21-item Hamilton Rating Scale for Depression was used to assess state measures of symptom severity in the 45 subjects. The standard deviation of the total scores for the

PTSD patients was 9.90, and for the patients with major depressive disorder the standard deviation was 6.30. State the necessary assumptions about the samples and the populations about which the sample data may be used to make inferences. Construct a 99 percent confidence interval for the ratio of the two population variances for the Hamilton Rating Scale for Depression scores.

6.10.3 Stroke index values were statistically analyzed for two samples of patients suffering from myocardial infarction. The sample variances were 12 and 10. There were 21 patients in each sample. Construct the 95 percent confidence interval for the ratio of the two population variances.

6.10.1 Thirty-two adult aphasics seeking speech therapy were divided equally into two groups. Group 1 received treatment 1, and group 2 received treatment 2. Statistical analysis of the treatment effectiveness scores yielded the following variances: $s_1^2 = 8$, $s_2^2 = 15$. Construct the 90 percent confidence interval for σ_2^2/σ_1^2.

6.10.5 Sample variances were computed for the tidal volumes (milliliters) of two groups of patients suffering from atrial septal defect. The results and sample sizes were as follows:

$$n_1 = 31, \quad s_1^2 = 35{,}000$$

$$n_2 = 41, \quad s_2^2 = 20{,}000$$

Construct the 95 percent confidence interval for the ratio of the two population variances.

6.10.6 Glucose responses to oral glucose were recorded for 11 patients with Huntington's disease (group 1) and 13 control subjects (group 2). Statistical analysis of the results yielded the following sample variances: $s_1^2 = 105$, $s_2^2 = 148$. Construct the 95 percent confidence interval for the ratio of the two population variances.

6.10.7 Measurements of gastric secretion of hydrochloric acid (milliequivalents per hour) in 16 normal subjects and 10 subjects with duodenal ulcer yielded the following results:

Normal subjects: 6.3, 2.0, 2.3, 0.5, 1.9, 3.2, 4.1, 4.0, 6.2, 6.1, 3.5, 1.3, 1.7, 4.5, 6.3, 6.2

Ulcer subjects: 13.7, 20.6, 15.9, 28.4, 29.4, 18.4, 21.1, 3.0, 26.2, 13.0

Construct a 95 percent confidence interval for the ratio of the two population variances. What assumptions must be met for this procedure to be valid?

6.11
Summary

This chapter is concerned with one of the major areas of statistical inference—estimation. Both point and interval estimation are covered. The concepts and methods involved in the construction of confidence intervals are illustrated for the following parameters: means, the difference between two means, proportions, the difference between two proportions, variances, and the ratio of two variances. In addition, we learned in this chapter how to determine the sample size needed to estimate a population mean and a population proportion at specified levels of precision.

We learned, also, in this chapter that interval estimates of population parameters are more desirable than point estimates because statements of confidence can be attached to interval estimates.

REVIEW QUESTIONS AND EXERCISES

1. What is statistical inference?

2. Why is estimation an important type of inference?

3. What is a point estimate?

4. Explain the meaning of unbiasedness.

5. Define the following:
   a. Reliability coefficient
   b. Confidence coefficient
   c. Precision
   d. Standard error
   e. Estimator
   f. Margin of error

6. Give the general formula for a confidence interval.

7. State the probabilistic and practical interpretations of a confidence interval.

8. Of what use is the central limit theorem in estimation?

9. Describe the t distribution.

10. What are the assumptions underlying the use of the t distribution in estimating a single population mean?

11. What is the finite population correction? When can it be ignored?

12. What are the assumptions underlying the use of the t distribution in estimating the difference between two population means?

13. Arterial blood gas analyses performed on a sample of 15 physically active adult males yielded the following resting PaO_2 values:

    75, 80, 80, 74, 84, 78, 89, 72, 83, 76, 75, 87, 78, 79, 88

    Compute the 95 percent confidence interval for the mean of the population.

14. What proportion of asthma patients are allergic to house dust? In a sample of 140, 35 percent had positive skin reactions. Construct the 95 percent confidence interval for the population proportion.

15. An industrial hygiene survey was conducted in a large metropolitan area. Of 70 manufacturing plants of a certain type visited, 21 received a "poor" rating with respect to absence of safety hazards. Construct a 95 percent confidence interval for the population proportion deserving a "poor" rating.

16. Refer to the previous problem. How large a sample would be required to estimate the population proportion to within .05 with 95 percent confidence (.30 is the best available estimate of p):

    a. If the finite population correction can be ignored?

    b. If the finite population correction is not ignored and $N = 1500$?

17. In a dental survey conducted by a county dental health team, 500 adults were asked to give the reason for their last visit to a dentist. Of the 220 who had less than a high school education, 44 said they went for preventive reasons. Of the remaining 280, who had a high school education or better, 150 stated that they went for preventive reasons. Construct a 95 percent confidence interval for the difference between the two population proportions.

18. A breast cancer research team collected the following data on tumor size:

Type of Tumor	n	$\bar{x}$	s
A	21	3.85 cm	1.95 cm
B	16	2.80 cm	1.70 cm

Construct a 95 percent confidence interval for the difference between population means.

19. A certain drug was found to be effective in the treatment of pulmonary disease in 180 of 200 cases treated. Construct the 90 percent confidence interval for the population proportion.

20. Seventy patients with stasis ulcers of the leg were randomly divided into two equal groups. Each group received a different treatment for edema. At the end of the experiment, treatment effectiveness was measured in terms of reduction in leg volume as determined by water displacement. The means and standard deviations for the two groups were as follows:

Group (Treatment)	$\bar{x}$	s
A	95 cc	25
B	125 cc	30

Construct a 95 percent confidence interval for the difference in population means.

21. What is the average serum bilirubin level of patients admitted to a hospital for treatment of hepatitis? A sample of 10 patients yielded the following results:

$$20.5, \ 14.8, \ 21.3, \ 12.7, \ 15.2, \ 26.6, \ 23.4, \ 22.9, \ 15.7, \ 19.2$$

Construct a 95 percent confidence interval for the population mean.

22. Determinations of saliva pH levels were made in two independent random samples of seventh grade schoolchildren. Sample A children were caries-free while sample B children had a high incidence of caries. The results were as follows:

    A: 7.14, 7.11, 7.61, 7.98, 7.21, 7.16, 7.89
          7.24, 7.86, 7.47, 7.82, 7.37, 7.66, 7.62, 7.65
    B: 7.36, 7.04, 7.19, 7.41, 7.10, 7.15, 7.36,
          7.57, 7.64, 7.00, 7.25, 7.19

    Construct a 90 percent confidence interval for the difference between the population means. Assume that the population variances are equal.

23. Drug A was prescribed for a random sample of 12 patients complaining of insomnia. An independent random sample of 16 patients with the same complaint received drug B. The numbers of hours of sleep experienced during the second night after treatment began were as follows:

    A: 3.5, 5.7, 3.4, 6.9, 17.8, 3.8, 3.0, 6.4, 6.8, 3.6, 6.9, 5.7
    B: 4.5, 11.7, 10.8, 4.5, 6.3, 3.8, 6.2, 6.6, 7.1, 6.4, 4.5,
          5.1, 3.2, 4.7, 4.5, 3.0

    Construct a 95 percent confidence interval for the difference between the population means. Assume that the population variances are equal.

24. Milliez et al. (A-27) conducted a study involving high-risk pregnancies. A sample of 23 nulliparous women delivered babies whose mean weight was 2958 grams with a standard deviation of 620. The mean and standard deviation of the weights of babies born to a sample of 26 multiparous women were 3085 and 704, respectively. State the necessary assumptions about the samples and the populations about which the sample data may be used to make inferences and construct a 95 percent confidence interval for the difference between the mean birth weights for the two populations.

25. The objective of a study by Martin et al. (A-28) was to compare the function of neutrophils in the pulmonary artery blood and lung lavage fluid of patients early in the course of adult respiratory distress syndrome. Of concern were three antibacterial functions: the release of reactive oxygen species, microbiocidal activity for a target organism, *Staphylococcus aureus*, and chemotaxis. For 18 of the subjects in the study the mean bronchoalveolar lavage fluid pH was 7.39 with a standard deviation of .39. Construct a 90 percent confidence interval for the population mean pH. State the assumptions necessary to make your procedure valid.

26. Harrison et al. (A-29) conducted a study of dependent elderly people in a London borough. Along with other characteristics, they collected data on the extent of depression among borough residents. In a sample of 158 subjects who had a previous diagnosis of depression, 48 were rated during the survey as having depression. In a sample of 745 subjects with no previous diagnosis of depression, 311 were rated by the survey as having depression. Construct a 99 percent confidence interval for the difference between population proportions. State the assumptions that make your procedure valid.

27. The purpose of a study by Thurnau et al. (A-30) was to evaluate the accuracy of the fetal–pelvic index disproportion and delivery outcome in gravid women attempting

vaginal birth after previous cesarean delivery. Among the data reported were the following on birth weight (grams):

Delivery Outcome	*n*	Mean	Standard Deviation
Cesarean delivery	18	3486	393
Vaginal delivery	47	3325	514

Construct a 95 percent confidence interval for the difference in population means. State the assumptions that make your procedure valid.

28. In a study of the role of dietary fats in the etiology of ischemic heart disease the subjects were 60 males between 40 and 60 years of age who had recently had a myocardial infarction and 50 apparently healthy males from the same age group and social class. One variable of interest in the study was the proportion of linoleic acid (L.A.) in the subjects' plasma triglyceride fatty acids. The data on this variable were as follows:

Subjects with Myocardial Infarction

Subject	L.A.	Subject	L.A.	Subject	L.A.	Subject	L.A.
1	18.0	2	17.6	3	9.6	4	5.5
5	16.8	6	12.9	7	14.0	8	8.0
9	8.9	10	15.0	11	9.3	12	5.8
13	8.3	14	4.8	15	6.9	16	18.3
17	24.0	18	16.8	19	12.1	20	12.9
21	16.9	22	15.1	23	6.1	24	16.6
25	8.7	26	15.6	27	12.3	28	14.9
29	16.9	30	5.7	31	14.3	32	14.1
33	14.1	34	15.1	35	10.6	36	13.6
37	16.4	38	10.7	39	18.1	40	14.3
41	6.9	42	6.5	43	17.7	44	13.4
45	15.6	46	10.9	47	13.0	48	10.6
49	7.9	50	2.8	51	15.2	52	22.3
53	9.7	54	15.2	55	10.1	56	11.5
57	15.4	58	17.8	59	12.6	60	7.2

Healthy Subjects

Subject	L.A.	Subject	L.A.	Subject	L.A.	Subject	L.A.
1	17.1	2	22.9	3	10.4	4	30.9
5	32.7	6	9.1	7	20.1	8	19.2
9	18.9	10	20.3	11	35.6	12	17.2
13	5.8	14	15.2	15	22.2	16	21.2
17	19.3	18	25.6	19	42.4	20	5.9
21	29.6	22	18.2	23	21.7	24	29.7
25	12.4	26	15.4	27	21.7	28	19.3
29	16.4	30	23.1	31	19.0	32	12.9
33	18.5	34	27.6	35	25.0	36	20.0
37	51.7	38	20.5	39	25.9	40	24.6
41	22.4	42	27.1	43	11.1	44	32.7
45	13.2	46	22.1	47	13.5	48	5.3
49	29.0	50	20.2				

Construct the 95 percent confidence interval for the difference between population means. What do these data suggest about the levels of linoleic acid in the two sampled populations?

29. Osberg et al. (A-31) conducted a study to identify factors that predict whether or not similarly impaired children treated at trauma centers are discharged to inpatient rehabilitation. Among other findings by the investigators were the following: In a sample of 115 subjects discharged from a trauma center to rehabilitation, 98.3 percent had head injuries; 68.5 percent of 200 subjects discharged to home had head injuries. Construct a 95 percent confidence interval for the difference between population proportions. State the assumptions that make your procedure valid.

30. The objectives of a study by Steinhardt et al. (A-32) were (1) to determine if level of physical activity and cardiovascular fitness were significantly related to absenteeism and medical care claims among law enforcement officers over a one-year period and (2) to determine if moderate levels of physical activity and fitness were inversely associated with reduced absenteeism and medical care claims. Subjects for the study were law enforcement officers in the city of Austin, Texas. Among other findings, the investigators reported that 65 subjects whose physical activity level was categorized as sedentary were absent, on the average, 10.04 days per year with a standard deviation of 9.65. The mean and standard deviation for 275 subjects who were physically active three times per week were 6.04 and 6.59, respectively. Construct a 95 percent confidence interval for the difference in population means. State the assumptions that make your procedure valid. What do you conclude from your findings?

31. In general, narrow confidence intervals are preferred over wide ones. We can make an interval narrow by using a small confidence coefficient. For a given set of other conditions, what happens to the level of confidence when we use a small confidence coefficient? What would happen to the interval width and the level of confidence if we were to use a confidence coefficient of zero?

32. In general, a high level of confidence is preferred over a low level of confidence. For a given set of other conditions, suppose we set our level of confidence at 100 percent. What would be the effect of such a choice on the width of the interval?

33. el Fiky et al. (A-33) measured shunt fraction invasively using a pulmonary artery catheter in 22 patients undergoing elective coronary artery surgery. From the results, the investigators computed a mean of 19.6 and constructed a 90 percent confidence interval for the population mean with endpoints of 18.8 and 20.4. Which would be the appropriate reliability factor for the interval, z or t? Justify your choice. What is the precision of the estimate? The margin of error?

34. Duncan et al. (A-34) report on a study designed to assess the relation of exclusive breastfeeding, independent of recognized risk factors, to acute and recurrent otitis media in the first 12 months of life. The subjects were 1220 infants who used a health maintenance organization. What was the target population? The sampled population?

35. The purpose of a study by Kay et al. (A-35) was to determine the safety and efficacy of radiofrequency ablation as definitive therapy for primary atrial tachycardias. Subjects were 15 consecutive patients with primary atrial arrhythmias that were refractory to medical management. The authors conclude that radiofrequency catheter ablation appears to be a safe and effective technique for the treatment of primary atrial arrhythmias that are refractory to antiarrhythmic medications. What was the target population? The sampled population?

36. Bellomo et al. (A-36) conducted a study to quantitate insulin losses and glucose absorption during acute continuous hemofiltration with dialysis and to assess the clinical importance of these changes. Subjects were 16 ICU patients with acute renal failure at a university medical center. The authors conclude that significant glucose absorption occurs during acute continuous hemofiltration with dialysis and is coupled with minor insulin losses through the filter. What was the target population? The sampled population? As part of their analysis, the authors constructed confidence intervals for several means. Based on the information given here, what is the appropriate numerical value of the reliability factor for the intervals?

Exercises for Use with Large Data Sets Available on Computer Disk from the Publisher

1. Refer to the serum cholesterol levels for 1000 subjects (CHOLEST, Disk 1). Select a simple random sample of size 15 from this population and construct a 95 percent confidence interval for the population mean. Compare your results with those of your classmates. What assumptions are necessary for your estimation procedure to be valid?

2. Refer to the serum cholesterol levels for 1000 subjects (CHOLEST, Disk 1). Select a simple random sample of size 50 from the population and construct a 95 percent confidence interval for the proportion of subjects in the population who have readings greater than 225. Compare your results with those of your classmates.

3. Refer to the weights of 1200 babies born in a community hospital (BABYWGTS, Disk 1). Draw a simple random sample of size 20 from this population and construct a 95 percent confidence interval for the population mean. Compare your results with those of your classmates. What assumptions are necessary for your estimation procedure to be valid?

4. Refer to the weights of 1200 babies born in a community hospital (BABYWGTS, Disk 1). Draw a simple random sample of size 35 from the population and construct a 95 percent confidence interval for the population mean. Compare this interval with the one constructed in Exercise 3.

5. Refer to the heights of 1000 twelve-year-old boys (BOYHGTS, Disk 1). Select a simple random sample of size 15 from this population and construct a 99 percent confidence interval for the population mean. What assumptions are necessary for this procedure to be valid?

6. Refer to the heights of 1000 twelve-year-old boys (BOYHGTS, Disk 1). Select a simple random sample of size 35 from the population and construct a 99 percent confidence interval for the population mean. Compare this interval with the one constructed in Exercise 5.

REFERENCES

References Cited

1. John E. Freund and Ronald E. Walpole, *Mathematical Statistics*, Third Edition, Prentice-Hall, Englewood Cliffs, N.J., 1980.

2. Alexander M. Mood, Franklin A. Graybill, and Duane C. Boes, *Introduction to the Theory of Statistics*, Third Edition, McGraw-Hill, New York, 1974.

3. Taro Yamane, *Statistics: An Introductory Analysis*, Second Edition, Harper & Row, New York, 1967.

4. John A. Rice, *Mathematical Statistics and Data Analysis*, Wadsworth & Brooks Cole, Pacific Grove, Calif., 1988.

5. W. S. Gosset ("Student"), "The Probable Error of a Mean," *Biometrika, 6* (1908), 1–25.

6. W. V. Behrens, "Ein Beitrag zu Fehlerberechnung bei wenige Beobachtungen," *Landwirtsschaftliche Jahrbücher, 68* (1929), 807–837.

7. R. A. Fisher, "The Comparison of Samples with Possibly Unequal Variances," *Annals of Eugenics, 9* (1939), 174–180.

8. R. A. Fisher, "The Asymptotic Approach to Behrens' Integral with Further Tables for the *d* Test of Significance," *Annals of Eugenics, 11* (1941), 141–172.

9. J. Neyman, "Fiducial Argument and the Theory of Confidence Intervals," *Biometrika, 32* (1941), 128–150.

10. H. Scheffé, "On Solutions of the Behrens-Fisher Problem Based on the *t*-Distribution," *The Annals of Mathematical Statistics, 14* (1943), 35–44.

11. H. Scheffé, "A Note on the Behrens-Fisher Problem," *The Annals of Mathematical Statistics, 15* (1944), 430–432.

12. B. L. Welch, "The Significance of the Difference Between Two Means When The Population Variances Are Unequal," *Biometrika, 29* (1937), 350–361.

13. B. L. Welch, "The Generalization of 'Student's' Problem When Several Different Population Variances Are Involved," *Biometrika, 34* (1947), 28–35.

14. Alice A. Aspin, "Tables for Use in Comparisons Whose Accuracy Involves Two Variances *s*, Separately Estimated," *Biometrika, 36* (1949), 290–296.

15. W. H. Trickett, B. L. Welch, and G. S. James, "Further Critical Values for the Two-Means Problem," *Biometrika, 43* (1956), 203–205.

16. William G. Cochran, "Approximate Significance Levels of the Behrens-Fisher Test," *Biometrics, 20* (1964), 191–195.

17. George W. Snedecor and William G. Cochran, *Statistical Methods*, Sixth Edition, The Iowa State University Press, Ames, 1967.

18. Edward E. Cureton, "Unbiased Estimation of the Standard Deviation," *The American Statistician, 22* (February 1968), 22.

19. John Gurland and Ran C. Tripathi, "A Simple Approximation for Unbiased Estimation of the Standard Deviation," *The American Statistician, 25* (October 1971), 30–32.

20. R. F. Tate and G. W. Klett, "Optimal Confidence Intervals for the Variance of a Normal Distribution," *Journal of the American Statistical Association, 54* (1959), 674–682.

21. Wayne W. Daniel, *Applied Nonparametric Statistics*, Second Edition, PWS-Kent, Boston, 1989.

Other References

1. H. A. Al-Bayyati, "A Rule of Thumb for Determining a Sample Size in Comparing Two Proportions," *Technometrics, 13* (1971), 675–677.

2. Jacob Cohen, *Statistical Power Analysis for the Behavioral Sciences*, Second Edition, Erlbaum, Hillsdale, N.J., 1988.

3. Armand J. Galfo, "Teaching Degrees of Freedom as a Concept in Inferential Statistics: An Elementary Approach," *School Science and Mathematics, 85* (1985), 240–247.

4. Helena Chmura Kraemer and Sue Thiemann, *How Many Subjects? Statistical Power Analysis in Research*, Sage, Newbury, Calif., 1987.

5. F. F. Ractliffe, "The Effect on the *t* Distribution of Nonnormality in the Sampled Population," *Applied Statistics, 17* (1968), 42–48.

Applications References

A-1. Maureen McCauley, "The Effect of Body Mechanics Instruction on Work Performance Among Young Workers," *The American Journal of Occupational Therapy, 44* (May 1990), 402–407. Copyright 1990 by the American Occupational Therapy Association, Inc. Reprinted with permission.

A-2. C. Tantucci, C. Corbeil, M. Chassé, J. Braidy, N. Matar, and J. Milic-Emili, "Flow Resistance in Patients with Chronic Obstructive Pulmonary Disease in Acute Respiratory Failure," *American Review of Respiratory Disease*, *144* (1991), 384–389.

A-3. Ricardo V. Lloyd and Joe Mailloux, "Analysis of S-100 Protein Positive Folliculo-Stellate Cells in Rat Pituitary Tissues," *American Journal of Pathology*, *133* (1988), 338–346.

A-4. Krzysztof Kaminski and Tomasz Rechberger, "Concentration of Digoxin-like Immunoreactive Substance in Patients With Preeclampsia and Its Relation to Severity of Pregnancy-induced Hypertension," *American Journal of Obstetrics and Gynecology*, *165* (1991), 733–736.

A-5. Jack M. Gorman, Robert Kertzner, Thomas Cooper, Raymond R. Goetz, Isabel Lagomasino, Hana Novacenko, Janet B. W. Williams, Yaakov Stern, Richard Mayeux, and Anke A. Ehrhardt, "Glucocorticoid Level and Neuropsychiatric Symptoms in Homosexual Men With HIV Positive Infection," *American Journal of Psychiatry*, *148* (1991), 41–45.

A-6. William J. Stone, Debra E. Rothstein, and Cynthia L. Shoenhair, "Coronary Health Disease Risk Factors and Health Related Fitness in Long-Term Exercising Versus Sedentary Corporate Executives," *American Journal of Health Promotion*, *5*, (1991), 169–173.

A-7. Phillip S. Buckner, David A. Todd, Kei Lui, and Elizabeth John, "Effect of Short-term Muscle Relaxation on Neonatal Plasma Volume," *Critical Care Medicine*, *19* (1991), 1357–1361. © Williams & Wilkins (1991).

A-8. Peter F. Zucker and Michael C. Archer, "Alterations in Pancreatic Islet Function Produced By Carcinogenic Nitrosamines in the Syrian Hamster," *American Journal of Pathology*, *133* (1988), 573–577.

A-9. Barbara L. Davies, Louise Matte-Lewis, Annette M. O'Connor, Corinne S. Dulberg, and Elizabeth R. Drake, "Evaluation of the 'Time to Quit' Self-Help Smoking Cessation Program," *Canadian Journal of Public Health*, *83* (1992), 19–23.

A-10. Ali A. Khraibi, "Direct Renal Interstitial Volume Expansion Causes Exaggerated Natriuresis in SHR," *American Journal of Physiology*, *30* (October 1991), F567–F570.

A-11. J. Scott Osberg and Carla Di Scala, "Morbidity Among Pediatric Motor Vehicle Crash Victims: The Effectiveness of Seat Belts," *American Journal of Public Health*, *82* (1992), 422–425.

A-12. D. C. Mathers, A. H. Ghodse, A. W. Caan, and S. A. Scott, "Cannabis Use in a Large Sample of Acute Psychiatric Admissions," *British Journal of Addiction*, *86* (1991), 779–784. © 1993, Society for the Study of Addiction to Alcohol and Other Drugs.

A-13. George R. Brown and Bradley Anderson, "Psychiatric Morbidity in Adult Inpatients With Childhood Histories of Sexual and Physical Abuse," *American Journal of Psychiatry*, *148* (1991), 55–61.

A-14. Joseph A. Catania, Thomas J. Coates, Susan Kegeles, Mindy Thompson Fullilove, John Peterson, Barbara Marin, David Siegel, and Stephen Hulley, "Condom Use in Multi-Ethnic Neighborhoods of San Francisco: The Population-Based AMEN (AIDS in Multi-Ethnic Neighborhoods) Study," *American Journal of Public Health*, *82* (1992), 284–287.

A-15. Alan D. Rothberg and Bernice Lits, "Psychosocial Support for Maternal Stress During Pregnancy: Effect on Birth Weight," *American Journal of Obstetrics and Gynecology*, *165* (1991), 403–407.

A-16. Sophie R. Borst, Gil G. Noam, and John A. Bartok, "Adolescent Suicidality: A Clinical-Development Approach," *Journal of the American Academy of Child and Adolescent Psychiatry*, *30* (1991), 796–803. © by Am. Acad. of Child & Adol. Psychiatry.

A-17. Christina Hartgers, Anneke (J. A. R.) van den Hoek, Pieta Krijnen, and Roel A. Coutinho, "HIV Prevalence and Risk Behavior Among Injecting Drug Users Who Participate in 'Low-Threshold' Methadone Programs in Amsterdam," *American Journal of Public Health*, *82* (1992), 547–551.

A-18. Dorothy S. Lane, Anthony P. Polednak, and Mary Ann Burg, "Breast Cancer Screening Practices Among Users of County-Funded Health Centers vs Women in the Entire Community," *American Journal of Public Health*, *82* (1992), 199–203.

A-19. Etta Williams, Leclair Bissell, and Eleanor Sullivan, "The Effects of Co-dependence on Physicians and Nurses," *British Journal of Addiction*, *86* (1991), 37–42. © 1993, Society for the Study of Addiction to Alcohol and Other Drugs.

A-20. Wilbert Aronow and Itzhak Kronzon, "Prevalence of Coronary Risk Factors in Elderly Blacks and Whites," *Journal of the American Geriatrics Society, 39* (1991), 567–570. © American Geriatrics Society.

A-21. Georgina Rassias, Mark Kestin, and Paul J. Nestel, "Linoleic Acid Lowers LDL Cholesterol Without a Proportionate Displacement of Saturated Fatty Acid," *European Journal of Clinical Nutrition, 45* (1991), 315–320.

A-22. Lorian E. Kennedy and Yagesh N. Bhambhani, "The Baltimore Therapeutic Equipment Work Simulator: Reliability and Validity at Three Work Intensities," *Archives of Physical Medicine and Rehabilitation, 72* (1991), 511–516.

A-23. Virginia L. Kubic, Paul T. Kubic, and Richard D. Brunning, "The Morphologic and Immunophenotypic Assessment of the Lymphocytosis Accompanying *Bordetella pertussis* Infection," *American Journal of Clinical Pathology, 95* (1991), 809–815.

A-24. Terry E. Goldberg, Llewellyn B. Bigelow, Daniel R. Weinberger, David G. Daniel, and Joel E. Kleinman, "Cognitive and Behavioral Effects of the Coadministration of Dextroamphetamine and Haloperidol in Schizophrenia," *American Journal of Psychiatry, 148* (1991), 78–84.

A-25. R. G. Hahn, A. W. Jones, B. Billing, and H. P. Stalberg, "Expired-Breath Ethanol Measurement in Chronic Obstructive Pulmonary Disease: Implications for Transurethral Surgery," *Acta Anaesthesiologica Scandinavica, 35* (1991), 393–397. © Munkagaard International Publishers Ltd., Copenhagen, Denmark.

A-26. Steven M. Southwick, Rachel Yehuda, and Earl L. Giller, Jr., "Characterization of Depression in War-Related Posttraumatic Stress Disorder," *American Journal of Psychiatry, 148* (1991), 179–183.

A-27. Jacques M. Milliez, Denis Jannet, Claudine Touboul, Mahfoudh El Medjadji, and Bernard J. Paniel, "Maturation of the Uterine Cervix by Repeated Intracervical Instillation of Prostaglandin E_2," *American Journal of Obstetrics and Gynecology, 165* (1991), 523–528.

A-28. Thomas R. Martin, Brent P. Pistorese, Leonard D. Hudson, and Richard J. Maunder, "The Function of Lung and Blood Neutrophils in Patients with the Adult Respiratory Distress Syndrome," *American Review of Respiratory Disease, 144* (1991), 254–262.

A-29. Robert Harrison, Navin Savla, and Kalman Kafetz, "Dementia, Depression and Physical Disability in a London Borough: A Survey of Elderly People in and out of Residential Care and Implications for Future Developments," *Age and Ageing, 19* (1990), 97–103. Used by permission of Oxford University Press.

A-30. Gary R. Thurnau, David H. Scates, and Mark A. Morgan, "The Fetal-pelvic Index: A Method of Identifying Fetal-pelvic Disproportion in Women Attempting Vaginal Birth After Previous Cesarean Delivery," *American Journal of Obstetrics and Gynecology, 165* (1991), 353–358.

A-31. J. Scott Osberg, Carla DiScala, and Bruce M. Gans, "Utilization of Inpatient Rehabilitation Services Among Traumatically Injured Children Discharged from Pediatric Trauma Centers," *American Journal of Physical Medicine & Rehabilitation, 69* (1990), 67–72.

A-32. Mary Steinhardt, Linda Greenhow, and Joy Stewart, "The Relationship of Physical Activity and Cardiovascular Fitness to Absenteeism and Medical Care Claims Among Law Enforcement Officers," *American Journal of Health Promotion, 5* (1991), 455–460.

A-33. M. M. el Fiky, D. P. Taggart, R. Carter, M. C. Stockwell, B. H. Maule, and D. J. Wheatley, "Respiratory Dysfunction Following Cardiopulmonary Bypass: Verification of a Non-invasive Technique to Measure Shunt Fraction," *Respiratory Medicine, 87* (April 1993), 193–198.

A-34. B. Duncan, J. Ey, C. J. Holberg, A. L. Wright, F. D. Martinez, and L. M. Taussig, "Exclusive Breast-feeding for at Least 4 Months Protects Against Otitis Media," *Pediatrics, 91* (May 1993), 867–872.

A-35. G. N. Kay, F. Chong, A. E. Epstein, S. M. Dailey, and V. J. Plumb, "Radiofrequency Ablation for Treatment of Primary Atrial Tachycardias," *Journal of the American College of Cardiology, 21* (March 15, 1993), 901–909.

A-36. R. Bellomo, P. G Colman, J. Caudwell, and N. Boyce, "Acute Continuous Hemofiltration With Dialysis: Effect on Insulin Concentrations and Glycemic Control in Critically Ill Patients," *Critical Care Medicine, 20* (December 1992), 1672–1676.

Hypothesis Testing

• •

CONTENTS

7.1
Introduction

One type of statistical inference, estimation, is discussed in the preceding chapter. The other type, hypothesis testing, is the subject of this chapter. As is true with estimation, the *purpose of hypothesis testing is to aid the clinician, researcher, or administrator in reaching a conclusion concerning a population by examining a sample from that population*. Estimation and hypothesis testing are not as different as they are made to appear by the fact that most textbooks devote a separate chapter to each. As we will explain later, one may use confidence intervals to arrive at the same conclusions that are reached by using the hypothesis testing procedures discussed in this chapter.

Basic Concepts   In this section some of the basic concepts essential to an understanding of hypothesis testing are presented. The specific details of particular tests will be given in succeeding sections.

DEFINITION

A *hypothesis* may be defined simply as *a statement about one or more populations*.

The hypothesis is frequently concerned with the parameters of the populations about which the statement is made. A hospital administrator may hypothesize that the average length of stay of patients admitted to the hospital is five days; a public health nurse may hypothesize that a particular educational program will result in improved communication between nurse and patient; a physician may hypothesize that a certain drug will be effective in 90 percent of the cases with which it is used. By means of hypothesis testing one determines whether or not such statements are compatible with available data.

Types of Hypotheses   Researchers are concerned with two types of hypotheses—*research hypotheses* and *statistical hypotheses*.

DEFINITION

The research hypothesis is the conjecture or supposition that motivates the research.

It may be the result of years of observation on the part of the researcher. A public health nurse, for example, may have noted that certain clients responded more readily to a particular type of health education program. A physician may recall numerous instances in which certain combinations of therapeutic measures were more effective than any one of them alone. Research projects often result from the desire of such health practitioners to determine whether or not their theories or suspicions can be supported when subjected to the rigors of scientific investigation.

Research hypotheses lead directly to statistical hypotheses.

DEFINITION

Statistical hypotheses are hypotheses that are stated in such a way that they may be evaluated by appropriate statistical techniques.

In this book the hypotheses that we will focus on are statistical hypotheses. We will assume that the research hypotheses for the examples and exercises have already been considered.

Hypothesis Testing Steps For convenience, hypothesis testing will be presented as a nine-step procedure. There is nothing magical or sacred about this particular format. It merely breaks the process down into a logical sequence of actions and decisions.

1. *Data* The nature of the data that form the basis of the testing procedures must be understood, since this determines the particular test to be employed. Whether the data consist of counts or measurements, for example, must be determined.

2. *Assumptions* As we learned in the chapter on estimation, different assumptions lead to modifications of confidence intervals. The same is true in hypothesis testing: A general procedure is modified depending on the assumptions. In fact, the same assumptions that are of importance in estimation are important in hypothesis testing. We have seen that these include, among others, assumptions about the normality of the population distribution, equality of variances, and independence of samples.

3. *Hypotheses* There are two statistical hypotheses involved in hypothesis testing, and these should be explicitly stated. The *null hypothesis* is the *hypothesis to be tested*. It is designated by the symbol H_0. The null hypothesis is sometimes referred to as a *hypothesis of no difference*, since it is a statement of agreement with (or no difference from) conditions presumed to be true in the population of interest. In general, the null hypothesis is set up for the express purpose of being discredited. Consequently, the complement of the conclusion that the researcher is seeking to reach becomes the statement of the null hypothesis. In the testing process the null hypothesis either is rejected or is not rejected. If the null hypothesis is not rejected, we will say that the data on which the test is based do not provide sufficient evidence to cause rejection. If the testing procedure leads to rejection, we will say that the data at hand are not compatible with the null hypothesis, but are supportive of some other hypothesis. The *alternative hypothesis* is a statement of what we will believe is true if our sample data causes us to reject the null hypothesis. Usually the alternative hypothesis and the research hypothesis are the same, and in fact the two terms are used interchangeably. We shall designate the alternative hypothesis by the symbol H_A.

Rules for Stating Statistical Hypotheses When hypotheses are of the type considered in this chapter an indication of equality (either $=$, $\leq$, or $\geq$) must appear in the null hypothesis. Suppose, for example, that we want to answer the question: Can we conclude that a certain population mean is not 50? The null hypothesis is

$$H_0: \mu = 50$$

and the alternative is

$$H_A: \mu \neq 50$$

Suppose we want to know if we can conclude that the population mean is greater than 50. Our hypotheses are

$$H_0: \mu \leq 50 \qquad H_A: \mu > 50$$

If we want to know if we can conclude that the population mean is less than 50, the hypotheses are

$$H_0: \mu \geq 50 \qquad H_A: \mu < 50$$

In summary, we may state the following rules of thumb for deciding what statement goes in the null hypothesis and what statement goes in the alternative hypothesis:

a. What you hope or expect to be able to conclude as a result of the test usually should be placed in the alternative hypothesis.

b. The null hypothesis should contain a statement of equality, either $=$, $\leq$, or $\geq$.

c. The null hypothesis is the hypothesis that is tested.

d. The null and alternative hypotheses are complementary. That is, the two together exhaust all possibilities regarding the value that the hypothesized parameter can assume.

A Precaution   It should be pointed out that neither hypothesis testing nor statistical inference, in general, leads to the proof of a hypothesis; it merely indicates whether the hypothesis is supported or is not supported by the available data. When we fail to reject a null hypothesis, therefore, we do not say that it is true, but that it may be true. When we speak of accepting a null hypothesis, we have this limitation in mind and do not wish to convey the idea that accepting implies proof.

4. *Test Statistic*   The test statistic is some statistic that may be computed from the data of the sample. As a rule, there are many possible values that the test statistic may assume, the particular value observed depending on the particular sample drawn. As we will see, the test statistic serves as a decision maker, since the decision to reject or not to reject the null hypothesis depends on the magnitude of the test statistic. An example of a test statistic is the quantity

$$z = \frac{\bar{x} - \mu_0}{\sigma/\sqrt{n}} \qquad (7.1.1)$$

where μ_0 is a hypothesized value of a population mean. This test statistic is related to the statistic

$$z = \frac{\bar{x} - \mu}{\sigma/\sqrt{n}} \qquad (7.1.2)$$

with which we are already familiar.

General Formula for Test Statistic The following is a general formula for a test statistic that will be applicable in many of the hypothesis tests discussed in this book:

$$\text{test statistic} = \frac{\text{relevant statistic} - \text{hypothesized parameter}}{\text{standard error of the relevant statistic}}$$

In Equation 7.1.1, $\bar{x}$ is the relevant statistic, μ_0 is the hypothesized parameter, and $\sigma/\sqrt{n}$ is the standard error of $\bar{x}$, the relevant statistic.

5. *Distribution of the Test Statistic* It has been pointed out that the key to statistical inference is the sampling distribution. We are reminded of this again when it becomes necessary to specify the probability distribution of the test statistic. The distribution of the test statistic

$$z = \frac{\bar{x} - \mu_0}{\sigma/\sqrt{n}}$$

for example, follows the standard normal distribution if the null hypothesis is true and the assumptions are met.

6. *Decision Rule* All possible values that the test statistic can assume are points on the horizontal axis of the graph of the distribution of the test statistic and are divided into two groups; one group constitutes what is known as the *rejection region* and the other group makes up the *nonrejection region*. The values of the test statistic forming the rejection region are those values that are less likely to occur if the null hypothesis is true, while the values making up the acceptance region are more likely to occur if the null hypothesis is true. *The decision rule tells us to reject the null hypothesis if the value of the test statistic that we compute from our sample is one of the values in the rejection region and to not reject the null hypothesis if the computed value of the test statistic is one of the values in the nonrejection region.*

Significance Level The decision as to which values go into the rejection region and which ones go into the nonrejection region is made on the basis of the desired *level of significance*, designated by α. The term *level of significance* reflects the fact that hypothesis tests are sometimes called significance tests, and a computed value of the test statistic that falls in the rejection region is said to be *significant*. The level of significance, α, specifies the area under the curve of the distribution of the test statistic that is above the values on the horizontal axis constituting the rejection region.

DEFINITION

The level of significance α is a probability and, in fact, is the *probability of rejecting a true null hypothesis.*

Since to reject a true null hypothesis would constitute an error, it seems only reasonable that we should make the probability of rejecting a true null hypothesis small and, in fact, that is what is done. We select a small value of α in order to make the probability of rejecting a true null hypothesis small. The more frequently encountered values of α are .01, .05, and .10.

Types of Errors   The error committed when a true null hypothesis is rejected is called the *type I error*. The *type II error* is the error committed when a false null hypothesis is not rejected. The probability of committing a type II error is designated by β.

Whenever we reject a null hypothesis there is always the concomitant risk of committing a type I error, rejecting a true null hypothesis. Whenever we fail to reject a null hypothesis the risk of failing to reject a false null hypothesis is always present. We make α small, but we generally exercise no control over β, although we know that in most practical situations it is larger than α.

We never know whether we have committed one of these errors when we reject or fail to reject a null hypothesis, since the true state of affairs is unknown. If the testing procedure leads to rejection of the null hypothesis, we can take comfort from the fact that we made α small and, therefore, the probability of committing a type I error was small. If we fail to reject the null hypothesis, we do not know the concurrent risk of committing a type II error, since β is usually unknown but, as has been pointed out, we do know that, in most practical situations, it is larger than α.

Figure 7.1.1 shows for various conditions of a hypothesis test the possible actions that an investigator may take and the conditions under which each of the two types of error will be made.

7. *Calculation of the Test Statistic*   From the data contained in the sample we compute a value of the test statistic and compare it with the rejection and nonrejection regions that have already been specified.

8. *Statistical Decision*   The statistical decision consists of rejecting or of not rejecting the null hypothesis. It is rejected if the computed value of the test statistic falls in the rejection region, and it is not rejected if the computed value of the test statistic falls in the nonrejection region.

9. *Conclusion*   If H_0 is rejected, we conclude that H_A is true. If H_0 is not rejected, we conclude that H_0 may be true.

CONDITION OF NULL HYPOTHESIS

		True	False
Possible Action	Fail to reject H_0	Correct action	Type II error
	Reject H_0	Type I error	Correct action

Figure 7.1.1 Conditions under which type I and type II errors may be committed.

We emphasize that when the null hypothesis is not rejected one should not say that the null hypothesis is accepted. We should say that the null hypothesis is "not rejected." We avoid using the word "accept" in this case because we may have committed a type II error. Since, frequently, the probability of committing a type II error can be quite high, we do not wish to commit ourselves to accepting the null hypothesis.

Figure 7.1.2 is a flowchart of the steps that we follow when we perform a hypothesis test.

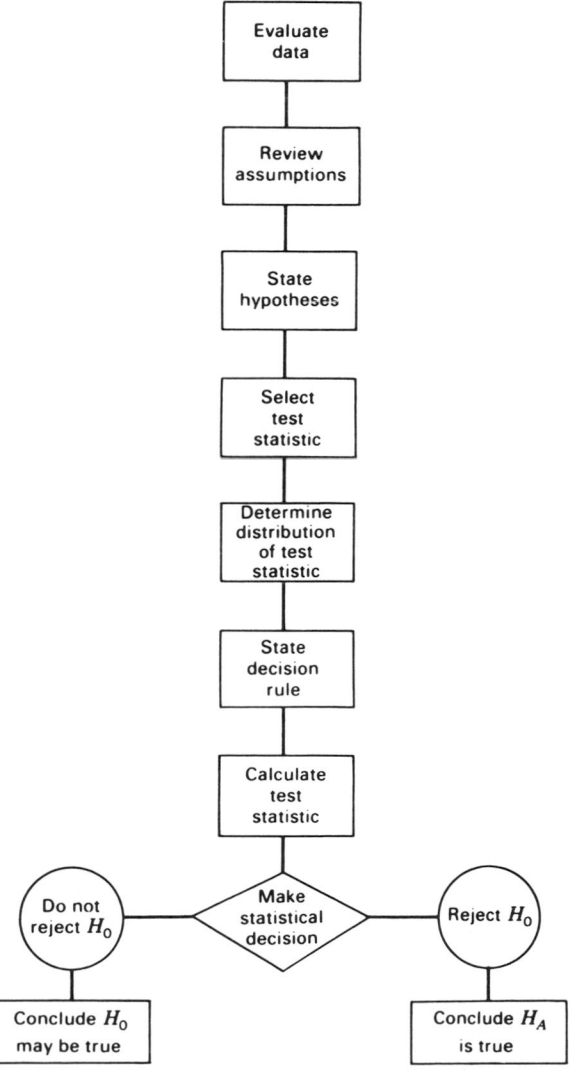

Figure 7.1.2 Steps in the hypothesis testing procedure.

Purpose of Hypothesis Testing   The purpose of hypothesis testing is to assist administrators and clinicians in making decisions. The administrative or clinical decision usually depends on the statistical decision. If the null hypothesis is rejected, the administrative or clinical decision usually reflects this, in that the decision is compatible with the alternative hypothesis. The reverse is usually true if the null hypothesis is not rejected. The administrative or clinical decision, however, may take other forms, such as a decision to gather more data.

We must emphasize at this point, however, that the outcome of the statistical test is only one piece of evidence that influences the administrative or clinical decision. The statistical decision should not be interpreted as definitive, but should be considered along with all the other relevant information available to the experimenter.

With these general comments as background, we now discuss specific hypothesis tests.

7.2
Hypothesis Testing: A Single Population Mean

In this section we consider the testing of a hypothesis about a population mean under three different conditions: (1) when sampling is from a normally distributed population of values with known variance, (2) when sampling is from a normally distributed population with unknown variance, and (3) when sampling is from a population that is not normally distributed. Although the theory for conditions 1 and 2 depends on normally distributed populations, it is common practice to make use of the theory when relevant populations are only approximately normally distributed. This is satisfactory as long as the departure from normality is not drastic. When sampling is from a normally distributed population and the population variance is known, the test statistic for testing H_0: $\mu = \mu_0$ is

$$z = \frac{\bar{x} - \mu_0}{\sigma/\sqrt{n}} \qquad (7.2.1)$$

which, when H_0 is true, is distributed as the standard normal. Examples 7.2.1 and 7.2.2 illustrate hypothesis testing under these conditions.

Sampling from Normally Distributed Populations: Population Variances Known   As we did in Chapter 6, we again emphasize that situations in which the variable of interest is normally distributed with a known variance are rare. The following example, however, will serve to illustrate the procedure.

Example 7.2.1   Researchers are interested in the mean age of a certain population. Let us say that they are asking the following question: Can we conclude that the mean age of this population is different from 30 years?

Solution: Based on our knowledge of hypothesis testing, we reply that they can conclude that the mean age is different from 30 if they can reject the null hypothesis that the mean is equal to 30. Let us use the nine-step hypothesis testing procedure given in the previous section to help the researchers reach a conclusion.

1. *Data* The data available to the researchers are the ages of a simple random sample of 10 individuals drawn from the population of interest. From this sample a mean of $\bar{x} = 27$ has been computed.

2. *Assumptions* It is assumed that the sample comes from a population whose ages are approximately normally distributed. Let us also assume that the population has a known variance of $\sigma^2 = 20$.

3. *Hypotheses* The hypothesis to be tested, or null hypothesis, is that the mean age of the population is equal to 30. The alternative hypothesis is that the mean age of the population is not equal to 30. Notice that we are identifying with the alternative hypothesis the conclusion the researchers wish to reach, so that if the data permit rejection of the null hypothesis, the researchers' conclusion will carry more weight, since the accompanying probability of rejecting a true null hypothesis will be small. We will make sure of this by assigning a small value to α, the probability of committing a type I error. We may present the relevant hypotheses in compact form as follows:

$$H_0: \mu = 30$$

$$H_A: \mu \neq 30$$

4. *Test Statistic* Since we are testing a hypothesis about a population mean, since we assume that the population is normally distributed, and since the population variance is known, our test statistic is give by Equation 7.2.1.

5. *Distribution of Test Statistic* Based on our knowledge of sampling distributions and the normal distribution, we know that the test statistic is normally distributed with a mean of 0 and a variance of 1, if H_0 is true. There are many possible values of the test statistic that the present situation can generate; one for every possible sample of size 10 that can be drawn from the population. Since we draw only one sample, we have only one of these possible values on which to base a decision.

6. *Decision Rule* The decision rule tells us to reject H_0 if the computed value of the test statistic falls in the rejection region and to fail to reject H_0 if it falls in the nonrejection region. We must now specify the rejection and nonrejection regions. We can begin by asking ourselves what magnitude of values of the test statistic will cause rejection of H_0. If the null hypothesis is false, it may be so either because the population mean is less than 30 or because the population mean is greater than 30. Therefore, either sufficiently small values or sufficiently large values of the test statistic will cause rejection of the null hypothesis. These extreme values we want to constitute the rejection region. How extreme must a possible value of the test statistic be to qualify for the

rejection region? The answer depends on the significance level we choose, that is, the size of the probability of committing a type I error. Let us say that we want the probability of rejecting a true null hypothesis to be $\alpha = .05$. Since our rejection region is to consist of two parts, sufficiently small values and sufficiently large values of the test statistic, part of α will have to be associated with the large values and part with the small values. It seems reasonable that we should divide α equally and let $\alpha/2 = .025$ be associated with small values and $\alpha/2 = .025$ be associated with large values.

Critical Value of Test Statistic   What value of the test statistic is so large that, when the null hypothesis is true, the probability of obtaining a value this large or larger is .025? In other words, what is the value of z to the right of which lies .025 of the area under the standard normal distribution? The value of z to the right of which lies .025 of the area is the same value that has .975 of the area between it and $-\infty$. We look in the body of Table D until we find .975 or its closest value and read the corresponding marginal entries to obtain our z value. In the present example the value of z is 1.96. Similar reasoning will lead us to find -1.96 as the value of the test statistic so small that when the null hypothesis is true, the probability of obtaining a value this small or smaller is .025. Our rejection region, then, consists of all values of the test statistic equal to or greater than 1.96 or less than or equal to -1.96. The nonrejection region consists of all values in between. We may state the decision rule for this test as follows: *Reject H_0 if the computed value of the test statistic is either ≥ 1.96 or ≤ -1.96.* Otherwise, do not reject H_0. The rejection and nonrejection regions are shown in Figure 7.2.1. The values of the test statistic that separate the rejection and nonrejection regions are called *critical values* of the test statistic, and the rejection region is sometimes referred to as the *critical region*.

The decision rule tells us to compute a value of the test statistic from the data of our sample and to reject H_0 if we get a value that is either equal to or greater than 1.96 or equal to or less than -1.96 and to fail to reject H_0 if we get any other value. The value of α and, hence, the decision rule should be decided on before

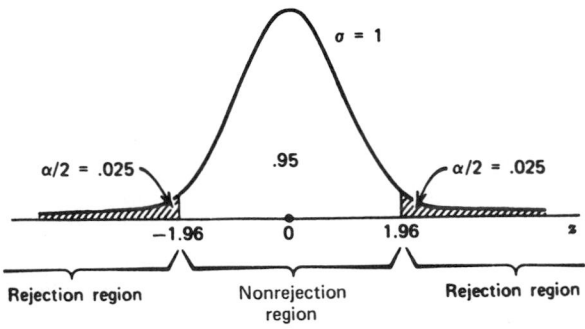

Figure 7.2.1 Rejection and nonrejection regions for Example 7.2.1.

gathering the data. This prevents our being accused of allowing the sample results to influence our choice of α. This condition of objectivity is highly desirable and should be preserved in all tests.

7. *Calculation of Test Statistic*   From our sample we compute

$$z = \frac{27 - 30}{\sqrt{20/10}} = \frac{-3}{1.4142} = -2.12$$

8. *Statistical Decision*   Abiding by the decision rule, we are able to reject the null hypothesis since -2.12 is in the rejection region. We can say that the computed value of the test statistic is significant at the .05 level.

9. *Conclusion*   We conclude that μ is not equal to 30 and let our administrative or clinical actions be in accordance with this conclusion.

---

p **Values**   Instead of saying that an observed value of the test statistic is significant or is not significant, most writers in the research literature prefer to report the exact probability of getting a value as extreme as or more extreme than that observed if the null hypothesis is true. In the present instance these writers would give the computed value of the test statistic along with the statement $p = .0340$. The statement $p = .0340$ means that the probability of getting a value as extreme as 2.12 in either direction, when the null hypothesis is true, is .0340. The value .0340 is obtained from Table D and is the probability of observing a $z \geq 2.12$ or a $z \leq -2.12$ when the null hypothesis is true. That is, when H_0 is true, the probability of obtaining a value of z as large as or larger than 2.12 is .0170, and the probability of observing a value of z as small as or smaller than -2.12 is .0170. The probability of one or the other of these events occurring, when H_0 is true, is equal to the sum of the two individual probabilities, and hence, in the present example, we say that $p = .0170 + .0170 = .0340$. The quantity p is referred to as the *p value* for the test.

DEFINITION

The *p* value for a hypothesis test is the probability of obtaining, when H_0 is true, a value of the test statistic as extreme as or more extreme (in the appropriate direction) than the one actually computed.

The *p* value for a test may be defined also as the smallest value of α for which the null hypothesis can be rejected. Since in Example 7.2.1, our *p* value is .0340, we know that we could have chosen an α value as small as .0340 and still have rejected the null hypothesis. If we had chosen an α smaller than .0340, we would not have been able to reject the null hypothesis. A general rule worth remembering then is this: *If the p value is less than or equal to α, we reject the null hypothesis. If the p value is greater than α, we do not reject the null hypothesis.*

The reporting of p values as part of the results of an investigation is more informative to the reader than such statements as "the null hypothesis is rejected at the .05 level of significance" or "the results were not significant at the .05 level." Reporting the p value associated with a test lets the reader know just how common or how rare is the computed value of the test statistic given that H_0 is true. Gibbons and Pratt (1), Bahn (2), and Daniel (3) may be consulted for a more extensive treatment of the subject of p values. Also of interest is a paper by Morgan and Morgan (4).

Testing H_0 by Means of a Confidence Interval   Earlier we stated that one can use confidence intervals to test hypotheses. In Example 7.2.1 we used a hypothesis testing procedure to test H_0: $\mu = 30$ against the alternative, H_A: $\mu \neq 30$. We were able to reject H_0 because the computed value of the test statistic fell in the rejection region.

Let us see how we might have arrived at this same conclusion by using a $100(1 - \alpha)$ percent confidence interval. The 95 percent confidence interval for μ is

$$27 \pm 1.96\sqrt{20/10}$$

$$27 \pm 1.96(1.4142)$$

$$27 \pm 2.7718$$

$$24.2282, 29.7718$$

Since this interval does not include 30, we say that 30 is not a candidate for the mean we are estimating and, therefore, μ is not equal to 30 and H_0 is rejected. This is the same conclusion reached by means of the hypothesis testing procedure.

If the hypothesized parameter, 30, had been within the 95 percent confidence interval, we would have said that H_0 is not rejected at the .05 level of signifance. In general, *when testing a null hypothesis by means of a two-sided confidence interval, we reject H_0 at the α level of significance if the hypothesized parameter is not contained within the $100(1 - \alpha)$ percent confidence interval. If the hypothesized parameter is contained within the interval, H_0 cannot be rejected at the α level of significance.*

One-Sided Hypothesis Tests   The hypothesis test illustrated by Example 7.2.1 is an example of a *two-sided test*, so called because the rejection region is split between the two sides or tails of the distribution of the test statistic. A hypothesis test may be *one-sided*, in which case all the rejection region is in one or the other tail of the distribution. Whether a one-sided or a two-sided test is used depends on the nature of the question being asked by the researcher.

If both large and small values will cause rejection of the null hypothesis, a two-sided test is indicated. When either sufficiently "small" values only or suffi-ciently "large" values only will cause rejection of the null hypothesis, a one-sided test is indicated.

Example 7.2.2

Refer to Exercise 7.2.1. Suppose, instead of asking if they could conclude that $\mu \neq 30$, the researchers had asked: Can we conclude that $\mu < 30$? To this question we would reply that they can so conclude if they can reject the null hypothesis that $\mu \geq 30$.

Solution: Let us go through the nine-step procedure to reach a decision based on a one-sided test.

1. *Data*   See the previous example.

2. *Assumptions*   See the previous example.

3. *Hypotheses*

$$H_0: \mu \geq 30$$

$$H_A: \mu < 30$$

The inequality in the null hypothesis implies that the null hypothesis consists of an infinite number of hypotheses. The test will be made only at the point of equality, since it can be shown that if H_0 is rejected when the test is made at the point of equality it would be rejected if the test were done for any other value of μ indicated in the null hypothesis.

4. *Test Statistic*

$$z = \frac{\bar{x} - \mu_0}{\sigma/\sqrt{n}}$$

5. *Distribution of Test Statistic*   See the previous example.

6. *Decision Rule*   Let us again let $\alpha = .05$. To determine where to place the rejection region, let us ask ourselves what magnitude of values would cause rejection of the null hypothesis. If we look at the hypotheses, we see that sufficiently small values would cause rejection and that large values would tend to reinforce the null hypothesis. We will want our rejection region to be where the small values are—at the lower tail of the distribution. This time, since we have a one-sided test, all of α will go in the one tail of the distribution. By consulting Table D, we find that the value of z to the left of which lies .05 of the area under the unit normal curve is -1.645 after interpolating. Our rejection and nonrejection regions are now specified and are shown in Figure 7.2.2.

Our decision rule tells us to reject H_0 if the computed value of the test statistic is less than or equal to -1.645.

7. *Calculation of Test Statistic*   From our data we compute

$$z = \frac{27 - 30}{\sqrt{20/10}} = -2.12$$

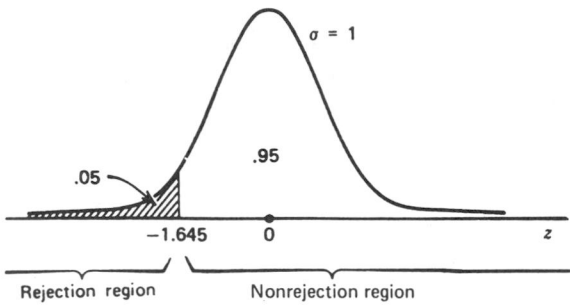

Figure 7.2.2 Rejection and nonrejection regions for Example 7.2.2.

---

8. *Statistical Decision*   We are able to reject the null hypothesis since $-2.12 <$ -1.645.

9. *Conclusion*   We conclude that the population mean is smaller than 30 and act accordingly.

The *p* Value   The *p* value for this test is .0170, since $P(z \leq -2.12)$, when H_0 is true, is .0170 as given by Table D when we determine the magnitude of the area to the left of -2.12 under the standard normal curve. One can test a one-sided null hypothesis by means of a one-sided confidence interval. However, we will not cover the construction and interpretation of this type of confidence interval in this book. The interested reader is referred to a discussion of the topic in the book by Daniel (5).

If the researcher's question had been, "Can we conclude that the mean is greater than 30?," following the above nine-step procedure would have led to a one-sided test with all the rejection region at the upper tail of the distribution of the test statistic and a critical value of $+1.645$.

Sampling from a Normally Distributed Population: Population Variance Unknown   As we have already noted, the population variance is usually unknown in actual situations involving statistical inference about a population mean. When sampling is from a normally distributed population with an unknown variance, the test statistic for testing $H_0: \mu = \mu_0$ is

$$t = \frac{\bar{x} - \mu_0}{s/\sqrt{n}} \qquad (7.2.2)$$

which, when H_0 is true, is distributed as Student's t with $n - 1$ degrees of freedom. The following example illustrates the hypothesis testing procedure when the population is assumed to be normally distributed and its variance is unknown. This is the usual situation encountered in practice.

Example 7.2.3

Castillo and Lillioja (A-1) describe a technique they developed for peripheral lymphatic cannulation in humans. The authors claim that their technique simplifies the procedure and enables the collection of adequate volumes of lymph for kinetic and metabolic studies. The investigators' subjects were 14 healthy adult males representing a wide range of body weight. One of the variables on which measurements were taken was body mass index (BMI) = weight (kg)/height^2 (m^2). The results are shown in Table 7.2.1. We wish to know if we can conclude that the mean BMI of the population from the sample was drawn is not 35.

Solution: We will be able to conclude that the mean BMI for the population is not 35 if we can reject the null hypothesis that the population mean is equal to 35.

1. *Data* The data consist of BMI measurements on 14 subjects as previously described.

2. *Assumptions* The 14 subjects constitute a simple random sample from a population of similar subjects. We assume that BMI measurements in this population are approximately normally distributed.

3. *Hypotheses*

$$H_0: \mu = 35$$

$$H_A: \mu \neq 35$$

4. *Test Statistic* Since the population variance is unknown, our test statistic is given by Equation 7.2.2.

5. *Distribution of Test Statistic* Our test statistic is distributed as Student's t with $n - 1 = 14 - 1 = 13$ degrees of freedom if H_0 is true.

6. *Decision Rule* Let $\alpha = .05$. Since we have a two-sided test, we put $\alpha/2 = .025$ in each tail of the distribution of our test statistic. The t values to the right and left of which .025 of the area lies are 2.1604 and -2.1604. These values

TABLE 7.2.1 Body Mass Index (BMI) Measurements for Male Subjects Described in Example 7.2.3

Subject	BMI	Subject	BMI	Subject	BMI
1	23	6	21	11	23
2	25	7	23	12	26
3	21	8	24	13	31
4	37	9	32	14	45
5	39	10	57		

Source: Charles E. Castillo and Stephen Lillioja, "Peripheral Lymphatic Cannulation for Physiological Analysis of Interstitial Fluid Compartment in Humans," *American Journal of Physiology*, 261 *(Heart and Circulation Phisiology, 30)*, (October 1991), H1324–H1328.

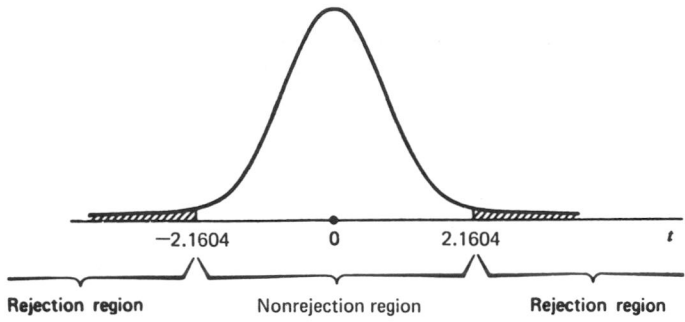

Figure 7.2.3 Rejection and nonrejection regions for Example 7.2.3.

are obtained from Table E. The rejection and nonrejection regions are shown in Figure 7.2.3.

The decision rule tells us to compute a value of the test statistic and reject H_0 if the computed t is either greater than or equal to 2.1604 or less than or equal to -2.1604.

7. *Calculation of Test Statistic*   From our sample data we compute a sample mean of 30.5 and a sample standard deviation of 10.6392. Substituting these statistics into Equation 7.2.2 gives

$$t = \frac{30.5 - 35}{10.6392/\sqrt{14}} = \frac{-4.5}{2.8434} = -1.58$$

8. *Statistical Decision*   Do not reject H_0, since -1.58 falls in the nonrejection region.

9. *Conclusion*   Our conclusion, based on these data, is that the mean of the population from which the sample came may be 35.

The *p* Value   The exact p value for this test cannot be obtained from Table E since it gives t values only for selected percentiles. The p value can be stated as an interval, however. We find that -1.58 is less than -1.350, the value of t to the left of which lies .10 of the area under the t with 13 degrees of freedom, but greater than -1.7709, to the left of which lies .05 of the area. Consequently, when H_0 is true, the probability of obtaining a value of t as small as or smaller than -1.58 is less than .10 but greater than .05. That is, $.05 < P\ (t \le -1.58) < .10$. Since the test was two-sided, we must allow for the possibility of a computed value of the test statistic as large in the opposite direction as that observed. Table E reveals that $.05 < P\ (t \ge 1.58) < .10$. The p value, then, is $.10 < p < .20$. Figure 7.2.4 shows the p value for this example.

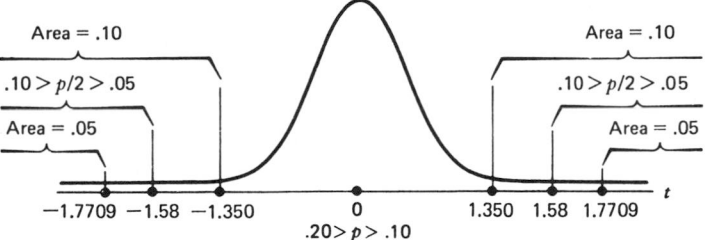

Figure 7.2.4 Determination of p value for Example 7.2.3.

If in the previous example the hypotheses had been

$$H_0: \mu \geq 35$$

$$H_A: \mu < 35$$

the testing procedure would have led to a one-sided test with all the rejection region at the lower tail of the distribution, and if the hypotheses had been

$$H_0: \mu \leq 35$$

$$H_A: \mu > 35$$

we would have had a one-sided test with all the rejection region at the upper tail of the distribution.

Sampling from a Population That Is Not Normally Distributed   If, as is frequently the case, the sample on which we base our hypothesis test about a population mean comes from a population that is not normally distributed, we may, if our sample is large (greater than or equal to 30), take advantage of the central limit theorem and use $z = (\bar{x} - \mu_0)/(\sigma/\sqrt{n})$ as the test statistic. If the population standard deviation is not known, the usual practice is to use the sample standard deviation as an estimate. The test statistic for testing $H_0: \mu = \mu_0$, then, is

$$z = \frac{\bar{x} - \mu_0}{s/\sqrt{n}} \qquad (7.2.3)$$

which, when H_0 is true, is distributed approximately as the standard normal distribution if n is large. The rationale for using s to replace σ is that the large sample, necessary for the central limit theorem to apply, will yield a sample standard deviation that closely approximates σ.

Example 7.2.4

The objectives of a study by Wilbur et al. (A-2) were to describe the menopausal status, menopausal symptoms, energy expenditure, and aerobic fitness of healthy midlife women and to determine relationships among these factors. Among the variables measured was maximum oxygen uptake ($VO_{2\,max}$). The mean $VO_{2\,max}$ score for a sample of 242 women was 33.3 with a standard deviation of 12.14. (*Source: Family and Community Health*, Vol. 13:3, p. 73, Aspen Publishers, Inc., © 1990.) We wish to know if, on the basis of these data, we may conclude that the mean score for a population of such women is greater than 30.

Solution: We will say that the data do provide sufficient evidence to conclude that the population mean is greater than 30 if we can reject the null hypothesis that the mean is less than or equal to 30. The following test may be carried out:

1. *Data* The data consist of $VO_{2\,max}$ scores for 242 women with $\bar{x} = 33.3$ and $s = 12.14$.

2. *Assumptions* The data constitute a simple random sample from a population of healthy midlife women similar to those in the sample. We are unwilling to assume that $VO_{2\,max}$ scores are normally distributed in such a population.

3. *Hypotheses*

$$H_0: \mu \le 30$$

$$H_A: \mu > 30$$

4. *Test Statistic* The test statistic is given by Equation 7.2.3, since σ is unknown.

5. *Distribution of Test Statistic* Because of the central limit theorem, the test statistic is at worst approximately normally distributed with $\mu = 0$ if H_0 is true.

6. *Decision Rule* Let $\alpha = .05$. The critical value of the test statistic is 1.645. The rejection and nonrejection regions are shown in Figure 7.2.5. Reject H_0 if computed $z \ge 1.645$.

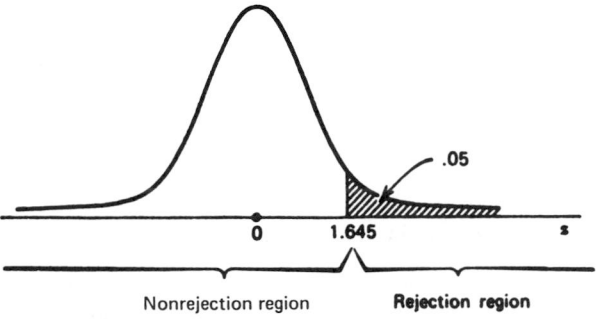

Figure 7.2.5 Rejection and nonrejection regions for Example 7.2.4.

7. *Calculation of Test Statistic*

$$z = \frac{33.3 - 30}{12.14/\sqrt{242}} = \frac{3.3}{.7804} = 4.23$$

8. *Statistical Decision* Reject H_0 since $4.23 > 1.645$.

9. *Conclusion* Conclude that the mean $Vo_{2\,max}$ score for the sampled population is greater than 30. The p value for this test is $< .001$, since 4.23 is greater than 3.89.

Procedures for Other Conditions If the population variance had been known, the procedure would have been identical to the above except that the known value of σ, instead of the sample value s, would have been used in the denominator of the computed test statistic.

Depending on what the investigators wished to conclude, either a two-sided test or a one-sided test, with the rejection region at the lower tail of the distribution, could have been made using the above data.

When testing a hypothesis about a single population mean, we may use Figure 6.3.3 to decide quickly whether the test statistic is z or t.

Computer Analysis To illustrate the use of computers in testing hypotheses we consider the following example.

Example 7.2.5

The following are the head circumferences (centimeters) at birth of 15 infants.

33.38	32.15	33.99	34.10	33.97
34.34	33.95	33.85	34.23	32.73
33.46	34.13	34.45	34.19	34.05

We wish to test H_0: $\mu = 34.5$ against H_A: $\mu \neq 34.5$.

Solution: We assume that the assumptions for use of the t statistic are met.

We enter the data into column 1 and issue the following MINITAB command.

```
TTEST 34.5 C1
```

We obtain the following printout.

```
TEST OF MU = 34.500 VS MU N.E. 34.500
N       MEAN      STDEV     SE MEAN     T        P VALUE
15      33.798    0.630     0.163       -4.31    0.0007
```

The MINITAB commands for one-sided tests each require a subcommand. The subcommand is $+1$ for a one-sided test with the rejection region in the right tail of the distribution of t and is -1 for a one-sided test with the rejection region in the left tail of the distribution. For example, if the alternative hypothesis for our example had been $\mu > 34.5$, the MINITAB command would have been

```
TTEST 34.5 C1;
ALTERNATIVE +1.
```

If the alternative hypothesis had been $\mu < 34.5$, the MINITAB command would have been

```
TTEST 34.5 C1;
ALTERNATIVE -1.
```

If z is the appropriate test statistic, the first word of the MINITAB commands is ZTEST. The remainder of the commands are the same as for the t test.

We learn from the printout that the computed value of the test statistic is -4.31 and the p value for the test is .0007. SAS® users may use the output from PROC MEANS or PROC UNIVARIATE to perform hypothesis tests.

When both the z statistic and the t statistic are inappropriate test statistics for use with the available data, one may wish to use a nonparametric technique to test a hypothesis about a single population measure of central tendency. One such procedure, the sign test, is discussed in Chapter 13.

EXERCISES

For each of the following exercises carry out the nine-step hypothesis testing procedure for the given significance level. Compute the p value for each test.

7.2.1 Bertino et al. (A-3) conducted a study to examine prospectively collected data on gentamicin in pharmacokinetics in three populations over 18 years of age: patients with acute leukemia, patients with other nonleukemic malignancies, and patients with no underlying malignancy or pathophysiology other than renal impairment known to alter gentamicin pharmacokinetics. Among other statistics reported by the investigators were a mean initial calculated creatinine clearance value of 59.1 with a standard deviation of 25.6 in a sample of 211 patients with malignancies other than leukemia. We wish to know if we may conclude that the mean for a population of similar subjects is less than 60. Let $\alpha = .10$.

7.2.2 The purpose of a study by Klesges et al. (A-4) was to investigate factors associated with discrepancies between self-reported smoking status and carboxyhemoglobin levels. A sample of 3918 self-reported nonsmokers had a mean carboxyhemoglobin level of .9 with a standard deviation of .96. We wish to know if we may conclude that the population mean is less than 1.0. Let $\alpha = .01$.

7.2.3 Dr. Jeffrey M. Barrett of Lakeland, Florida, reported data on eight cases of umbilical cord prolapse (A-5). The maternal ages were 25, 28, 17, 26, 27, 22, 25, and 30. We wish to know if we may conclude that the mean age of the population from which the sample may be presumed to have been drawn is greater than 20 years. Let $\alpha = .01$.

7.2.4 A study was made of a sample of 25 records of patients seen at a chronic disease hospital on an outpatient basis. The mean number of outpatient visits per patient was 4.8, and the sample standard deviation was 2. Can it be concluded from these data that the population mean is greater than four visits per patient? Let the probability of committing a type I error be .05. What assumptions are necessary?

7.2.5 In a sample of 49 adolescents who served as the subjects in an immunologic study, one variable of interest was the diameter of skin test reaction to an antigen. The sample mean and standard deviation were 21 and 11 mm erythema, respectively. Can it be concluded from these data that the population mean is less than 30? Let $\alpha = .05$.

7.2.6 Nine laboratory animals were infected with a certain bacterium and then immuno-suppressed. The mean number of organisms later recovered from tissue specimens was 6.5 (coded data) with a standard deviation of .6. Can one conclude from these data that the population mean is greater than 6? Let $\alpha = .05$. What assumptions are necessary?

7.2.7 A sample of 25 freshman nursing students made a mean score of 77 on a test designed to measure attitude toward the dying patient. The sample standard deviation was 10. Do these data provide sufficient evidence to indicate, at the .05 level of significance, that the population mean is less than 80? What assumptions are necessary?

7.2.8 We wish to know if we can conclude that the mean daily caloric intake in the adult rural population of a developing country is less than 2000. A sample of 500 had a mean of 1985 and a standard deviation of 210. Let $\alpha = .05$.

7.2.9 A survey of 100 similar-sized hospitals revealed a mean daily census in the pediatrics service of 27 with a standard deviation of 6.5. Do these data provide sufficient evidence to indicate that the population mean is greater than 25? Let $\alpha = .05$.

7.2.10 Following a week-long hospital supervisory training program, 16 assistant hospital administrators made a mean score of 74 on a test administered as part of the evaluation of the training program. The sample standard deviation was 12. Can it be concluded from these data that the population mean is greater than 70? Let $\alpha = .05$. What assumptions are necessary?

7.2.11 A random sample of 16 emergency reports was selected from the files of an ambulance service. The mean time (computed from the sample data) required for ambulances to reach their destinations was 13 minutes. Assume that the population of times is normally distributed with a variance of 9. Can we conclude at the .05 level of significance that the population mean is greater than 10 minutes?

7.2.12 The following data are the oxygen uptakes (milliliters) during incubation of a random sample of 15 cell suspensions.

14.0, 14.1, 14.5, 13.2, 11.2, 14.0, 14.1, 12.2
11.1, 13.7, 13.2, 16.0, 12.8, 14.4, 12.9

Do these data provide sufficient evidence at the .05 level of significance that the population mean is not 12 ml? What assumptions are necessary?

7.2.13 Can we conclude that the mean maximum voluntary ventilation value for apparently healthy college seniors is not 110 liters per minute? A sample of 20 yielded the following values:

132, 33, 91, 108, 67, 169, 54, 203, 190, 133
96, 30, 187, 21, 63, 166, 84, 110, 157, 138

Let $\alpha = .01$. What assumptions are necessary?

7.2.14 The following are the systolic blood pressures (mm Hg) of 12 patients undergoing drug therapy for hypertension:

183, 152, 178, 157, 194, 163, 144, 114, 178, 152, 118, 158

Can we conclude on the basis of these data that the population mean is less than 165? Let $\alpha = .05$. What assumptions are necessary?

7.2.15 Can we conclude that the mean age at death of patients with homozygous sickle-cell disease is less than 30 years? A sample of 50 patients yielded the following ages in years:

15.5,	2.0,	45.1,	1.7,	.8,	1.1,	18.2,	9.7,	28.1,	18.2
27.6,	45.0,	1.0,	66.4,	2.0,	67.4,	2.5,	61.7,	16.2,	31.7
6.9,	13.5,	1.9,	31.2,	9.0,	2.6,	29.7,	13.5,	2.6,	14.4,
20.7,	30.9,	36.6,	1.1,	23.6,	.9,	7.6,	23.5,	6.3,	40.2
23.7,	4.8,	33.2,	27.1,	36.7,	3.2,	38.0,	3.5,	21.8,	2.4

Let $\alpha = .05$. What assumptions are necessary?

7.2.16 The following are intraocular pressure (mm Hg) values recorded for a sample of 21 elderly subjects.

14.5,	12.9,	14.0,	16.1,	12.0,	17.5,	14.1,	12.9,	17.9,	12.0
16.4,	24.2,	12.2,	14.4,	17.0,	10.0,	18.5,	20.8,	16.2,	14.9
19.6									

Can we conclude from these data that the mean of the population from which the sample was drawn is greater than 14? Let $\alpha = .05$. What assumptions are necessary?

7.2.17 Suppose it is known that the IQ scores of a certain population of adults are approximately normally distributed with a standard deviation of 15. A simple random sample of 25 adults drawn from this population had a mean IQ score of 105. On the basis of these data can we conclude that the mean IQ score for the population is not 100? Let the probability of committing a type I error be .05.

7.2.18 A research team is willing to assume that systolic blood pressures in a certain population of males is approximately normally distributed with a standard deviation of 16. A simple random sample of 64 males from the population had a mean systolic blood pressure reading of 133. At the .05 level of significance, do these data provide sufficient evidence for us to conclude that the population mean is greater than 130?

7.2.19 A simple random sample of 16 adults drawn from a certain population of adults yielded a mean weight of 63 kg. Assume that weights in the population are approximately normally distributed with a variance of 49. Do the sample data provide sufficient evidence for us to conclude that the mean weight for the population is less than 70 kg? Let the probability of committing a type I error be .01.

7.3
Hypothesis Testing: The Difference Between Two Population Means

Hypothesis testing involving the difference between two population means is most frequently employed to determine whether or not it is reasonable to conclude that the two population means are unequal. In such cases, one or the other of the following hypotheses may be formulated:

1. $H_0: \mu_1 - \mu_2 = 0,$ $H_A: \mu_1 - \mu_2 \neq 0$
2. $H_0: \mu_1 - \mu_2 \geq 0,$ $H_A: \mu_1 - \mu_2 < 0$
3. $H_0: \mu_1 - \mu_2 \leq 0,$ $H_A: \mu_1 - \mu_2 > 0$

It is possible, however, to test the hypothesis that the difference is equal to, greater than or equal to, or less than or equal to some value other than zero.

As was done in the previous section, hypothesis testing involving the difference between two population means will be discussed in three different contexts: (1) when sampling is from normally distributed populations with known population variances, (2) when sampling is from normally distributed populations with unknown population variances, and (3) when sampling is from populations that are not normally distributed.

Sampling from Normally Distributed Populations: Population Variances Known   When each of two independent simple random samples has been drawn from a normally distributed population with a known variance, the test statistic for testing the null hypothesis of equal population means is

$$z = \frac{(\bar{x}_1 - \bar{x}_2) - (\mu_1 - \mu_2)_0}{\sqrt{\dfrac{\sigma_1^2}{n_1} + \dfrac{\sigma_2^2}{n_2}}} \qquad (7.3.1)$$

where the subscript 0 indicates that the difference is a hypothesized parameter. When H_0 is true the test statistic of Equation 7.3.1 is distributed as the standard normal.

Example 7.3.1

Researchers wish to know if the data they have collected provide sufficient evidence to indicate a difference in mean serum uric acid levels between normal individuals and individuals with Down's syndrome. The data consist of serum uric acid readings on 12 individuals with Down's syndrome and 15 normal individuals. The means are $\bar{x}_1 = 4.5$ mg/100 ml and $\bar{x}_2 = 3.4$ mg/ml.

Solution: We will say that the sample data do provide evidence that the population means are not equal if we can reject the null hypothesis that the population means are equal. Let us reach a conclusion by means of the nine-step hypothesis testing procedure.

1. *Data* See problem statement.

2. *Assumptions* The data constitute two independent simple random samples each drawn from a normally distributed population with a variance equal to 1 for the Down's syndrome population and 1.5 for the normal population.

3. *Hypotheses*

$$H_0: \mu_1 - \mu_2 = 0$$

$$H_A: \mu_1 - \mu_2 \neq 0$$

An alternative way of stating the hypotheses is as follows:

$$H_0: \mu_1 = \mu_2$$

$$H_A: \mu_1 \neq \mu_2$$

4. *Test Statistic* The test statistic is given by Equation 7.3.1.

5. *Distribution of Test Statistic* When the null hypothesis is true, the test statistic follows the standard normal distribution.

6. *Decision Rule* Let $\alpha = .05$. The critical values of z are ± 1.96. Reject H_0 unless $-1.96 < z_{computed} < 1.96$. The rejection and nonrejection regions are shown in Figure 7.3.1.

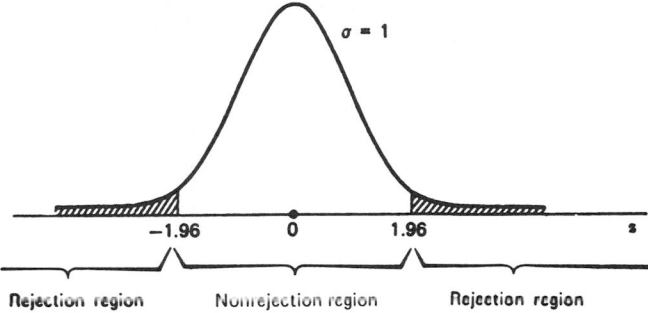

Figure 7.3.1 Rejection and nonrejection regions for Example 7.3.1.

7. *Calculation of Test Statistic*

$$z = \frac{(4.5 - 3.4) - 0}{\sqrt{1/12 + 1.5/15}} = \frac{1.1}{.4282} = 2.57$$

8. *Statistical Decision*   Reject H_0, since $2.57 > 1.96$.

9. *Conclusion*   Conclude that, on the basis of these data, there is an indication that the two population means are not equal. For this test, $p = .0102$.

A 95 Percent Confidence Interval for μ   In the previous chapter the 95 percent confidence interval for $\mu_1 - \mu_2$, computed from the same data, was found to be .26 to 1.94. Since this interval does not include 0, we say that 0 is not a candidate for the difference between population means, and we conclude that the difference is not zero. Thus we arrive at the same conclusion by means of a confidence interval.

Sampling from Normally Distributed Populations: Population Variances Unknown   As we have learned, when the population variances are unknown, two possibilities exist. The two population variances may be equal or they may be unequal. We consider first the case where it is known, or it is reasonable to assume, that they are equal.

Population Variances Equal   When the population variances are unknown, but assumed to be equal, we recall from Chapter 6 that it is appropriate to pool the sample variances by means of the following formula:

$$s_p^2 = \frac{(n_1 - 1)s_1^2 + (n_2 - 1)s_2^2}{n_1 + n_2 - 2}$$

TABLE 7.3.1 Lung Destructive Index Scores for Example 7.3.2

Nonsmokers:	18.1,	6.0,	10.8,	11.0,	7.7,	17.9,	8.5,	13.0,	18.9
Smokers:	16.6,	13.9,	11.3,	26.5,	17.4,	15.3,	15.8,	12.3,	18.6,
	12.0,	24.1,	16.5,	21.8,	16.3,	23.4,	18.8		

SOURCE: D. H. Eidelman, H. Ghezzo, W. D. Kim, and M. G. Cosio, "The Destructive Index and Early Lung Destruction in Smokers," *American Review of Respiratory Disease*, *144* (1991), 156–159.

When each of two independent simple random samples has been drawn from a normally distributed population and the two populations have equal but unknown variances, the test statistic for testing $H_0: \mu_1 = \mu_2$ is given by

$$t = \frac{(\bar{x}_1 - \bar{x}_2) - (\mu_1 - \mu_2)_0}{\sqrt{\dfrac{s_p^2}{n_1} + \dfrac{s_p^2}{n_2}}} \qquad (7.3.2)$$

which, when H_0 is true, is distributed as Student's t with $n_1 + n_2 - 2$ degrees of freedom.

Example 7.3.2

The purpose of a study by Eidelman et al. (A-6) was to investigate the nature of lung destruction in the lungs of cigarette smokers before the development of marked emphysema. Three lung destructive index measurements were made on the lungs of lifelong nonsmokers and smokers who died suddenly outside the hospital of nonrespiratory causes. A larger score indicates greater lung damage. For one of the indexes the scores yielded by the lungs of a sample of nine nonsmokers and a sample of 16 smokers are shown in Table 7.3.1. We wish to know if we may conclude, on the basis of these data, that smokers, in general, have greater lung damage as measured by this destructive index than do nonsmokers.

Solution:

1. *Data*   See statement of problem.

2. *Assumptions*   The data constitute two independent simple random samples of lungs, one sample from a population of nonsmokers (NS) and the other sample from a population of smokers (S). The lung destructive index scores in both populations are approximately normally distributed. The population variances are unknown but are assumed to be equal.

3. *Hypotheses* $H_0: \mu_S \leq \mu_{NS}$, $H_A: \mu_S > \mu_{NS}$.

4. *Test Statistic*   The test statistic is given by Equation 7.3.2.

5. *Distribution of Test Statistic*   When the null hypothesis is true, the test statistic follows Student's t distribution with $n_1 + n_2 - 2$ degrees of freedom.

6. *Decision Rule*   Let $\alpha = .05$. The critical values of t are ± 2.0687. Reject H_0 unless $-2.0687 < t_{computed} < 2.0687$.

7. *Calculation of Test Statistic*   From the sample data we compute

$$\bar{x}_S = 17.5, \quad s_S = 4.4711, \quad \bar{x}_{NS} = 12.4, \quad s_{NS} = 4.8492$$

Next we pool the sample variances to obtain

$$s_p^2 = \frac{15(4.4711)^2 + 8(4.8492)^2}{15 + 8} = 21.2165$$

We now compute

$$t = \frac{(17.5 - 12.4) - 0}{\sqrt{\dfrac{21.2165}{16} + \dfrac{21.2165}{9}}} = 2.6573$$

8. *Statistical Decision*   We reject H_0, since $2.6573 > 2.0687$; that is, 2.6573 falls in the rejection region.

9. *Conclusion*   On the basis of these data we conclude that the two population means are different; that is, we conclude that, as measured by the index used in the study, smokers have greater lung damage than nonsmokers. For this test $.01 > p > .005$, since $2.500 < 2.6573 < 2.8073$.

Population Variances Unequal   When two independent simple random samples have been drawn from normally distributed populations with unknown and unequal variances, the test statistic for testing $H_0: \mu_1 = \mu_2$ is

$$t' = \frac{(\bar{x}_1 - \bar{x}_2) - (\mu_1 - \mu_2)_0}{\sqrt{\dfrac{s_1^2}{n_1} + \dfrac{s_2^2}{n_2}}} \tag{7.3.3}$$

The critical value of t' for an α level of significance and a two-sided test is approximately

$$t'_{1-(\alpha/2)} = \frac{w_1 t_1 + w_2 t_2}{w_1 + w_2} \tag{7.3.4}$$

where $w_1 = s_1^2/n_1$, $w_2 = s_2^2/n_2$, $t_1 = t_{1-(\alpha/2)}$ for $n_1 - 1$ degrees of freedom, and $t_2 = t_{1-(\alpha/2)}$ for $n_2 - 1$ degrees of freedom. The critical value of t' for a one-sided test is found by computing $t'_{1-\alpha}$ by Equation 7.3.4, using $t_1 = t_{1-\alpha}$ for $n_1 - 1$ degrees of freedom and $t_2 = t_{1-\alpha}$ for $n_2 - 1$ degrees of freedom.

For a two-sided test reject H_0 if the computed value of t' is either greater than or equal to the critical value given by Equation 7.3.4 or less than or equal to the negative of that value.

For a one-sided test with the rejection region in the right tail of the sampling distribution, reject H_0 if the computed t' is equal to or greater than the critical t'. For a one-sided test with a left-tail rejection region, reject H_0 if the computed value of t' is equal to or smaller than the negative of the critical t' computed by the indicated adaptation of Equation 7.3.4.

Example 7.3.3

Researchers wish to know if two populations differ with respect to the mean value of total serum complement activity (C_{H50}). The data consist of C_{H50} determinations on $n_2 = 20$ apparently normal subjects and $n_1 = 10$ subjects with disease. The sample means and standard deviations are

$$\bar{x}_1 = 62.6, \qquad s_1 = 33.8$$

$$\bar{x}_2 = 47.2, \qquad s_2 = 10.1$$

Solution:

1. *Data*   See statement of problem.

2. *Assumptions*   The data constitute two independent random samples, one from a population of apparently normal subjects and the other from a population of subjects with disease. We assume that C_{H50} values are approximately normally distributed in both populations. The population variances are unknown and unequal.

3. *Hypotheses*

$$H_0: \mu_1 - \mu_2 = 0$$

$$H_A: \mu_1 - \mu_2 \neq 0$$

4. *Test Statistic*   The test statistic is given by Equation 7.3.3.

5. *Distribution of the Test Statistic*   The statistic given by Equation 7.3.3 does not follow Student's t distribution. We, therefore, obtain its critical values by Equation 7.3.4.

6. *Decision Rule*   Let $\alpha = .05$. Before computing t' we calculate $w_1 = (33.8)^2/10 = 114.244$ and $w_2 = (10.1)^2/20 = 5.1005$. In Table E we find that $t_1 = 2.2622$ and $t_2 = 2.0930$. By Equation 7.3.4 we compute

$$t' = \frac{114.244(2.2622) + 5.1005(2.0930)}{114.244 + 5.1005} = 2.255$$

Our decision rule, then, is reject H_0 if the computed t is either ≥ 2.255 or ≤ -2.255.

7. *Calculations of the Test Statistic*   By Equation 7.3.3 we compute

$$t' = \frac{(62.6 - 47.2) - 0}{\sqrt{\dfrac{(33.8)^2}{10} + \dfrac{(10.1)^2}{20}}} = \frac{15.4}{10.92} = 1.41$$

8. *Statistical Decision*   Since $-2.255 < 1.41 < 2.255$, we cannot reject H_0.

9. *Conclusion*   On the basis of these results we cannot conclude that the two population means are different.

Sampling from Populations That Are Not Normally Distributed   When sampling is from populations that are not normally distributed, the results of the central limit theorem may be employed if sample sizes are large (say ≥ 30). This will allow the use of normal theory since the distribution of the difference between sample means will be approximately normal. When each of two large independent simple random samples has been drawn from a population that is not normally distributed, the test statistic for testing $H_0: \mu_1 = \mu_2$ is

$$z = \frac{(\bar{x}_1 - \bar{x}_2) - (\mu_1 - \mu_2)_0}{\sqrt{\dfrac{\sigma_1^2}{n_1} + \dfrac{\sigma_2^2}{n_2}}} \qquad (7.3.5)$$

which, when H_0 is true, follows the standard normal distribution. If the population variances are known, they are used; but if they are unknown, as is the usual case, the sample variances, which are necessarily based on large samples, are used as estimates. Sample variances are not pooled, since equality of population variances is not a necessary assumption when the z statistic is used.

Example 7.3.4   An article by Becker et al. in the *American Journal of Health Promotion* (A-7) describes the development of a tool to measure barriers to health promotion among persons with disabilities. The authors state that the issue of barriers is especially salient for disabled persons who experience barriers in such contexts as employment, transportation, housing, education, insurance, architectural access, entitlement programs, and society's attitudes. Studies suggest that measurement of barriers can enhance health workers' understanding of the likelihood of people engaging in various health-promoting behaviors and may be a relevant construct in assessing the health behaviors of disabled persons. To measure this construct the authors developed the Barriers to Health Promotion Activities for Disabled Persons Scale

(BHADP). The scale was administered to a sample of 132 disabled (D) and 137 nondisabled (ND) subjects with the following results:

Sample	Mean Score	Standard Deviation
D	31.83	7.93
ND	25.07	4.80

SOURCE: Heather Becker, Alexa K. Stuifbergen, and Dolores Sands, "Development of a Scale to Measure Barriers to Health Promotion Activities Among Persons with Disabilities," *American Journal of Health Promotion*, 5 (1991), 449–454. Used by permission.

We wish to know if we may conclude, on the basis of these results, that, in general, disabled persons, on the average, score higher on the BHADP scale.

Solution:

1. *Data* See statement of example.

2. *Assumption* The statistics were computed from two independent samples that behave as simple random samples from a population of disabled persons and a population of nondisabled persons. Since the population variances are unknown, we will use the sample variances in the calculation of the test statistic.

3. *Hypotheses*

$$H_0: \mu_D - \mu_{ND} \leq 0$$

$$H_A: \mu_D - \mu_{ND} > 0$$

or, alternatively,

$$H_0: \mu_D \leq \mu_{ND}$$

$$H_A: \mu_D > \mu_{ND}$$

4. *Test Statistic* Since we have large samples, the central limit theorem allows us to use Equation 7.3.5 as the test statistic.

5. *Distribution of Test Statistic* When the null hypothesis is true, the test statistic is distributed approximately as the standard normal.

6. *Decision Rule* Let $\alpha = .01$. This is a one-sided test with a critical value of z equal to 2.33. Reject H_0 if $z_{computed} \geq 2.33$.

7. *Calculation of Test Statistic*

$$z = \frac{(31.83 - 25.07) - 0}{\sqrt{\dfrac{(7.93)^2}{132} + \dfrac{(4.80)^2}{137}}} = 8.42$$

8. *Statistical Decision* Reject H_0, since $z = 8.42$ is in the rejection region.

9. *Conclusion* These data indicate that on the average disabled persons score higher on the BHADP scale than do nondisabled persons. For this test $p < .0001$, since $8.42 > 3.89$. When testing a hypothesis about the difference between two population means, we may use Figure 6.4.1 to decide quickly whether the test statistic should be z or t.

Alternatives to z and t Sometimes neither the z statistic nor the t statistic is an appropriate test statistic for use with the available data. When such is the case, one may wish to use a nonparametric technique for testing a hypothesis about the difference between two population measures of central tendency. The Mann–Whitney test statistic and the median test, discussed in Chapter 13, are frequently used alternatives to the z and t statistics.

EXERCISES

In each of the following exercises complete the nine-step hypothesis testing procedure and compute the p value for each test. State the assumptions that are necessary for your procedure to be valid.

7.3.1 Evans et al. (A-8) conducted a study to determine if the prevalence and nature of podiatric problems in elderly diabetic patients are different from those found in a similarly aged group of nondiabetic patients. Subjects, who were seen in outpatient clinics, were 70 to 90 years old. Among the investigators' findings were the following statistics with respect to scores on the measurement of deep tendon reflexes:

Sample	n	Mean	Standard Deviation
Nondiabetic patients	79	2.1	1.1
Diabetic patients	74	1.6	1.2

SOURCE: Scott L. Evans, Brent P. Nixon, Irvin Lee, David Yee, and Arshag D. Mooradian, "The Prevalence and Nature of Podiatric Problems in Elderly Diabetic Patients," *Journal of the American Geriatrics Society*, **39** (1991), 241–245. ©American Geriatrics Society, 1991.

We wish to know if we can conclude, on the basis of these data, that, on the average, diabetic patients have reduced deep tendon reflexes when compared to nondiabetic patients of the same age. Let $\alpha = .01$.

7.3.2 The twofold purpose of a study by Hommes et al. (A-9) was (1) to investigate whether resting energy expenditure (REE) is increased in the early asymptomatic stage of HIV infection and (2) to study the relative contributions of carbohydrate and fat oxidation to REE in these patients. Subjects consisted of 11 clinically asymptomatic male HIV-infected outpatients between the ages of 23 and 50 years. A control group was made up of 11 healthy, male volunteers aged 25 to 51 years who had normal physical examinations and medical histories. Among other findings were the following statistics on the measurement of REE:

Sample	Mean	Standard Error of the Mean
HIV subjects	7116	173
Controls	7058	205

SOURCE: Mirjam J. T. Hommes, Johannes A. Romijn, Erik Endert, and Hans P. Sauerwein, "Resting Energy Expenditure and Substrate Oxidation in Human Immunodeficiency Virus (HIV)-infected Asymptomatic Men: HIV Affects Host Metabolism in the Early Asymptomatic Stage," *American Journal of Clinical Nutrition*, *54* (1991), 311–315.

Do these data provide sufficient evidence to allow you to conclude that REE is increased in the early asymptomatic stage of HIV infection? Let $\alpha = .05$.

7.3.3 Frigerio et al. (A-10) measured the energy intake in 32 Gambian women. Sixteen of the subjects were lactating (L) and the remainder were nonpregnant and nonlactating (NPNL). The following data were reported:

Sample	Energy Intake (kJ / d)
L	5289, 6209, 6054, 6665, 6343, 7699, 5678, 6954 6916, 4770, 5979, 6305, 6502, 6113, 6347, 5657
NPNL	9920, 8581, 9305, 10765, 8079, 9046, 7134, 8736, 10230, 7121, 8665, 5167, 8527, 7791, 8782, 6883

SOURCE: Christian Frigerio, Yves Schutz, Roger Whitehead, and Eric Jéquier, "A New Procedure to Assess the Energy Requirements of Lactation in Gambian Women," *American Journal of Clinical Nutrition*, *54* (1991), 526–533. © *Am. J. Clin. Nut.* American Society for Clinical Nutrition.

Do these data provide sufficient evidence to allow us to conclude that the two sampled populations differ with respect to mean energy intake? Let $\alpha = .01$. Do these data provide sufficient evidence to indicate that the means of the populations represented by the samples differ? Let $\alpha = .05$.

7.3.4 Can we conclude that chronically ill children tend, on the average, to be less self-confident than healthy children? A test designed to measure self-confidence was administered to 16 chronically ill and 21 healthy children. The mean scores and standard deviations were as follows:

	$\bar{x}$	s
Ill group	22.5	4.1
Well group	26.9	3.2

Let $\alpha = .05$.

7.3.5 A nurse researcher wished to know if graduates of baccalaureate nursing programs and graduates of associate degree nursing programs differ with respect to mean scores on a personality inventory. A sample of 50 associate degree graduates (sample

A) and a sample of 60 baccalaureate graduates (sample B) yielded the following means and standard deviations.

Sample	$\bar{x}$	s
A	52.5	10.5
B	49.6	11.2

On the basis of these data, what should the researcher conclude? Let $\alpha = .05$.

7.3.6 A test designed to measure mothers' attitudes toward their labor and delivery experiences was given to two groups of new mothers. Sample 1 (attenders) had attended prenatal classes held at the local health department. Sample 2 (nonattenders) did not attend the classes. The sample sizes and means and standard deviations of the test scores were as follows:

Sample	n	$\bar{x}$	s
1	15	4.75	1.0
2	22	3.00	1.5

Do these data provide sufficient evidence to indicate that attenders, on the average, score higher than nonattenders? Let $\alpha = .05$.

7.3.7 Cortisol level determinations were made on two samples of women at childbirth. Group 1 subjects underwent emergency cesarean section following induced labor. Group 2 subjects delivered by either cesarean section or the vaginal route following spontaneous labor. The sample sizes, mean cortisol levels, and standard deviations were as follows:

Sample	n	$\bar{x}$	s
1	10	435	65
2	12	645	80

Do these data provide sufficient evidence to indicate a difference in the mean cortisol levels in the populations represented? Let $\alpha = .05$.

7.3.8 Protoporphyrin levels were measured in two samples of subjects. Sample 1 consisted of 50 adult male alcoholics with ring sideroblasts in the bone marrow. Sample 2 consisted of 40 apparently healthy adult nonalcoholic males. The mean protoporphyrin levels and standard deviations for the two samples were as follows:

Sample	$\bar{x}$	s
1	340	250
2	45	25

Can one conclude on the basis of these data that protoporphyrin levels are higher in the represented alcoholic population than in the nonalcoholic population? Let $\alpha = .01$.

7.3.9 A researcher was interested in knowing if preterm infants with late metabolic acidosis and preterm infants without the condition differ with respect to urine levels of a certain chemical. The mean levels, standard deviations, and sample sizes for the two samples studied were as follows:

Sample	n	$\bar{x}$	s
With condition	35	8.5	5.5
Without condition	40	4.8	3.6

What should the researcher conclude on the basis of these results? Let $\alpha = .05$.

7.3.10 Researchers wished to know if they could conclude that two populations of infants differ with respect to mean age at which they walked alone. The following data (ages in months) were collected:

Sample from population A:

9.5, 10.5, 9.0, 9.75, 10.0, 13.0, 10.0, 13.5, 10.0, 9.5, 10.0, 9.75

Sample from population B:

12.5, 9.5, 13.5, 13.75, 12.0, 13.75, 12.5, 9.5, 12.0, 13.5, 12.0, 12.0

What should the researchers conclude? Let $\alpha = .05$.

7.3.11 Does sensory deprivation have an effect on a person's alpha-wave frequency? Twenty volunteer subjects were randomly divided into two groups. Subjects in group A were subjected to a 10-day period of sensory deprivation, while subjects in group B served as controls. At the end of the experimental period the alpha-wave frequency component of subjects' electroencephalograms were measured. The results were as follows:

Group A: 10.2, 9.5, 10.1, 10.0, 9.8, 10.9, 11.4, 10.8, 9.7, 10.4
Group B: 11.0, 11.2, 10.1, 11.4, 11.7, 11.2, 10.8, 11.6, 10.9, 10.9

Let $\alpha = .05$.

7.3.12 Can we conclude that, on the average, lymphocytes and tumor cells differ in size? The following are the cell diameters (μm) of 40 lymphocytes and 50 tumor cells obtained from biopsies of tissue from patients with melanoma.

Lymphocytes							
9.0	9.4	4.7	4.8	8.9	4.9	8.4	5.9
6.3	5.7	5.0	3.5	7.8	10.4	8.0	8.0
8.6	7.0	6.8	7.1	5.7	7.6	6.2	7.1
7.4	8.7	4.9	7.4	6.4	7.1	6.3	8.8
8.8	5.2	7.1	5.3	4.7	8.4	6.4	8.3

Tumor Cells									
12.6	14.6	16.2	23.9	23.3	17.1	20.0	21.0	19.1	19.4
16.7	15.9	15.8	16.0	17.9	13.4	19.1	16.6	18.9	18.7
20.0	17.8	13.9	22.1	13.9	18.3	22.8	13.0	17.9	15.2
17.7	15.1	16.9	16.4	22.8	19.4	19.6	18.4	18.2	20.7
16.3	17.7	18.1	24.3	11.2	19.5	18.6	16.4	16.1	21.5

Let $\alpha = .05$.

7.4
Paired Comparisons

In our previous discussion involving the difference between two population means, it was assumed that the samples were independent. A method frequently employed for assessing the effectiveness of a treatment or experimental procedure is one that makes use of related observations resulting from nonindependent samples. A hypothesis test based on this type of data is known as a *paired comparisons* test.

Reasons for Pairing It frequently happens that true differences do not exist between two populations with respect to the variable of interest, but the presence of extraneous sources of variation may cause rejection of the null hypothesis of no difference. On the other hand, true differences also may be masked by the presence of extraneous factors.

Suppose, for example, that we wish to compare two sunscreens. There are at least two ways in which the experiment may be carried out. One method would be to select a simple random sample of subjects to receive sunscreen A and an independent simple random sample of subjects to receive sunscreen B. We send the subjects out into the sunshine for a specified length of time, after which we will measure the amount of damage from the rays of the sun. Suppose we employ this method, but inadvertently, most of the subjects receiving sunscreen A have darker complexions that are naturally less sensitive to sunlight. Let us say that after the experiment has been completed we find that subjects receiving sunscreen A had less sun damage. We would not know if they had less sun damage because sunscreen A was more protective than sunscreen B or because the subjects were naturally less sensitive to the sun.

A better way to design the experiment would be to select just one simple random sample of subjects and let each member of the sample receive both sunscreens. We could, for example, randomly assign the sunscreens to the left or the right side of each subject's back with each subject receiving both sunscreens. After a specified length of exposure to the sun, we would measure the amount of sun damage to each half of the back. If the half of the back receiving sunscreen A tended to be less damaged, we could more confidently attribute the result to the sunscreen, since in each instance both sunscreens were applied to equally pigmented skin.

The objective in paired comparisons tests is to eliminate a maximum number of sources of extraneous variation by making the pairs similar with respect to as many variables as possible.

Related or paired observations may be obtained in a number of ways. The same subjects may be measured before and after receiving some treatment. Litter mates of the same sex may be randomly assigned to receive either a treatment or a placebo. Pairs of twins or siblings may be randomly assigned to two treatments in such a way that members of a single pair receive different treatments. In comparing two methods of analysis, the material to be analyzed may be equally divided so that one half is analyzed by one method and one half is analyzed by the other. Or pairs may be formed by matching individuals on some characteristic, for example, digital dexterity, which is closely related to the measurement of interest, say, posttreatment scores on some test requiring digital manipulation.

Instead of performing the analysis with individual observations, we use d_i, the difference between pairs of observations, as the variable of interest.

When the n sample differences computed from the n pairs of measurements constitute a simple random sample from a normally distributed population of differences, the test statistic for testing hypotheses about the population mean difference μ_d is

$$t = \frac{\bar{d} - \mu_{d_0}}{s_{\bar{d}}} \tag{7.4.1}$$

where $\bar{d}$ is the sample mean difference, μ_{d_0} is the hypothesized population mean difference, $s_{\bar{d}} = s_d / \sqrt{n}$, n is the number of sample differences, and s_d is the standard deviation of the sample differences. When H_0 is true the test statistic is distributed as Student's t with $n - 1$ degrees of freedom.

Although, to begin with we have two samples—say, before levels and after levels—we do not have to worry about equality of variances, as with independent samples, since our variable is the difference between readings in the same individual, or matched individuals, and, hence, only one variable is involved. The arithmetic involved in performing a paired comparisons test, therefore, is the same as for performing a test involving a single sample as described in Section 7.2.

The following example illustrates the procedures involved in a paired comparisons test.

Example 7.4.1

Nancy Stearns Burgess (A-11) conducted a study to determine weight loss, body composition, body fat distribution, and resting metabolic rate in obese subjects before and after 12 weeks of treatment with a very-low-calorie diet (VLCD) and to compare hydrodensitometry with bioelectrical impedance analysis. The 17 subjects (9 women and 8 men) participating in the study were from an outpatient, hospital-based treatment program for obesity. The women's weights before and after the 12-week VLCD treatment are shown in Table 7.4.1. We wish to know if these data provide sufficient evidence to allow us to conclude that the treatment is effective in causing weight reduction in obese women.

Solution: We will say that sufficient evidence is provided for us to conclude that the diet program is effective if we can reject the null hypothesis that the population

TABLE 7.4.1 Weights (kg) of Obese Women Before and After 12-Week VLCD Treatment

B:	117.3	111.4	98.6	104.3	105.4	100.4	81.7	89.5	78.2
A:	83.3	85.9	75.8	82.9	82.3	77.7	62.7	69.0	63.9

SOURCE: Nancy Stearns Burgess. Used by permission.

mean change μ_d is zero or positive. We may reach a conclusion by means of the nine-step hypothesis testing procedure.

1. *Data*   The data consist of the weights of nine individuals, before and after an experimental diet program. We shall perform the statistical analysis on the differences between the before and after weights. We may obtain the differences in one of two ways: by subtracting the before weights from the after weights ($A - B$), or by subtracting the after weights from the before weights ($B - A$). Let us obtain the differences by subtracting the before weights from the after weights. The $d_i = A - B$ differences are $-34.0, -25.5, -22.8, -21.4, -23.1, -22.7, -19.0, -20.5, -14.3$.

2. *Assumptions*   The observed differences constitute a simple random sample from a normally distributed population of differences that could be generated under the same circumstances.

3. *Hypotheses*   The way we state our null and alternative hypotheses must be consistent with the way in which we subtract measurements to obtain the differences. In the present example, we want to know if we can conclude that the VLCD program is effective in reducing weight. If it is effective in reducing weight, we would expect the after weights to tend to be less than the before weights. If, therefore, we subtract the before weights from the after weights ($A - B$), we would expect the differences to tend to be negative. Furthermore, we would expect the mean of a population of such differences to be negative. So, under these conditions, asking if we can conclude that the VLCD program is effective is the same as asking if we can conclude that the population mean difference is negative (less than zero).

   The null and alternative hypotheses are as follows:

$$H_0: \mu_d \geq 0$$

$$H_A: \mu_d < 0$$

If we had obtained the differences by subtracting the after weights from the before weights ($B - A$) our hypotheses would have been

$$H_0: \mu_d \leq 0$$

$$H_A: \mu_d > 0$$

If the question had been such that a two-sided test was indicated, the hypotheses would have been

$$H_0: \mu_d = 0$$

$$H_A: \mu_d \neq 0$$

regardless of the way we subtracted to obtain the differences.

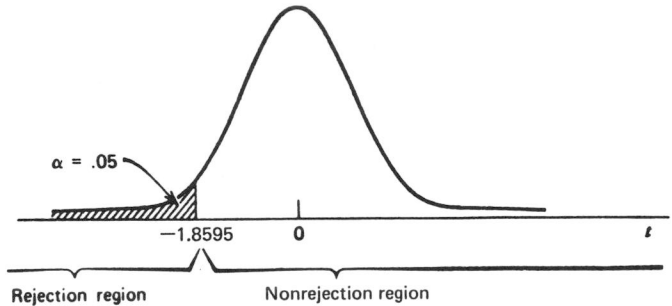

Figure 7.4.1   Rejection and nonrejection regions for Example 7.4.1.

4. *Test Statistic*   The appropriate test statistic is given by Equation 7.4.1.

5. *Distribution of Test Statistic*   If the null hypothesis is true, the test statistic is distributed as Student's t with $n - 1$ degrees of freedom.

6. *Decision Rule*   Let $\alpha = .05$. The critical value of t is -1.8595. Reject H_0 if computed t is less than or equal to the critical value. The rejection and nonrejection regions are shown in Figure 7.4.1.

7. *Calculation of Test Statistic*   From the $n = 9$ differences d_i, we compute the following descriptive measures:

$$\bar{d} = \frac{\Sigma d_i}{n} = \frac{(-34.0) + (-25.5) + \cdots + (-14.3)}{9} = \frac{-203.3}{9} = -22.5889$$

$$s_d^2 = \frac{\Sigma(d_i - \bar{d})^2}{n - 1} = \frac{n\Sigma d_i^2 - (\Sigma d_i)^2}{n(n - 1)} = \frac{9(4818.69) - (-203.3)^2}{9(8)} = 28.2961$$

$$t = \frac{-22.5889 - 0}{\sqrt{28.2961/9}} = \frac{-22.5889}{1.77314} = -12.7395$$

8. *Statistical Decision*   Reject H_0, since -12.7395 is in the rejection region.

9. *Conclusion*   We may conclude that the diet program is effective. For this test, $p < .005$, since $-12.7395 < -3.3554$.

A Confidence Interval for μ_d   A 95 percent confidence interval for μ_d may be obtained as follows:

$$\bar{d} \pm t_{1-(\alpha/2)} s_{\bar{d}}$$

$$-22.5889 \pm 2.3060\sqrt{28.2961/9}$$

$$-22.5889 \pm 4.0888$$

$$-26.68, -18.50$$

The Use of z If, in the analysis of paired data, the population variance of the differences is known, the appropriate test statistic is

$$z = \frac{\bar{d} - \mu_d}{\sigma_d / \sqrt{n}} \qquad (7.4.2)$$

It is unlikely that σ_d will be known in practice.

If the assumption of normally distributed d_i's cannot be made, the central limit theorem may be employed if n is large. In such cases, the test statistic is Equation 7.4.2, with s_d used to estimate σ_d when, as is generally the case, the latter is unknown.

Disadvantages The use of the paired comparisons test is not without its problems. If different subjects are used and randomly assigned to two treatments, considerable time and expense may be involved in our trying to match individuals on one or more relevant variables. A further price we pay for using paired comparisons is a loss of degrees of freedom. If we do not use paired observations we have $2n - 2$ degrees of freedom available as compared to $n - 1$ when we use the paired comparisons procedure.

In general, in deciding whether or not to use the paired comparisons procedure, one should be guided by the economics involved as well as by a consideration of the gains to be realized in terms of controlling extraneous variation.

Alternatives If neither z nor t is an appropriate test statistic for use with available data, one may wish to consider using some nonparametric technique to test a hypothesis about a median difference. The sign test, discussed in Chapter 13, is a candidate for use in such cases.

EXERCISES

In the following exercises carry out the nine-step hypothesis testing procedure at the specified significance level. Determine the p value for each test.

7.4.1 A journal article by Kashima et al. (A-12) describes research with parents of mentally retarded children in which a media-based program presented, primarily through videotapes and instructional manuals, information on self-help skill teaching. As part of the study 17 families participated in a training program led by experienced staff members of a parent training project. Before and after the training program the Behavioral Vignettes Test was administered to the primary parent in each family. The test assesses knowledge of behavior modification principles. A higher score indicates greater knowledge. The following are the pre- and post-training scores made by the primary parent on the test:

Pre:	7	6	10	16	8	13	8	14	16	11	12	13	9	10	17	8	5
Post:	11	14	16	17	9	15	9	17	20	12	14	15	14	15	18	15	9

SOURCE: Bruce L. Baker, Ph.D. Used by permission.

May we conclude, on the basis of these data, that the training program increases knowledge of behavior modification principles? Let $\alpha = .01$.

7.4.2 Schwartz et al. (A-13) conducted a study to test the hypotheses that weight loss in apneic patients results in decreases in upper airway critical pressure (Pcrit) and that these decreases are associated with reductions in apnea severity. The study subjects were patients referred to the Johns Hopkins Sleep Disorder Center and in whom obstructive sleep apnea was newly diagnosed. Patients were invited to participate in either a weight loss program (experimental group) or a "usual care" program (control group). Among the data collected during the course of the study were the following before and after Pcrit (cm H_2O) scores for the weight-loss subjects:

Before:	−2.3	5.4	4.1	12.5	.4	−.6	2.7	2.7	−.3	3.1	4.9	8.9	−1.5
After:	−6.3	.2	−5.1	6.6	−6.8	−6.9	−2.0	−6.6	−5.2	3.5	2.2	−1.5	−3.2

SOURCE: Alan R. Schwartz, M.D. Used by permission.

May we conclude on the basis of these data that the weight-loss program was effective in decreasing upper airway Pcrit? Let $\alpha = .01$.

7.4.3. The purpose of an investigation by Alahuhta et al. (A-14) was to evaluate the influence of extradural block for elective caesarean section simultaneously on several maternal and fetal hemodynamic variables and to determine if the block modified fetal myocardial function. The study subjects were eight healthy parturients in gestational weeks 38–42 with uncomplicated singleton pregnancies undergoing elective caesarean section under extradural anesthesia. Among the measurements taken were maternal diastolic arterial pressures during two stages of the study. The following are the lowest values of this variable at the two stages.

Stage 1:	70	87	72	70	73	66	63	57
Stage 2:	79	87	73	77	80	64	64	60

SOURCE: Seppo Alahuhta, M.D. Used by permission.

Do these data provide sufficient evidence, at the .05 level, to indicate that, in general under similar conditions, mean maternal diastolic arterial pressure is different at the two stages?

7.4.4. Wolin et al. (A-15) demonstrated that long-wavelength ultraviolet (UV) light promotes relaxation, promotes increased metabolism of H_2O_2 via catalase, and stimulates nonmitochondrial consumption of O_2 in the vascular smooth muscle of the bovine pulmonary artery. They also demonstrate that hypoxia and cyanide inhibit UV light-elicited relaxation and catalase-dependent H_2O_2 metabolism by bovine pulmonary arterial smooth muscle. Among the measurements made by the investigators were the following measurements (nmoles/g/min) of formaldehyde production from methanol by pulmonary arterial smooth muscle during irradiation with UV light in the absence (A) and presence (P) of cyanide (1 mM NaCN).

A:	1.850	.177	.564	.140	.128	.500	.000	.759	.332
P:	.000	.000	.000	.140	.000	.000	.000	.000	.332

SOURCE: Michael S. Wolin, Ph.D. Used by permission.

Do these data provide sufficient evidence, at the .05 level, to support the investigators' claim that cyanide inhibits UV light-elicited relaxation?

7.4.5. The purposes of an investigation by Mancebo et al. (A-16) were (1) to evaluate the acute effects of β_2-agonist bronchodilator albuterol inhalation on the work of breathing (WOB), gas exchange, and ventilatory pattern in spontaneously breathing intubated patients during weaning from mechanical ventilation and (2) to ascertain whether or not the changes in WOB induced by such inhalation are related to a specific bronchodilator effect. Subjects were intubated adult patients (mean age, 59.5 years) recovering from acute respiratory failure and meeting other technical criteria. The following WOB values (Joules/min) were obtained from the subjects before (1) and after (2) inhalation of albuterol:

Patient	COND	WOB
1	1	6.972
1	2	5.642
2	1	4.850
2	2	3.634
3	1	8.280
3	2	5.904
4	1	19.437
4	2	18.865
5	1	14.500
5	2	13.400
6	1	10.404
6	2	8.832
7	1	9.856
7	2	7.560
8	1	4.531
8	2	4.546
9	1	6.732
9	2	5.893
10	1	7.371
10	2	5.512
11	1	6.037
11	2	4.239
12	1	12.600
12	2	11.784
13	1	11.067
13	2	12.621
14	1	5.959
14	2	4.978
15	1	11.739
15	2	11.590

SOURCE: Dr. Jorge Mancebo. Used by permission.

Do these data provide sufficient evidence to allow us to conclude that, in general under similar conditions, albuterol inhalation has an effect on mean WOB? Let $\alpha = .01$.

7.5
Hypothesis Testing: A Single Population Proportion

Testing hypotheses about population proportions is carried out in much the same way as for means when the conditions necessary for using the normal curve are met. One-sided or two-sided tests may be made, depending on the question being asked. When a sample sufficiently large for application of the central limit theorem is available for analysis, the test statistic is

$$z = \frac{\hat{p} - p_0}{\sqrt{\dfrac{p_0 q_0}{n}}} \tag{7.5.1}$$

which, when H_0 is true, is distributed approximately as the standard normal.

Example 7.5.1   In a survey of injection drug users in a large city, Coates et al. (A-17) found that 18 out of 423 were HIV positive. We wish to know if we can conclude that fewer than 5 percent of the injection drug users in the sampled population are HIV positive.

Solution:

1. *Data*   The data are obtained from the responses of 423 individuals of which 18 possessed the characteristic of interest, that is, $\hat{p} = 18/423 = .0426$.

2. *Assumptions*   The sampling distribution of $\hat{p}$ is approximately normally distributed in accordance with the central limit theorem.

3. *Hypotheses*

$$H_0: p \geq .05$$
$$H_A: p < .05$$

We conduct the test at the point of equality. The conclusion we reach will be the same that we would reach if we conducted the test using any other hypothesized value of p greater than .05. If H_0 is true, $p = .05$ and the standard error, $\sigma_{\hat{p}} = \sqrt{(.05)(.95)/423}$. Note that we use the hypothesized value of p in computing $\sigma_{\hat{p}}$. We do this because the entire test is based on the assumption that the null hypothesis is true. To use the sample proportion, $\hat{p}$, in computing $\sigma_{\hat{p}}$ would not be consistent with this concept.

4. *Test Statistic*   The test statistic is given by Equation 7.5.1.

5. *Distribution of Test Statistic*   If the null hypothesis is true, the test statistic is approximately normally distributed with a mean of zero.

6. *Decision Rule* Let $\alpha = .05$. The critical value of z is -1.645. Reject H_0 if the computed z is ≤ -1.645.

7. *Calculation of Test Statistic*

$$z = \frac{.0426 - .05}{\sqrt{\dfrac{(.05)(.95)}{423}}} = -.70$$

8. *Statistical Decision* Do not reject H_0 since $-.70 > -1.645$.

9. *Conclusion* We conclude that in the population the proportion who are HIV positive may be .05 or more.

EXERCISES

For each of the following exercises, carry out the nine-step hypothesis testing procedure at the designated level of significance. Compute the p value for each test.

7.5.1 Diana M. Bailey conducted a study to examine the reasons why occupational therapists have left the field of occupational therapy (A-18). Her sample consisted of female certified occupational therapists who had left the profession either permanently or temporarily. Out of 696 subjects who responded to the data-gathering survey, 63 percent had planned to take time off from their jobs to have and raise children. On the basis of these data can we conclude that, in general, more than 60 percent of the subjects in the sampled population had planned to take time off to have and raise children? Let $\alpha = .05$. What is the sampled population? What assumptions are necessary to make your procedure valid?

7.5.2 In an article in the *American Journal of Public Health*, Colsher et al. (A-19) describe the results of a health survey of 119 male inmates 50 years of age and older residing in a state's correctional facilities. They found that 21.6 percent of the respondents reported a history of venereal disease. On the basis of these findings, can we conclude that in the sampled population more than 15 percent have a history of a venereal disease? Let $\alpha = .05$.

7.5.3 Henning et al. (A-20) found that 66 percent of a sample of 670 infants had completed the hepatitis B vaccine series. Can we conclude on the basis of these data that, in the sampled population, more than 60 percent have completed the series? Let $\alpha = .05$.

7.5.4 The following questionnaire was completed by a simple random sample of 250 gynecologists. The number checking each response is shown in the appropriate box.

1. When you have a choice, which procedure do you prefer for obtaining samples of endometrium?

   a. Dilation and curettage | 175 |

   b. Vobra aspiration | 75 |

2. Have you seen one or more pregnant women during the past year whom you knew to have elevated blood lead levels?

a. Yes `25`

b. No `225`

3. Do you routinely acquaint your pregnant patients who smoke with the suspected hazards of smoking to the fetus?

a. Yes `238`

b. No `12`

Can we conclude from these data that in the sampled population more than 60 percent prefer dilation and curettage for obtaining samples of endometrium? Let $\alpha = .01$.

7.5.5 Refer to Exercise 7.5.4. Can we conclude from these data that in the sampled population fewer than 15 percent have seen (during the past year) one or more pregnant women with elevated blood lead levels? Let $\alpha = .05$.

7.5.6 Refer to Exercise 7.5.4. Can we conclude from these data that more than 90 percent acquaint their pregnant patients who smoke with the suspected hazards of smoking to the fetus? Let $\alpha = .05$.

7.6
Hypothesis Testing: The Difference Between Two Population Proportions

The most frequent test employed relative to the difference between two population proportions is that their difference is zero. It is possible, however, to test that the difference is equal to some other value. Both one-sided and two-sided tests may be made.

When the null hypothesis to be tested is $p_1 - p_2 = 0$, we are hypothesizing that the two population proportions are equal. We use this as justification for combining the results of the two samples to come up with a pooled estimate of the hypothesized common proportion. If this procedure is adopted, one computes

$$\bar{p} = \frac{x_1 + x_2}{n_1 + n_2}$$

where x_1 and x_2 are the numbers in the first and second samples, respectively, possessing the characteristic of interest. This pooled estimate of $p = p_1 = p_2$ is used in computing $\hat{\sigma}_{\hat{p}_1 - \hat{p}_2}$, the estimated standard error of the estimator, as follows

$$\hat{\sigma}_{\hat{p}_1 - \hat{p}_2} = \sqrt{\frac{\bar{p}(1 - \bar{p})}{n_1} + \frac{\bar{p}(1 - \bar{p})}{n_2}} \qquad (7.6.1)$$

The test statistic becomes

$$z = \frac{(\hat{p}_1 - \hat{p}_2) - (p_1 - p_2)_0}{\hat{\sigma}_{\hat{p}_1 - \hat{p}_2}} \tag{7.6.2}$$

which is distributed approximately as the standard normal if the null hypothesis is true.

Example 7.6.1

In a study of nutrition care in nursing homes Lan and Justice (A-21) found that among 55 patients with hypertension, 24 were on sodium-restricted diets. Of 149 patients without hypertension, 36 were on sodium-restricted diets. May we conclude that in the sampled populations the proportion of patients on sodium-restricted diets is higher among patients with hypertension than among patients without hypertension?

Solution:

1. *Data* The data consist of information regarding the sodium status of the diets of nursing-home patients with and without hypertension as described in the statement of the example.

2. *Assumptions* We assume that the patients in the study constitute independent simple random samples from populations of patients with and without hypertension.

3. *Hypotheses*

$$H_0: p_H \leq p_{\overline{H}} \quad \text{or} \quad p_H - p_{\overline{H}} \leq 0$$

$$H_A: p_H > p_{\overline{H}} \quad \text{or} \quad p_H - p_{\overline{H}} > 0$$

where p_H is the proportion on sodium-restricted diets in the population of hypertensive patients and $p_{\overline{H}}$ is the proportion on sodium-restricted diets in the population of patients without hypertension.

4. *Test Statistic* The test statistic is given by Equation 7.6.2.

5. *Distribution of the Test Statistic* If the null hypothesis is true, the test statistic is distributed approximately as the standard normal.

6. *Decision Rule* Let $\alpha = .05$. The critical value of z is 1.645. Reject H_0 if computed z is greater than 1.645.

7. *Calculation of Test Statistic* From the sample data we compute $\hat{p}_H = 24/55 = .4364$, $\hat{p}_{\overline{H}} = 36/149 = .2416$, and $\bar{p} = (24 + 36)/(55 + 149) = .2941$. The computed value of the test statistic, then, is

$$z = \frac{(.4364 - .2416)}{\sqrt{\dfrac{(.2941)(.7059)}{55} + \dfrac{(.2941)(.7059)}{149}}} = 2.71$$

8. *Statistical Decision*   Reject H_0 since $2.71 > 1.645$.

9. *Conclusion*   The proportion of patients on sodium-restricted diets is higher among hypertensive patients than among patients without hypertension ($p = .0034$).

EXERCISES

In each of the following exercises use the nine-step hypothesis testing procedure. Determine the p value for each test.

7.6.1   Babaian and Camps (A-22) state that prostate-specific antigen (PSA), found in the ductal epithelial cells of the prostate, is specific for prostatic tissue and is detectable in serum from men with normal prostates and men with either benign or malignant diseases of this gland. They determined the PSA values in a sample of 124 men who underwent a prostate biopsy. Sixty-seven of the men had elevated PSA values ($> 4 \, \text{ng/ml}$). Of these, 46 were diagnosed as having cancer. Ten of the 57 men with PSA values $\leq 4 \, \text{ng/ml}$ had cancer. On the basis of these data may we conclude that, in general, men with elevated PSA values are more likely to have prostate cancer? Let $\alpha = .01$.

7.6.2   Most people who quit smoking complain of subsequent weight gain. Hall et al. (A-23) designed an innovative intervention for weight gain prevention, which they compared to two other conditions including a standard treatment control condition designed to represent standard care of cessation-induced weight gain. One of the investigators' hypotheses was that smoking abstinence rates in the innovative intervention would be greater than those in the other two conditions. Of 53 subjects assigned to the innovative condition, 11 were not smoking at the end of 52 weeks. Nineteen of the 54 subjects assigned to the control condition were abstinent at the end of the same time period. Do these data provide sufficient evidence to support, at the .05 level, the investigators' hypothesis?

7.6.3   Research has suggested a high rate of alcoholism among patients with primary unipolar depression. An investigation by Winokur and Coryell (A-24) further explores this possible relationship. In 210 families of females with primary unipolar major depression, they found that alcoholism was present in 89. Of 299 control families, alcoholism was present in 94. Do these data provide sufficient evidence for us to conclude that alcoholism is more likely to be present in families of subjects with unipolar depression? Let $\alpha = .05$.

7.6.4   In a study of obesity the following results were obtained from samples of males and females between the ages of 20 and 75:

	n	Number Overweight
Males	150	21
Females	200	48

Can we conclude from these data that in the sampled populations there is a difference in the proportions who are overweight? Let $\alpha = .05$.

7.7
Hypothesis Testing: A Single Population Variance

In Section 6.9 we examined how it is possible to construct a confidence interval for the variance of a normally distributed population. The general principles presented in that section may be employed to test a hypothesis about a population variance. When the data available for analysis consist of a simple random sample drawn from a normally distributed population, the test statistic for testing hypotheses about a population variance is

$$\chi^2 = (n - 1)s^2/\sigma^2 \qquad (7.7.1)$$

which, when H_0 is true, is distributed as χ^2 with $n - 1$ degrees of freedom.

**Example
7.7.1**

The purpose of a study by Gundel et al. (A-25) was to examine the release of preformed and newly generated mediators in the immediate response to allergen inhalation in allergic primates. Subjects were 12 wild-caught, adult male cynomolgus monkeys meeting certain criteria of the study. Among the data reported by the investigators was a standard error of the sample mean of .4 for one of the mediators recovered from the subjects by bronchoalveolar lavage (BAL). We wish to know if we may conclude from these data that the population variance is not 4.

Solution:

1. *Data*   See statement in the example.

2. *Assumptions*   The study sample constitutes a simple random sample from a population of similar animals. The values of the mediator are normally distributed.

3. *Hypotheses*

$$H_0: \sigma^2 = 4$$
$$H_A: \sigma^2 \neq 4$$

4. *Test Statistic*   The test statistic is given by Equation 7.7.1

5. *Distribution of Test Statistic*   When the null hypothesis is true, the test statistic is distributed as χ^2 with $n - 1$ degrees of freedom.

6. *Decision Rule*   Let $\alpha = .05$. Critical values of χ^2 are 3.816 and 21.920. Reject H_0 unless the computed value of the test statistic is between 3.816 and 21.920. The rejection and nonrejection regions are shown in Figure 7.7.1.

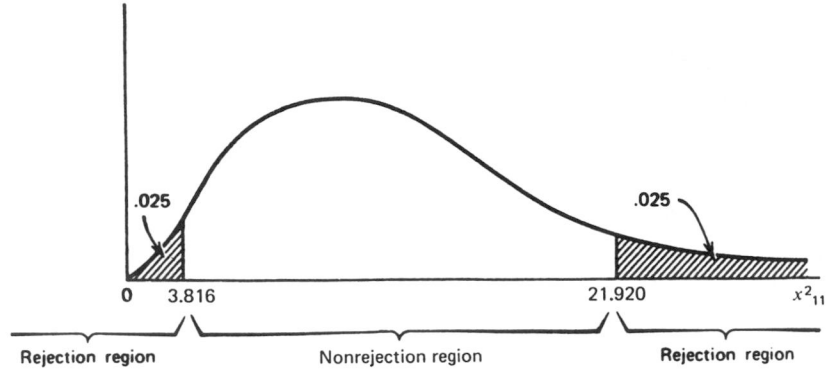

Figure 7.7.1   Rejection and nonrejection regions for Example 7.7.1.

7. *Calculation of Test Statistic*

$$s^2 = 12(.4)^2 = 1.92$$

$$\chi^2 = \frac{(11)(1.92)}{4} = 5.28$$

8. *Statistical Decision*   Do not reject H_0 since $3.816 < 5.28 < 21.920$.

9. *Conclusion*   Based on these data we are unable to conclude that the population variance is not 4.

One-Sided Tests   Although this was an example of a two-sided test, one-sided tests may also be made by logical modification of the procedure given here.

For $H_A: \sigma^2 > \sigma_0^2$, reject H_0 if computed $\chi^2 \geq \chi_{1-\alpha}^2$.

For $H_A: \sigma_2 < \sigma_0^2$, reject H_0 if computed $\chi^2 \leq \chi_{\alpha}^2$.

Determining the *p* Value   The determination of the p value for this test is complicated by the fact that we have a two-sided test and an asymmetric sampling distribution. When we have a two-sided test and a symmetric sampling distribution such as the standard normal or t, we may, as we have seen, double the one-sided p value. Problems arise when we attempt to do this with an asymmetric sampling distribution such as the chi-square distribution. Gibbons and Pratt (1) suggest that in this situation the one-sided p value be reported along with the direction of the observed departure from the null hypothesis. In fact, this procedure may be followed in the case of symmetric sampling distributions. Precedent, however, seems to favor doubling the one-sided p value when the test is two-sided and involves a symmetric sampling distribution.

For the present example, then, we may report the p value as follows:

$p > .05$ (two-sided test). A population variance less than 4 is suggested by the sample data, but this hypothesis is not strongly supported by the test.

If the problem is stated in terms of the population standard deviation, one may square the sample standard deviation and perform the test as indicated above.

EXERCISES

In each of the following exercises carry out the nine-step testing procedure. Determine the p value for each test.

7.7.1 Infante et al. (A-26) carried out a validation study of the dose-to-mother deuterium dilution method to measure breastmilk intake. Subjects were 10 infants hospitalized in a Nutrition Recovery Centre in Santiago, Chile. Among the data collected and analyzed was a measure of water intake from which the investigators computed a standard deviation of 124 (ml/day). We wish to know if we may conclude that the population standard deviation is less than 175? Let $\alpha = .05$.

7.7.2 Greenwald and Henke (A-27) compared treatment and mortality risks between prostate cancer patients receiving care in fee-for-service settings and those receiving care in a health maintenance organization (HMO). Among other findings, the investigators reported, for a sample of 44 HMO patients, a value of 2.33 for the standard error of the sample mean income. Do these data provide sufficient evidence to indicate that the population standard deviation is less than 18? Let $\alpha = .01$.

7.7.3 Vital capacity values were recorded for a sample of 10 patients with severe chronic airway obstruction. The variance of the 10 observations was .75. Test the null hypothesis that the population variance is 1.00. Let $\alpha = .05$.

7.7.4 Hemoglobin (gm %) values were recorded for a sample of 20 children who were part of a study of acute leukemia. The variance of the observations was 5. Do these data provide sufficient evidence to indicate that the population variance is greater than 4? Let $\alpha = .05$.

7.7.5 A sample of 25 administrators of large hospitals participated in a study to investigate the nature and extent of frustration and emotional tension associated with the job. Each participant was given a test designed to measure the extent of emotional tension he or she experienced as a result of the duties and responsibilities associated with the job. The variance of the scores was 30. Can it be concluded from these data that the population variance is greater than 25? Let $\alpha = .05$.

7.7.6 In a study in which the subjects were 15 patients suffering from pulmonary sarcoid disease, blood gas determinations were made. The variance of the Pa_{O_2} (mm Hg) values was 450. Test the null hypothesis that the population variance is greater than 250. Let $\alpha = .05$.

7.7.7   Analysis of the amniotic fluid from a simple random sample of 15 pregnant women yielded the following measurements on total protein (grams per 100 ml) present:

$$.69, 1.04, .39, .37, .64, .73, .69, 1.04$$
$$.83, 1.00, .19, .61, .42, .20, .79$$

Do these data provide sufficient evidence to indicate that the population variance is greater than .05? Let $\alpha = .05$. What assumptions are necessary?

7.8
Hypothesis Testing: The Ratio of Two Population Variances

As we have seen, the use of the t distribution in constructing confidence intervals and in testing hypotheses for the difference between two population means assume that the population variances are equal. As a rule, the only hints available about the magnitudes of the respective variances are the variances computed from samples taken from the populations. We would like to know if the difference that, undoubtedly, will exist between the sample variances is indicative of a real difference in population variances, or if the difference is of such magnitude that it could have come about as a result of chance alone when the population variances are equal.

Two methods of chemical analysis may give the same results on the average. It may be, however, that the results produced by one method are more variable than the results of the other. We would like some method of determining whether this is likely to be true.

Variance Ratio Test   Decisions regarding the comparability of two population variances are usually based on the *variance ratio test*, which is a test of the null hypothesis that two population variances are equal. When we test the hypothesis that two population variances are equal, we are, in effect, testing the hypothesis that their ratio is equal to 1.

We learned in the preceding chapter that, when certain assumptions are met, the quantity $(s_1^2/\sigma_1^2)/(s_2^2/\sigma_2^2)$ is distributed as F with $n_1 - 1$ numerator degrees of freedom and $n_2 - 1$ denominator degrees of freedom. If we are hypothesizing that $\sigma_1^2 = \sigma_2^2$, we assume that the hypothesis is true, and the two variances cancel out in the above expression leaving s_1^2/s_2^2, which follows the same F distribution. The ratio s_1^2/s_2^2 will be designated V.R. for variance ratio.

For a two-sided test, we follow the convention of placing the larger sample variance in the numerator and obtaining the critical value of F for $\alpha/2$ and the appropriate degrees of freedom. However, for a one-sided test, which of the two sample variances is to be placed in the numerator is predetermined by the statement of the null hypothesis. For example, for the null hypothesis that $\sigma_1^2 \leq \sigma_2^2$, the appropriate test statistic is V.R. $= s_1^2/s_2^2$. The critical value of F is obtained for α (not $\alpha/2$) and the appropriate degrees of freedom. In like manner, if the null hypothesis is that $\sigma_1^2 \geq \sigma_2^2$, the appropriate test statistic is V.R. $= s_2^2/s_1^2$. In all cases, the decision rule is to reject the null hypothesis if the computed V.R. is equal to or greater than the critical value of F.

Example 7.8.1

Behr et al. (A-28) investigated alterations of thermoregulation in patients with certain pituitary adenomas (P). The standard deviation of the weights of a sample of 12 patients was 21.4 kg. The weights of a sample of five control subjects (C) yielded a standard deviation of 12.4 kg. We wish to know if we may conclude that the weights of the population represented by the sample of patients are more variable than the weights of the population represented by the sample of control subjects.

Solution

1. *Data*   See the statement of the example.

2. *Assumptions*   Each sample constitutes a simple random sample of a population of similar subjects. The samples are independent. The weights in both populations are approximately normally distributed.

3. *Hypotheses*

$$H_0: \sigma_P^2 \leq \sigma_C^2$$
$$H_A: \sigma_P^2 > \sigma_C^2$$

4. *Test Statistic*

$$\text{V.R.} = s_P^2/s_C^2$$

5. *Distribution of Test Statistic*   When the null hypothesis is true, the test statistic is distributed as F with $n_P - 1$ numerator and $n_C - 1$ denominator degrees of freedom.

6. *Decision Rule*   Let $\alpha = .05$. The critical value of F, from Table G, is 5.91. Note that Table G does not contain an entry for 11 numerator degrees of freedom and, therefore, 5.91 is obtained by using 12, the closest value to 11 in the table. Reject H_0 if V.R. ≥ 5.91. The rejection and nonrejection regions are shown in Figure 7.8.1.

7. *Calculation of Test Statistic*

$$\text{V.R.} \frac{(21.4)^2}{(12.4)^2} = 2.98$$

8. *Statistical Decision*   We cannot reject H_0, since $2.98 < 5.91$; that is, the computed ratio falls in the nonrejection region.

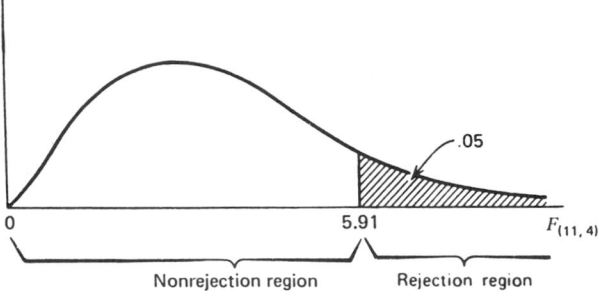

Figure 7.8.1 Rejection and nonrejection regions, Example 7.8.1.

---

9. *Conclusion*   The weights of the population of patients may not be any more variable than the weights of control subjects. Since the computed V.R. of 2.98 is less than 3.90, the p value for this test is greater than .10.

EXERCISES

In the following exercises perform the nine-step test. Determine the p value for each test.

7.8.1 Perry et al. (A-29) conducted a study to determine whether a correlation exists between clozapine concentrations and therapeutic response. The subjects were patients with a diagnosis of schizophrenia who met other criteria. At the end of four weeks of clozapine treatment they were classified as responders or nonresponders. The standard deviation of scores on the Brief Psychiatric Rating Scale (BPRS) was 2.6 among 11 responders and 7.7 among 18 nonresponders at the end of the treatment period. May we conclude on the basis of these data that, in general, the variance of BPRS scores among nonresponders is greater than among responsers? Let $\alpha = .05$.

7.8.2 Studenski et al. (A-30) conducted a study in which the subjects were older persons with unexplained falls (fallers) and well elderly persons (controls). Among the findings reported by the investigators were statistics on tibialis anterior (TA) latency (msec). The standard deviation was 23.7 for a sample of 10 fallers and 15.7 for a sample of 24 controls. Do these data provide sufficient evidence for us to conclude that the variability of the scores on this variable differ between the populations represented by the fallers and the controls? Let $\alpha = .05$.

7.8.3 A test designed to measure level of anxiety was administered to a sample of male and a sample of female patients just prior to undergoing the same surgical procedure. The sample sizes and the variances computed from the scores were as follows:

$$\text{Males:} \quad n = 16, \quad s^2 = 150$$
$$\text{Females:} \quad n = 21, \quad s^2 = 275$$

Do these data provide sufficient evidence to indicate that in the represented populations the scores made by females are more variable than those made by males? Let $\alpha = .05$.

7.8.4 In an experiment to assess the effects on rats of exposure to cigarette smoke, 11 animals were exposed and 11 control animals were not exposed to smoke from unfiltered cigarettes. At the end of the experiment measurements were made of the frequency of the ciliary beat (beats/min at $20° C$) in each animal. The variance for the exposed group was 3400 and 1200 for the unexposed group. Do these data indicate that in the populations represented the variances are different? Let $\alpha = .05$.

7.8.5 Two pain-relieving drugs were compared for effectiveness on the basis of length of time elapsing between administration of the drug and cessation of pain. Thirteen patients received drug 1 and 13 received drug 2. The sample variances were $s_1^2 = 64$ and $s_2^2 = 16$. Test the null hypothesis that the two population variances are equal. Let $\alpha = .05$.

7.8.6 Packed cell volume determinations were made on two groups of children with cyanotic congenital heart disease. The sample sizes and variances were as follows:

Group	n	s^2
1	10	40
2	16	84

Do these data provide sufficient evidence to indicate that the variance of population 2 is larger than the variance of population 1? Let $\alpha = .05$.

7.8.7. Independent simple random samples from two strains of mice used in an experiment yielded the following measurements on plasma glucose levels following a traumatic experience:

Strain A: 54, 99, 105, 46, 70, 87, 55, 58, 139, 91

Strain B: 93, 91, 93, 150, 80, 104, 128, 83, 88, 95, 94, 97

Do these data provide sufficient evidence to indicate that the variance is larger in the population of strain A mice than in the population of strain B mice? Let $\alpha = .05$. What assumptions are necessary?

7.9
The Type II Error and the Power
of a Test

In our discussion of hypothesis testing our focus has been on α, the probability of committing a type I error (rejecting a true null hypothesis). We have paid scant attention to β, the probability of committing a type II error (failing to reject a false null hypothesis). There is a reason for this difference in emphasis. For a given test, α is a single number assigned by the investigator in advance of performing the test. It is a measure of the acceptable risk of rejecting a true null hypothesis. On the other hand, β may assume one of many values. Suppose we wish to test the null hypothesis that some population parameter is equal to some specified value. If H_0 is false and we fail to reject it, we commit a type II error. If the hypothesized value of the parameter is not the true value, the value of β (the probability of committing a type II error) depends on several factors: (1) the true value of the parameter of interest, (2) the hypothesized value of the parameter, (3) the value of α, and (4) the sample size, n. For fixed α and n, then, we may, before performing a hypothesis test, compute many values of β by postulating many values for the parameter of interest given that the hypothesized value is false.

For a given hypothesis test it is of interest to know how well the test controls type II errors. If H_0 is in fact false, we would like to know the probability that we will reject it. The *power* of a test, designated $1 - \beta$, provides this desired information. The quantity $1 - \beta$ is the probability that we will reject a false null hypothesis; it may be computed for any alternative value of the parameter about which we are testing a hypothesis. Therefore, $1 - \beta$ is the probability that we will take the correct action when H_0 is false because the true parameter value is equal to the one for which we computed $1 - \beta$. For a given test we may specify any number of possible values of the parameter of interest and for each compute the value of $1 - \beta$. The result is called a *power function*. The graph of a power function, called a *power curve*, is a helpful device for quickly assessing the nature of the power of a given test. The following example illustrates the procedures we use to analyze the power of a test.

Example 7.9.1

Suppose we have a variable whose values yield a population standard deviation of 3.6. From the population we select a simple random sample of size $n = 100$. We select a value of $\alpha = .05$ for the following hypotheses

$$H_0: \mu = 17.5, \qquad H_A: \mu \neq 17.5$$

Solution: When we study the power of a test, we locate the rejection and nonrejection regions on the $\bar{x}$ scale rather than the z scale. We find the critical values of $\bar{x}$ for a two-sided test using the following formulas:

$$\bar{x}_U = \mu_0 + z\frac{\sigma}{\sqrt{n}} \qquad (7.9.1)$$

and

$$\bar{x}_L = \mu_0 - z\frac{\sigma}{\sqrt{n}} \qquad (7.9.2)$$

where $\bar{x}_U$ and $\bar{x}_L$ are the upper and lower critical values, respectively, of $\bar{x}$; $+z$ and $-z$ are the critical values of z; and μ_0 is the hypothesized value of μ. For our example, we have

$$\bar{x}_U = 17.50 + 1.96\frac{(3.6)}{(10)} = 17.50 + 1.96(.36)$$

$$= 17.50 + .7056 = 18.21$$

and

$$\bar{x}_L = 17.50 - 1.96(.36) = 17.50 - .7056 = 16.79$$

Suppose that H_0 is false, that is, that μ is not equal to 17.5. In that case, μ is equal to some value other than 17.5. We do not know the actual value of μ. But if H_0 is false, μ is one of the many values that are greater than or smaller than 17.5. Suppose that the true population mean is $\mu_1 = 16.5$. Then the sampling distribution of $\bar{x}_1$ is also approximately normal, with $\mu_{\bar{x}} = \mu = 16.5$. We call this sampling distribution $f(\bar{x}_1)$, and we call the sampling distribution under the null hypothesis $f(\bar{x}_0)$.

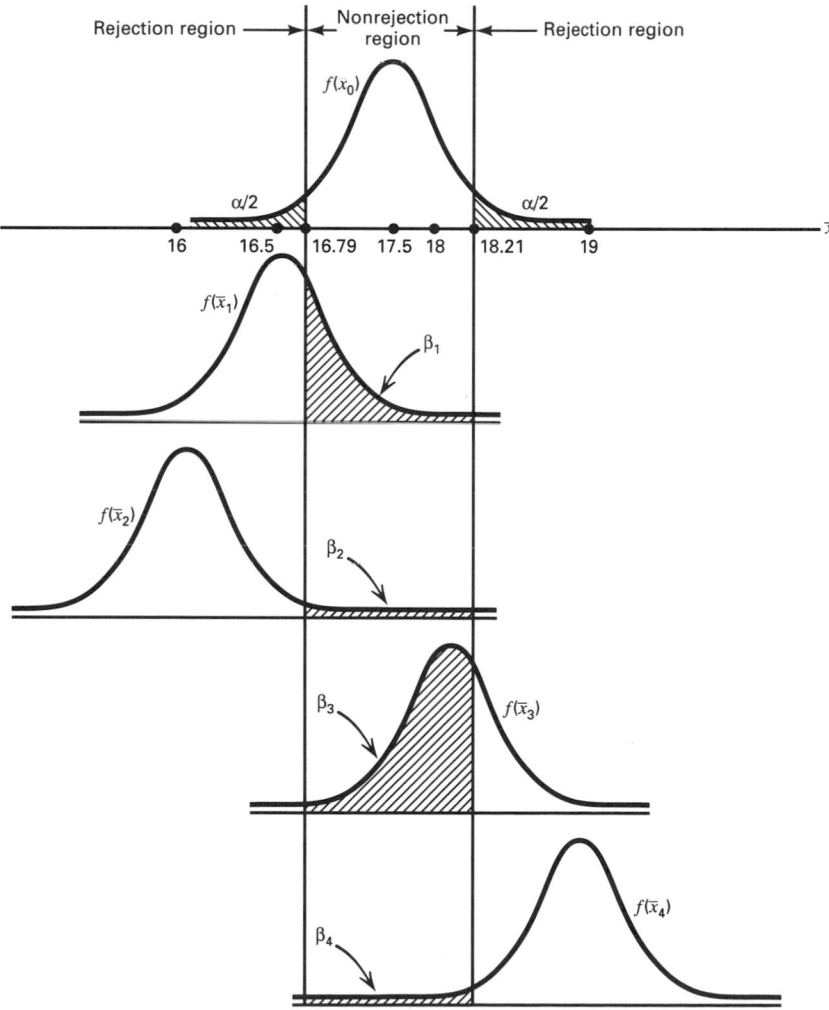

Figure 7.9.1 Size of β for selected values for H_1 for Example 7.9.1.

TABLE 7.9.1 Values of β and $1 - \beta$ for Selected Alternative Values of μ_1, Example 7.9.1

Possible Values of μ Under H_1 When H_0 is False	β	$1 - \beta$
16.0	0.0143	0.9857
16.5	0.2090	0.7910
17.0	0.7190	0.2810
18.0	0.7190	0.2810
18.5	0.2090	0.7910
19.0	0.0143	0.9857

β, the probability of the type II error of failing to reject a false null hypothesis, is the area under the curve of $f(\bar{x}_1)$ that overlaps the nonrejection region specified under H_0. To determine the value of β, we find the area under $f(\bar{x}_1)$, above the $\bar{x}$ axis, and between $\bar{x} = 16.79$ and $\bar{x} = 18.21$. The value of β is equal to $P(16.79 \leq \bar{x} \leq 18.21)$ when $\mu = 16.5$. This is the same as

$$P\left(\frac{16.79 - 16.5}{.36} \leq z \leq \frac{18.21 - 16.5}{.36} \right) = P\left(\frac{.29}{.36} \leq z \leq \frac{1.71}{.36} \right)$$

$$= P(.81 \leq z \leq 4.75)$$

$$\approx 1 - .7910 - .2090$$

Thus the probability of taking an appropriate action (that is, rejecting H_0) when the null hypothesis states that $\mu = 17.5$, but in fact $\mu = 16.5$, is $1 - .2090 = .7910$. As we noted, μ may be one of a large number of possible values when H_0 is false. Figure 7.9.1 shows a graph of several such possibilities. Table 7.9.1 shows the corresponding values of β and $1 - \beta$ (which are approximate), along with the values of β for some additional alternatives.

Note that in Figure 7.9.1 and Table 7.9.1 those values of μ under the alternative hypothesis that are closer to the value of μ specified by H_0 have larger associated β values. For example, when $\mu = 18$ under the alternative hypothesis, $\beta = .7190$; and when $\mu = 19.0$ under H_1, $\beta = .0143$. The power of the test for these two alternatives, then, is $1 - .7190 = .2810$ and $1 - .0143 = .9857$, respectively. We show the power of the test graphically in a power curve, as in Figure 7.9.2. Note that the higher the curve, the greater the power.

Although only one value of α is associated with a given hypothesis test, there are many values of β, one for each possible value of μ if μ_0 is not the true value of μ as hypothesized. Unless alternative values of μ are much larger or smaller than μ_0, β is relatively large compared with α. Typically, we use hypothesis-testing procedures more often in those cases in which, when H_0 is false, the true value of the parameter is fairly close to the hypothesized value. In most cases, β, the computed probability of failing to reject a false null hypothesis, is larger than α,

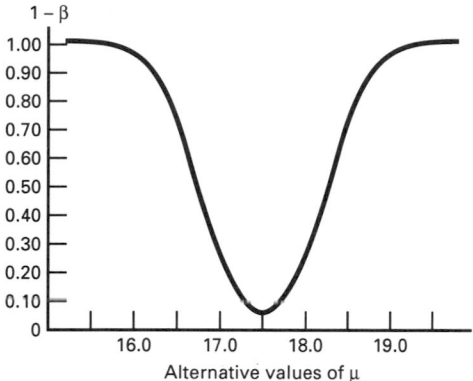

Figure 7.9.2 Power curve for Example 7.9.1.

the probability of rejecting a true null hypothesis. These facts are compatible with our statement that a decision based on a rejected null hypothesis is more conclusive than a decision based on a null hypothesis that is not rejected. The probability of being wrong in the latter case is generally larger than the probability of being wrong in the former case.

Figure 7.9.2 shows the V-shaped appearance of a power curve for a two-sided test. In general, a two-sided test that discriminates well between the value of the parameter in H_0 and values in H_1 results in a narrow V-shaped power curve. A wide V-shaped curve indicates that the test discriminates poorly over a relatively wide interval of alternative values of the parameter.

Power Curves for One-Sided Tests   The shape of a power curve for a one-sided test with the rejection region in the upper tail is an elongated S. If the rejection of a one-sided test is located in the lower tail of the distribution, the power curve takes the form of a reverse elongated S. The following example shows the nature of the power curve for a one-sided test.

Example 7.9.2   The mean time laboratory employees now take to do a certain task on a machine is 65 seconds, with a standard deviation of 15 seconds. The times are approximately normally distributed. The manufacturers of a new machine claim that their machine will reduce the mean time required to perform the task. The quality-control supervisor designs a test to determine whether or not she should believe the claim of the makers of the new machine. She chooses a significance level of $\alpha = 0.01$ and randomly selects 20 employees to perform the task on the new machine. The hypotheses are

$$H_0: \mu \geq 65, \qquad H_A: \mu < 65$$

The quality-control supervisor also wishes to construct a power curve for the test.

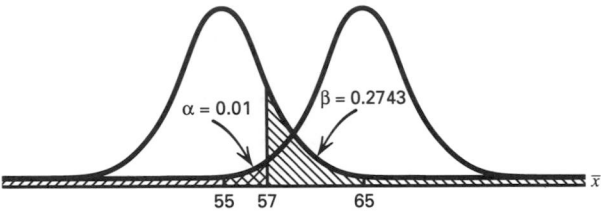

Figure 7.9.3 β calculated for $\mu = 55$.

Solution: The quality control supervisor computes, for example, the following value of $1 - \beta$ for the alternative $\mu = 55$. The critical value of $\bar{x}$ for the test is

$$65 - 2.33\left(\frac{15}{\sqrt{20}}\right) = 57$$

We find β as follows:

$$\beta = P(\bar{x} > 57 | \mu = 55) = P\left(z > \frac{57 - 55}{15/\sqrt{20}}\right) = P(z > .60)$$

$$= 1 - .7257 = .2743$$

Consequently, $1 - \beta = 1 - .2743 = .7257$. Figure 7.9.3 shows the calculation of β. Similar calculations for other alternative values of μ also yield values of $1 - \beta$. When plotted against the values of μ, these give the power curve shown in Figure 7.9.4.

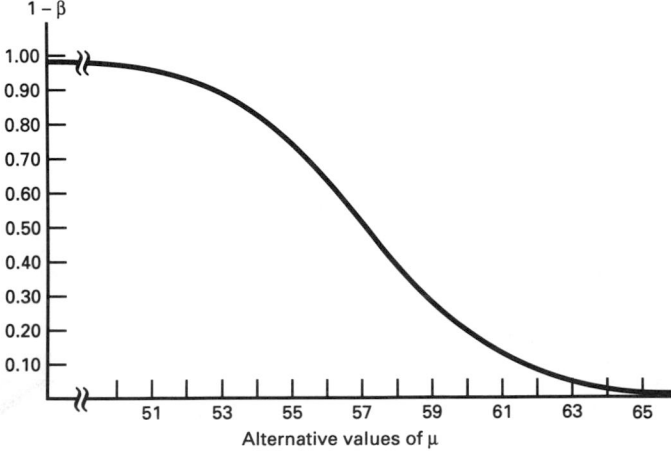

Figure 7.9.4 Power curve for Example 7.9.2.

Operating Characteristic Curves Another way of evaluating a test is to look at its *operating characteristic* (OC) *curve*. To construct an OC curve, we plot values of β, rather than $1 - \beta$, along the vertical axis. Thus an OC curve is the complement of the corresponding power curve.

EXERCISES

Construct and graph the power function for each of the following situations.

7.9.1 $H_0. \ \mu \leq 516,$ $H_A. \ \mu > 516,$ $n = 16, \ \sigma = 32, \ \alpha = 0.05.$

7.9.2 $H_0: \mu = 3,$ $H_A: \mu \neq 3,$ $n = 100, \ \sigma = 1, \ \alpha = 0.05.$

7.9.3 $H_0: \mu \leq 4.25,$ $H_A: \mu > 4.25,$ $n = 81, \ \sigma = 1.8, \ \alpha = 0.01.$

7.10
Determining Sample Size to Control Both Type I and Type II Errors

You learned in Chapter 6 how to find the sample sizes needed to construct confidence intervals for population means and proportions for specified levels of confidence. You learned in Chapter 7 that confidence intervals may be used to test hypotheses. The method of determining sample size presented in Chapter 6 takes into account the probability of a type I error, but not a type II error since the level of confidence is determined by the confidence coefficient, $1 - \alpha$.

In many statistical inference procedures, the investigator wishes to consider the type II error as well as the type I error when determining the sample size. To illustrate the procedure, we refer again to Example 7.9.2.

Example 7.10.1

In Example 7.9.2, the hypotheses are

$$H_0: \mu \geq 65, \qquad H_A: \mu < 65$$

The population standard deviation is 15, and the probability of a type I error is set at .01. Suppose that we want the probability of failing to reject H_0 (β) to be .05 if H_0 is false because the true mean is 55 rather than the hypothesized 65. How large a sample do we need in order to realize, simultaneously, the desired levels of α and β.

Solution: For $\alpha = .01$ and $n = 20$, β is equal to .2743. The critical value is 57. Under the new conditions, the critical value is unknown. Let us call this new critical value C. Let μ_0 be the hypothesized mean and μ_1 the mean under the

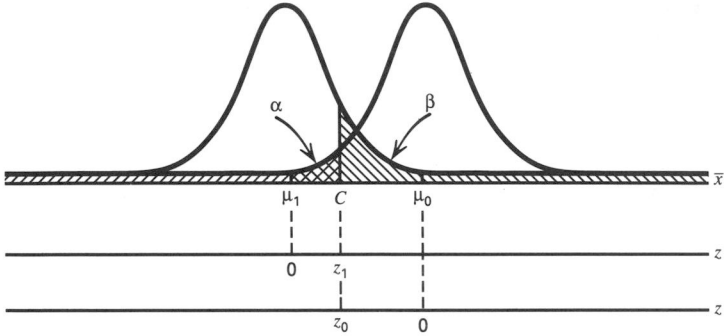

Figure 7.10.1   Graphic representation of relationships in determination of sample size to control both type I and type II errors.

alternative hypothesis. We can transform each of the relevant sampling distributions of $\bar{x}$, the one with a mean of μ_0 and the one with a mean of μ_1, to a z distribution. Therefore we can convert C to a z value on the horizontal scale of each of the two standard normal distributions. When we transform the sampling distribution of $\bar{x}$ that has a mean of μ_0 to the standard normal distribution, we call the z that results z_0. When we transform the sampling distribution of $\bar{x}$ that has a mean of μ_1 to the standard normal distribution, we call the z that results z_1. Figure 7.10.1 represents the situation described so far.

We can express the critical value C as a function of z_0 and μ_0 and also as a function of z_1 and μ_1. This gives the following equations:

$$C = \mu_0 - z_0 \frac{\sigma}{\sqrt{n}} \tag{7.10.1}$$

$$C = \mu_1 + z_1 \frac{\sigma}{\sqrt{n}} \tag{7.10.2}$$

We set the right-hand sides of these equations equal to each other and solve for n, to obtain

$$n = \left[\frac{(z_0 + z_1)\sigma}{(\mu_0 - \mu_1)} \right]^2 \tag{7.10.3}$$

To find n for our illustrative example, we substitute appropriate quantities into Equation 7.10.3. We have $\mu_0 = 65$, $\mu_1 = 55$, and $\sigma = 15$. From Table D of Appendix II, the value of z that has .01 of the area to its left is -2.33. The value of z that has .05 of the area to its right is 1.645. Both z_0 and z_1 are taken as positive. We determine whether C lies above or below either μ_0 or μ_1 when we substitute into Equations 7.10.1 and 7.10.2. Thus, we compute

$$n = \left[\frac{(2.33 + 1.645)(15)}{(65 - 55)} \right]^2 = 35.55$$

We would need a sample of size 36 to achieve the desired levels of α and β when we choose $\mu_1 = 55$ as the alternative value of μ.

We now compute C, the critical value for the test, and state an appropriate decision rule. To find C, we may substitute known numerical values into either Equation 7.10.1 or Equation 7.10.2. For illustrative purposes, we solve both equations for C. First we have

$$C = 65 - 2.33\left(\frac{15}{\sqrt{36}}\right) = 59.175$$

From Equation 7.10.2, we have

$$C = 55 + 1.645\left(\frac{15}{\sqrt{36}}\right) = 59.1125$$

The difference between the two results is due to rounding error.

The decision rule, when we use the first value of C, is as follows.

Select a sample of size 36 *and compute* $\bar{x}$. *If* $\bar{x} \leq 59.175$, *reject* H_0. *If* $\bar{x} > 59.175$, *do not reject* H_0.

We have limited our discussion of the type II error and the power of a test to the case involving a population mean. The concepts extend to cases involving other parameters.

EXERCISES

7.10.1 Given H_0: $\mu \leq 516$, H_A: $\mu > 516$, $n = 16$, $\sigma = 32$, $\alpha = .05$. Let $\beta = .10$ and $\mu_1 = 520$, and find n and C. State the appropriate decision rule.

7.10.2 Given H_0: $\mu \leq 4.500$, H_A: $\mu > 4.500$, $n = 16$, $\sigma = .020$, $\alpha = .01$. Let $\beta = .05$ and $\mu_1 = 4.52$, and find n and C. State the appropriate decision rule.

7.10.3 Given H_0: $\mu \leq 4.25$, H_A: $\mu > 4.25$, $n = 81$, $\sigma = 1.8$, $\alpha = .01$. Let $\beta = .03$ and $\mu_1 = 5.00$, and find n and C. State the appropriate decision rule.

7.11
Summary

In this chapter the general concepts of hypothesis testing are discussed. A general procedure for carrying out a hypothesis test consisting of the following nine steps is suggested.

1. Description of data.

2. Statement of necessary assumptions.

3. Statement of null and alternative hypotheses.

4. Specification of the test statistic.

5. Specification of the distribution of the test statistic.

6. Statement of the decision rule.

7. Calculation of test statistic from sample data.

8. The statistical decision based on sample results.

9. Conclusion.

A number of specific hypothesis tests are described in detail and are illustrated with appropriate examples. These include tests concerning population means, the difference between two population means, paired comparisons, population proportions, the difference between two population proportions, a population variance, and the ratio of two population variances. In addition we discuss the power of a test and the determination of sample size for controlling both type I and type II errors.

REVIEW QUESTIONS AND EXERCISES

1. What is the purpose of hypothesis testing?

2. What is a hypothesis?

3. List and explain each step in the nine-step hypothesis testing procedure.

4. Define
   a. Type I error
   b. Type II error
   c. The power of a test
   d. Power function
   e. Power curve
   f. Operating characteristic curve

5. Explain the difference between the power curves for one-sided tests and two-sided tests.

6. Explain how one decides what statement goes into the null hypothesis and what statement goes into the alternative hypothesis.

7. What are the assumptions underlying the use of the t statistic in testing hypotheses about a single mean? The difference between two means?

8. When may the z statistic be used in testing hypotheses about
   a. A single population mean?
   b. The difference between two population means?
   c. A single population proportion?
   d. The difference between two population proportions?

9. In testing a hypothesis about the difference between two population means, what is the rationale behind pooling the sample variances?

10. Explain the rationale behind the use of the paired comparisons test.

11. Give an example from your field of interest where a paired comparisons test would be appropriate. Use real or realistic data and perform an appropriate hypothesis test.

12. Give an example from your field of interest where it would be appropriate to test a hypothesis about the difference between two population means. Use real or realistic data and carry out the nine-step hypothesis testing procedure.

13. Do Exercise 12 for a single population mean.

14. Do Exercise 12 for a single population proportion.

15. Do Exercise 12 for the difference between two population proportions.

16. Do Exercise 12 for a population variance.

17. Do Exercise 12 for the ratio of two population variances.

18. Dr. Yue Chen (A-31), in an article in the *American Journal of Public Health*, presents information on some factors associated with the infant-feeding practices of mothers in Shanghai. This investigator found that, among 1706 male infants, 35.9 percent were artificially fed. Among 1579 female infants, 32.9 percent were artificially fed. Is the proportion of artificially fed infants significantly higher among males than females? Let $\alpha = .10$.

19. Rodriguez-Roisin et al. (A-32) state that methacholine (MTH) inhalation challenge is by far one of the most widely used tools for the diagnosis of asthma. They investigated the pattern and time course of ventilation-profusion ($\dot{V}A/\dot{Q}$) inequality after challenge to better define the model of MTH bronchial challenge in patients with asymptomatic mild asthma. Among the data collected from the 16 subjects in the study were the following Pa_{O_2} measurements before (B) and after (A) challenge by MTH.

Case#	B	A
1	88.2	70.6
2	100.9	70.0
3	96.0	71.0
4	99.1	64.1
5	86.9	79.5
6	103.7	79.5
7	76.0	72.2
8	81.8	70.6
9	72.1	66.9
10	93.7	67.0
11	98.3	67.2
12	77.5	71.6
13	73.5	71.5
14	91.7	71.1
15	97.4	77.0
16	73.5	66.4

SOURCE: Robert Rodriguez-Roisin, M.D.
Used with permission.

Do these data provide sufficient evidence to indicate that MTH causes a decrease in Pa_{O_2}? Let $\alpha = .05$.

20. Darko et al. (A-33) evaluated the utility of mitogen-induced lymphocyte proliferation assays in clinical research in psychoimmunology. Study respondents were patients with a diagnosis of major depressive disorder who met other study criteria and medically and psychiatrically healthy comparison subjects. Among the data collected were scores on the Brief Psychiatric Rating Scale (BPRS) by two groups of subjects. Group A patients fit the hypothesis of lessened immune response in depression and group B patients responded better than their matched comparison subjects. The BPRS depression subscales scores by subjects in the two groups were as follows:

Group A	Group B
12	17
13	14
12	19
12	15
9	8
7	19
8	12
5	20
10	9
13	10
15	12
11	
7	

SOURCE: Denis F. Darko, M. D.
Used with permission.

May we conclude on the basis of these data that, in general, group B patients, on the average, score higher on the BPRS depression subscale? Let $\alpha = .05$.

21. Nace et al. (A-34) conducted a study to assess the complex relationship between substance abuse and personality disorders. The authors determined the prevalence of personality disorders in a group of middle-class substance abusers and compared the subjects who had personality disorders with those who did not. Among the data reported were the following statistics on the depression component of the Minnesota Multiphasic Personality Inventory (MMPI).

With Personality Disorders			Without Personality Disorders		
n	$\bar{x}$	s	n	$\bar{x}$	s
57	70.63	16.27	43	64.33	12.99

SOURCE: Edgar P. Nace, Carlos W. Davis, and Joseph P. Gaspari, "Axis I Comorbidity in Substance Abusers," *American Journal of Psychiatry*, *148* (1991), 118–120.

May we conclude on the basis of these data that, in general, substance abusers with and without personality disorders differ with respect to their mean scores on the depression component of the MMPI? Let $\alpha = .05$.

22. Researchers wish to know if urban and rural adult residents of a developing country differ with respect to the prevalence of blindness. A survey revealed the following

information:

Group	Number in Sample	Number Blind
Rural	300	24
Urban	500	15

Do these data provide sufficient evidence to indicate a difference in the prevalence of blindness in the two populations? Let $\alpha = .05$. Determine the p value.

23. During an experiment using laboratory animals the following data on renal cortical blood flow during control conditions and during the administration of a certain anesthetic were recorded.

Animal Number	Renal Cortical Blood Flow (ml / g / min)	
	Control	**During Administration of Anesthetic**
1	2.35	2.00
2	2.55	1.71
3	1.95	2.22
4	2.79	2.71
5	3.21	1.83
6	2.97	2.14
7	3.44	3.72
8	2.58	2.10
9	2.66	2.58
10	2.31	1.32
11	3.43	3.70
12	2.37	1.59
13	1.82	2.07
14	2.98	2.15
15	2.53	2.05

Can one conclude on the basis of these data that the anesthetic retards renal cortical blood flow? Let $\alpha = .05$. Determine the p value.

24. An allergy research team conducted a study in which two groups of subjects were used. As part of the research, blood eosinophil determinations were made on each subject with the following results:

Sample	n	Eosinophil Value (no./ mm^3)	
		$\bar{x}$	s
A	14	584	225
B	16	695	185

Do these data provide sufficient evidence to indicate that the population means are different? Let $\alpha = .05$. Determine the p value.

25. A survey of 90 recently delivered women on the rolls of a county welfare department revealed that 27 had a history of intrapartum or postpartum infection. Test the null hypothesis that the population proportion with a history of intrapartum or postpartum infection is less than or equal to .25. Let $\alpha = .05$. Determine the p value.

26. In a sample of 150 hospital emergency admissions with a certain diagnosis, 128 listed vomiting as a presenting symptom. Do these data provide sufficient evidence to indicate, at the .01 level of significance, that the population proportion is less than .92? Determine the p value.

27. A research team measured tidal volume in 15 experimental animals. The mean and standard deviation were 45 and 5 cc, respectively. Do these data provide sufficient evidence to indicate that the population mean is greater than 40 cc? Let $\alpha = .05$.

28. A sample of eight patients admitted to a hospital with a diagnosis of biliary cirrhosis had a mean IgM level of 160.55 units per milliliter. The sample standard deviation was 50. Do these data provide sufficient evidence to indicate that the population mean is greater than 150? Let $\alpha = .05$. Determine the p value.

29. Some researchers have observed a greater airway resistance in smokers than in non-smokers. Suppose a study, conducted to compare the percent tracheobronchial retention of particles in smoking-discordant monozygotic twins, yielded the following results:

Percent Retention	
Smoking Twin	**Nonsmoking Twin**
60.6	47.5
12.0	13.3
56.0	33.0
75.2	55.2
12.5	21.9
29.7	27.9
57.2	54.3
62.7	13.9
28.7	8.9
66.0	46.1
25.2	29.8
40.1	36.2

Do these data support the hypothesis that tracheobronchial clearance is slower in smokers? Let $\alpha = .05$. Determine the p value for this test.

30. Circulating levels of estrone were measured in a sample of 25 postmenopausal women following estrogen treatment. The sample mean and standard deviation were 73 and 16, respectively. At the .05 significance level can one conclude on the basis of these data that the population mean is higher than 70?

31. Systemic vascular resistance determinations were made on a sample of 16 patients with chronic, congestive heart failure while receiving a particular treatment. The sample mean and standard deviation were 1600 and 700, respectively. At the .05 level of significance do these data provide sufficient evidence to indicate that the population mean is less than 2000?

32. The mean length at birth of 14 male infants was 53 cm with a standard deviation of 9 cm. Can one conclude on the basis of these data that the population mean is not 50 cm? Let the probability of committing a type I error be .10.

For each of the studies described in Exercises 33 through 38, answer as many of the following questions as possible: (a) What is the variable of interest? (b) Is the parameter of interest a mean, the difference between two means (independent samples), a mean difference (paired data), a proportion, or the difference between two proportions (independent samples)? (c) What is the sampled population? (d) What is the target population? (e) What are the null and alternative hypotheses? (f) Is the alternative hypothesis one-sided (left tail), one-sided (right tail), or two-sided? (g) What type I and type II errors are possible? (h) Do you think the null hypothesis was rejected? Explain why or why not.

33. Jara et al. (A-35) conducted a study in which they found that the potassium concentration in the saliva from Down's syndrome patients was significantly lower than that of control individuals.

34. In a study by Hemming et al. (A-36), 50 consecutive patients undergoing segmental hepatic resection during a three-year time period were reviewed. Student's t tests were used to analyze the data. Among the findings was the fact that cirrhotic patients showed a significantly increased transfusion requirement of 2.0 ± 1.3 U versus 0.7 ± 1.3 U.

35. Sokas et al. (A-37) reported on a study in which second-year medical students participated in a training program that focused on the risks of bloodborne-disease exposure and the techniques of phlebotomy and intravenous insertion using universal precautions. The students answered pre- and posttraining knowledge questions and rated their preparedness on a five-point scale. The researchers found that the students' knowledge and self-assessed preparedness scores increased.

36. Wu et al. (A-38) conducted a study to determine the effect of zidovudine on functional status and well-being in patients with early symptomatic human immunodeficiency virus (HIV). Thirty-four subjects were assigned at random to placebo and 36 subjects to zidovudine. The mean changes from baseline for zidovudine versus placebo groups were compared. Subjects receiving a placebo reported better quality of life compared to baseline than subjects receiving zidovudine at 24 weeks for all dimensions of well-being, including overall health, energy, mental health, health distress, pain, and quality of life.

37. Stockwell et al. (A-39) categorized 15 establishments licensed to sell alcohol in metropolitan Perth, Western Australia, as either high risk (seven establishments) or low risk (eight establishments) on the basis of incidence of customers involved in road traffic accidents and drunk-driving offences. Subjects were 414 customers exiting from the chosen establishments between 8 P.M. and midnight on Friday and Saturday nights. They found that high-risk establishments had three times more customers whose breathalyser readings were in excess of 0.15 mg/ml ($p < 0.01$). They also found that significantly more patrons from high-risk establishments than from low-risk establishments were rated as appearing moderately or severely intoxicated but refused to be breath-tested.

38. Is the frequency of biotinidase deficiency greater in children with unexplained developmental delay or neurologic abnormalities than in the general population? This question was investigated by Sutherland et al. (A-40). They studied 274 children seen at a large outpatient clinic over a four-year period who had one or more of these neurologic abnormalities and for whom no specific cause for their abnormalities could be found. None of the patients with nonclassic biotinidase-deficiency findings had a deficiency of biotinidase activity.

39. For each of the following situations, identify the type I and type II errors and the correct actions.

    (a) H_0: A new treatment is not more effective than the traditional one.

        (1) Adopt the new treatment when the new one is more effective.

        (2) Continue with the traditional treatment when the new one is more effective.

        (3) Continue with the traditional treatment when the new one is not more effective.

        (4) Adopt the new treatment when the new one is not more effective.

    (b) H_0: A new physical therapy procedure is satisfactory.

        (1) Employ a new procedure when it is unsatisfactory.

        (2) Do not employ a new procedure when it is unsatisfactory.

        (3) Do not employ a new procedure when it is satisfactory.

        (4) Employ a new procedure when it is satisfactory.

    (c) H_0: A production run of a drug is of satisfactory quality.

        (1) Reject a run of satisfactory quality.

        (2) Accept a run of satisfactory quality.

        (3) Reject a run of unsatisfactory quality.

        (4) Accept a run of unsatisfactory quality.

Exercises for Use With Large Data Sets Available on Computer Disk from the Publisher

1. Refer to the creatine phosphokinase data on 1005 subjects (PCKDATA, Disk 1). Researchers would like to know if psychologically stressful situations cause an increase in serum creatine phosphokinase (CPK) levels among apparently healthy individuals. To help the researchers reach a decision, select a simple random sample from this population, perform an appropriate analysis of the sample data, and give a narrative report of your findings and conclusions. Compare your results with those of your classmates.

2. Refer to the prothrombin time data on 1000 infants (PROTHROM, Disk 1). Select a simple random sample of size 16 from each of these populations and conduct an appropriate hypothesis test to determine whether one should conclude that the two populations differ with respect to mean prothrombin time. Let $\alpha = .05$. Compare your results with those of your classmates. What assumptions are necessary for the validity of the test?

3. Refer to the head circumference data of 1000 matched subjects (HEADCIRC, Disk 1). Select a simple random sample of size 20 from the population and perform an appropriate hypothesis test to determine if one can conclude that subjects with the sex chromosome abnormality tend to have smaller heads than normal subjects. Let $\alpha = .05$. Construct a 95 percent confidence interval for the population mean difference. What assumptions are necessary? Compare your results with those of your classmates.

4. Refer to the hemoglobin data on 500 children with iron deficiency anemia and 500 apparently healthy children (HEMOGLOB, Disk 1). Select a simple random sample of size 16 from population A and an independent simple random sample of size 16 from population B. Do your sample data provide sufficient evidence to indicate that the two populations differ with respect to mean Hb value? Let $\alpha = .05$. What assumptions are necessary for your procedure to be valid? Compare your results with those of your classmates.

5. Refer to the manual dexterity scores of 500 children with learning disabilities and 500 children with no known learning disabilities (MANDEXT, Disk 1). Select a simple random sample of size 10 from population A and an independent simple random sample of size 15 from population B. Do your samples provide sufficient evidence for you to conclude that learning-disabled children, on the average, have lower manual dexterity scores than children without a learning disability? Let $\alpha = .05$. What assumptions are necessary in order for your procedure to be valid? Compare your results with those of your classmates.

REFERENCES

References Cited

1. Jean D. Gibbons and John W. Pratt, "*P*-values: Interpretation and Methodology," *The American Statistician, 29* (1975), 20–25.

2. Anita K. Bahn, "*P* and the Null Hypothesis," *Annals of Internal Medicine, 76* (1972), 674.

3. Wayne W. Daniel, "What are *p*-values? How Are They Calculated? How Are They Related to Levels of Significance?" *Nursing Research, 26* (1977), 304–306.

4. Larry A. Morgan and Frank W. Morgan, "Personal Computers, *p*-values and Hypotheses Testing," *Mathematics Teacher, 77* (1984), 473–478.

5. Wayne W. Daniel, *Introductory Statistics with Applications*, Houghton Mifflin, Boston, 1977.

Other References, Journal Articles

1. Arnold Binder, "Further Considerations of Testing the Null Hypothesis and the Strategy and Tactics of Investigating Theoretical Models," *Psychological Review, 70* (1963), 107–115.

2. C. Allen Boneau, "The Effects of Violations of Assumptions Underlying the *t* Test," *Psychological Bulletin, 57* (1960), 49–64.

3. Donna R. Brogan, "Choosing an Appropriate Statistical Test of Significance for a Nursing Research Hypothesis or Question," *Western Journal of Nursing, 3* (1981), 337–363.

4. C. J. Burke, "A Brief Note on One-tailed Tests," *Psychological Bulletin, 50* (1953), 384–387.

5. C. J. Burke, "Further Remarks on One-tailed Tests," *Psychological Bulletin, 51* (1954), 587–590.

6. Wayne W. Daniel, "Statistical Significance versus Practical Significance," *Science Education, 61* (1977) 423–427.

7. Eugene S. Edgington, "Statistical Inference and Nonrandom Samples," *Psychological Bulletin, 66* (1966), 485–487.

8. Ward Edwards, "Tactical Note on the Relation Between Scientific and Statistical Hypotheses," *Psychological Bulletin, 63* (1965), 400–402.

9. William E. Feinberg, "Teaching the Type I and II Errors: The Judicial Process," *The American Statistician*, 25 (June 1971), 30–32.

10. I. J. Good, "What Are Degrees of Freedom?" *The American Statistician, 27* (1973), 227–228.

11. David A. Grant, "Testing the Null Hypothesis and the Strategy and Tactics of Investigating Theoretical Models," *Psychological Review, 69* (1962), 54–61.

12. W. E. Hick, "A Note on One-tailed and Two-tailed Tests," *Psychological Review, 59* (1952), 316–318.

13. L. V. Jones, "Tests of Hypotheses: One-sided vs. Two-sided Alternatives," *Psychological Bulletin, 46* (1949), 43–46.

14. L. V. Jones, "A Rejoinder on One-tailed Tests," *Psychological Bulletin, 51* (1954), 585–586.

15. Sanford Labovitz, "Criteria for Selecting a Significance Level: A Note on the Sacredness of .05," *The American Sociologist, 3* (1968), 220–222.

16. William Lurie, "The Impertinent Questioner: The Scientist's Guide to the Statistician's Mind," *American Scientist*, *46* (1958), 57–61.

17. M. R. Marks, "One- and Two-tailed Tests," *Psychological Review*, *60* (1953), 207–208.

18. C. A. McGilchrist and J. Y. Harrison, "Testing of Means with Different Alternatives," *Technometrics*, *10* (1968), 195–198.

19. Mary G. Natrella, "The Relation Between Confidence Intervals and Tests of Significance," *American Statistician*, *14* (1960), 20–22, 33.

20. O. B. Ross, Jr., "Use of Controls in Medical Research," *Journal of the American Medical Association*, *145*, (1951), 72–75.

21. William W. Rozeboom, "The Fallacy of the Null-Hypothesis Significance Test," *Psychological Bulletin*, *57* (1960), 416–428.

22. H. C. Selvin, "A Critique of Tests of Significance in Survey Research," *American Sociological Review*, *22* (1957), 519–527.

23. James K. Skipper, Anthony L. Guenther, and Gilbert Nass, "The Sacredness of .05: A Note Concerning the Uses of Significance in Social Science," *The American Sociologist*, *2* (1967), 16–18.

24. Warren R. Wilson and Howard Miller, "A Note on the Inconclusiveness of Accepting the Null Hypothesis," *Psychological Review*, *71* (1964), 238–242.

25. Warren Wilson, Howard L. Miller, and Jerold S. Lower, "Much Ado About the Null Hypothesis," *Psychological Bulletin*, *67* (1967), 188–196.

26. R. F. Winch and D. T. Campbell, "Proof? No. Evidence? Yes. The Significance of Tests of Significance," *American Sociologist*, *4* (1969), 140–143.

Other References, Books

1. W. I. B. Beveridge, *The Art of Scientific Investigation*, Third Edition, W. W. Norton, New York, 1957.

2. Herbert A. David, *The Method of Paired Comparisons*, Second Edition, Oxford University Press, New York, 1988.

3. Dwight J. Ingle, *Principles of Research in Biology and Medicine*, J. B. Lippincott, Philadelphia, 1958.

4. E. L. Lehman, *Testing Statistical Hypotheses*, Wiley, New York, 1959.

5. Stanley Lemeshow, David W. Hosmer, Jr., Janelle Klar, and Stephen K. Lwanga, *Adequacy of Sample Size in Health Studies*, John Wiley & Sons, Ltd., Chichester, 1990.

Other References, Other Publications

1. David Bakan, "The Test of Significance in Psychological Research," in *One Method: Toward a Reconstruction of Psychological Investigation*, Jossey-Bass, San Francisco, 1967.

2. William H. Kruskal, "Tests of Significance," in *International Encyclopedia of the Social Sciences*, *14* (1968), 238–250.

Applications References

A-1. Charles E. Castillo and Stephen Lillioja, "Peripheral Lymphatic Cannulation for Physiological Analysis of Interstitial Fluid Compartment in Humans," *American Journal of Physiology*, 261 (*Heart and Circulation Physiology*, *30*), (October 1991), H1324–H1328.

A-2. JoEllen Wilbur, Alice Dan, Cynthia Hedricks, and Karyn Holm, "The Relationship Among Menopausal Status, Menopausal Symptoms, and Physical Activity in Midlife Women," *Family & Community Health*, *13* (November 1990), 67–78.

A-3. Joseph S. Bertino, Jr., Leigh Ann Booker, Patrick Franck, and Benjamin Rybicki, "Gentamicin Pharmacokinetics in Patients with Malignancies," *Antimicrobial Agents and Chemotherapy*, *35* (1991), 1501–1503.

A-4. Lisa M. Klesges, Robert C. Klesges, and Jeffrey A. Cigrang, "Discrepancies Between Self-reported Smoking and Carboxyhemoglobin: An Analysis of the Second National Health and Nutrition Survey," *American Journal of Public Health*, *82* (1992), 1026–1029.

A-5. Jeffrey M. Barrett, "Funic Reduction for the Management of Umbilical Cord Prolapse," *American Journal of Obstetrics and Gynecology*, *165* (1991), 654–657.

A-6. D. H. Eidelman, H. Ghezzo, W. D. Kim, and M. G. Cosio, "The Destructive Index and Early Lung Destruction in Smokers," *American Review of Respiratory Disease*, *144* (1991), 156–159.

A-7. Heather Becker, Alexa K. Stuifbergen, and Dolores Sands, "Development of a Scale to Measure Barriers to Health Promotion Activities Among Persons with Disabilities," *American Journal of Health Promotion*, *5* (1991), 449–454.

A-8. Scott L. Evans, Brent P. Nixon, Irvin Lee, David Yee, and Arshag D. Mooradian, "The Prevalence and Nature of Podiatric Problems in Elderly Diabetic Patients," *Journal of the American Geriatrics Society*, *39* (1991), 241–245.

A-9. Mirjam J. T. Hommes, Johannes A. Romijn, Erik Endert, and Hans P. Sauerwein, "Resting Energy Expenditure and Substrate Oxidation in Human Immunodeficiency Virus (HIV)-infected Asymptomatic Men: HIV Affects Host Metabolism in the Early Asymptomatic Stage," *American Journal of Clinical Nutrition*, *54* (1991), 311–315.

A-10. Christian Frigerio, Yves Schutz, Roger Whitehead, and Eric Jéquier, "A New Procedure to Assess the Energy Requirements of Lactation in Gambian Women," *American Journal of Clinical Nutrition*, *54* (1991), 526–533.

A-11. Nancy Stearns Burgess, "Effect of a Very-Low-Calorie Diet on Body Composition and Resting Metabolic Rate in Obese Men and Women," *Journal of the American Dietetic Association*, *91* (1991), 430–434.

A-12. Kathleen J. Kashima, Bruce L. Baker, and Sandra J. Landen, "Media-Based Versus Professionally Led Training for Parents of Mentally Retarded Children," *American Journal on Mental Retardation*, *93* (1988), 209–217.

A-13. Alan R. Schwartz, Avram R. Gold, Norman Schubert, Alexandra Stryzak, Robert A. Wise, Solbert Permutt, and Philip L. Smith, "Effect of Weight Loss on Upper Airway Collapsibility in Obstructive Sleep Apnea," *American Review of Respiratory Disease*, *144* (1991), 494–498.

A-14. S. Alahuhta, J. Räsänen, R. Jouppila, P. Jouppila, T. Kangas-Saarela, and A. I. Hollmen, "Uteroplacental and Fetal Haemodynamics During Extradural Anaesthesia for Caesarean Section," *British Journal of Anaesthesia*, *66* (1991), 319–323.

A-15. Michael S. Wolin, Hatim A. Omar, Michael P. Mortelliti, and Peter D. Cherry, "Association of Pulmonary Artery Photorelaxation with H_2O_2 Metabolism by Catalase," *American Journal of Physiology*, *261* (*Heart Circulation Physiology*, *30*), 1991, H1141–H1147.

A-16. Jorge Mancebo, Piedade Amaro, Hubert Lorino, FranÇois Lemaire, Alain Harf, and Laurent Brochard, "Effects of Albuterol Inhalation on the Work of Breathing During Weaning from Mechanical Ventilation," *American Review of Respiratory Disease*, *144* (1991), 95–100.

A-17. Randall Coates, Margaret Millson, Ted Myers, James Rankin, Bernadette McLaughlin, Carol Major, Janet Rigby, and William Mindell, "The Benefits of HIV Antibody Testing of Saliva in Field Research," *Canadian Journal of Public Health*, *82* (1991), 397–398.

A-18. Diana M. Bailey, "Reasons for Attrition from Occupational Therapy," *The American Journal of Occupational Therapy*, *44* (1990), 23–29. Copyright 1990 by the American Occupational Therapy Association, Inc. Reprinted with permission.

A-19. Patricia L. Colsher, Robert B. Wallace, Paul L. Loeffelholz, and Marilyn Sales, "Health Status of Older Male Prisoners: A Comprehensive Survey," *American Journal of Public Health*, *82* (1992), 881–884.

A-20. Kelly J. Henning, Daphna M. Pollack, and Stephen M. Friedman, "A Neonatal Hepatitis B Surveillance and Vaccination Program: New York City, 1987 to 1988," *American Journal of Public Health*, *82* (1992), 885–888.

A-21. Shu-Jan J. Lan and Catherine L. Justice, "Use of Modified Diets in Nursing Homes," Copyright The American Dietetic Association. Reprinted by permission from *Journal of the American Dietetic Association*, *91* (1991), 46–51.

A-22. R. Joseph Babaian and Joseph L. Camps, "The Role of Prostate-Specific Antigen as Part of the Diagnostic Triad and as a Guide When to Perform a Biopsy," *Cancer*, *68* (1991), 2060–2063.

A-23. Sharon M. Hall, Chrystal D. Tunstall, Katharine L. Vila, and Joanne Duffy, "Weight Gain Prevention and Smoking Cessation: Cautionary Findings," *American Journal of Public Health*, *82* (1992), 799–803.

A-24. George Winokur and William Coryell, "Familial Alcoholism in Primary Unipolar Major Depressive Disorder," *American Journal of Psychiatry*, *148* (1991), 184–188.

A-25. Robert H. Gundel, Peter Kinkade, Carol A. Torcellini, Cosmos C. Clarke, Jane Watrous, Sudha Desai, Carol A. Homon, Peter R. Farina, and Craig D. Wegner, "Antigen-Induced Mediator Release in Primates," *American Review of Respiratory Disease*, *144* (1991), 76–82.

A-26. C. Infante, J. Hurtado, G. Salazar, A. Pollastri, E. Aguirre, and F. Vío, "The Dose-to-Mother Method to Measure Milk Intake in Infants by Deuterium Dilution: A Validation Study," *European Journal of Clinical Nutrition*, *45* (1991), 121–129.

A-27. Howard P. Greenwald and Curtis J. Henke, "HMO Membership, Treatment, and Mortalilty Risk Among Prostatic Cancer Patients," *American Journal of Public Health*, *82* (1992), 1099–1104.

A-28. R. Behr, G. Hildebrandt, M. Koca, and K. Brück, "Modifications of Thermoregulation in Patients with Suprasellar Pituitary Adenomas," *Brain*, *114* (1991), 697–708. Used by permission of Oxford University Press.

A-29. Paul J. Perry, Del D. Miller, Stephan V. Arndt, and Remi J. Cadoret, "Clozapine and Norclozapine Plasma Concentrations and Clinical Response of Treatment-Refractory Schizophrenic Patients," *American Journal of Psychiatry*, *148* (1991), 231–235.

A-30. Stephanie Studenski, Pamela W. Duncan, and Julie Chandler, "Postural Responses and Effector Factors in Persons with Unexplained Falls: Results and Methodologic Issues," *Journal of the American Geriatrics Society*, *39* (1991), 229–235. © American Geriatrics Society, 1991.

A-31. Yue Chen, "Factors Associated with Artificial Feeding in Shanghai," *American Journal of Public Health*, *82* (1992), 264–266.

A-32. Robert Rodriguez-Roisin, Antoni Ferrer, Daniel Navajas, Alvar G. N. Agusti, Peter D. Wagner, and Josep Roca, "Ventilation-Perfusion Mismatch after Methacholine Challenge in Patients with Mild Bronchial Asthma," *American Review of Respiratory Disease*, *144* (1991), 88–94.

A-33. Denis F. Darko, Nevin W. Wilson, J. Christian Gillin, and Shahrokh Golshan, "A Critical Appraisal of Mitogen-Induced Lymphocyte Proliferation in Depressed Patients," *American Journal of Psychiatry*, *148* (1991), 337–344.

A-34. Edgar P. Nace, Carlos W. Davis, and Joseph P. Gaspari, "Axis II Comorbidity in Substance Abusers," *American Journal of Psychiatry*, *148* (1991), 118–120.

A-35. L. Jara, A. Ondarza, R. Blanco, and L. Rivera, "Composition of the Parotid Saliva in Chilean Children With Down's Syndrome," *Archivos de Biologia Medicina Experimentales* (*Santiago*), *24* (1991), 57–60.

A-36. A. W. Hemming, C. H. Scudamore, A. Davidson, and S. R. Erb, "Evaluation of 50 Consecutive Segmental Hepatic Resections," *American Journal of Surgery*, *165* (May 1993), 621–624.

A-37. R. K. Sokas, S. Simmens, and J. Scott, "A Training Program in Universal Precautions for Second-year Medical Students," *Academic Medicine*, *68* (May 1993), 374–376.

A-38. A. W. Wu, H. R. Rubin, W. C. Mathews, L. M. Brysk, S. A. Bozzette, W. D. Hardy, J. H. Atkinson, I. Grant, S. A. Spector, J. A. McCutchan, and D. D. Richman, "Functional Status and Well-being in a Placebo-Controlled Trial of Zidovudine in Early Symptomatic HIV Infection," *Journal of Acquired Immune Deficiency Syndrome*, *6* (May 1993), 452–458.

A-39. T. Stockwell, P. Rydon, S. Gianatti, E. Jenkins, C. Ovenden, and D. Syed, "Levels of Drunkenness of Customers Leaving Licensed Premises in Perth, Western Australia: A Comparison of High and Low 'Risk' Premises," *British Journal of Addiction*, *87* (June 1992), 873–881.

A-40. S. J. Sutherland, R. D. Olsen, V. Michels, M. A. Schmidt, and J. F. O'Brien, "Screening for Biotinidase Deficiency in Children With Unexplained Neurologic or Developmental Abnormalities," *Clinical Pediatrics Philadelphia*, *30* (February 1991), 81–84.

CHAPTER 8

Analysis of Variance

. . . .

CONTENTS

8.1
Introduction

In the preceding chapters the basic concepts of statistics have been examined, and they provide a foundation for the present and succeeding chapters.

This chapter is concerned with *analysis of variance*, which may be defined as *a technique whereby the total variation present in a set of data is partitioned into two or more components. Associated with each of these components is a specific source of variation, so that in the analysis it is possible to ascertain the magnitude of the contributions of each of these sources to the total variation.*

The development of analysis of variance (ANOVA) is due mainly to the work of R. A. Fisher (1), whose contributions to statistics, spanning the years 1912 to 1962, have had a tremendous influence on modern statistical thought (2, 3).

Applications Analysis of variance finds its widest application in the analysis of data derived from experiments. The principles of the design of experiments are well covered in several books, including those of Cochran and Cox (4), Cox (5), Davies (6), Federer (7), Finney (8), Fisher (1), John (9), Kempthorne (10), Li (11), and Mendenhall (12). We do not study this topic in detail, since to do it justice would require a minimum of an additional chapter. Some of the important concepts in experimental design, however, will become apparent as we discuss analysis of variance.

Analysis of variance is used for two different purposes: (1) to estimate and test hypotheses about population variances and (2) to estimate and test hypotheses about population means. We are concerned here with the latter use. However, as we will see, our conclusions regarding the means will depend on the magnitudes of the observed variances.

As we shall see the concepts and techniques that we cover under the heading of analysis of variance are extensions of the concepts and techniques covered in Chapter 7. In Chapter 7 we learned to test the null hypothesis that two means are equal. In this chapter we learn to test the null hypothesis that three or more means are equal. Whereas, for example, what we learned in Chapter 7 enables us to determine if we can conclude that two treatments differ in effectiveness, what we learn in this chapter enables us to determine if we can conclude that three or more treatments differ in effectiveness. The following example illustrates some basic ideas involved in the application of analysis of variance. These will be extended and elaborated on later in this chapter.

Example 8.1.1

Suppose we wish to know if three drugs differ in their effectiveness in lowering serum cholesterol in human subjects. Some subjects receive drug A, some drug B, and some drug C. After a specified period of time measurements are taken to determine the extent to which serum cholesterol was reduced in each subject. We find that the amount by which serum cholesterol was lowered is not the same in all subjects. In other words, there is *variability* among the measurements. Why, we ask ourselves, are the measurements not all the same? Presumably, one reason they are not the same is that the subjects received different drugs. We now look at the measurements of those subjects who received drug A. We find that the amount by which serum cholesterol was lowered is not the same among these subjects. We find this to be the case when we look at the measurements for subjects who received drug B and those subjects who received drug C. We see that there is *variability* among the measurements within the treatment groups. Why, we ask ourselves again, are these measurements not the same? Among the reasons that come to mind are differences in the genetic makeup of the subjects and differences in their diets. Through an analysis of the *variability* that we have observed we will be able to reach a conclusion regarding the equality of the effectiveness of the three drugs. To do this we employ the techniques and concepts of analysis of variance.

Variables   In our example we alluded to three kinds of variables. We find these variables to be present in all situations in which the use of analysis of variance is appropriate. First we have the *treatment variable*, which in our example was "drug." We had three "values" of this variable, drug A, drug B, and drug C.

The second kind of variable we referred to is the *response variable*. In the example it is change in serum cholesterol. The response variable is the variable that we expect to exhibit different values when different "values" of the treatment variable are employed. Finally, we have the other variables that we mentioned—genetic composition and diet. These are called *extraneous variables*. These variables may have an effect on the response variable, but they are not the focus of our attention in the experiment. The treatment variable is the variable of primary concern, and the question to be answered is do the different "values" of the treatment variable result in differences, on the average, in the response variable?

Assumptions Underlying the valid use of analysis of variance as a tool of statistical inference are a set of fundamental assumptions. For a detailed discussion of these assumptions, refer to the paper by Eisenhart (13). Although an experimenter must not expect to find all the assumptions met to perfection, it is important that the user of analysis of variance techniques be aware of the underlying assumptions and be able to recognize when they are substantially unsatisfied. The consequences of the failure to meet the assumptions are discussed by Cochran (14) in a companion paper to that of Eisenhart. Because experiments in which all the assumptions are perfectly met are rare, Cochran suggests that analysis of variance results be considered as approximate rather than exact. These assumptions are pointed out at appropriate points in the following sections.

We discuss analysis of variance as it is used to analyze the results of two different experimental designs, the completely randomized and the randomized complete block designs. In addition to these, the concept of a factorial experiment is given through its use in a completely randomized design. These do not exhaust the possibilities. A discussion of additional designs will be found in the references (4–12).

The ANOVA Procedure In our presentation of the analysis of variance for the different designs, we follow the nine-step procedure presented in Chapter 7. The following is a restatement of the steps of the procedure, including some new concepts necessary for its adaptation to analysis of variance.

1. *Description of Data* In addition to describing the data in the usual way, we display the sample data in tabular form.

2. *Assumptions* Along with the assumptions underlying the analysis, we present the model for each design we discuss. The model consists of a symbolic representation of a typical value from the data being analyzed.

3. *Hypotheses*

4. *Test Statistic*

5. *Distribution of the Test Statistic*

6. *Decision Rule*

7. *Calculation of Test Statistic* The results of the arithmetic calculations will be summarized in a table called the analysis of variance (ANOVA) table. The entries in the table make it easy to evaluate the results of the analysis.

8. *Statistical Decision*

9. *Conclusion*

We discuss these steps in greater detail in Section 8.2.

The Use of Computers   The calculations required by analysis of variance are lengthier and more complicated than those we have encountered in preceding chapters. For this reason the computer assumes an important role in analysis of variance. All the exercises appearing in this chapter are suitable for computer analysis and may be used with the statistical packages mentioned in Chapter 1. The output of the statistical packages may vary slightly from that presented in this chapter, but this should pose no major problem to those who use a computer to analyze the data of the exercises. The basic concepts of analysis of variance that we present here should provide the necessary background for understanding the description of the programs and their output in any of the statistical packages.

8.2
The Completely Randomized Design

We saw in Chapter 7 how it is possible to test the null hypothesis of no difference between two population means. It is not unusual for the investigator to be interested in testing the null hypothesis of no difference among several population means. The student first encountering this problem might be inclined to suggest that all possible pairs of sample means be tested separately by means of the Student t test. Suppose there are five populations involved. The number of possible pairs of sample means is $_5C_2 = 10$. As the amount of work involved in carrying out this many t tests is substantial, it would be worthwhile if a more efficient alternative for analysis were available. A more important consequence of performing all possible t tests, however, is that it is very likely to lead to a false conclusion.

Suppose we draw five samples from populations having equal means. As we have seen, there would be 10 tests if we were to do each of the possible tests separately. If we select a significance level of $\alpha = .05$ for each test, the probability of failing to reject a hypothesis of no difference in each case would be .95. By the multiplication rule of probability, if the tests were independent of one another, the probability of failing to reject a hypothesis of no difference in all 10 cases would be $(.95)^{10} = .5987$. The probability of rejecting at least one hypothesis of no difference, then, would be $1 - .5987 = .4013$. Since we know that the null hypothesis is true in every case in this illustrative example, rejecting the null hypothesis constitutes the committing of a type I error. In the long run, then, in testing all possible pairs of means from five samples, we would commit a type I error 40 percent of the time.

The problem becomes even more complicated in practice, since three or more t tests based on the same data would not be independent of one another.

It becomes clear, then, that some other method for testing for a significant difference among several means is needed. Analysis of variance provides such a method.

One-Way ANOVA The simplest type of analysis of variance is that known as *one-way analysis of variance*, in which only one source of variation, or *factor*, is investigated. It is an extension to three or more samples of the t-test procedure (discussed in Chapter 7) for use with two independent samples. Stated another way, we can say that the t test for use with two independent samples is a special case of one-way analysis of variance.

In a typical situation we want to use one-way analysis of variance to test the null hypothesis that three or more treatments are equally effective. The necessary experiment is designed in such a way that the treatments of interest are assigned completely at random to the subjects or objects on which the measurements to determine treatment effectiveness are to be made. For this reason the design is called the *completely randomized experimental design*.

We may randomly allocate subjects to treatments as follows. Suppose we have 16 subjects available to participate in an experiment in which we wish to compare four drugs. We number the subjects from 01 through 16. We then go to a table of random numbers and select 16 consecutive, unduplicated, numbers between 01 and 16. To illustrate, let us use Table D and a random starting point which, say, is at the intersection of row 4 and columns 11 and 12. The two-digit number at this intersection is 98. The succeeding (moving downward) 16 consecutive two digit numbers between 01 and 16 are 16, 09, 06, 15, 14, 11, 02, 04, 10, 07, 05, 13, 03, 12, 01, and 08. We allocate subjects 16, 09, 06, and 15 to drug A; subjects 14, 11, 02, and 04 to drug B; subjects 10, 07, 05, and 13 to drug C; and subjects 03, 12, 01, and 08 to drug D. We emphasize that the number of subjects in each treatment group does not have to be the same. Figure 8.2.1 illustrates the scheme of random allocation.

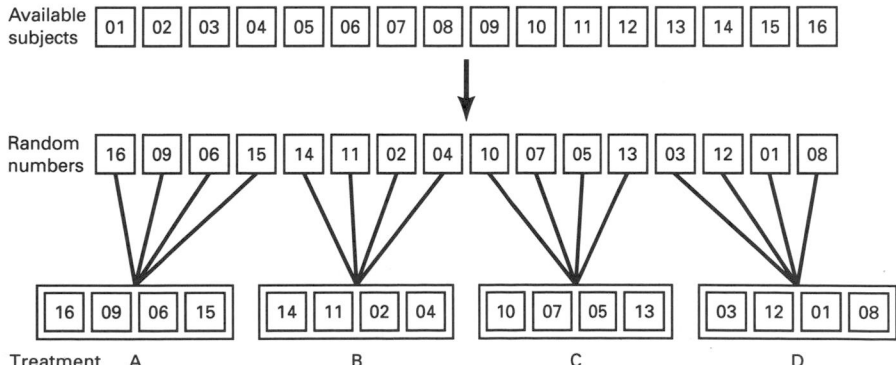

Figure 8.2.1 Allocation of subjects to treatments, completely randomized design.

Hypothesis Testing Steps   Once we decide that the completely randomized design is the appropriate design we may proceed with the hypothesis testing steps. We discuss these in detail first, and follow with an example.

1. *Description of Data*   The measurements (or observations) resulting from a completely randomized experimental design, along with the means and totals that can be computed from them, may be displayed for convenience as in Table 8.2.1. The symbols used in Table 8.2.1 are defined as follows:

$$x_{ij} = \text{the } i\text{th observation resulting from the } j\text{th treatment}$$
$$(\text{there are a total of } k \text{ treatments})$$

$$i = 1, 2, \ldots, n_j, \, j = 1, 2, \ldots, k$$

$$T_{.j} = \sum_{i=1}^{n_j} x_{ij} = \text{total of the } j\text{th treatment}$$

$$\bar{x}_{.j} = \frac{T_{.j}}{n_j} = \text{mean of the } j\text{th treatment}$$

$$T_{..} = \sum_{j=1}^{k} T_{.j} = \sum_{j=1}^{k} \sum_{i=1}^{n_j} x_{ij} = \text{total of all observations}$$

$$\bar{x}_{..} = \frac{T_{..}}{N}, \qquad N = \sum_{j=1}^{k} n_j$$

2. *Assumptions*   Before stating the assumptions, let us specify the model for the experiment described here.

TABLE 8.2.1 Table of Sample Values for the Completely Randomized Design

	Treatment					
	1	**2**	**3**	$\cdots$	**k**	
	x_{11}	x_{12}	x_{13}	$\cdots$	x_{1k}	
	x_{21}	x_{22}	x_{23}	$\cdots$	x_{2k}	
	x_{31}	x_{32}	x_{33}	$\cdots$	x_{3k}	
	$\vdots$	$\vdots$	$\vdots$	$\vdots$	$\vdots$	
	$x_{n_1 1}$	$x_{n_2 2}$	$x_{n_3 3}$	$\cdots$	$x_{n_k k}$	
Total	$T_{.1}$	$T_{.2}$	$T_{.3}$		$T_{.k}$	$T_{..}$
Mean	$\bar{x}_{.1}$	$\bar{x}_{.2}$	$\bar{x}_{.3}$		$\bar{x}_{.k}$	$\bar{x}_{..}$

The Model As already noted, a model is a symbolic representation of a typical value of a data set. To write down the model for the completely randomized experimental design, let us begin by identifying a typical value from the set of data represented by the sample displayed in Table 8.2.1. We use the symbol x_{ij} to represent this typical value.

Within each treatment group (or population) represented by our data, any particular value bears this relationship to the true mean, μ_j, of that group: it is equal to the true group mean plus some amount that is either zero, a positive amount, or a negative amount. This means that a particular value in a given group may be equal to the group mean, larger than the group mean, or smaller than the group mean. Let us call the amount by which any value differs from its group mean the *error* and represent this error by the symbol e_{ij}. By the term error, we do not mean a mistake. The term is used to refer to the extraneous variation that exists among members of any population. Given a population of adult males, for example, we know that the heights of some individuals are above the true mean height of the population, while some heights are below the population mean. This variation is caused by a myriad of hereditary and environmental factors. If to any group mean, μ_j, we add a given error, e_{ij}, the result will be x_{ij}, the observation that deviates from the group mean by the amount e_{ij}.

We may write this relationship symbolically as

$$x_{ij} = \mu_j + e_{ij} \qquad (8.2.1)$$

Solving for e_{ij} we have

$$e_{ij} = x_{ij} + \mu_j \qquad (8.2.2)$$

If we have in mind k populations, we may refer to the grand mean of all the observations in all the populations as μ. Given k populations of equal size, we could compute μ by taking the average of the k population means, that is,

$$\mu = \frac{\sum \mu_j}{k} \qquad (8.2.3)$$

Just as a particular observation within a group, in general, differs from its group mean by some amount, a particular group mean differs from the grand mean by some amount. The amount by which a group mean differs from the grand mean we refer to as the *treatment effect*. We may write the jth treatment effect as

$$\tau_j = \mu_j - \mu \qquad (8.2.4)$$

τ_j is a measure of the effect on μ_j of having been computed from observations receiving the jth treatment.

We may solve Equation 8.2.4 for μ_j to obtain

$$\mu_j = \mu + \tau_j \qquad (8.2.5)$$

If we substitute the right-hand portion of Equation 8.2.5 for μ_j in Equation 8.2.1 we have

$$x_{ij} = \mu + \tau_j + e_{ij}; \qquad i = 1, 2, \ldots, n_j, \qquad j = 1, 2, \ldots, k \qquad (8.2.6)$$

and our model is specified.

Components of the Model   By looking at our model we can see that a typical observation from the total set of data under study is composed of (1) the grand mean, (2) a treatment effect, and (3) an error term representing the deviation of the observation from its group mean.

In most situations we are interested only in the k treatments represented in our experiment. Any inferences that we make apply only to these treatments. We do not wish to extend our inference to any larger collection of treatments. When we place such a restriction on our inference goals, we refer to our model as the *fixed-effects model*, or *model I*. The discussion in this book is limited to this model.

Information on other models will be found in the articles by Eisenhart (13), Wilk and Kempthorne (15), Crump (16), Cunningham and Henderson (17), Henderson (18), Rutherford (19), Schultz (20), and Searle (21).

Assumptions of the Model   The assumptions for the fixed effects model are as follows:

a. The k sets of observed data constitute k independent random samples from the respective populations.
b. Each of the populations from which the samples come is normally distributed with mean μ_j and variance σ_j^2.
c. Each of the populations has the same variance. That is, $\sigma_1^2 = \sigma_2^2 = \cdots = \sigma_k^2 = \sigma^2$, the common variance.
d. The τ_j's are unknown constants and $\Sigma\tau_j = 0$, since the sum of all deviations of the μ_j from their mean, μ, is zero.

Three consequences of the relationship

$$e_{ij} = x_{ij} - \mu_j$$

specified in Equation 8.2.2 are

a. The e_{ij} have a mean of 0, since the mean of x_{ij} is μ_j.
b. The e_{ij} have a variance equal to the variance of the x_{ij}, since the e_{ij} and x_{ij} differ only by a constant; that is, the error variance is equal to σ^2, the common variance specified in assumption c.
c. The e_{ij} are normally (and independently) distributed.

3. *Hypotheses*   We test the null hypothesis that all population or treatment means are equal against the alternative that the members of at least one pair are not equal. We may state the hypotheses formally as follows:

$$H_0: \mu_1 = \mu_2 = \cdots = \mu_k$$

$$H_A: \text{not all } \mu_j \text{ are equal}$$

If the population means are equal, each treatment effect is equal to zero, so that, alternatively, the hypotheses may be stated as

$$H_0: \tau_j = 0, \qquad j = 1, 2, \ldots, k$$

$$H_A: \text{not all } \tau_j = 0$$

If H_0 is true and the assumption of equal variances and normally distributed populations are met, a picture of the populations will look like Figure 8.2.2. When H_0 is true the population means are all equal, and the populations are centered at the same point (the common mean) on the horizontal axis. If the populations are all normally distributed with equal variances the distributions will be identical, so that in drawing their pictures each is superimposed on each of the others, and a single picture sufficiently represents them all.

When H_0 is false it may be false because one of the population means is different from the others, which are all equal. Or, perhaps, all the population means are different. These are only two of the possibilities when H_0 is false. There are many other possible combinations of equal and unequal means. Figure 8.2.3 shows a picture of the populations when the assumptions are met, but H_0 is false because no two population means are equal.

4. *Test Statistic*   The test statistic for one-way analysis of variance is a computed variance ratio, which we designate by V.R. as we did in Chapter 7. The two variances from which V.R. is calculated are themselves computed from the

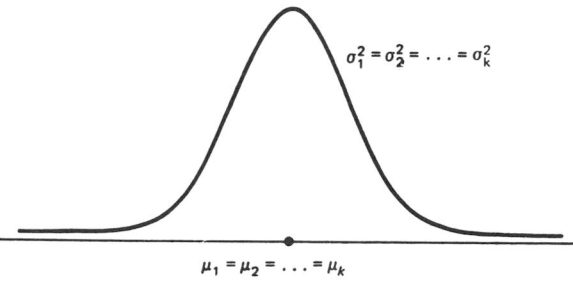

Figure 8.2.2 Picture of the populations represented in a completely randomized design when H_0 is true and the assumptions are met.

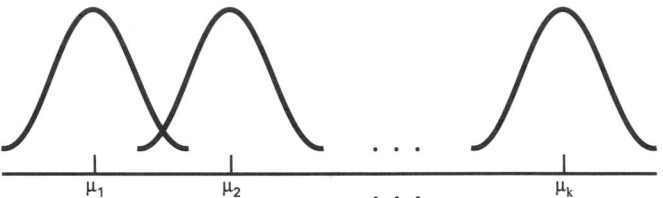

Figure 8.2.3 Picture of the populations represented in a completely randomized design when the assumptions of equal variances and normally distributed populations are met, but H_0 is false because none of the population means are equal.

sample data. The methods by which they are calculated will be given in the discussion that follows.

5. *Distribution of the Test Statistic*   As discussed in Section 7.8, V.R. is distributed as the F distribution when H_0 is true and the assumptions are met.

6. *Decision Rule*   In general, the decision rule is: Reject the null hypothesis if the computed value of V.R. is equal to or greater than the critical value of F for the chosen α level.

7. *Calculation of the Test Statistic*   We have defined analysis of variance as a process whereby the total variation present in a set of data is partitioned into components that are attributable to different sources. The term *variation* used in this context refers to the *sum of squared deviations of observations from their mean*, or *sum of squares* for short.

Those who use a computer for calculations may wish to skip the following discussion of the computations involved in obtaining the test statistic.

The Total Sum of Squares   Before we can do any partitioning, we must first obtain the total sum of squares. The total sum of squares is the sum of the squares of the deviations of individual observations from the mean of all the observations taken together. This *total sum of squares* is defined as

$$SST = \sum_{j=1}^{k} \sum_{i=1}^{n_j} \left(x_{ij} - \bar{x}.. \right)^2 \tag{8.2.7}$$

where $\sum_{i=1}^{n_j}$ tells us to sum the squared deviations for each treatment group, and $\sum_{j=1}^{k}$ tells us to add the k group totals obtained by applying $\sum_{i=1}^{n_j}$. The reader will recognize Equation 8.2.7 as the numerator of the variance that may be computed from the complete set of observations taken together.

We may rewrite Equation 8.2.7 as

$$SST = \sum_{j=1}^{k} \sum_{i=1}^{n_j} x_{ij}^2 - \frac{T_{..}^2}{N} \tag{8.2.8}$$

which is more convenient for computational purposes.

We now proceed with the partitioning of the total sum of squares. We may, without changing its value, insert $-\bar{x}_{.j} + \bar{x}_{.j}$ in the parentheses of Equation 8.2.7. The reader will recognize this added quantity as a well-chosen zero that does not change the value of the expression. The result of this addition is

$$SST = \sum_{j=1}^{k} \sum_{i=1}^{n_j} \left(x_{ij} - \bar{x}_{.j} + \bar{x}_{.j} - \bar{x}_{..} \right)^2 \qquad (8.2.9)$$

If we group terms and expand, we have

$$SST = \sum_{j=1}^{k} \sum_{i=1}^{n_j} \left[\left(x_{ij} - \bar{x}_{.j} \right) + \left(\bar{x}_{.j} - \bar{x}_{..} \right) \right]^2$$

$$= \sum_{j=1}^{k} \sum_{i=1}^{n_j} \left(x_{ij} - \bar{x}_{.j} \right)^2 + 2 \sum_{j=1}^{k} \sum_{i=1}^{n_j} \left(x_{ij} - \bar{x}_{.j} \right)\left(\bar{x}_{.j} - \bar{x}_{..} \right)$$

$$+ \sum_{j=1}^{k} \sum_{i=1}^{n_j} \left(\bar{x}_{.j} - \bar{x}_{..} \right)^2 \qquad (8.2.10)$$

The middle term may be written as

$$2 \sum_{j=1}^{k} \left(\bar{x}_{.j} - \bar{x}_{..} \right) \sum_{i=1}^{n_j} \left(x_{ij} - \bar{x}_{.j} \right) \qquad (8.2.11)$$

Examination of Equation 8.2.11 reveals that this term is equal to zero, since the sum of the deviations of a set of values from their mean as in $\sum_{i=1}^{n_j}(x_{ij} - \bar{x}_{.j})$ is equal to zero.

We now may write Equation 8.2.10 as

$$SST = \sum_{j=1}^{k} \sum_{i=1}^{n_j} \left(x_{ij} - \bar{x}_{.j} \right)^2 + \sum_{j=1}^{k} \sum_{i=1}^{n_j} \left(\bar{x}_{.j} - \bar{x}_{..} \right)^2$$

$$= \sum_{j=1}^{k} \sum_{i=1}^{n_j} \left(x_{ij} - \bar{x}_{.j} \right)^2 + \sum_{j=1}^{k} n_j \left(\bar{x}_{.j} - \bar{x}_{..} \right)^2 \qquad (8.2.12)$$

When the number of observations is the same in each group the last term on the right may be rewritten to give

$$SST = \sum_{j=1}^{k} \sum_{i=1}^{n_j} \left(x_{ij} - \bar{x}_{.j} \right)^2 + n \sum_{j=1}^{k} \left(\bar{x}_{.j} - \bar{x}_{..} \right)^2 \qquad (8.2.13)$$

where $n = n_1 = n_2 = \cdots = n_k$.

The Within Groups Sum of Squares   The partitioning of the total sum of squares is now complete, and we see that in the present case there are two components. Let us now investigate the nature and source of these two components of variation.

If we look at the first term on the right of the Equation 8.2.12, we see that the first step in the indicated computation calls for performing certain calculations *within* each group. These calculations involve computing within each group the sum of the squared deviations of the individual observations from their mean. When these calculations have been performed within each group, the symbol $\sum_{j=1}^{k}$ tells us to obtain the sum of the individual group results. This component of variation is called the *within groups sum of squares* and may be designated *SSW*. This quantity is sometimes referred to as the *residual* or *error* sum of squares. The expression may be written in a computationally more convenient form as follows:

$$SSW = \sum_{j=1}^{k} \sum_{i=1}^{n_j} \left(x_{ij} - \bar{x}_{.j} \right)^2 = \sum_{j=1}^{k} \sum_{i=1}^{n_j} x_{ij}^2 - \sum_{j=1}^{k} \frac{\left(T_{.j} \right)^2}{n_j} \qquad (8.2.14)$$

The Among Groups Sum of Squares   Now let us examine the second term on the right in Equation 8.2.12. The operation called for by this term is to obtain for each group the squared deviation of the group mean from the grand mean and to multiply the result by the size of the group. Finally, we must add these results over all groups. This quantity is a measure of the variation among groups and is referred to as the *sum of squares among groups* or *SSA*. The computing formula is as follows:

$$SSA = \sum_{j=1}^{k} n_j \left(\bar{x}_{.j} - \bar{x}_{..} \right)^2 = \sum_{j=1}^{k} \frac{T_{.j}^2}{n_j} - T_{..}^2/N \qquad (8.2.15)$$

In summary, then, we have found that the total sum of squares is equal to the sum of the among and the within sum of squares. We express this relationship as follows:

$$SST = SSA + SSW$$

From the sums of squares that we have now learned to compute, it is possible to obtain two estimates of the common population variance, σ^2. It can be shown that when the assumptions are met and the population means are all equal, both the among sum of squares and the within sum of squares, when divided by their respective degrees of freedom, yield independent and unbiased estimates of σ^2.

The First Estimate of σ^2 Within any sample

$$\frac{\sum_{i=1}^{n_j} \left(x_{ij} - \bar{x}_{.j}\right)^2}{n_j - 1}$$

provides an unbiased estimate of the true variance of the population from which the sample came. Under the assumption that the population variances are all equal, we may pool the k estimates to obtain

$$\frac{\sum_{j=1}^{k} \sum_{i=1}^{n_j} \left(x_{ij} - \bar{x}_{.j}\right)^2}{\sum_{j=1}^{k} \left(n_j - 1\right)} \tag{8.2.16}$$

This is our first estimate of σ^2 and may be called the *within groups variance*, since it is the within groups sum of squares of Equation 8.2.14 divided by the appropriate degrees of freedom. The student will recognize this as an extension to k samples of the pooling of variances procedure encountered in Chapters 6 and 7 when the variances from two samples were pooled in order to use the t distribution. The quantity in Equation 8.2.16 is customarily referred to as the within groups *mean square* rather than the within groups variance.

The within groups mean square is a valid estimate of σ^2 only if the population variances are equal. It is not necessary, however, for H_0 to be true in order for the within groups mean square to be a valid estimate of σ^2. That is, the within groups mean square estimates σ^2 regardless of whether H_0 is true or false, as long as the population variances are equal.

The Second Estimate of σ^2 The second estimate of σ^2 may be obtained from the familiar formula for the variance of sample means, $\sigma_{\bar{x}}^2 = \sigma^2/n$. If we solve this equation for σ^2, the variance of the population from which the samples were drawn, we have

$$\sigma^2 = n\sigma_{\bar{x}}^2 \tag{8.2.17}$$

An unbiased estimate of $\sigma_{\bar{x}}^2$, computed from sample data, is provided by

$$\frac{\sum_{j=1}^{k} \left(\bar{x}_{.j} - \bar{x}_{..}\right)^2}{k - 1}$$

If we substitute this quantity into Equation 8.2.17, we obtain the desired estimate of σ^2,

$$\frac{n \sum_{j=1}^{k} \left(\bar{x}_{.j} - \bar{x}_{..}\right)^2}{k - 1} \tag{8.2.18}$$

The reader will recognize the numerator of Equation 8.2.18 as the among groups sum of squares for the special case when all sample sizes are equal. This sum of squares when divided by the associated degrees of freedom $k - 1$ is referred to as the *among groups mean square.*

When the sample sizes are not all equal, an estimate of σ^2 based on the variability among sample means is provided by

$$\frac{\sum_{j=1}^{k} n_j \left(\bar{x}_{.j} - \bar{x}_{..} \right)^2}{k - 1} \tag{8.2.19}$$

If, indeed, the null hypothesis is true we would expect these two estimates of σ^2 to be fairly close in magnitude. If the null hypothesis is false, that is, if all population means are not equal, we would expect the among groups mean square, which is computed by using the squared deviations of the sample means from the overall mean, to be larger than the within groups mean square.

In order to understand analysis of variance we must realize that the among groups mean square provides a valid estimate of σ^2 when the assumption of equal population variances is met *and when H_0 is true.* Both conditions, a true null hypothesis and equal population variances, must be met in order for the among groups mean square to be a valid estimate of σ^2.

The Variance Ratio What we need to do now is to compare these two estimates of σ^2, and we do this by computing the following variance ratio, which is the desired test statistic:

$$\text{V.R.} = \frac{\text{among groups mean square}}{\text{within groups mean square}}$$

If the two estimates are about equal, V.R. will be close to 1. A ratio close to 1 tends to support the hypothesis of equal population means. If, on the other hand, the among groups mean square is considerably larger than the within groups mean square, V.R. will be considerably greater than 1. A value of V.R. sufficiently greater than 1 will cast doubt on the hypothesis of equal population means.

We know that because of the vagaries of sampling, even when the null hypothesis is true, it is unlikely that the among and within groups mean squares will be equal. We must decide, then, how big the observed difference has to be before we can conclude that the difference is due to something other than sampling fluctuation. In other words, how large a value of V.R. is required for us to be willing to conclude that the observed difference between our two estimates of σ^2 is not the result of chance alone?

The *F* Test To answer the question just posed, we must consider the sampling distribution of the ratio of two sample variances. In Chapter 6 we learned that the quantity $(s_1^2/\sigma_1^2)/(s_2^2/\sigma_2^2)$ follows a distribution known as the F distribution when the sample variances are computed from random and independently drawn samples from normal populations. The F distribution, introduced by R. A. Fisher in the early 1920s, has become one of the most widely used distributions in modern statistics. We have already become acquainted with its use in constructing confidence intervals for, and testing hypotheses about, population variances. In this chapter, we will see that it is the distribution fundamental to analysis of variance.

In Chapter 7 we learned that when the population variances are the same, they cancel in the expression $(s_1^2/\sigma_1^2)/(s_2^2/\sigma_2^2)$, leaving s_1^2/s_2^2, which is itself distributed as F. The F distribution is really a family of distributions, and the particular F distribution we use in a given situation depends on the number of degrees of freedom associated with the sample variance in the numerator (*numerator degrees of freedom*) and the number of degrees of freedom associated with the sample variance in the denominator (*denominator degrees of freedom*).

Once the appropriate F distribution has been determined, the size of the observed V.R. that will cause rejection of the hypothesis of equal population variances depends on the significance level chosen. The significance level chosen determines the critical value of F, the value that separates the nonrejection region from the rejection region.

As we have seen, we compute V.R. in situations of this type by placing the among groups mean square in the numerator and the within groups mean square in the denominator, so that the numerator degrees of freedom is equal to the number of groups minus 1, $(k-1)$, and the denominator degrees of freedom value is equal to

$$\sum_{j=1}^{k}\left(n_j-1\right) = \sum_{j=1}^{k}n_j - k = N - k.$$

The ANOVA table The calculations that we perform may be summarized and displayed in a table such as Table 8.2.2, which is called the ANOVA table.

Notice that in Table 8.2.2 the term $\sum_{j=1}^{k}\sum_{i=1}^{n_j}x_{ij}^2/N = T_{..}^2/N$ occurs in the expression for both SSA and SST. A savings in computational time and labor may be realized if we take advantage of this fact. We need only to compute this quantity, which is called the *correction term* and designated by the letter C, once and use it as needed.

The computational burden may be lightened in still another way. Since SST is equal to the sum of SSA and SSW, and since SSA is easier to compute than SSW, we may compute SST and SSA and subtract the latter from the former to obtain SSW.

8. *Statistical Decision* To reach a decision we must compare our computed V.R. with the critical value of F, which we obtain by entering Table G with $k-1$ numerator degrees of freedom and $N-k$ denominator degrees of freedom.

TABLE 8.2.2 Analysis of Variance Table for the Completely Randomized Design

Source of Variation	Sum of Squares	Degrees of Freedom	Mean Square	Variance Ratio
Among samples	$SSA = \sum\limits_{j=1}^{k} n_j(\bar{x}_{.j} - \bar{x}_{..})^2$ $= \sum\limits_{j=1}^{k} \dfrac{T_{.j}^2}{n_j} - \dfrac{T_{..}^2}{N}$	$k - 1$	MSA $= SSA/(k - 1)$	$\text{V.R.} = \dfrac{MSA}{MSW}$
Within samples	$SSW = \sum\limits_{j=1}^{k} \sum\limits_{i=1}^{n_j} (x_{ij} - \bar{x}_{.j})^2$ $= \sum\limits_{j=1}^{k} \sum\limits_{i=1}^{n_j} x_{ij}^2 - \sum\limits_{j=1}^{k} \dfrac{(T_{.j})^2}{n_j}$	$N - k$	MSW $= SSW/(N - k)$	
Total	$SST = \sum\limits_{j=1}^{k} \sum\limits_{i=1}^{n_j} (x_{ij} - \bar{x}_{..})^2$ $= \sum\limits_{j=1}^{k} \sum\limits_{i=1}^{n_j} x_{ij}^2 - \dfrac{T_{..}^2}{N}$	$N - 1$		

If the computed V.R. is equal to or greater than the critical value of F, we reject the null hypothesis. If the computed value of V.R. is smaller than the critical value of F, we do not reject the null hypothesis.

Explaining a Rejected Null Hypothesis   There are two possible explanations for a rejected null hypothesis. If the null hypothesis is true, that is, if the two sample variances are estimates of a common variance, we know that the probability of getting a value of V.R. as large as or larger than the critical F is equal to our chosen level of significance. When we reject H_0 we may, if we wish, conclude that the null hypothesis is true and assume that because of chance we got a set of data that gave rise to a rare event. On the other hand, we may prefer to take the position that our large computed V.R. value does not represent a rare event brought about by chance but, instead, reflects the fact that something other than chance is operative. This other something we conclude to be a false null hypothesis.

It is this latter explanation that we usually give for computed values of V.R. that exceed the critical value of F. In other words, if the computed value of V.R. is greater than the critical value of F, we reject the null hypothesis.

It will be recalled that the original hypothesis we set out to test was

$$H_0: \mu_1 = \mu_2 = \cdots = \mu_k$$

Does rejection of the hypothesis about variances imply a rejection of the hypothesis of equal population means? The answer is, yes. A large value of V.R. resulted from the fact that the among groups mean square was considerably larger than the within groups mean square. Since the among groups mean square is based on the dispersion of the sample means about their mean, this quantity will be large when there is a large discrepancy among the sizes of the sample means. Because of this, then, a significant value of V.R. tells us to reject the null hypothesis that all population means are equal.

9.   *Conclusion*   When we reject H_0 we conclude that not all population means are equal. When we fail to reject H_0, we conclude that the population means may all be equal.

Example 8.2.1   Miller and Vanhoutte (A-1) conducted experiments in which adult ovariectomized female mongrel dogs were treated with estrogen, progesterone, or estrogen plus progesterone. Five untreated animals served as controls. A variable of interest was concentration of progesterone in the serum of the animals 14 to 21 days after treatment. We wish to know if the treatments have different effects on the mean serum concentration of progesterone.

Solution:

1.   *Description of Data*   Four dogs were treated with estrogen, four with progesterone, and five with estrogen plus progesterone. Five dogs were not treated. The serum progesterone levels (ng/dl) following treatment, along with treatment totals and means are shown in Table 8.2.3. A graph of the data in the form of a *dotplot* is shown in Figure 8.2.4. Such a graph highlights the main features of the data and brings into clear focus differences in response by treatment.

2.   *Assumptions*   We assume that the four sets of data constitute independent simple random samples from four populations that are similar except for the treatment received. We assume that the four populations of measurements are normally distributed with equal variances.

TABLE 8.2.3 Concentration of Serum Progesterone (ng / dl) in Dogs Treated with Estrogen, Progesterone, Estrogen Plus Progesterone, and in Untreated Controls

			Treatment		
	Untreated	**Estrogen**	**Progesterone**	**Estrogen + Progesterone**	
	117	440	605	2664	
	124	264	626	2078	
	40	221	385	3584	
	88	136	475	1540	
	40			1840	
Total	409	1061	2091	11706	15267
Mean	81.80	265.25	522.75	2341.20	848.1667

SOURCE: Virginia M. Miller, Ph.D. Used by permission.

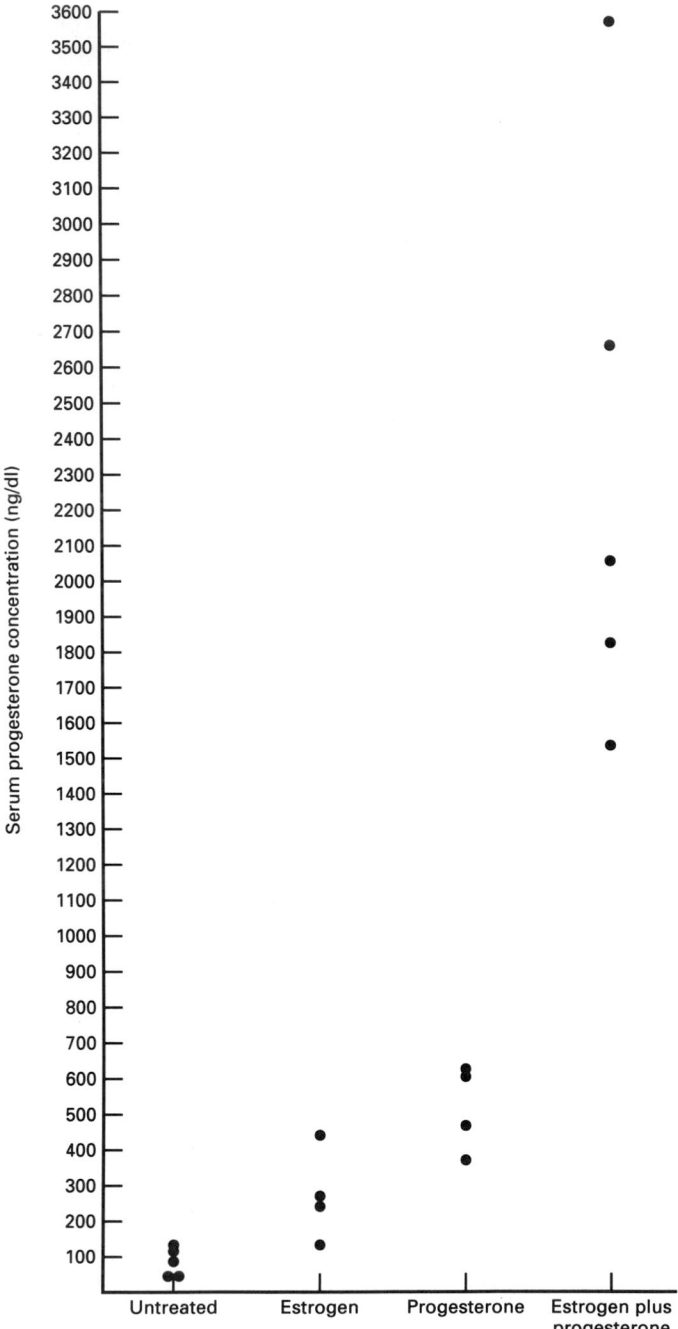

Figure 8.2.4   Plot of serum progesterone concentration (ng / dl) by treatment.

3. *Hypotheses*

H_0: $\mu_1 = \mu_2 = \mu_3 = \mu_4$ (On the average the four treatments elicit the same response)

H_A: Not all μ's are equal (At least one treatment has an average response different from the average response of at least one other treatment)

4. *Test Statistic*   The test statistic is V.R. $= MSA/MSW$.

5. *Distribution of the Test Statistic*   If H_0 is true and the assumptions are met, V.R. follows the F distribution with $4 - 1 = 3$ numerator degrees of freedom and $18 - 4 = 14$ denominator degrees of freedom.

6. *Decision Rule*   Suppose we let $\alpha = .05$. The critical value of F from Table G is 3.34. The decision rule, then, is reject H_0 if the computed V.R. is equal to or greater than 3.34.

7. *Calculation of the Test Statistic*   By Equation 8.2.8 we compute

$$SST = (117)^2 + (124)^2 + \cdots + (1840)^2 - (15267)^2/18$$

$$= 31519629 - 12948960.5 = 18570668.5$$

By Equation 8.2.15 we compute

$$SSA = \frac{409^2}{5} + \frac{1061^2}{4} + \frac{2091^2}{4} + \frac{11706^2}{5} - \frac{15267^2}{18} = 28814043.9$$

$$- 12948960.5 = 15865083.4$$

$$SSW = 18570668.5 - 15865083.4 = 2705585.1$$

The results of our calculations are displayed in the Table 8.2.4.

8. *Statistical Decision*   Since our computed V.R. of 27.3645 is greater than the critical F of 3.34, we reject H_0.

TABLE 8.2.4 ANOVA Table for Example 8.2.1

Source	SS	d.f.	MS	V.R.
Among samples	15865083.4	3	5288361.133	27.3645
Within samples	2705585.1	14	193256.0786	
Total	18570668.5	17		

9. *Conclusion*   Since we reject H_0, we conclude that the alternative hypothesis is true. That is, we conclude that the four treatments do not all have the same average effect.

A Word of Caution   The completely randomized design is simple and, therefore, widely used. It should be used, however, only when the units receiving the treatments are homogeneous. If the experimental units are not homogeneous, the researcher should consider an alternative design such as one of those to be discussed later in this chapter.

In our illustrative example the treatments are treatments in the usual sense of the word. This is not always the case, however, as the term "treatment" as used in experimental design is quite general. We might, for example, wish to study the response to the same treatment (in the usual sense of the word) of several breeds of animals. We would, however, refer to the breed of animal as the "treatment."

We must also point out that, although the techniques of analysis of variance are more often applied to data resulting from controlled experiments, the techniques also may be used to analyze data collected by a survey, provided that the underlying assumptions are reasonably well met.

Computer Analysis   Figure 8.2.6 shows the computer output for Example 8.2.1 provided by a one-way analysis of variance program found in the MINITAB package. The data were entered into columns 1 through 4 and the command

```
AOVONEWAY C1, C2, C3, C4
```

was issued. When you compare the ANOVA table on this printout with the one given in Table 8.2.4, you see that the printout uses the label "factor" instead of "among samples." The different treatments are referred to on the printout as

```
ANALYSIS OF VARIANCE
SOURCE    DF       SS        MS        F       p
FACTOR     3   15865083   5288361   27.36   0.000
ERROR     14    2705585    193256
TOTAL     17   18570668
                                  INDIVIDUAL 95 PCT CI'S FOR MEAN
                                  BASED ON POOLED STDEV
 LEVEL    N      MEAN      STDEV   ----+---------+---------+---------+
C1        5      81.8       40.5   (---*---)
C2        4     265.2      128.1   (----*---)
C3        4     522.8      113.5      (---*----)
C4        5    2341.2      808.0                          (---*----)
                                  ----+---------+---------+---------+
POOLED STDEV =   439.6            0       1000      2000      30l
```

Figure 8.2.6 MINITAB output for Example 8.2.1.

```
                                    SAS
                    ANALYSIS OF VARIANCE PROCEDURE
DEPENDENT VARIABLE: SERUM
SOURCE                    DF      SUM OF SQUARES          MEAN SQUARE
MODEL                      3   15865083.40000000   5288361.13333333
ERROR                     14    2705585.10000000    193256.07857143
CORRECTED TOTAL           17   18570668.50000000

MODEL F =              27.36                        PR>F = 0.0001
```

Figure 8.2.7 *Partial SAS® printout for Example 8.2.1.*

levels. Thus level 1 = treatment 1, level 2 = treatment 2, and so on. The printout gives the four sample means and standard deviations as well as the pooled standard deviation. This last quantity is equal to the square root of the error mean square shown in the ANOVA table. Finally, the computer output gives graphic representations of the 95 percent confidence intervals for the mean of each of the four populations represented by the sample data. The MINITAB package can provide additional analyses through the use of appropriate commands. The package also contains programs for two-way analysis of variance, to be discussed in the following sections. Figure 8.2.7 contains a partial SAS® printout resulting from analysis of the data of Example 8.2.1 through use of the SAS® statement PROC ANOVA.

A useful device for displaying important characteristics of a set of data analyzed by one-way analysis of variance is a graph consisting of side-by-side boxplots. For each sample a boxplot is constructed using the method described in Chapter 2. Figure 8.2.8 shows the side-by-side boxplots for Example 8.2.1. Note that in Figure 8.2.8 the variable of interest is represented by the vertical axis rather than the horizontal axis.

Alternatives   If the data available for analysis do not meet the assumptions for one-way analysis of variance as discussed here, one may wish to consider the use of the Kruskal–Wallis procedure, a nonparametric technique discussed in Chapter 13. Since, for example, the sample variances in Example 8.2.1 vary so greatly, we might question whether the data satisfy the assumption of equal population variances and wish to use the Kruskal–Wallis procedure to analyze the data.

Testing for Significant Differences Between Individual Pairs of Means
When the analysis of variance leads to a rejection of the null hypothesis of no difference among population means, the question naturally arises regarding just which pairs of means are different. In fact, the desire, more often than not, is to carry out a significance test on each and every pair of treatment means. For instance, in Example 8.2.1, where there are four treatments, we may wish to know,

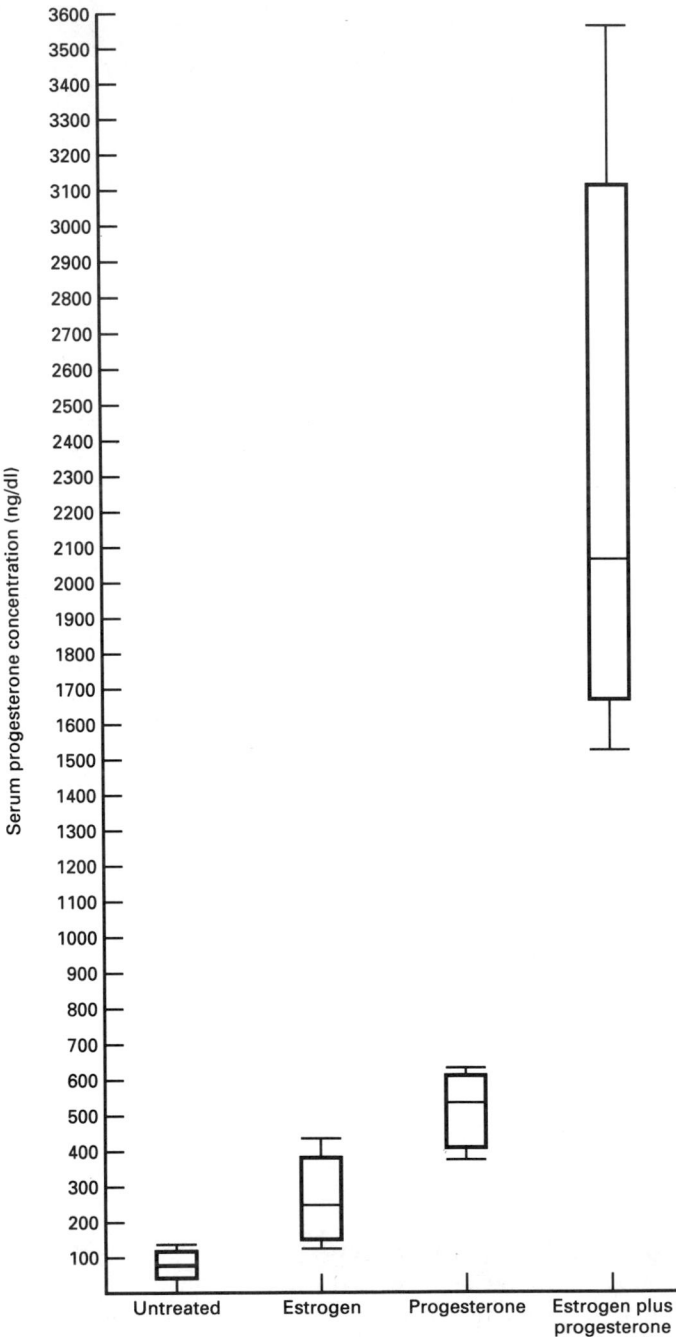

Figure 8.2.8   Side-by-side boxplots for Example 8.2.1.

after rejecting H_0: $\mu_1 = \mu_2 = \mu_3 = \mu_4$, which of the 6 possible individual hypotheses should be rejected. The experimenter, however, must exercise caution in testing for significant differences between individual means and must always make certain that the procedure is valid. The critical issue in the procedure is the level of significance. Although the probability, α, of rejecting a true null hypothesis for the test as a whole is made small, the probability of rejecting at least one true hypothesis when several pairs of means are tested is, as we have seen, greater than α.

Multiple Comparison Procedure Over the years several procedures for making multiple comparisons have been suggested. The oldest procedure, and perhaps the one most widely used in the past, is the *least significant difference* (LSD) procedure of Fisher, who first discussed it in the 1935 edition of his book *The Design of Experiments* (1). The LSD procedure, which is a Student's *t* test using a pooled error variance, is valid only when making independent comparisons or comparisons planned before the data are analyzed. A difference between any two means that exceeds a least significant difference is considered significant at the level of significance used in computing the LSD. The LSD procedure usually is used only when the overall analysis of variance leads to a significant V.R. For an example of the use of the LSD, see Steel and Torrie (22).

Duncan (23–26) has contributed a considerable amount of research to the subject of multiple comparisons with the result that at present a widely used procedure is *Duncan's new multiple range test*. The extension of the test to the case of unequal sample sizes is discussed by Kramer (27).

When the objective of an experiment is to compare several treatments with a control, and not with each other, a procedure due to Dunnet (28, 29) for comparing the control against each of the other treatments is usually followed.

Other multiple comparison procedures in use are those proposed by Tukey (30, 31), Newman (32), Keuls (33), and Scheffé (34, 35). The advantages and disadvantages of the various procedures are discussed by Bancroft (36), Daniel and Coogler (37), and Winer (38). Daniel (39) has prepared a bibliography on multiple comparison procedures.

Tukey's HSD Test A multiple comparison procedure developed by Tukey (31) is frequently used for testing the null hypotheses that all possible pairs of treatment means are equal when the samples are all of the same size. When this test is employed we select an overall significance level of α. The probability is α, then, that one or more of the null hypotheses is false.

Tukey's test, which is usually referred to as the HSD (*honestly significant difference*) test, makes use of a single value against which all differences are compared. This value, called the HSD, is given by

$$\text{HSD} = q_{\alpha, k, N-k} \sqrt{\frac{\text{MSE}}{n}} \qquad (8.2.20)$$

where α is the chosen level of significance, k is the number of means in the experiment, N is the total number of observations in the experiment, n is the number of observations in a treatment, MSE is the error or within mean square from the ANOVA table, and q is obtained by entering Appendix I Table H with α, k, and $N - k$.

All possible differences between pairs of means are computed, and any difference that yields an absolute value that exceeds HSD is declared to be significant.

Tukey's Test for Unequal Sample Sizes When the samples are not all the same size, as is the case in Example 8.2.1, Tukey's HSD test given by Equation 8.2.20 is not applicable. Spjøtvoll and Stoline (40), however, have extended the Tukey procedure to the case where the sample sizes are different. Their procedure, which is applicable for experiments involving three or more treatments and significance levels of .05 or less, consists of replacing n in Equation 8.2.20 with n_j^*, the smallest of the two sample sizes associated with the two sample means that are to be compared. If we designate the new quantity by HSD*, we have as the new test criterion

$$\text{HSD}^* = q_{\alpha, k, N-k} \sqrt{\frac{\text{MSE}}{n_j^*}} \qquad (8.2.21)$$

Any absolute value of the difference between two sample means, one of which is computed from a sample of size n_j^* (which is smaller than the sample from which the other mean is computed), that exceeds HSD* is declared to be significant.

Example 8.2.2

Let us illustrate the use of the HSD test with the data from Example 8.2.1.

Solution: The first step is to prepare a table of all possible (ordered) differences between means. The results of this step for the present example are displayed in Table 8.2.5.

Suppose we let $\alpha = .05$. Entering Table H with $\alpha = .05$, $k = 4$, and $N - k = 14$, we find that q is 4.11. In Table 8.2.4 we have MSE = 193256.0786.

The hypotheses that can be tested, the value of HSD*, and the statistical decision for each test are shown in Table 8.2.6.

TABLE 8.2.5 Differences Between Sample Means (Absolute Value) for Example 8.2.2

	Untreated	Estrogen	Progesterone	Estrogen + Progesterone
Untreated (u)	—	183.45	440.95	2259.40
Estrogen (e)	—	—	257.50	2075.95
Progesterone (p)	—	—	—	1818.45
Estrogen + Progesterone (pe)	—	—	—	—

TABLE 8.2.6 Multiple Comparison Tests Using Data of Example 8.2.1 and HSD*

Hypotheses	HSD*	Statistical Decision
$H_0: \mu_u = \mu_e$	$\text{HSD*} = 4.11\sqrt{\dfrac{193256.0786}{4}} = 903.40$	Do not reject H_0 since $183.45 < 903.40$
$H_0: \mu_u = \mu_p$	$\text{HSD*} = 4.11\sqrt{\dfrac{193256.0786}{4}} = 903.40$	Do not reject H_0 since $440.95 < 903.40$
$H_0: \mu_u = \mu_{pe}$	$\text{HSD*} = 4.11\sqrt{\dfrac{193256.0786}{5}} = 808.02$	Reject H_0 since $2259.4 > 808.02$
$H_0: \mu_e = \mu_p$	$\text{HSD*} = 4.11\sqrt{\dfrac{193256.0786}{4}} = 903.40$	Do not reject H_0 since $257.5 < 903.40$
$H_0: \mu_e = \mu_{pe}$	$\text{HSD*} = 4.11\sqrt{\dfrac{193256.0786}{4}} = 903.40$	Reject H_0 since $2075.95 > 903.40$
$H_0: \mu_p = \mu_{pe}$	$\text{HSD*} = 4.11\sqrt{\dfrac{193256.0786}{4}} = 903.40$	Reject H_0 since $1818.45 > 903.40$

```
                              SAS
                 ANALYSIS OF VARIANCE PROCEDURE
     TUKEY 'S STUDENTIZED RANGE (HSD) TEST FOR VARIABLE: SERUM
     NOTE: THIS TEST CONTROLS THE TYPE I EXPERIMENTWISE ERROR RATE
               ALPHA = 0.05 CONFIDENCE = 0.95   DF = 14   MSE = 193256
               CRITICAL VALUE OF STUDENTIZED RANGE = 4.111
     COMPARISONS SIGNIFICANT AT THE 0.05 LEVEL ARE INDICATED BY  '***
                         SIMULTANEOUS                SIMULTANEOUS
                            LOWER       DIFFERENCE      UPPER
            TREAT         CONFIDENCE     BETWEEN      CONFIDENCE
          COMPARISON       LIMIT         MEANS          LIMIT
           pe  - p          961.3        1818.4        2675.6      ***
           pe  - e         1218.8        2075.9        2933.1      ***
           pe  - u         1451.3        2259.4        3067.5      ***
           p   - pe       -2675.6       -1818.4        -961.3      ***
           p   - e         -646.0         257.5        1161.0
           p   - u         -416.2         440.9        1298.1
           e   - pe       -2933.1       -2075.9       -1218.8      ***
           e   - p        -1161.0        -257.5         646.0
           e   - u         -673.7         183.5        1040.8
           u   - pe       -3067.5       -2259.4       -1451.3      ***
           u   - p        -1298.1        -440.9         416.2
           u   - e        -1040.6        -183.5         673.7
```

Figure 8.2.9 SAS® multiple comparisons for Example 8.2.1.

The results of the hypothesis tests displayed in Table 8.2.6 may be summarized by a technique suggested by Duncan (26). The sample means are displayed in a line approximately to scale. Any two that are not significantly different are underscored by the same line. Any two sample means that are not underscored by the same line are significantly different. Thus, for the present example, we may write

81.8   265.25
<u>   </u>
                                                   522.75   2341.2
<u>   </u>

SAS® uses Tukey's procedure to test the hypothesis of no difference between population means for all possible pairs of sample means. The output also contains confidence intervals for the difference between all possible pairs of population means. This SAS output for Example 8.2.1 is displayed in Figure 8.2.9.

EXERCISES

In Exercises 8.2.1–8.2.7 go through the nine steps of analysis of variance hypothesis testing to see if you can conclude that there is a difference among population means. Let $\alpha = .05$ for each test. Determine the p value for each test. Use Tukey's HSD procedure to test for significant differences among individual pairs of means. Use the same α value as for the F test. Construct a dotplot and side-by-side boxplots of the data.

8.2.1 Research by Singh et al. (A-2) as reported in the journal *Clinical Immunology and Immunopathology* is concerned with immune abnormalities in autistic children. As part of their research they took measurements on the serum concentration of an antigen in three samples of children, all of whom were 10 years old or younger. The results in units per milliliter of serum follow.

Autistic children ($n = 23$): 755, 385, 380, 215, 400, 343, 415, 360, 345, 450, 410, 435, 460, 360, 225, 900, 365, 440, 820, 400, 170, 300, 325
Normal children ($n = 33$): 165, 390, 290, 435, 235, 345, 320, 330, 205, 375, 345, 305, 220, 270, 355, 360, 335, 305, 325, 245, 285, 370, 345, 345, 230, 370, 285, 315, 195, 270, 305, 375, 220
Mentally retarded children (non-Down's syndrome) ($n = 15$): 380, 510, 315, 565, 715, 380, 390, 245, 155, 335, 295, 200, 105, 105, 245

Source: Vijendra K. Singh, Ph.D. Used by permission.

8.2.2 The purpose of an investigation by Schwartz et al. (A-3) was to quantify the effect of cigarette smoking on standard measures of lung function in patients with idiopathic pulmonary fibrosis. Among the measurements taken were percent predicted residual volume. The results by smoking history were as follows:

Never ($n = 21$)	Former ($n = 44$)		Current ($n = 7$)
35.0	62.0	95.0	96.0
120.0	73.0	82.0	107.0
90.0	60.0	141.0	63.0
109.0	77.0	64.0	134.0
82.0	52.0	124.0	140.0
40.0	115.0	65.0	103.0
68.0	82.0	42.0	158.0
84.0	52.0	53.0	
124.0	105.0	67.0	
77.0	143.0	95.0	
140.0	80.0	99.0	
127.0	78.0	69.0	
58.0	47.0	118.0	
110.0	85.0	131.0	
42.0	105.0	76.0	
57.0	46.0	69.0	
93.0	66.0	69.0	
70.0	91.0	97.0	
51.0	151.0	137.0	
74.0	40.0	103.0	
74.0	80.0	108.0	
	57.0	56.0	

SOURCE: David A. Schwartz, M.D., M.P.H. Used by permission.

8.2.3 Szádóczky et al. (A-4) examined the characteristics of ^{3}H-imipramine binding sites in seasonal (SAD) and nonseasonal (non-SAD) depressed patients and in healthy individuals (Control). One of the variables on which they took measurements was the density of binding sites for ^{3}H-imipramine on blood platelets (B_{max}). The results were as follows:

SAD	Non-SAD	Control
634	771	1067
585	546	1176
520	552	1040
525	557	1218
693	976	942
660	204	845
520	807	
573	526	
731		
788		
736		
1007		
846		
701		
584		
867		
691		

SOURCE: Erika Szádóczky. Used by permission.

8.2.4 Meg Gulanick (A-5) compared the effects of teaching plus exercise testing, both with and without exercise training, on self-efficacy and on activity performance during early recovery in subjects who had had myocardial infarction or cardiac surgery. Self-efficacy (confidence) to perform physical activity is defined as one's judgment of one's capability to perform a range of physical activities frequently encountered in daily living. Subjects were randomly assigned to one of three groups. Group 1 received teaching, treadmill exercise testing, and exercise training three times per week. Group 2 received only teaching and exercise testing. Group 3 received only routine care without supervised exercise or teaching. The following are the total self-efficacy scores by group at four weeks after the cardiac event.

Group 1: 156, 119, 107, 108, 100, 170, 130, 154, 107, 137, 107
Group 2: 132, 105, 144, 136, 136, 132, 159, 152, 117, 89, 142, 151, 82
Group 3: 110, 117, 124, 106, 113, 94, 113, 121, 101, 119, 77, 90, 66

SOURCE: Meg Gulanick, Ph.D., R. N. Used by permission.

8.2.5 Azoulay-Dupuis et al. (A-6) studied the efficacy of five drugs on the clearance of *Streptococcus pneumoniae* in the lung of female mice at various times after infection. The following are measurements of viable bacteria in lungs ($\log_{10}$ cfu/ml of lung homogenate) 24 hours after six injections. Dosages are given per injection.

Drug Dosage (mg / kg)	Viable Bacteria
Controls	8.80
	8.60
	8.10
	8.40
	8.80
Amoxicyllin, 50	2.60
	2.60
	2.60
Erythromycin, 50	2.60
	2.60
	2.60
Temafloxacin, 50	2.60
	2.60
	2.60
Ofloxacin, 100	7.30
	5.30
	7.48
Ciprofloxacin, 100	7.86
	4.60
	6.45

SOURCE: Esther Azoulay-Dupuis. Used by permission.

8.2.6 The purpose of a study by Robert D. Budd (A-7) was to explore the relationship between cocaine use and violent behavior in coroners' cases. The following are the cocaine concentrations (μg/ml) in victims of violent death by type of death.

Homicide						
.78	1.71	.19	1.55	.27	4.08	.16
1.88	4.10	.14	3.11	.42	1.52	.35
.25	.38	2.38	2.49	.35	.41	1.49
.81	2.50	.21	4.70	2.39	.35	1.18
.04	1.80	.13	1.81	4.38	1.79	2.26
.04	.12	1.32	1.15	.10	.27	.19
.09	.30	3.58	3.49	1.24	2.77	.47
1.88						

Accident						
1.18	1.46	.03	.65	.40	7.62	.04
.05	3.85	.46	.47	2.96		

Suicide						
1.15	.54	.92	.35	3.22	.21	.54
1.82						

SOURCE: Robert D. Budd. Used by permission.

8.2.7 A study by Rosen et al. (A-8) was designed to test the hypothesis that survivors of the Nazi Holocaust have more and different sleep problems than depressed and healthy comparison subjects and that the severity of the survivors' problems correlate with length of time spent in a concentration camp. Subjects consisted of survivors of the Nazi Holocaust, depressed patients, and healthy subjects. The subjects described their sleep patterns over the preceding month on the Pittsburgh Sleep Quality Index, a self-rating instrument that inquires about quality, latency, duration, efficiency, and disturbances of sleep, use of sleep medication, and daytime dysfunction. The following are the subjects' global scores on the index by type of subject.

Survivors		Depressed Patients		Healthy Controls		
5	4	16	16	2	2	1
9	1	12	13	0	3	2
12	12	10	12	5	3	1
3	12	12	11	4	1	4
15	15	11	5	8	1	3
7	20	17	13	4	2	3
5	8	17	10	2	3	
4	5	16	15	2	1	
21	3	10	16	3	1	
12	15	6	19	2	3	
2	0	7		1	3	
10	1	16		2	9	
8	12	14		1	5	
8	5	7		2	1	
10	16	12		1	5	
8	3	8		2	1	
6	6	10		2	2	
13	2	12		1	2	
3		9		6	4	
6		9		3	1	
11		6		2	2	
					4	
					4	

SOURCE: Jules Rosen, M. D. Used by permission.

8.2.8 The objective of a study by Regenstein et al. (A-9) was to determine whether there is an increased incidence of glucose intolerance in association with chronic terbutaline therapy, administered either orally or as a continuous subcutaneous infusion. Thirty-eight and 31 women, respectively, received terbutaline orally or as a continuous subcutaneous infusion. Their gestational diabetes screening results were compared to the results in 82 women not receiving therapy. What is the treatment variable in this study? The response variable? What extraneous variables can you think of whose effects would be included in the error term? What are the "values" of the treatment variable? Construct an analysis of variance table in which you specify for this study the sources of variation and the degrees of freedom.

8.2.9 Jessee and Cecil (A-10) conducted a study to compare the abilities, as measured by a test and a ranking procedure, of variously trained females to suggest and prioritize solutions to a medical dilemma. The 77 females fell into one of four groups: trained home visitors with 0 to 6 months of experience, trained home visitors with more than 6 months of experience, professionally trained nurses, and women with no training or experience. What is the treatment variable? The response variable? What are the "values" of the treatment variable? Who are the subjects? What extraneous variables whose effects would be included in the error term can you think of? What was the purpose of including the untrained and inexperienced females in the study? Construct an ANOVA table in which you specify the sources of variation and the degrees of freedom for each. The authors reported a computed V.R. of 11.79. What is the p value for the test?

8.3
The Randomized Complete Block Design

Of all the experimental designs that are in use, the *randomized complete block* design appears to be the most widely used. This design was developed about 1925 by R. A. Fisher (3, 41), who was seeking methods of improving agricultural field experiments.

The randomized complete block design is a design in which the units (called *experimental units*) to which the treatments are applied are subdivided into homogeneous groups called *blocks*, so that the number of experimental units in a block is equal to the number (or some multiple of the number) of treatments being studied. The treatments are then assigned at random to the experimental units within each block. It should be emphasized that each treatment appears in every block, and each block receives every treatment.

Objective   The objective in using the randomized complete block design is to isolate and remove from the error term the variation attributable to the blocks, while assuring that treatment means will be free of block effects. The effectiveness of the design depends on the ability to achieve homogeneous blocks of experimental units. The ability to form homogeneous blocks depends on the researcher's knowledge of the experimental material. When blocking is used effectively, the error mean square in the ANOVA table will be reduced, the V.R. will be increased, and the chance of rejecting the null hypothesis will be improved.

In animal experiments, if it is believed that different breeds of animal will respond differently to the same treatment, the breed of animal may be used as a blocking factor. Litters may also be used as blocks, in which case an animal from each litter receives a treatment. In experiments involving human beings, if it is desired that differences resulting from age be eliminated, then subjects may be grouped according to age so that one person of each age receives each treatment. The randomized complete block design also may be employed effectively when an experiment must be carried out in more than one laboratory (block) or when several days (blocks) are required for completion.

Advantages Some of the advantages of the randomized complete block design include the fact that it is both easily understood and computationally simple. Furthermore, certain complications that may arise in the course of an experiment are easily handled when this design is employed.

It is instructive here to point out that the paired comparisons analysis presented in Chapter 7 is a special case of the randomized complete block design. Example 7.4.1, for example, may be treated as a randomized complete block design in which the two points in time (Before and After) are the treatments and the individuals on whom the measurements were taken are the blocks.

Data Display In general, the data from an experiment utilizing the randomized complete block design may be displayed in a table such as Table 8.3.1. The following new notation in this table should be observed:

$$\text{the total of the } i\text{th block} = T_{i.} = \sum_{j=1}^{k} x_{ij}$$

$$\text{the mean of the } i\text{th block} = \bar{x}_{i.} = \frac{\sum_{j=1}^{k} x_{ij}}{k} = \frac{T_{i.}}{k}$$

$$\text{and the grand total} = T_{..} = \sum_{j=1}^{k} T_{.j} = \sum_{i=1}^{n} T_{i.}$$

TABLE 8.3.1 Table of Sample Values for the Randomized Complete Block Design

Blocks	Treatments 1	2	3	$\cdots$	k	Total	Mean
1	x_{11}	x_{12}	x_{13}	$\cdots$	x_{1k}	$T_{1.}$	$\bar{x}_{1.}$
2	x_{21}	x_{22}	x_{23}	$\cdots$	x_{2k}	$T_{2.}$	$\bar{x}_{2.}$
3	x_{31}	x_{32}	x_{33}	$\cdots$	x_{3k}	$T_{3.}$	$\bar{x}_{3.}$
$\vdots$	$\vdots$	$\vdots$	$\vdots$	$\vdots$	$\vdots$	$\vdots$	$\vdots$
n	x_{n1}	x_{n2}	x_{n3}	$\cdots$	x_{nk}	$T_{n.}$	$\bar{x}_{n.}$
Total	$T_{.1}$	$T_{.2}$	$T_{.3}$	$\cdots$	$T_{.k}$	$T_{..}$	
Mean	$\bar{x}_{.1}$	$\bar{x}_{.2}$	$\bar{x}_{.3}$	$\cdots$	$\bar{x}_{.k}$		$\bar{x}_{..}$

indicating that the grand total may be obtained either by adding row totals or by adding column totals.

Two-Way ANOVA   The technique for analyzing the data from a randomized complete block design is called *two-way analysis of variance* since an observation is categorized on the basis of two criteria—the block to which it belongs as well as the treatment group to which it belongs.

The steps for hypothesis testing when the randomized complete block design is used are as follows:

1. *Data*   After identifying the treatments, the blocks, and the experimental units, the data, for convenience, may be displayed as in Table 8.3.1.

2. *Assumptions*   The model for the randomized complete block design and its underlying assumptions are as follows:

The Model

$$x_{ij} = \mu + \beta_i + \tau_j + e_{ij} \tag{8.3.1}$$

$$i = 1, 2, \ldots, n; \qquad j = 1, 2, \ldots, k$$

In this model

x_{ij} is a typical value from the overall population.

μ is an unknown constant.

β_i represents a block effect reflecting the fact that the experimental unit fell in the ith block.

τ_j represents a treatment effect, reflecting the fact that the experimental unit received the jth treatment.

e_{ij} is a residual component representing all sources of variation other than treatments and blocks.

Assumptions of the Model

a. Each x_{ij} that is observed constitutes a random independent sample of size 1 from one of the kn populations represented.
b. Each of these kn populations is normally distributed with mean μ_{ij} and the same variance σ^2. This implies that the e_{ij} are independently and normally distributed with mean 0 and variance σ^2.
c. The block and treatment effects are additive. This assumption may be interpreted to mean that there is no *interaction* between treatments and blocks. In other words, a particular block-treatment combination does not produce an effect that is greater or less than the sum of their individual

effects. It can be shown that when this assumption is met

$$\sum_{j=1}^{k} \tau_j = \sum_{i=1}^{n} \beta_i = 0$$

The consequences of a violation of this assumption are misleading results. Anderson and Bancroft (42) suggest that one need not become concerned with the violation of the additivity assumption unless the largest mean is more than 50 percent greater than the smallest. The nonadditivity problem is also dealt with by Tukey (43) and Mandel (44).

When these assumptions hold true, the τ_j and β_i are a set of fixed constants, and we have a situation that fits the fixed-effects model.

3. *Hypotheses*   We may test

$$H_0: \tau_j = 0, \qquad j = 1, 2, \ldots, k$$

against the alternative

$$H_A: \text{not all } \tau_j = 0$$

A hypothesis test regarding block effects is not usually carried out under the assumptions of the fixed-effects model for two reasons. First, the primary interest is in treatment effects, the usual purpose of the blocks being to provide a means of eliminating an extraneous source of variation. Second, although the experimental units are randomly assigned to the treatments, the blocks are obtained in a nonrandom manner.

4. *Test Statistic*   The test statistic is V.R.

5. *Distribution of the Test Statistic*   When H_0 is true and the assumptions are met, V.R. follows an F distribution.

6. *Decision Rule*   Reject the null hypothesis if the computed value of the test statistic V.R. is equal to or greater than the critical value of F.

7. *Calculation of Test Statistic*   It can be shown that the total sum of squares for the randomized complete block design can be partitioned into three components, one each attributable to treatments (SST_r), blocks ($SSBl$), and error (SSE). The algebra is somewhat tedious and will be omitted. The partitioned sum of squares may be expressed by the following equation:

$$\sum_{j=1}^{k} \sum_{i=1}^{n} \left(x_{ij} - \bar{x}_{..}\right)^2 = \sum_{j=1}^{k} \sum_{i=1}^{n} \left(\bar{x}_{i.} - \bar{x}_{..}\right)^2 + \sum_{j=1}^{k} \sum_{i=1}^{n} \left(\bar{x}_{.j} - \bar{x}_{..}\right)^2$$

$$+ \sum_{j=1}^{k} \sum_{i=1}^{n} \left(x_{ij} - \bar{x}_{i.} - \bar{x}_{.j} + \bar{x}_{..}\right)^2 \qquad (8.3.2)$$

that is,

$$SST = SSBl + SSTr + SSE \qquad (8.3.3)$$

The computing formulas for the quantities in Equations 8.3.2 and 8.3.3 are as follows:

$$SST = \sum_{j=1}^{k} \sum_{i=1}^{n} x_{ij}^2 - C \qquad (8.3.4)$$

$$SSBl = \sum_{i=1}^{n} \frac{T_{i.}^2}{k} - C \qquad (8.3.5)$$

$$SSTr = \sum_{j=1}^{k} \frac{T_{.j}^2}{n} - C \qquad (8.3.6)$$

$$SSE = SST - SSBl - SSTr \qquad (8.3.7)$$

It will be recalled that C is a correction term, and in the present situation it is computed as follows:

$$C = \left(\sum_{j=1}^{k} \sum_{i=1}^{n} x_{ij}\right)^2 \bigg/ kn$$

$$= T_{..}^2 / kn \qquad (8.3.8)$$

The appropriate degrees of freedom for each component of Equation 8.3.3 are:

$$\begin{array}{cccc} \text{total} & \text{blocks} & \text{treatments} & \text{residual (error)} \\ kn - 1 = & (n - 1) + & (k - 1) & + (n - 1)(k - 1) \end{array}$$

The residual degrees of freedom, like the residual sum of squares, may be obtained by subtraction as follows:

$$(kn - 1) - (n - 1) - (k - 1) = kn - 1 - n + 1 - k + 1$$

$$= n(k - 1) - 1(k - 1) = (n - 1)(k - 1)$$

The ANOVA Table   The results of the calculations for the randomized complete block design may be displayed in an ANOVA table such as Table 8.3.2.

TABLE 8.3.2 ANOVA Table for the Randomized Complete Block Design

Source	SS	d.f.	MS	V.R.
Treatments	SSTr	$(k - 1)$	$MSTr = SSTr/(k - 1)$	$MSTr/MSE$
Blocks	SSBl	$(n - 1)$	$MSBl = SSBl/(n - 1)$	
Residual	SSE	$(n - 1)(k - 1)$	$MSE = SSE/(n - 1)(k - 1)$	
Total	SST	$kn - 1$		

8. *Statistical Decision* It can be shown that when the fixed-effects model applies and the null hypothesis of no treatment effects (all $\tau_i = 0$) is true, both the error, or residual, mean square and the treatments mean square are estimates of the common variance σ^2. When the null hypothesis is true, therefore, the quantity

$$MSTr/MSE$$

is distributed as F with $k - 1$ numerator degrees of freedom and $(n - 1) \times (k - 1)$ denominator degrees of freedom. The computed variance ratio, therefore, is compared with the critical value of F.

9. *Conclusion* If we reject H_0, we conclude that the alternative hypothesis is true. If we fail to reject H_0, we conclude that H_0 may be true.

The following example illustrates the use of the randomized complete block design.

Example 8.3.1

A physical therapist wished to compare three methods for teaching patients to use a certain prosthetic device. He felt that the rate of learning would be different for patients of different ages and wished to design an experiment in which the influence of age could be taken into account.

Solution: The randomized complete block design is the appropriate design for this physical therapist.

1. *Data* Three patients in each of five age groups were selected to participate in the experiment, and one patient in each age group was randomly assigned to each of the teaching methods. The methods of instruction constitute our three treatments, and the five age groups are the blocks. The data shown in Table 8.3.3 were obtained.

2. *Assumptions* We assume that each of the 15 observations constitutes a simple random sample of size 1 from one of the 15 populations defined by a block–treatment combination. For example, we assume that the number 7 in the table constitutes a randomly selected response from a population of responses that would result if a population of subjects under the age of 20 received teaching method A. We assume that the responses in the 15 represented populations are normally distributed with equal variances.

TABLE 8.3.3 Time (In Days) Required to Learn the Use of a Certain Prosthetic Device

Age Group	Teaching Method			Total	Mean
	A	**B**	**C**		
Under 20	7	9	10	26	8.67
20 to 29	8	9	10	27	9.00
30 to 39	9	9	12	30	10.00
40 to 49	10	9	12	31	10.33
50 and over	11	12	14	37	12.33
Total	45	48	58	151	
Mean	9.0	9.6	11.6		10.07

3. *Hypotheses*

$$H_0: \tau_j = 0, \qquad j = 1, 2, 3$$

$$H_A: \text{not all } \tau_j = 0$$

Let $\alpha = .05$.

4. *Test Statistic*   The test statistic is V.R. $= MSTr/MSE$.

5. *Distribution of the Test Statistic*   When H_0 is true and the assumptions are met, V.R. follows an F distribution with 2 degrees of freedom.

6. *Decision Rule*   Reject the null hypothesis if the computed V.R. is equal to or greater than the critical F, which we find in Appendix Table G to be 4.46.

7. *Calculation of Test Statistic*   We compute the following sums of squares:

$$C = \frac{(151)^2}{(3)(5)} = \frac{22801}{15} = 1520.0667$$

$$SST = 7^2 + 9^2 + \cdots + 14^2 - 1520.0667 = 46.9333$$

$$SSBl = \frac{26^2 + 27^2 + \cdots + 37^2}{3} - 1520.0667 = 24.9333$$

$$SSTr = \frac{45^2 + 48^2 + 58^2}{5} - 1520.0667 = 18.5333$$

$$SSE = 46.9333 - 24.9333 - 18.5333 = 3.4667$$

The degrees of freedom are total $= (3)(5) - 1 = 14$, blocks $= 5 - 1 = 4$, treatments $= 3 - 1 = 2$, and residual $= (5 - 1)(3 - 1) = 8$. The results of the calculations may be displayed in an ANOVA table as in Table 8.3.4.

TABLE 8.3.4 ANOVA Table for Example 8.3.1

Source	SS	*d.f.*	MS	V.R.
Treatments	18.5333	2	9.26665	21.38
Blocks	24.9333	4	6.233325	
Residual	3.4667	8	.4333375	
Total	46.9333	14		

ROW	C1	C2	C3
1	7	1	1
2	9	1	2
3	10	1	3
4	8	2	1
5	9	2	2
6	10	2	3
7	9	3	1
8	9	3	2
9	12	3	3
10	10	4	1
11	9	4	2
12	12	4	3
13	11	5	1
14	12	5	2
15	14	5	3

Figure 8.3.1 MINITAB worksheet for the data in Figure 8.3.2.

8. *Statistical Decision* Since our computed variance ratio, 21.38, is greater than 4.46, we reject the null hypothesis of no treatment effects on the assumption that such a large V.R. reflects the fact that the two sample mean squares are not estimating the same quantity. The only other explanation for this large V.R. would be that the null hypothesis is really true, and we have just observed an unusual set of results. We rule out the second explanation in favor of the first.

9. *Conclusion* We conclude that not all treatment effects are equal to zero, or equivalently, that not all treatment means are equal. For this test $p < .005$.

Computer Analysis Most statistics software packages will analyze data from a randomized complete block design. We illustrate the input and output for MINITAB. We use the data from the experiment to set up a MINITAB worksheet consisting of three columns. Column 1 contains the observations, column 2 contains numbers that identify the block to which each observation belongs, and column 3 contains numbers that identify the treatment to which each observation belongs. Figure 8.3.1 shows the MINITAB worksheet for Exercise 8.3.1. Figure 8.3.2 contains the MINTAB command that initiates the analysis and the resulting ANOVA table.

Alternatives When the data available for analysis do not meet the assumptions of the randomized complete block design as discussed here, the Friedman procedure discussed in Chapter 13 may prove to be a suitable nonparametric alternative.

```
MTB > twoway c1, c2, c3
ANALYSIS OF VARIANCE   C1
SOURCE      DF        SS        MS
C2           4    24.933     6.233
C3           2    18.533     9.267
ERROR        8     3.467     0.433
TOTAL       14    46.933
```

Figure 8.3.2 MINITAB command and printout for two-way analysis of variance, Example 8.3.1.

EXERCISES

For Exercises 8.3.1–8.35 perform the nine-step hypothesis testing procedure for analysis of variance. Determine the p value for each exercise.

8.3.1 The objective of a study by Druml et al. (A-11) was to evaluate the impact of respiratory alkalosis on the elimination of intravenously infused lactate. Subjects were eight patients treated by ventilatory support for neurologic or neuromuscular diseases. Plasma lactate concentration measurements were taken on two randomly assigned occasions: during normoventilation and during respiratory alkalosis induced by controlled hyperventilation. Lactate elimination was evaluated after infusing 1 mmol/kg body weight of L-lactic acid within five minutes. The following are the plasma lactate values (mmol/l) 90 minutes after infusion for each subject for each occasion.

Subject	Normoventilation	Hyperventilation
1	1.3	2.8
2	1.4	2.0
3	1.2	1.7
4	1.1	2.7
5	1.8	2.1
6	1.4	1.8
7	1.3	2.0
8	1.9	2.8

SOURCE: Wilfred Druml, Georg Grimm, Anton N. Laggner, Kurt Lenz, and Bruno Schneeweiß, "Lactic Acid Kinetics in Respiratory Alkalosis," *Critical Care Medicine*, *19* (1991), 1120–1124. © by Williams & Wilkins, 1991.

After eliminating subject effects, can we conclude that the mean plasma lactate value is different for normoventilation and hyperventilation? Let $\alpha = .05$.

8.3.2 McConville et al. (A-12) report the effects of chewing one piece of nicotine gum (containing 2 mg of nicotine) on tic frequency in patients whose Tourette's disorder was inadequately controlled by haloperidol. The following are the tic frequencies under four conditions.

| | | | **Number of Tics During 30-Minute Period** | |
| | | | **After End of Chewing** | |
Patient	**Baseline**	**Gum Chewing**	**0–30 Minutes**	**30–60 Minutes**
1	249	108	93	59
2	1095	593	600	861
3	83	27	32	61
4	569	363	342	312
5	368	141	167	180
6	326	134	144	158
7	324	126	312	260
8	95	41	63	71
9	413	365	282	321
10	332	293	525	455

SOURCE: Brian J. McConville, M. Harold Fogelson, Andrew B. Norman, William M. Klykylo, Pat Z. Manderscheid, Karen W. Parker, and Paul R. Sanberg, "Nicotine Potentiation of Haloperidol in Reducing Tic Frequency in Tourette's Disorder," *American Journal of Psychiatry*, *148* (1991), 793–794. Copyright 1991, The American Psychiatric Association. Reprinted by permission.

After eliminating patient effects can we conclude that the mean number of tics differs among the four conditions? Let $\alpha = .01$.

8.3.3 A remotivation team in a psychiatric hospital conducted an experiment to compare five methods for remotivating patients. Patients were grouped according to level of initial motivation. Patients in each group were randomly assigned to the five methods. At the end of the experimental period the patients were evaluated by a team composed of a psychiatrist, a psychologist, a nurse, and a social worker, none of whom was aware of the method to which patients had been assigned. The team assigned each patient a composite score as a measure of his or her level of motivation. The results were as follows.

| **Level of Initial Motivation** | **Remotivation Method** | | | | |
	A	**B**	**C**	**D**	**E**
Nil	58	68	60	68	64
Very low	62	70	65	80	69
Low	67	78	68	81	70
Average	70	81	70	89	74

Do these data provide sufficient evidence to indicate a difference in mean scores among methods? Let $\alpha = .05$.

8.3.4 The nursing supervisor in a local health department wished to study the influence of time of day on length of home visits by the nursing staff. It was thought that individual differences among nurses might be large, so the nurse was used as a blocking factor. The nursing supervisor collected the following data.

	Length of Home Visit by Time of Day			
Nurse	Early Morning	Late Morning	Early Afternoon	Late Afternoon
A	27	28	30	23
B	31	30	27	20
C	35	38	34	30
D	20	18	20	14

Do these data provide sufficient evidence to indicate a difference in length of home visit among the different times of day? Let $\alpha = .05$.

8.3.5 Four subjects participated in an experiment to compare three methods of relieving stress. Each subject was placed in a stressful situation on three different occasions. Each time a different method for reducing stress was used with the subject. The response variable is the amount of decrease in stress level as measured before and after treatment application. The results were as follows.

	Treatment		
Subject	A	B	C
1	16	26	22
2	16	20	23
3	17	21	22
4	28	29	36

Can we conclude from these data that the three methods differ in effectiveness? Let $\alpha = .05$.

8.3.6 In a study by Valencia et al. (A-13) the effects of environmental temperature and humidity on 24-hour energy expenditure were measured using whole-body indirect calorimetry in eight normal-weight young men who wore standardized light clothing and followed a controlled activity regimen. Temperature effects were assessed by measurements at 20, 23, 26, and 30 degrees at ambient humidity and at 20 and 30 degrees with high humidity. What is the blocking variable? The treatment variable? How many blocks are there? How many treatments? Construct an ANOVA table in which you specify the sources of variability and the degrees of freedom for each. What are the experimental units? What extraneous variables can you think of whose effects would be included in the error term?

8.3.7 Hodgson et al. (A-14) conducted a study in which they induced gastric dilatation in six anesthetized dogs maintained with constant-dose isoflurane in oxygen. Cardiopulmonary measurements prior to stomach distension (baseline) were compared with measurements taken during .1, .5, 1.0, 1.5, 2.5, and 3.5 hours of stomach distension by analyzing the change from baseline. After distending the stomach, cardiac index increased from 1.5 to 3.5 hours. Stroke volume did not change. During inflation, increases were observed in systemic arterial, pulmonary arterial, and right atrial pressure. Respiratory frequency was unchanged. Pa_{O_2} tended to decrease during gastric dilatation. What are the experimental units? The blocks? Treatment variable? Response variable(s)? Can you think of any extraneous variable whose effect would contribute to the error term? Construct an ANOVA table for this study in which you identify the sources of variability and specify the degrees of freedom.

8.4
The Repeated Measures Design

One of the most frequently used experimental designs in the health sciences field is the *repeated measures* design.

DEFINITION

A *repeated measures* design is one in which measurements of the same variable are made on each subject on two or more different occasions.

The different occasions during which measurements are taken may be either points in time or different conditions such as different treatments.

When to Use Repeated Measures   The usual motivation for using a repeated measures design is a desire to control for variability among subjects. In such a design each subject serves as its own control. When measurements are taken on only two occasions we have the paired comparisons design that we discussed in Chapter 7. One of the most frequently encountered situations in which the repeated measures design is used is the situation in which the investigator is concerned with responses over time.

Advantages   The major advantage of the repeated measures design is, as previously mentioned, its ability to control for extraneous variation among subjects. An additional advantage is the fact that fewer subjects are needed for the repeated measures design than for a design in which different subjects are used for each occasion on which measurements are made. Suppose, for example, that we have four treatments (in the usual sense) or four points in time on each of which we would like to have 10 measurements. If a different sample of subjects is used for each of the four treatments or points in time, 40 subjects would be required. If we are able to take measurements on the same subject for each treatment or point in time—that is, if we can use a repeated measures design—only 10 subjects would be required. This can be a very attractive advantage if subjects are scarce or expensive to recruit.

Disadvantages   A major potential problem to be on the alert for is what is known as the *carry-over effect*. When two or more treatments are being evaluated, the investigator should make sure that a subject's response to one treatment does not reflect a residual effect from previous treatments. This problem can frequently be solved by allowing a sufficient length of time between treatments.

Another possible problem is the *position effect*. A subject's response to a treatment experienced last in a sequence may be different from the response that would have occurred if the treatment had been first in the sequence. In certain studies, such as those involving physical participation on the part of the subjects, enthusiasm that is high at the beginning of the study may give way to boredom toward the end. A way around this problem is to randomize the sequence of treatments independently for each subject.

Single-Factor Repeated Measures Design   The simplest repeated measures design is the one in which, in addition to the treatment variable, one additional variable is considered. The reason for introducing this additional variable is to measure and isolate its contribution to the total variability among the observations. We refer to this additional variable as a *factor*.

DEFINITION

The repeated measures design in which one additional factor is introduced into the experiment is called a *single-factor repeated measures design*.

We refer to the additional factor as subjects. In the single-factor repeated measures design, each subject receives each of the treatments. The order in which the subjects are exposed to the treatments, when possible, is random, and the randomization is carried out independently for each subject.

Assumptions   The following are the assumptions of the single-factor repeated measures design that we consider in this text. A design in which these assumptions are met is called a *fixed-effects additive* design.

1. The subjects under study constitute a simple random sample from a population of similar subjects.
2. Each observation is an independent simple random sample of size 1 from each of kn populations, where n is the number of subjects and k is the number of treatments to which each subject is exposed.
3. The kn populations have potentially different means, but they all have the same variance.
4. The k treatments are fixed, that is, they are the only treatments about which we have an interest in the current situation. We do not wish to make inferences to some larger collection of treatments.
5. There is no interaction between treatments and subjects. That is, the treatment and subject effects are additive.

Experimenters may find frequently that their data do not conform to the assumptions of fixed treatments and/or additive treatment and subject effects. For such cases the references at the end of this chapter may be consulted for guidance.

TABLE 8.4.1 Daily (24-h) Respiratory Quotients at Three Different Points in Time

Subject	Baseline	Day 3	Day 7	Total
1	0.800	0.809	0.832	2.441
2	0.819	0.858	0.835	2.512
3	0.886	0.865	0.837	2.588
4	0.824	0.876	0.900	2.600
5	0.820	0.903	0.877	2.600
6	0.906	0.820	0.865	2.591
7	0.800	0.867	0.857	2.524
8	0.837	0.852	0.847	2.536
Total	6.692	6.850	6.850	20.392

SOURCE: James O. Hill, John C. Peters, George W. Reed, David G. Schlundt, Teresa Sharp, and Harry L. Greene, "Nutrient Balance in Humans: Effect of Diet Composition," *American Journal of Clinical Nutrition*, *54* (1991), 10–17. © *American Journal of Clinical Nutrition*.

The Model The model for the fixed-effects additive single-factor repeated measures design is

$$x_{ij} = \mu + \beta_i + \tau_j + e_{ij} \qquad (8.4.1)$$

$$i = 1, 2, \ldots, n; \qquad j = 1, 2, \ldots, k$$

The reader will recognize this model as the model for the randomized complete block design discussed in Section 8.3. The subjects are the blocks. Consequently the notation, data display, and hypothesis testing procedure are the same as for the randomized complete block design as presented earlier. The following is an example of a repeated measures design.

Example 8.4.1

Hill, et al. (A-15) examined the effect of alterations in diet composition on energy expenditure and nutrient balance in humans. One measure of energy expenditure employed was a quantity called the respiratory quotient (RQ). Table 8.4.1 shows, for three different points in time, the daily (24-h) respiratory quotients following a high calorie diet of the eight subjects who participated in the study. We wish to know if there is a difference in the mean RQ values among the three points in time.

Solution:

1. *Data* See Table 8.4.1.

2. *Assumptions* We assume that the assumptions for the fixed-effects, additive single-factor repeated measures design are met.

3. *Hypotheses*

$$H_0: \mu_B = \mu_{D3} = \mu_{D7}$$

$$H_A: \text{not all } \mu\text{'s are equal}$$

4. *Test Statistic*   V.R. = Treatment MS/Error MS.

5. *Distribution of Test Statistic* F with $3 - 1 = 2$ numerator degrees of freedom and $23 - 2 - 7 = 14$ denominator degrees of freedom.

6. *Decision Rule*   Let $\alpha = .05$. The critical value of F is 3.74. Reject H_0 if computed V.R. is equal to or greater than 3.74.

7. *Calculation of Test Statistic*   By Equation 8.3.4

$$SST = [.800^2 + .819^2 + \cdots + .847^2] - 20.392^2/24 = .023013$$

By Equation 8.3.5

$$SSBl = \frac{2.441^2 + 2.512^2 + \cdots + 2.536^2}{3} - 20.392^2/24 = .007438$$

By Equation 8.3.6

$$SSTr = \frac{6.692^2 + 6.850^2 + 6.850^2}{7} - 20.392^2 = .002080$$

By Equation 8.3.7

$$SSE = .023013 - .007438 - .002080 = .013495$$

The results of the calculations are displayed in Table 8.4.2.

8. *Statistical Decision*   Since 1.0788 is less than 3.74, we are unable to reject the null hypothesis.

9. *Conclusion*   We conclude that there may be no difference in the three population means. Since 1.0788 is less than 2.73, the critical F for $\alpha = .10$, the p value is greater than .10.

TABLE 8.4.2 ANOVA Table for Example 8.4.1

Source	SS	df	MS	V.R.
Treatments	.002080	2	.001040	1.0788
Blocks	.007438	7	.001063	
Error	.013495	14	.000964	
Total	.023013	23		

EXERCISES

For Exercises 8.4.1–8.4.3 perform the nine-step hypothesis testing procedure. Let $\alpha = .05$ and find the p value for each test.

8.4.1 One of the purposes of a study by Blum et al. (A-16) was to determine the pharmacokinetics of phenytoin in the presence and absence of concomitant fluconazole therapy. Among the data collected during the course of the study were the following trough serum concentrations of fluconazole for 10 healthy male subjects at three different points in time.

Subject	Day 14 C_{min} (μg / ml)	Day 18 C_{min} (μg / ml)	Day 21 C_{min} (μg / ml)
001	8.28	9.55	11.21
004	4.71	5.05	5.20
005	9.48	11.33	8.45
007	6.04	8.08	8.42
008	6.02	6.32	6.93
012	7.34	7.44	8.12
013	5.86	6.19	5.98
016	6.08	6.03	6.45
017	7.50	8.04	6.26
020	4.92	5.28	6.17

SOURCE: Robert A. Blum, John H. Wilton, Donald M. Hilligoss, Mark J. Gardner, Eugenia B. Henry, Nedra J. Harrison, and Jerome J. Schentag, "Effect of Fluconazole on the Disposition of Phenytoin," *Clinical Pharmacology and Therapeutics*, *49* (1991), 420–425.

8.4.2 Abbrecht et al. (A-17) examined the respiratory effects of exercise and various degrees of airway resistance. The five subjects, who were healthy nonsmoking men, engaged in prolonged submaximal exercise while breathing through different flow-resistive loads. Among the measurements taken were the following inspired ventilation values (l/min) at five successive points in time under one of the resistive-load conditions.

Subject	Time Interval				
	1	**2**	**3**	**4**	**5**
1	39.65	36.60	39.96	40.37	37.82
2	44.88	40.84	43.96	44.10	45.41
3	32.98	33.79	34.32	33.89	32.81
4	38.49	35.50	39.63	35.21	37.51
5	39.71	41.90	36.50	40.36	42.48

SOURCE: Peter H. Abbrecht, M.D., Ph.D. Used by permission.

8.4.3 Kabat-Zinn et al. (A-18) designed a study to determine the effectiveness of a group stress reduction program based on mindfulness meditation for patients with anxiety disorders. The subjects were selected from those referred to a stress reduction and relaxation program. Among the data collected were the scores made on the Hamilton Rating Scale for Anxiety at three different points in time: initial recruitment (IR), pretreatment (Pre), posttreatment (Post), and three-month followup (3-M). The results for 14 subjects were as follows:

IR	Pre	Post	3-M
21	21	16	19
30	38	10	21
38	19	15	6
43	33	30	24
35	34	25	10
40	40	31	30
27	15	11	6
18	11	4	7
31	42	23	27
21	23	21	17
18	24	16	13
28	8	5	2
40	37	31	19
35	32	12	21

SOURCE: Kenneth E. Fletcher, Ph.D. Used with permission.

8.4.4. The purpose of a study by Speechley et al. (A-19) was to compare changes in self-assessed clinical confidence over a two-year residency between two groups of family practice residents, one starting in a family practice center and the other starting in a hospital. Forty-two residents participated at baseline, and 24 provided completed responses after two years. Confidence regarding 177 topics in 19 general topic areas was assessed using self-completed questionnaires administered at baseline and after 6, 12, and 24 months. Residents rotated every 6 months between sites, with approximately half starting in each site. Assignment to starting site included consideration of the residents' stated preferences. Who are the subjects in this study? What is the treatment variable? The response variable(s)? Comment on carry-over effect and position effect as they may or may not be of concern in this study. Construct an ANOVA table for this study in which you identify the sources of variability and specify the degrees of freedom for each.

8.4.5. Barnett and Maughan (A-20) conducted a study to determine if there is an acclimation effect when unacclimatized males exercise in the heat at weekly intervals. Five subjects exercised for one hour at 55 percent Vo_{2max} on four different occasions. The first exercise was in moderate conditions. The subsequent three were performed at weekly intervals in the heat. There were no significant differences between trials in the heat for heart rate, rectal temperature or Vo_2. Who are the subjects for this study? What is the treatment variable? The response variable(s)? Comment on carry-over effect and position effect as they may or may not be of concern in this study. Construct an ANOVA table for this study in which you identify the sources of variability and specify the degrees of freedom for each.

8.5
The Factorial Experiment

In the experimental designs that we have considered up to this point we have been interested in the effects of only one variable, the treatments. Frequently, however, we may be interested in studying, simultaneously, the effects of two or more variables. We refer to the variables in which we are interested as *factors*. The experiment in which two or more factors are investigated simultaneously is called a *factorial experiment*.

The different designated categories of the factors are called *levels*. Suppose, for example, that we are studying the effect on reaction time of three dosages of some drug. The drug factor, then, is said to occur at three levels. Suppose the second factor of interest in the study is age, and it is thought that two age groups, under 65 years and 65 years and over, should be included. We then have two levels of the age factor. In general, we say that factor A occurs at a levels and factor B occurs at b levels.

In a factorial experiment we may study not only the effects of individual factors but also, if the experiment is properly conducted, the *interaction* between factors. To illustrate the concept of interaction let us consider the following example.

Example 8.5.1

Suppose, in terms of effect on reaction time, that the true relationship between three dosage levels of some drug and the age of human subjects taking the drug is known. Suppose further that age occurs at two levels—"young" (under 65) and "old" (65 and over). If the true relationship between the two factors is known, we will know, for the three dosage levels, the mean effect on reaction time of subjects in the two age groups. Let us assume that effect is measured in terms of reduction in reaction time to some stimulus. Suppose these means are as shown in Table 8.5.1.

The following important features of the data in Table 8.5.1 should be noted.

1. For both levels of factor A the difference between the means for any two levels of factor B is the same. That is, for both levels of factor A, the difference between means for levels 1 and 2 is 5, for levels 2 and 3 the difference is 10, and for levels 1 and 3 the difference is 15.

TABLE 8.5.1 Mean Reduction in Reaction Time (Milliseconds) of Subjects in Two Age Groups at Three Drug Dosage Levels

Factor A—Age	Factor B—Drug Dosage		
	$j = 1$	$j = 2$	$j = 3$
Young ($i = 1$)	$\mu_{11} = 5$	$\mu_{12} = 10$	$\mu_{13} = 20$
Old ($i = 2$)	$\mu_{21} = 10$	$\mu_{22} = 15$	$\mu_{23} = 25$

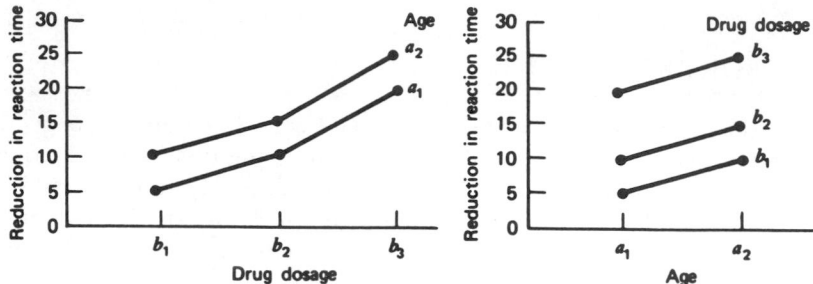

Figure 8.5.1 Age and drug effects, no interaction present.

2. For all levels of factor B the difference between means for the two levels of factor A is the same. In the present case the difference is 5 at all three levels of factor B.

3. A third characteristic is revealed when the data are plotted as in Figure 8.5.1. We note that the curves corresponding to the different levels of a factor are all parallel.

When population data possess the three characteristics listed above, we say that there is no interaction present.

The presence of interaction between two factors can affect the characteristics of the data in a variety of ways depending on the nature of the interaction. We illustrate the effect of one type of interaction by altering the data of Table 8.5.1 as shown in Table 8.5.2.

The important characteristics of the data in Table 8.5.2 are as follows.

1. The difference between means for any two levels of factor B is not the same for both levels of factor A. We note in Table 8.5.2, for example, that the difference between levels 1 and 2 of factor B is -5 for the young age group and $+5$ for the old age group.

2. The difference between means for both levels of factor A is not the same at all levels of factor B. The differences between factor A means are -10, 0, and 15 for levels 1, 2, and 3, respectively, of factor B.

3. The factor level curves are not parallel, as shown in Figure 8.5.2.

TABLE 8.5.2 Data of Table 8.5.1 Altered to Show the Effect of One Type of Interaction

| | Factor B—Drug Dosage | | |
Factor A—Age	$j = 1$	$j = 2$	$j = 3$
Young ($i = 1$)	$\mu_{11} = 5$	$\mu_{12} = 10$	$\mu_{13} = 20$
Old ($i = 2$)	$\mu_{21} = 15$	$\mu_{22} = 10$	$\mu_{23} = 5$

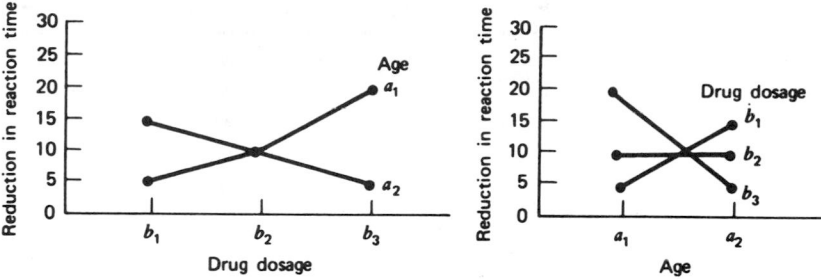

Figure 8.5.2 Age and drug effects, interaction present.

When population data exhibit the characteristics illustrated in Table 8.5.2 and Figure 8.5.2 we say that there is interaction between the two factors. We emphasize that the kind of interaction illustrated by the present example is only one of many types of interaction that may occur between two factors.

In summary, then, we can say that *there is interaction between two factors if a change in one of the factors produces a change in response at one level of the other factor different from that produced at other levels of this factor.*

Advantages   The advantages of the factorial experiment include the following.

1. The interaction of the factors may be studied.
2. There is a saving of time and effort.

In the factorial experiment all the observations may be used to study the effects of each of the factors under investigation. The alternative, when two factors are being investigated, would be to conduct two different experiments, one to study each of the two factors. If this were done, some of the observations would yield information only on one of the factors, and the remainder would yield information only on the other factor. To achieve the level of accuracy of the factorial experiment, more experimental units would be needed if the factors were studied through two experiments. It is seen, then, that 1 two-factor experiment is more economical than 2 one-factor experiments.

3. Since the various factors are combined in one experiment, the results have a wider range of application.

The Two-Factor Completely Randomized Design   A factorial arrangement may be studied with either of the designs that have been discussed. We illustrate the analysis of a factorial experiment by means of a two-factor completely randomized design.

TABLE 8.5.3 Table of Sample Data From a Two-Factor Completely Randomized Experiment

Factor A	Factor B 1	2	$\cdots$	b	Totals	Means
1	x_{111} $\vdots$ x_{11n}	x_{121} $\vdots$ x_{12n}	$\cdots$ $\vdots$ $\cdots$	x_{1b1} $\vdots$ x_{1bn}	$T_{1..}$	$\bar{x}_{1..}$
2	x_{211} $\vdots$ x_{21n}	x_{221} $\vdots$ x_{22n}	$\cdots$ $\vdots$ $\cdots$	x_{2b1} $\vdots$ x_{2bn}	$T_{2..}$	$\bar{x}_{2..}$
$\vdots$	$\vdots$	$\vdots$	$\vdots$	$\vdots$	$\vdots$	$\vdots$
a	x_{a11} $\vdots$ x_{a1n}	x_{a21} $\vdots$ x_{a2n}	$\cdots$ $\vdots$ $\cdots$	x_{ab1} $\vdots$ x_{abn}	$T_{a..}$	$\bar{x}_{a..}$
Totals	$T_{.1.}$	$T_{.2.}$	$\cdots$	$T_{.b.}$	$T_{...}$	
Means	$\bar{x}_{.1.}$	$\bar{x}_{.2.}$	$\cdots$	$\bar{x}_{.b.}$		$\bar{x}_{...}$

1. *Data* The results from a two-factor completely randomized design may be presented in tabular form as shown in Table 8.5.3.

Here we have a levels of factor A, b levels of factor B, and n observations for each combination of levels. Each of the ab combinations of levels of factor A with levels of factor B is a treatment. In addition to the totals and means shown in Table 8.5.3, we note that the total and mean of the ijth cell are

$$T_{ij} = \sum_{k=1}^{n} x_{ijk} \quad \text{and} \quad \bar{x}_{ij} = T_{ij.}/n$$

respectively. The subscript i runs from 1 to a and j runs from 1 to b. The total number of observations is nab.

To show that Table 8.5.3 represents data from a completely randomized design, we consider that each combination of factor levels is a treatment and that we have n observations for each treatment. An alternative arrangement of the data would be obtained by listing the observations of each treatment in a separate column. Table 8.5.3 may also be used to display data from a two-factor randomized block design if we consider the first observation in each cell as belonging to block 1, the second observation in each cell as belonging to block 2, and so on to the nth observation in each cell, which may be considered as belonging to block n.

Note the similarity of the data display for the factorial experiment as shown in Table 8.5.3 to the randomized complete block data display of Table 8.3.1. The factorial experiment, in order that the experimenter may test for interaction, requires at least two observations per cell, whereas the randomized complete block design only requires one observation per cell. We use two-way analysis of variance to analyze the data from a factorial experiment of the type presented here.

2. *Assumptions*   We assume a fixed-effects model and a two-factor completely randomized design. For a discussion of other designs consult the references at the end of this chapter.

   The Model   The fixed-effects model for the two-factor completely randomized design may be written as

$$x_{ijk} = \mu + \alpha_i + \beta_j + (\alpha\beta)_{ij} + e_{ijk}$$

$$i = 1, 2, \ldots, a; \qquad j = 1, 2, \ldots, b; \qquad k = 1, 2, \ldots, n \qquad (8.5.1)$$

where x_{ijk} is a typical observation, μ is a constant, α represents an effect due to factor A, β represents an effect due to factor B, $(\alpha\beta)$ represents an effect due to the interaction of factors A and B, and e_{ijk} represents the experimental error.

Assumptions of the Model

a. The observations in each of the ab cells constitute a random independent sample of size n drawn from the population defined by the particular combination of the levels of the two factors.

b. Each of the ab populations is normally distributed.

c. The populations all have the same variance.

3. *Hypotheses*   The following hypotheses may be tested.

   a. $H_0: \alpha_i = 0$ $\qquad\qquad\qquad$ $i = 1, 2, \ldots, a$
   $\quad\ H_A:$ not all $\alpha_i = 0$
   b. $H_0: \beta_j = 0$ $\qquad\qquad\qquad$ $j = 1, 2, \ldots, b$
   $\quad\ H_A:$ not all $\beta_j = 0$
   c. $H_0: (\alpha\beta)_{ij} = 0$ $\qquad\qquad$ $i = 1, 2, \ldots, a; \quad j = 1, 2, \ldots, b$
   $\quad\ H_A:$ not all $(\alpha\beta)_{ij} = 0$

Before collecting data, the researchers may decide to test only one of the possible hypotheses. In this case they select the hypothesis they wish to test, choose a significance level α, and proceed in the familiar, straightforward fashion. This procedure is free of the complications that arise if the researchers wish to test all three hypotheses.

When all three hypotheses are tested, the situation is complicated by the fact that the three tests are not independent in the probability sense. If we let α be the significance level associated with the test as a whole, and α', α'', and α''' the significance levels associated with hypotheses 1, 2, and 3, respectively, Kimball (45) has shown that

$$\alpha < 1 - (1 - \alpha')(1 - \alpha'')(1 - \alpha''') \qquad (8.5.2)$$

If $\alpha' = \alpha'' = \alpha''' = .05$, then $\alpha < 1 - (.95)^3$, or $\alpha < .143$. This means that the probability of rejecting one or more of the three hypotheses is something less than .143 when a significance level of .05 has been chosen for the hypotheses and all are true. To demonstrate the hypothesis testing procedure for each case, we perform all three tests. The reader, however, should be aware of the problem involved in interpreting the results. The problem is discussed by Dixon and Massey (46) and Guenther (47).

4. *Test Statistic*   The test statistic for each hypothesis set is V.R.

5. *Distribution of Test Statistic*   When H_0 is true and the assumptions are met each of the test statistics is distributed as F.

6. *Decision Rule*   Reject H_0 if the computed value of the test statistic is equal to or greater than the critical value of F.

7. *Calculation of Test Statistic*   By an adaptation of the procedure used in partitioning the total sum of squares for the completely randomized design, it can be shown that the total sum of squares under the present model can be partitioned into two parts as follows:

$$\sum_{i=1}^{a}\sum_{j=1}^{b}\sum_{k=1}^{n}\left(x_{ijk}-\bar{x}_{...}\right)^2 = \sum_{i=1}^{a}\sum_{j=1}^{b}\sum_{k=1}^{n}\left(\bar{x}_{ij.}-\bar{x}_{...}\right)^2$$

$$+\sum_{i=1}^{a}\sum_{j=1}^{b}\sum_{k=1}^{n}\left(x_{ijk}-\bar{x}_{ij.}\right)^2 \qquad (8.5.3)$$

or

$$SST = SSTr + SSE \qquad (8.5.4)$$

The sum of squares for treatments can be partitioned into three parts as follows:

$$\sum_{i=1}^{a}\sum_{j=1}^{b}\sum_{k=1}^{n}\left(\bar{x}_{ij.}-\bar{x}_{...}\right)^2 = \sum_{i=1}^{a}\sum_{j=1}^{b}\sum_{k=1}^{n}\left(\bar{x}_{i..}-\bar{x}_{...}\right)^2$$

$$+\sum_{i=1}^{a}\sum_{j=1}^{b}\sum_{k=1}^{n}\left(\bar{x}_{.j.}-\bar{x}_{...}\right)^2$$

$$+\sum_{i=1}^{a}\sum_{j=1}^{b}\sum_{k=1}^{n}\left(\bar{x}_{ij.}-\bar{x}_{i..}-\bar{x}_{.j.}+\bar{x}_{...}\right)^2 \qquad (8.5.5)$$

or

$$SSTr = SSA + SSB + SSAB$$

The computing formulas for the various components are as follows:

$$SST = \sum_{i=1}^{a} \sum_{j=1}^{b} \sum_{k=1}^{n} x_{ijk}^2 - C \qquad (8.5.6)$$

$$SSTr = \frac{\sum_{i=1}^{a} \sum_{j=1}^{b} T_{ij.}^2}{n} - C \qquad (8.5.7)$$

$$SSE = SST - SSTr \qquad (8.5.8)$$

$$SSA = \frac{\sum_{i=1}^{a} T_{i..}^2}{bn} - C \qquad (8.5.9)$$

$$SSB = \frac{\sum_{j=1}^{b} T_{.j.}^2}{an} - C \qquad (8.5.10)$$

and

$$SSAB = SSTr - SSA - SSB \qquad (8.5.11)$$

In the above equations

$$C = \left(\sum_{i=1}^{a} \sum_{j=1}^{b} \sum_{k=1}^{n} x_{ijk} \right)^2 \Big/ abn \qquad (8.5.12)$$

The ANOVA Table The results of the calculations for the fixed-effects model for a two-factor completely randomized experiment may, in general, be displayed as shown in Table 8.5.4.

8. *Statistical Decision* If the assumptions stated earlier hold true, and if each hypothesis is true, it can be shown that each of the variance ratios shown in Table 8.5.4 follows an F distribution with the indicated degrees of freedom. We reject H_0 if the computed V.R. values are equal to or greater than the corresponding critical values as determined by the degrees of freedom and the chosen significance levels.

9. *Conclusion* If we reject H_0, we conclude that H_A is true. If we fail to reject H_0, we conclude that H_0 may be true.

TABLE 8.5.4 Analysis of Variance Table for a Two-Factor Completely Randomized Experiment (Fixed-Effects Model)

Source	SS	d.f.	MS	V.R.
A	SSA	$a - 1$	$MSA = SSA/(a - 1)$	MSA/MSE
B	SSB	$b - 1$	$MSB = SSB/(b - 1)$	MSB/MSE
AB	$SSAB$	$(a - 1)(b - 1)$	$MSAB = SSAB/(a - 1)(b - 1)$	$MSAB/MSE$
Treatments	$SSTr$	$ab - 1$		
Residual	SSE	$ab(n - 1)$	$MSE = \dfrac{SSE}{ab(n - 1)}$	
Total	SST	$abn - 1$		

Example 8.5.2

In a study of length of time spent on individual home visits by public health nurses, data were reported on length of home visit, in minutes, by a sample of 80 nurses. A record was made also of each nurse's age and the type of illness of each patient visited. The researchers wished to obtain from their investigation answers to the following questions:

1. Does the mean length of home visit differ among different age groups of nurses?

2. Does the type of patient affect the mean length of home visit?

3. Is there interaction between nurse's age and type of patient?

Solution:

1. *Data*   The data on length of home visit that were obtained during the study are shown in Table 8.5.5.

2. *Assumptions*   To analyze these data we assume a fixed-effects model and a two-factor completely randomized design.

For our illustrative example we may test the following hypotheses subject to the conditions mentioned above.

   a. H_0: $\alpha_1 = \alpha_2 = \alpha_3 = \alpha_4 = 0$
       H_A: not all $\alpha_i = 0$

   b. H_0: $\beta_1 = \beta_2 = \beta_3 = \beta_4 = 0$
       H_A: not all $\beta_j = 0$

TABLE 8.5.5 Length of Home Visit in Minutes by Public Health Nurses by Nurse's Age Group and Type of Patient

	Factor B (Nurse's Age Group) Levels					
Factor A (Type of Patient) Levels	1 (20 to 29)	2 (30 to 39)	3 (40 to 49)	4 (50 and over)	Totals	Means
1 (Cardiac)	20	25	24	28		
	25	30	28	31		
	22	29	24	26	534	26.70
	27	28	25	29		
	21	30	30	32		
2 (Cancer)	30	30	39	40		
	45	29	42	45		
	30	31	36	50	765	38.25
	35	30	42	45		
	36	30	40	60		
3 (C.V.A.)	31	32	41	42		
	30	35	45	50		
	40	30	40	40	766	38.30
	35	40	40	55		
	30	30	35	45		
4 (Tuberculosis)	20	23	24	29		
	21	25	25	30		
	20	28	30	28	509	25.45
	20	30	26	27		
	19	31	23	30		
Totals	557	596	659	762	2574	
Means	27.85	29.8	32.95	38.10		32.18

Cell	a_1b_1	a_1b_2	a_1b_3	a_1b_4	a_2b_1	a_2b_2	a_2b_3	a_2b_4
Totals	115	142	131	146	176	150	199	240
Means	23.0	28.4	26.2	29.2	35.2	30.0	39.8	48.0

Cell	a_3b_1	a_3b_2	a_3b_3	a_3b_4	a_4b_1	a_4b_2	a_4b_3	a_4b_4
Totals	166	167	201	232	100	137	128	144
Means	33.2	33.4	40.2	46.4	20.0	27.4	25.6	28.8

    c. H_0: all $(\alpha\beta)_{ij} = 0$

       H_A: not all $(\alpha\beta)_{ij} = 0$

       Let $\alpha = .05$

4. *Test Statistic*　The test statistic for each hypothesis set is V.R.

5. *Distribution of Test Statistic* When H_0 is true and the assumptions are met each of the test statistics is distributed as F.

6. *Decision Rule* Reject H_0 if the computed value of the test statistic is equal to or greater than the critical value of F. The critical values of F for testing the three hypotheses of our illustrative example are 2.76, 2.76, and 2.04, respectively. Since denominator degrees of freedom equal to 64 are not shown in Table G, 60 was used as the denominator degrees of freedom.

7. *Calculation of Test Statistic* We use the data in Table 8.5.5 to perform the following calculations.

$$C = (2574)^2/80 = 82818.45$$

$$SST = (20^2 + 25^2 + \cdots + 30^2) - 82818.45 = 5741.55$$

$$SSTr = \frac{115^2 + 142^2 + \cdots + 144^2}{5} - 82818.45 = 4801.95$$

$$SSA = \frac{534^2 + 765^2 + 766^2 + 509^2}{20} - 82818.45 = 2992.45$$

$$SSB = \frac{557^2 + 596^2 + 659^2 + 762^2}{20} - 82818.45 = 1201.05$$

$$SSAB = 4801.95 - 2992.45 - 1201.05 = 608.45$$

$$SSE = 5741.55 - 4801.95 = 939.60$$

We display the results in Table 8.5.6.

8. *Statistical Decision* Since the three computed values of V.R. are all greater than the corresponding critical values, we reject all three null hypotheses.

TABLE 8.5.6 ANOVA Table for Example 8.5.2

Source	SS	d.f.	MS	V.R.
A	2992.45	3	997.48	67.95
B	1201.05	3	400.35	27.27
AB	608.45	9	67.61	4.61
Treatments	4801.95	15		
Residual	939.60	64	14.68	
Total	5741.55	79		

9. *Conclusion* When H_0: $\alpha_1 = \alpha_2 = \alpha_3 = \alpha_4$ is rejected, we conclude that there are differences among the levels of A, that is, differences in the average amount of time spent in home visits with different types of patients. Similarly, when H_0: $\beta_1 = \beta_2 = \beta_3 = \beta_4$ is rejected, we conclude that there are differences among the levels of B, or differences in the average amount of time spent on home visits among the different nurses when grouped by age. When H_0: $(\alpha\beta)_{ij} = 0$ is rejected, we conclude that factors A and B interact; that is, different combinations of levels of the two factors produce different effects. When the hypothesis of no interaction is rejected, interest in the levels of factors A and B usually become subordinate to interest in the interaction effects. In other words, we are more interested in learning what combinations of levels are significantly different.

We have treated only the case where the number of observations in each cell is the same. When the number of observations per cell is not the same for every cell the analysis becomes more complex. Many of the references that have been cited cover the analysis appropriate to such a situation, and the reader is referred to them for further information.

Computer Analysis Most statistical software packages, such as MINITAB and SAS®, will allow you to use a computer to analyze data generated by a factorial experiment. When MINITAB is used the response variable is entered in one column, the levels of the first factor in another column, the levels of the second factor in a third column, and so on. The resulting table will have for each observation a row containing the value of the response variable and the level of each factor at which the value was observed. The command is TWOWAY. MINITAB requires an equal number of observations in each cell. Some of the other software packages such as SAS® will accommodate unequal cell sizes.

EXERCISES

For Exercises 8.5.1–8.5.4 perform the analysis of variance, test appropriate hypotheses at the .05 level of significance, and determine the p value associated with each test.

8.5.1 Orth et al. (A-21) studied the effect of excessive levels of cysteine and homocysteine on tibial dyschondroplasia (TD) in broiler chicks. In one experiment, the researchers investigated the interaction between DL-homocystine and copper supplementation in the animals' diet. Among the variables on which they collected data were body weight at three weeks (WT1), severity of TD (TDS), and incidence of TD (TDI). There were two levels of homocysteine (HOMO): 1 = no added homocysteine, 2 = .48 percent homocysteine. The two levels of copper (CU) were 1 = no added copper, 2 = 250 ppm copper added. The results were as follows: (The authors used SAS to analyze their data.)

HOMO	CU	WT1	TDS	TDI	HOMO	CU	WT1	TDS	TDI
1	1	503	1	0	2	1	426	4	1
1	1	465	1	0	2	1	392	4	1
1	1	513	1	0	2	1	520	3	1
1	1	453	1	0	2	1	367	4	1
1	1	574	1	0	2	1	545	4	1
1	1	433	1	0	2	1	523	4	1
1	1	526	2	1	2	1	304	4	1
1	1	505	1	0	2	1	437	4	1
1	1	487	1	0	2	1	357	4	1
1	1	483	1	0	2	1	420	3	1
1	1	459	1	0	2	1	448	4	1
1	1	505	1	0	2	1	346	4	1
1	1	648	1	0	2	1	382	4	1
1	1	472	1	0	2	1	331	4	1
1	1	469	1	0	2	1	532	2	1
1	1	506	1	0	2	1	536	4	1
1	1	507	1	0	2	1	508	1	0
1	1	523	1	0	2	1	492	4	1
1	1	554	4	1	2	1	426	1	0
1	1	518	1	0	2	1	437	4	1
1	1	614	1	0	2	1	496	4	1
1	1	552	1	0	2	1	594	3	1
1	1	580	4	1	2	1	466	4	1
1	1	531	4	1	2	1	463	4	1
1	2	544	1	0	2	2	551	1	0
1	2	592	1	0	2	2	443	4	1
1	2	485	1	0	2	2	517	4	1
1	2	578	4	1	2	2	442	4	1
1	2	514	1	0	2	2	516	2	1
1	2	482	3	1	2	2	433	3	1
1	2	653	4	1	2	2	383	4	1
1	2	462	1	0	2	2	506	1	0
1	2	577	1	0	2	2	336	1	0
1	2	462	4	1	2	2	491	1	0
1	2	524	3	1	2	2	531	4	1
1	2	484	1	0	2	2	572	1	0
1	2	571	1	0	2	2	512	4	1
1	2	586	1	0	2	2	465	2	1
1	2	426	1	0	2	2	497	3	1
1	2	546	4	1	2	2	617	3	1
1	2	503	1	0	2	2	456	2	1
1	2	468	2	1	2	2	487	4	1
1	2	570	1	0	2	2	448	4	1
1	2	554	1	0	2	2	440	4	1
1	2	455	1	0	2	2	484	3	1
1	2	507	1	0	2	2	431	4	1
1	2	460	1	0	2	2	493	2	1
1	2	550	1	0	2	2	553	4	1

SOURCE: Michael Orth. Used with permission.

8.5.2. Researchers at a trauma center wished to develop a program to help brain-damaged trauma victims regain an acceptable level of independence. An experiment involving 72 subjects with the same degree of brain damage was conducted. The objective was to compare different combinations of psychiatric treatment and physical therapy. Each subject was assigned to one of 24 different combinations of four types of psychiatric treatment and six physical therapy programs. There were three subjects in each combination. The response variable is the number of months elapsing between initiation of therapy and time at which the patient was able to function independently. The results were as follows:

Physical Therapy Program	Psychiatric Treatment			
	A	B	C	D
I	11.0	9.4	12.5	13.2
	9.6	9.6	11.5	13.2
	10.8	9.6	10.5	13.5
II	10.5	10.8	10.5	15.0
	11.5	10.5	11.8	14.6
	12.0	10.5	11.5	14.0
III	12.0	11.5	11.8	12.8
	11.5	11.5	11.8	13.7
	11.8	12.3	12.3	13.1
IV	11.5	9.4	13.7	14.0
	11.8	9.1	13.5	15.0
	10.5	10.8	12.5	14.0
V	11.0	11.2	14.4	13.0
	11.2	11.8	14.2	14.2
	10.0	10.2	13.5	13.7
VI	11.2	10.8	11.5	11.8
	10.8	11.5	10.2	12.8
	11.8	10.2	11.5	12.0

Can one conclude on the basis of these data that the different psychiatric treatment programs have different effects? Can one conclude that the physical therapy programs differ in effectiveness? Can one conclude that there is interaction between psychiatric treatment programs and physical therapy programs? Let $\alpha = .05$ for each test.

Exercises 8.5.3 and 8.5.4 are optional since they have unequal cell sizes. It is recommended that the data for these be analyzed using SAS® or some other software package that will accept unequal cell sizes.

8.5.3 The effects of printed factual information and three augmentative communication techniques on attitudes of nondisabled individuals toward nonspeaking persons with physical disabilities were investigated by Gorenflo and Gorenflo (A-22). Subjects were undergraduates enrolled in an introductory psychology course at a large southwestern university. The variable of interest was scores on the Attitudes Toward Nonspeaking Persons Scale (ATNP). Higher scores indicated more favorable attitudes. The independent variables (factors) were information (INFO) and augmentative techniques (AID). The levels of INFO were as follows: 1 = presence of a sheet containing information about the nonspeaking person, 2 = absence of the sheet. The scores (levels) of AID were: 1 = no aid, 2 = alphabet board, 3 = computer-based voice output communication aid (VOCA). Subjects viewed a videotape depicting a nonspeaking adult having a conversation with a normal-speaking individual under one of the three AID conditions. The following data were collected and analyzed by SPSS/PC + :

INFO	AID	ATNP	INFO	AID	ATNP	INFO	AID	ATNP
1	1	82.00	1	3	109.00	2	1	33.00
1	1	92.00	1	3	96.00	2	1	34.00
1	1	100.00	1	3	127.00	2	1	29.00
1	1	110.00	1	3	124.00	2	2	118.00
1	1	99.00	1	3	93.00	2	2	110.00
1	1	96.00	1	3	112.00	2	2	74.00
1	1	92.00	1	3	95.00	2	2	106.00
1	1	95.00	1	3	107.00	2	2	107.00
1	1	126.00	1	3	102.00	2	2	83.00
1	1	93.00	1	3	102.00	2	2	82.00
1	1	103.00	1	3	112.00	2	2	92.00
1	1	101.00	1	3	105.00	2	2	89.00
1	1	120.00	1	3	109.00	2	2	108.00
1	1	94.00	1	3	111.00	2	2	106.00
1	1	94.00	1	3	116.00	2	2	95.00
1	1	93.00	1	3	112.00	2	2	97.00
1	1	101.00	1	3	112.00	2	2	98.00
1	1	65.00	1	3	84.00	2	2	108.00
1	1	29.00	1	3	107.00	2	2	120.00
1	2	112.00	1	3	123.00	2	2	94.00
1	2	100.00	1	3	97.00	2	2	99.00
1	2	88.00	1	3	108.00	2	2	99.00
1	2	99.00	1	3	105.00	2	2	104.00
1	2	97.00	1	3	129.00	2	2	110.00
1	2	107.00	1	3	140.00	2	2	33.00
1	2	110.00	1	3	141.00	2	3	99.00
1	2	91.00	1	3	145.00	2	3	112.00
1	2	123.00	2	1	107.00	2	3	98.00
1	2	97.00	2	1	82.00	2	3	84.00
1	2	115.00	2	1	78.00	2	3	100.00
1	2	107.00	2	1	98.00	2	3	101.00
1	2	107.00	2	1	88.00	2	3	94.00
1	2	101.00	2	1	95.00	2	3	101.00
1	2	122.00	2	1	95.00	2	3	97.00
1	2	114.00	2	1	93.00	2	3	95.00
1	2	101.00	2	1	108.00	2	3	98.00
1	2	125.00	2	1	102.00	2	3	116.00
1	2	104.00	2	1	83.00	2	3	99.00
1	2	102.00	2	1	111.00	2	3	97.00
1	2	113.00	2	1	97.00	2	3	84.00
1	2	88.00	2	1	90.00	2	3	91.00
1	2	116.00	2	1	90.00	2	3	106.00
1	2	114.00	2	1	85.00	2	3	100.00
1	2	108.00	2	1	95.00	2	3	104.00
1	2	95.00	2	1	97.00	2	3	79.00
1	2	84.00	2	1	78.00	2	3	84.00
1	2	83.00	2	1	98.00	2	3	110.00
1	2	134.00	2	1	91.00	2	3	141.00
1	2	96.00	2	1	99.00	2	3	141.00
1	2	37.00	2	1	102.00			
1	2	36.00	2	1	102.00			

SOURCE: Carole Wood Gorenflo, Ph.D. Used with permission.

8.5.4 The individual and combined influences of castration and adrenalectomy (ADX) on energy balance in rats were investigated by Ouerghi et al. (A-23). The following data on two dependent variables, gross energy (GE) intake and energy gain, by adrenalectomy and castration status were obtained:

Rat#	ADX	Castration	GE Intake	Energy Gain
1	No	No	3824	740.3
2	No	No	4069	1113.8
3	No	No	3782	331.42
4	No	No	3887	323.6
5	No	No	3670	259.02
6	No	No	3740	294.74
7	No	No	4356	336.14
8	No	No	4026	342.3
9	No	No	4367	261.47
10	No	No	4006	166.45
11	No	No	4251	385.98
12	No	No	4585	749.09
13	Yes	No	3557	253
14	Yes	No	3831	−106
15	Yes	No	3528	192
16	Yes	No	3270	−21
17	Yes	No	3078	−47
18	Yes	No	3314	39
19	Yes	No	3525	95
20	Yes	No	2953	−116
21	Yes	No	3351	−27
22	Yes	No	4197	496
23	Yes	No	4978	123
24	Yes	No	3269	78
25	No	Yes	4571	1012
26	No	Yes	3994	742
27	No	Yes	4138	481
28	No	Yes	5175	1179
29	No	Yes	5049	1399
30	No	Yes	5042	1017
31	No	Yes	5058	966
32	No	Yes	4267	662
33	No	Yes	5205	830
34	No	Yes	4541	638
35	No	Yes	5453	1732
36	No	Yes	4753	936
37	Yes	Yes	3924	189
38	Yes	Yes	3497	215
39	Yes	Yes	3417	304
40	Yes	Yes	3785	37
41	Yes	Yes	4157	360
42	Yes	Yes	4073	73
43	Yes	Yes	4510	483
44	Yes	Yes	3828	112
45	Yes	Yes	3530	154
46	Yes	Yes	3996	77

SOURCE: Denis Richard, Department of Physiology, Laval University. Used with permission.

8.5.5 Niaura et al. (A-24) examined 56 smokers' reactions to smoking cues and interpersonal interaction. Subjects participated in role play either with a confederate present or with a confederate absent. In each role-play situation, the subjects were exposed to either no smoking cues, visual cues, or visual plus olfactory cues. Measures of reactivity included changes from resting baseline on blood pressure, heart rate, self-reported smoking urge, and a measure of ad lib smoking behavior obtained after exposure to the experimental procedures. What are the factors in this study? At how many levels does each occur? Who are the subjects? What is (are) the response variable(s)? Comment on the number of subjects per cell in this experiment. Can you think of any extraneous variables whose effects are included in the error term?

8.5.6 Max et al. (A-25) randomized 62 inpatients with pain following major surgery to receive either desipramine or placebo at 6 A.M. on the first day after surgery. At their first request of pain medication after 8 A.M., they were given intravenous morphine, either 0.033 mg/kg or 0.10 mg/kg. Pain relief (measured on the visual analog scale), side effect scores, and time to remediation were determined for each subject. What are the factors in this study? At how many levels does each occur? Comment on the number of subjects per cell. What is (are) the response variable(s)?

8.6
Summary

The purpose of this chapter is to introduce the student to the basic ideas and techniques of analysis of variance. Two experimental designs, the completely randomized and the randomized complete block, are discussed in considerable detail. In addition, the concept of repeated measures designs and a factorial experiment as used with the completely randomized design are introduced. Individuals who wish to pursue further any aspect of analysis of variance will find the references at the end of the chapter most helpful. The extensive bibliography by Herzberg and Cox (48) indicates further readings.

REVIEW QUESTIONS AND EXERCISES

1. Define analysis of variance.

2. Describe the completely randomized design.

3. Describe the randomized block design.

4. Describe the repeated measures design.

5. Describe the factorial experiment as used in the completely randomized design.

6. What is the purpose of Tukey's HSD test?

7. What is an experimental unit?

8. What is the objective of the randomized complete block design?

9. What is interaction?

10. What is a mean square?

11. What is an ANOVA table?

12. For each of the following designs describe a situation in your particular field of interest where the design would be an appropriate experimental design. Use real or realistic data and do the appropriate analysis of variance for each one:

   a. Completely randomized design.
   b. Randomized complete block design.
   c. Completely randomized design with a factorial experiment.
   d. Repeated measures designs.

13. Maes et al. (A-26) conducted a study to determine whether depression might be associated with serologic indices of autoimmune processes or active virus infections. Four categories of subjects participated in the study: Healthy controls (1), patients with minor depression (2), patients with major depression without melancholia (3), and patients with major depression with melancholia (4). Among the measurements obtained for each subject were soluble interleukin-2 receptor circulating levels in serum (sIL-2R). The results by subject by category of subject were as follows. We wish to know if we can conclude that, on the average, sIL-2R values differ among the four categories of patients represented in this study. Let $\alpha = .01$ and find the p value. Use Tukey's procedure to test for significant differences among individual pairs of sample means.

Subject	sIL-2R (U / ml)	Subject Category	Subject	sIL-2R (U / ml)	Subject Category
1	92.00	1.00	26	230.00	2.00
2	259.00	1.00	27	253.00	3.00
3	157.00	1.00	28	271.00	3.00
4	220.00	1.00	29	254.00	3.00
5	240.00	1.00	30	316.00	3.00
6	203.00	1.00	31	303.00	3.00
7	190.00	1.00	32	225.00	3.00
8	244.00	1.00	33	363.00	3.00
9	182.00	1.00	34	288.00	3.00
10	192.00	1.00	35	349.00	3.00
11	157.00	1.00	36	237.00	3.00
12	164.00	1.00	37	361.00	3.00
13	196.00	1.00	38	273.00	3.00
14	74.00	1.00	39	262.00	3.00
15	634.00	2.00	40	242.00	4.00
16	305.00	2.00	41	283.00	4.00
17	324.00	2.00	42	354.00	4.00
18	250.00	2.00	43	517.00	4.00
19	306.00	2.00	44	292.00	4.00
20	369.00	2.00	45	439.00	4.00
21	428.00	2.00	46	444.00	4.00
22	324.00	2.00	47	348.00	4.00
23	655.00	2.00	48	230.00	4.00
24	395.00	2.00	49	255.00	4.00
25	270.00	2.00	50	270.00	4.00

SOURCE: Dr. M. Maes. Used by permission.

14. Graveley and Littlefield (A-27) conducted a study to determine the relationship between the cost and effectiveness of three prenatal clinic staffing models: physician based (1),

mixed (M.D., R.N.) staffing (2), and clinical nurse specialist with physicians available for consultation (3). Subjects were women who met the following criteria: (a) 18 years of age or older or emancipated minors, (b) obtained prenatal care at one of the three clinics with a minimum of three prenatal visits, (c) delivered within 48 hours of the interview. Maternal satisfaction with access to care was assessed by means of a patient satisfaction tool (PST) that addressed five categories of satisfaction: accessibility, affordability, availability, acceptability, and accommodation. The following are the subjects' total PST scores by clinic. Can we conclude, on the basis of these data, that, on the average, subject satisfaction differs among the three clinics? Let $\alpha = .05$ and find the p value. Use Tukey's procedure to test for differences between individual pairs of sample means.

Clinic 1		Clinic 2		Clinic 3	
119	133	132	115	131	132
126	135	121	92	109	135
125	125	79	126	127	125
111	135	127	107	124	130
127	130	133	108	135	135
123	122	127	125	131	135
119	135	121	130	131	135
119	116	127	121	126	133
125	126	130	124	132	131
106	129	111	112	128	131
124	133	117	131	129	126
131	126	101	118	128	132
131	102	111	109	114	133
117	131	121	116	120	135
105	128	109	112	120	132
129	128	131	110	135	131
130	130	129	117	127	132
131	116	126	118	124	126
119	121	124	120	129	135
98	121	126	113	125	135
120	131	97	114	135	135
125	135	104	107	122	134
128	127	121	119	117	127
126	125	114	124	126	131
130	133	95	98	130	131
127	128	128	114	131	131

Source: Elaine Graveley, D.B.A., R.N. Used by permission.

15. Respiratory rate (breaths per minute) was measured in eight experimental animals under three levels of exposure to carbon monoxide. The results were as follows.

Animal	Exposure Level		
	Low	Moderate	High
1	36	43	45
2	33	38	39
3	35	41	33
4	39	34	39
5	41	28	33
6	41	44	26
7	44	30	39
8	45	31	29

Can one conclude on the basis of these data that the three exposure levels, on the average, have a different effect on respiratory rate? Let $\alpha = .05$. Determine the p value.

16. An experiment was designed to study the effects of three different drugs and three types of stressful situation in producing anxiety in adolescent subjects. The table shows the difference between the pre- and posttreatment scores of 18 subjects who participated in the experiment.

Stressful Situation (Factor A)	Drug (Factor B)		
	A	B	C
I	4	1	1
	5	3	0
II	6	6	6
	6	6	3
III	5	7	4
	4	4	5

Perform an analysis of variance of these data and test the three possible hypotheses. Let $\alpha' = \alpha'' = \alpha''' = .05$. Determine the p values.

17. The following table shows the emotional maturity scores of 27 young adult males cross-classified by age and the extent to which they use marijuana.

Age (Factor A)	Marijuana Usage (Factor B)		
	Never	Occasionally	Daily
15–19	25	18	17
	28	23	24
	22	19	19
20–24	28	16	18
	32	24	22
	30	20	20
25–29	25	14	10
	35	16	8
	30	15	12

Perform an analysis of variance of these data. Let $\alpha' = \alpha'' = \alpha''' = .05$. Compute the p values.

18. The effects of cigarette smoking on maternal airway function during pregnancy were investigated by Das et al. (A-28). The subjects were women in each of the three trimesters of pregnancy. Among the data collected were the following measurements on forced vital capacity (FVC), which are shown by smoking status of the women. May we conclude, on the basis of these data, that mean FVC measurements differ according to smoking status? Let $\alpha = .01$ and find the p value. Use Tukey's procedure to test for significant differences among individual pairs of sample means.

Nonsmokers			Light Smokers			Heavy Smokers	
3.45	4.05	3.15	4.03	3.95	4.29	3.04	3.02
4.00	4.66	3.86	3.69	3.78	4.38	4.34	3.12
4.00	3.45	3.85	3.83	3.63		3.50	4.05
2.74	3.49	4.94	3.99	3.74		2.68	4.33
3.95	4.75	3.10	3.12	4.84		3.10	3.39
4.03	3.55	3.65	3.43	3.20		3.60	4.24
3.80	4.14	4.44	3.58	3.65		4.93	4.37
3.99	3.82	3.24	2.93	4.78		4.21	3.64
4.13	4.20	3.68	4.77	4.36		4.87	4.62
4.54	3.86	3.94	4.03	4.37		4.02	4.64
4.60	4.34	4.10	4.48	3.20		3.31	2.74
3.73	4.45	4.22	4.26	3.29		4.25	4.34
3.94	4.05	3.63	3.45	3.40		4.37	4.10
3.90	3.60	3.42	3.99	4.40		2.97	3.75
3.20	4.21	4.31	3.78	3.36		3.89	4.06
3.74	3.72	4.24	2.90	2.72		3.80	3.67
3.87	4.73	2.92	3.94	4.21		2.87	3.07
3.44	3.45	4.05	3.84	3.53		3.89	4.59
4.44	4.78	3.94	3.33	3.48		4.07	3.60
3.70	4.54	4.10	4.18	3.62			
3.10	3.86		2.70	3.51			
4.81	4.04		3.74	3.73			
3.41	4.46		3.65	3.40			
3.38	3.90		3.72	3.63			
3.39	3.66		4.69	3.68			
3.50	4.08		2.84	4.07			
3.62	3.84		3.34	3.95			
4.27	2.82		3.47	4.25			
3.55			4.14				

SOURCE: Jean-Marie Moutquin, M.D. Used by permission.

19. An experiment was conducted to test the effect of four different drugs on blood coagulation time (in minutes). Specimens of blood drawn from 10 subjects were divided equally into four parts that were randomly assigned to one of the four drugs. The results were as follows:

Subject	Drug			
	W	X	Y	Z
A	1.5	1.8	1.7	1.9
B	1.4	1.4	1.3	1.5
C	1.8	1.6	1.5	1.9
D	1.3	1.2	1.2	1.4
E	2.0	2.1	2.2	2.3
F	1.1	1.0	1.0	1.2
G	1.5	1.6	1.5	1.7
H	1.5	1.5	1.5	1.7
I	1.2	1.0	1.3	1.5
J	1.5	1.6	1.6	1.9

Can we conclude on the basis of these data that the drugs have different effects? Let $\alpha = .05$.

20. In a study of the Marfan syndrome, Pyeritz et al. (A-29) reported the following severity scores of patients with none, mild, and marked dural ectasia. May we conclude, on the basis of these data, that mean severity scores differ among the three populations represented in the study? Let $\alpha = .05$ and find the p value. Use Tukey's procedure to test for significant differences among individual pairs of sample means.

No dural ectasia: 18, 18, 20, 21, 23, 23, 24, 26, 26, 27, 28, 29, 29, 29, 30, 30, 30, 30, 32, 34, 34, 38.

Mild dural ectasia: 10, 16, 22, 22, 23, 26, 28, 28, 28, 29, 29, 30, 31, 32, 32, 33, 33, 38, 39, 40, 47.

Marked dural ectasia: 17, 24, 26, 27, 29, 30, 30, 33, 34, 35, 35, 36, 39.

SOURCE: Reed E. Pyeritz, M.D., Ph.D. Used by permission.

21. The following table shows the arterial plasma epinephrine concentrations (nanograms per milliliter) found in 10 laboratory animals during three types of anesthesia.

Anes-thesia	Animal									
	1	2	3	4	5	6	7	8	9	10
A	.28	.50	.68	.27	.31	.99	.26	.35	.38	.34
B	.20	.38	.50	.29	.38	.62	.42	.87	.37	.43
C	1.23	1.34	.55	1.06	.48	.68	1.12	1.52	.27	.35

Can we conclude from these data that the three types of anesthesia, on the average, have different effects? Let $\alpha = .05$.

22. The nutritive value of a certain edible fruit was measured in a total of 72 specimens representing 6 specimens of each of four varieties grown in each of the three geographic regions. The results were as follows.

Geographic Region	Variety			
	W	X	Y	Z
A	6.9	11.0	13.1	13.4
	11.8	7.8	12.1	14.1
	6.2	7.3	9.9	13.5
	9.2	9.1	12.4	13.0
	9.2	7.9	11.3	12.3
	6.2	6.9	11.0	13.7
B	8.9	5.8	12.1	9.1
	9.2	5.1	7.1	13.1
	5.2	5.0	13.0	13.2
	7.7	9.4	13.7	8.6
	7.8	8.3	12.9	9.8
	5.7	5.7	7.5	9.9
C	6.8	7.8	8.7	11.8
	5.2	6.5	10.5	13.5
	5.0	7.0	10.0	14.0
	5.2	9.3	8.1	10.8
	5.5	6.6	10.6	12.3
	7.3	10.8	10.5	14.0

Test for a difference among varieties, a difference among regions, and interaction. Let $\alpha = .05$ for all tests.

23. A random sample of the records of single births was selected from each of four populations. The weights (grams) of the babies at birth were as follows:

Sample			
A	B	C	D
2946	3186	2300	2286
2913	2857	2903	2938
2280	3099	2572	2952
3685	2761	2584	2348
2310	3290	2675	2691
2582	2937	2571	2858
3002	3347		2414
2408			2008
			2850
			2762

Do these data provide sufficient evidence to indicate, at the .05 level of significance, that the four populations differ with respect to mean birth weight? Test for a significant difference between all possible pairs of means.

24. The following table shows the aggression scores of 30 laboratory animals reared under three different conditions. One animal from each of 10 litters was randomly assigned to each of the three rearing conditions.

	Rearing Condition		
Litter	Extremely Crowded	Moderately Crowded	Not Crowded
1	30	20	10
2	30	10	20
3	30	20	10
4	25	15	10
5	35	25	20
6	30	20	10
7	20	20	10
8	30	30	10
9	25	25	10
10	30	20	20

Do these data provide sufficient evidence to indicate that level of crowding has an effect on aggression? Let $\alpha = .05$.

25. The following table shows the vital capacity measurements of 60 adult males classified by occupation and age group.

Age Group	Occupation			
	A	**B**	**C**	**D**
	4.31	4.68	4.17	5.75
	4.89	6.18	3.77	5.70
1	4.05	4.48	5.20	5.53
	4.44	4.23	5.28	5.97
	4.59	5.92	4.44	5.52
	4.13	3.41	3.89	4.58
	4.61	3.64	3.64	5.21
2	3.91	3.32	4.18	5.50
	4.52	3.51	4.48	5.18
	4.43	3.75	4.27	4.15
	3.79	4.63	5.81	6.89
	4.17	4.59	5.20	6.18
3	4.47	4.90	5.34	6.21
	4.35	5.31	5.94	7.56
	3.59	4.81	5.56	6.73

Test for differences among occupations, for differences among age groups, and for interaction. Let $\alpha = .05$ for all tests.

26. Complete the following ANOVA table and state which design was used.

Source	SS	d.f.	MS	VR	p
Treatments	154.9199	4			
Error					
Total	200.4773	39			

27. Complete the following ANOVA table and state which design was used.

Source	SS	d.f.	MS	VR	p
Treatments		3			
Blocks	183.5	3			
Error	26.0				
Total	709.0	15			

28. Consider the following ANOVA table.

Source	SS	d.f.	MS	VR	p
A	12.3152	2	6.15759	29.4021	< .005
B	19.7844	3	6.59481	31.4898	< .005
AB	8.94165	6	1.49027	7.11596	< .005
Treatments	41.0413	11			
Error	10.0525	48	0.209427		
Total	51.0938	59			

a. What sort of analysis was employed?

b. What can one conclude from the analysis? Let $\alpha = .05$.

29. Consider the following ANOVA table.

Source	SS	d.f.	MS	VR
Treatments	5.05835	2	2.52917	1.0438
Error	65.42090	27	2.4230	

a. What design was employed?

b. How many treatments were compared?

c. How many observations were analyzed?

d. At the .05 level of significance, can one conclude that there is a difference among treatments? Why?

30. Consider the following ANOVA table.

Source	SS	d.f.	MS	VR
Treatments	231.5054	2	115.7527	2.824
Blocks	98.5000	7	14.0714	
Error	573.7500	14	40.9821	

a. What design was employed?

b. How many treatments were compared?

c. How many observations were analyzed?

d. At the .05 level of significance, can one conclude that the treatments have different effects? Why?

31. In a study of the relationship between smoking and serum concentrations of high-density lipoprotein cholesterol (HDL-C) the following data (coded for ease of calculation) were collected from samples of adult males who were nonsmokers, light smokers, moderate smokers, and heavy smokers. We wish to know if these data provide sufficient evidence to indicate that the four populations differ with respect to mean serum concentration of HDL-C. Let the probability of committing a type I error be .05. If an overall significant difference is found, determine which pairs of individual sample means are significantly different.

Smoking Status			
Nonsmokers	**Light**	**Moderate**	**Heavy**
12	9	5	3
10	8	4	2
11	5	7	1
13	9	9	5
9	9	5	4
9	10	7	6
12	8	6	2

32. The purpose of a study by Nehlsen-Cannarella et al. (A-30) was to examine the relationship between moderate exercise training and changes in circulating numbers of immune system variables. Subjects were nonsmoking, premenopausal women who were divided into two groups (1 = exercise, 2 = nonexercise). Data were collected on three dependent variables: serum levels of the immunoglobulins IgG, IgA, and IgM. Determinations were made at three points in time: baseline (B), at the end of 6 weeks (M), and at the end of 15 weeks (E). The following data were obtained. (The authors analyzed the data with SPSS/PC + .)

Group	BIGG	MIGG	EIGG
1	797.00	956.00	855.00
1	1030.00	1050.00	1020.00
1	981.00	1340.00	1300.00
1	775.00	1100.00	1060.00
1	823.00	1220.00	1140.00
1	1080.00	1120.00	1100.00
1	613.00	958.00	960.00
1	1020.00	1320.00	1200.00
1	956.00	1020.00	1020.00
1	1140.00	1580.00	1520.00
1	872.00	935.00	1000.00
1	1270.00	1290.00	1520.00
1	798.00	1050.00	1130.00
1	643.00	801.00	847.00
1	772.00	1110.00	1150.00
1	1480.00	1590.00	1470.00
1	1250.00	1720.00	1690.00
1	968.00	1150.00	1090.00
2	1470.00	1470.00	560.00
2	962.00	1260.00	1020.00
2	881.00	797.00	828.00
2	1040.00	1040.00	931.00
2	1160.00	1280.00	1300.00
2	1460.00	1440.00	1570.00
2	1010.00	974.00	1080.00
2	549.00	1030.00	1030.00
2	1610.00	1510.00	1560.00
2	1060.00	966.00	1020.00
2	1400.00	1320.00	1260.00
2	1330.00	1320.00	1240.00
2	874.00	1000.00	970.00
2	828.00	1140.00	1240.00
2	1210.00	1160.00	1080.00
2	1220.00	1150.00	1160.00
2	981.00	979.00	943.00
2	1140.00	1220.00	1550.00

Group	BIGA	MIGA	EIGA
1	97.70	126.00	110.00
1	173.00	182.00	179.00
1	122.00	151.00	160.00
1	74.30	123.00	113.00
1	118.00	162.00	164.00
1	264.00	306.00	292.00
1	113.00	173.00	188.00
1	239.00	310.00	295.00

Group	BIGA	MIGA	EIGA
1	231.00	258.00	245.00
1	219.00	320.00	320.00
1	137.00	177.00	183.00
1	94.30	99.10	134.00
1	94.70	143.00	142.00
1	102.00	135.00	146.00
1	127.00	192.00	195.00
1	434.00	472.00	480.00
1	187.00	236.00	255.00
1	80.80	98.50	89.70
2	262.00	290.00	249.00
2	142.00	201.00	160.00
2	113.00	107.00	112.00
2	176.00	194.00	181.00
2	154.00	147.00	144.00
2	286.00	300.00	308.00
2	138.00	148.00	160.00
2	73.40	164.00	166.00
2	123.00	127.00	122.00
2	218.00	198.00	198.00
2	220.00	245.00	220.00
2	210.00	219.00	190.00
2	207.00	237.00	239.00
2	124.00	189.00	204.00
2	194.00	184.00	178.00
2	344.00	356.00	335.00
2	117.00	125.00	135.00
2	259.00	307.00	296.00

Group	BIGM	MIGM	EIGM
1	128.00	150.00	139.00
1	145.00	139.00	146.00
1	155.00	169.00	166.00
1	78.10	124.00	119.00
1	143.00	186.00	183.00
1	273.00	273.00	270.00
1	154.00	234.00	245.00
1	113.00	139.00	130.00
1	124.00	127.00	128.00
1	102.00	142.00	133.00
1	134.00	139.00	146.00
1	146.00	141.00	173.00
1	119.00	124.00	141.00
1	141.00	181.00	195.00
1	115.00	194.00	200.00
1	187.00	224.00	196.00
1	234.00	306.00	295.00
1	83.80	94.60	98.20
2	279.00	286.00	263.00
2	154.00	201.00	147.00
2	167.00	180.00	165.00
2	157.00	175.00	152.00
2	223.00	252.00	250.00

Group	BIGM	MIGM	EIGM
2	189.00	199.00	166.00
2	103.00	117.00	110.00
2	104.00	173.00	150.00
2	185.00	190.00	157.00
2	101.00	81.10	91.50
2	156.00	153.00	140.00
2	217.00	187.00	152.00
2	190.00	202.00	223.00
2	110.00	176.00	188.00
2	123.00	123.00	113.00
2	179.00	189.00	170.00
2	115.00	114.00	113.00
2	297.00	297.00	308.00

SOURCE: David C. Nieman. Used with permission.

a. Perform a repeated measures analysis for each immunoglobulin/exercise group combination.
b. Analyze the data as a factorial experiment for each immunoglobulin in which the factors are exercise group (2 levels) and time period (3 levels). Let $\alpha = .05$ for all tests.

33. The purpose of a study by Roodenburg et al. (A-31) was the classification and quantitative description of various fetal movement patterns during the second half of pregnancy. The following are the number of incidents of general fetal movements per hour experienced by nine pregnant women at four-week intervals. May we conclude from these data that the average number of general movements per hour differs among the time periods? Let $\alpha = .05$.

Patient No.	Weeks of Gestation				
	20	24	28	32	36
1	66	57	52	37	40
2	47	65	44	34	24
3	57	63	57	34	10
4	39	49	58	27	26
5	54	46	54	22	35
6	53	62	45	37	40
7	96	46	64	43	41
8	60	47	50	62	26
9	63	47	44	42	39

SOURCE: J. W. Wladimiroff, M.D., Ph.D. Used with permission.

For Exercises 34–38 do the following:
a. Indicate which technique studied in this chapter (the completely randomized design, the randomized block design, the repeated measures design, or the factorial experiment) is appropriate.
b. Identify the response variable and treatment variables.
c. As appropriate, identify the factors and the number of levels of each, the blocking variables, and the subjects.
d. List any extraneous variables whose effects you think might be included in the error term.

    e. As appropriate, comment on carry-over and position effects.

    f. Construct an ANOVA table in which you indicate the sources of variability and the number of degrees of freedom for each.

34. In a study by Vasterling et al. (A-32) 60 cancer chemotherapy patients who were categorized as exhibiting either high or low anxiety were randomly assigned to one of three conditions: cognitive distraction, relaxation training, or no intervention. Patients were followed for five consecutive chemotherapy sessions. Data were collected on such variables as nausea and both systolic and diastolic blood pressure.

35. In a double-blind placebo-controlled study involving 30 patients with acute ischemic stroke, Huber et al. (A-33) investigated the effect of the adenosine uptake blocker propentofylline on regional brain glucose metabolism.

36. The purpose of a study by Smith et al. (A-34) was to determine if static and ballistic stretching would induce significant amounts of delayed onset muscle soreness (DOMS) and increases in creatine kinase (CK). Twenty males were randomly assigned to a static (STATIC) or ballistic (BALLISTIC) stretching group. All subjects performed three sets of 17 stretches during a 90-minute period with STATIC remaining stationary during each 60-second stretch while BALLISTIC performed bouncing movements. Subjective ratings of DOMS and serum CK levels were assessed before and every 24 hours poststretching for five days.

37. A study by Cimprich (A-35) tested the effects of an experimental intervention aimed at maintaining or restoring attentional capacity in 32 women during the three months after surgery for localized breast cancer. Attentional capacity was assessed using objective and subjective measures at four time points after breast cancer surgery. After the first observation, subjects were divided equally into two groups by random assignment either to receive intervention or not to receive intervention.

38. Paradis et al. (A-36) compared the pharmacokinetics and the serum bactericidal activities of five bactericidal agents. Fifteen healthy volunteers received each of the agents.

REFERENCES

References Cited

1. R. A. Fisher, *The Design of Experiments*, Eighth Edition, Oliver and Boyd, Edinburgh, 1966.
2. R. A. Fisher, *Contributions to Mathematical Statistics*, Wiley, New York, 1950.
3. Ronald A. Fisher, *Statistical Methods for Research Workers*, Thirteenth Edition, Hafner, New York, 1958.
4. William G. Cochran and Gertrude M. Cox, *Experimental Designs*, Wiley, New York, 1957.
5. D. R. Cox, *Planning of Experiments*, Wiley, New York, 1958.
6. Owen L. Davies (ed.), *The Design and Analysis of Experiments*, Hafner, New York, 1960.
7. Walter T. Federer, *Experimental Design*, Macmillan, New York, 1955.
8. D. J. Finney, *Experimental Design and Its Statistical Basis*, The University of Chicago Press, Chicago, 1955.
9. Peter W. M. John, *Statistical Design and Analysis of Experiments*, Macmillan, New York, 1971.
10. Oscar Kempthorne, *The Design and Analysis of Experiments*, Wiley, New York, 1952.
11. C. C. Li, *Introduction to Experimental Statistics*, McGraw-Hill, New York, 1964.

12. William Mendenhall, *Introduction to Linear Models and the Design and Analysis of Experiments*, Wadsworth, Belmont, Cal., 1968.

13. Churchill Eisenhart, "The Assumptions Underlying the Analysis of Variance," *Biometrics*, *21* (1947), 1–21.

14. W. G. Cochran, "Some Consequences When the Assumptions for the Analysis of Variance Are Not Satisfied," *Biometrics*, *3* (1947), 22–38.

15. M. B. Wilk and O. Kempthorne, "Fixed, Mixed and Random Models," *Journal of the American Statistical Association*, *50* (1955), 1144–1167.

16. S. L. Crump, "The Estimation of Variance Components in Analysis of Variance," *Biometrics*, *2* (1946), 7–11.

17. E. P. Cunningham and C. R. Henderson, "An Iterative Procedure for Estimating Fixed Effects and Variance Components in Mixed Model Situations," *Biometrics*, *24* (1968), 13–25.

18. C. R. Henderson, "Estimation of Variance and Covariance Components," *Biometrics*, *9* (1953), 226–252.

19. J. R. Rutherford, "A Note on Variances in the Components of Variance Model," *The American Statistician*, *25* (June 1971), 1, 2.

20. E. F. Schultz, Jr., "Rules of Thumb for Determining Expectations of Mean Squares in Analysis of Variance," *Biometrics*, *11* (1955), 123–135.

21. S. R. Searle, "Topics in Variance Component Estimation," *Biometrics*, *27* (1971), 1–76.

22. Robert G. D. Steel and James H. Torrie, *Principles and Procedures of Statistics*, McGraw-Hill, New York, 1960.

23. David B. Duncan, *Significance Tests for Differences Between Ranked Variates Drawn from Normal Populations*, Ph.D. Thesis (1949), Iowa State College, Ames, 117 pp.

24. David B. Duncan, "A Significance Test for Differences Between Ranked Treatments in an Analysis of Variance," *Virginia Journal of Science*, *2* (1951), 171–189.

25. David B. Duncan, "On the Properties of the Multiple Comparisons Test," *Virginia Journal of Science*, *3* (1952), 50–67.

26. David B. Duncan, "Multiple Range and Multiple-*F* Tests," *Biometrics*, *11* (1955), 1–42.

27. C. Y. Kramer, "Extension of Multiple Range Tests to Group Means with Unequal Numbers of Replications," *Biometrics*, *12* (1956) 307–310.

28. C. W. Dunnett, "A Multiple Comparisons Procedure for Comparing Several Treatments with a Control," *Journal of the American Statistical Association*, *50* (1955), 1096–1121.

29. C. W. Dunnett, "New Tables for Multiple Comparisons with a Control," *Biometrics*, *20* (1964), 482–491.

30. J. W. Tukey, "Comparing Individual Means in the Analysis of Variance," *Biometrics*, *5* (1949), 99–114.

31. J. W. Tukey, "The Problem of Multiple Comparisons," Ditto, Princeton University, 1953; cited in Roger E. Kirk, *Experimental Design: Procedures for the Behavioral Sciences*, Brooks/Cole, Belmont, Cal., 1968.

32. D. Newman, "The Distribution of the Range in Samples from a Normal Population in Terms of an Independent Estimate of Standard Deviation," *Biometrika*, *31* (1939), 20–30.

33. M. Keuls, "The Use of the Studentized Range in Connection with the Analysis of Variance," *Euphytica*, *1* (1952), 112–122.

34. Henry Scheffé, "A Method for Judging All Contrasts in the Analysis of Variance," *Biometrika*, *40* (1953), 87–104.

35. Henry Scheffé, *Analysis of Variance*, Wiley, New York (1959).

36. T. A. Bancroft, *Topics in Intermediate Statistical Methods*, Volume I, The Iowa State University Press, Ames, 1968.

37. Wayne W. Daniel and Carol E. Coogler, "Beyond Analysis of Variance: A Comparison of Some Multiple Comparison Procedures," *Physical Therapy*, *55* (1975), 144–150.

38. B. J. Winer, *Statistical Principles in Experimental Design*, Second Edition, McGraw-Hill, New York, 1971.

39. Wayne W. Daniel, *Multiple Comparison Procedures: A Selected Bibliography*, Vance Bibliographies, Monticello, Ill., June 1980.

40. Emil Spjøtvoll and Michael R. Stoline, "An Extension of the T-Method of Multiple Comparison to Include the Cases with Unequal Sample Sizes," *Journal of the American Statistical Association*, *68* (1973), 975–978.

41. R. A. Fisher, "The Arrangement of Field Experiments," *Journal of Ministry of Agriculture*, *33* (1926), 503–513.

42. R. L. Anderson and T. A. Bancroft, *Statistical Theory in Research*, McGraw-Hill, New York, 1952.

43. J. W. Tukey, "One Degree of Freedom for Non-Additivity," *Biometrics*, *5* (1949), 232–242.

44. John Mandel, "A New Analysis of Variance Model for Non-Additive Data," *Technometrics*, *13* (1971), 1–18.

45. A. W. Kimball, "On Dependent Tests of Significance in the Analysis of Variance," *Annals of Mathematical Statistics*, *22* (1951), 600–602.

46. Wilfred J. Dixon and Frank J. Massey, *Introduction to Statistical Analysis*, Fourth Edition, McGraw-Hill, New York, 1983.

47. William C. Guenther, *Analysis of Variance*, Prentice-Hall, Englewood Cliffs, N.J., 1964.

48. Agnes M. Herzberg and D. R. Cox, "Recent Work on the Design of Experiments: A Bibliography and a Review," *Journal of the Royal Statistical Society* (Series A), *132* (1969), 29–67.

Other References, Books

1. Geoffrey M. Clarke, *Statistics and Experimental Design*, American Elsevier, New York, 1969.

2. M. J. Crowder and D. J. Hand, *Analysis of Repeated Measures*, Chapman and Hall, New York, 1990.

3. Richard A. Damon, Jr., and Walter R. Harvey, *Experimental Design, ANOVA, and Regression*, Harper & Row, New York, 1967.

4. M. N. Das and N. C. Giri, *Design and Analysis of Experiments*, Second Edition, Wiley, New York, 1986.

5. Janet D. Elashoff, *Analysis of Repeated Measures Designs*, *BMDP Technical Report #83*, BMDP Statistical Software, Los Angeles, 1986.

6. D. J. Finney, *An Introduction to the Theory of Experimental Design*, The University of Chicago Press, Chicago, 1960.

7. Charles P. Hicks, *Fundamental Concepts in the Design of Experiments*, Second Edition, Holt, Rinehart & Winston, New York, 1973.

8. David C. Hoaglin, Frederick Mosteller, and John W. Tukey, *Fundamentals of Exploratory Analysis of Variance*, Wiley, New York, 1991.

9. Yosef Hochberg and Ajit C. Tamhane, *Multiple Comparison Procedures*, Wiley, New York, 1987.

10. Geoffrey Keppel, *Design and Analysis: A Researcher's Handbook*, Prentice-Hall, Englewood Cliffs, N.J., 1973.

11. Alan J. Klockars and Gilbert Sax, *Multiple Comparisons*, Sage, Beverly Hills, Cal., 1986.

12. Wayne Lee, *Experimental Design and Analysis*, W. H. Freeman, San Francisco, 1975.

13. Harold R. Lindman, *Analysis of Variance in Complex Experimental Designs*, W. H. Freeman, San Francisco, 1974.

14. Rupert G. Miller, Jr., *Simultaneous Statistical Inference*, Second Edition, Springer-Verlag, New York, 1981.

15. Douglas C. Montgomery, *Design and Analysis of Experiments*, Wiley, New York, 1976.

16. John Neter and William Wasserman, *Applied Linear Statistical Models*, Irwin, Homewood, Ill., 1974.

17. E. G. Olds, T. B. Mattson, and R. E. Odeh: *Notes on the Use of Transformations in the Analysis of Variance*, WADC Tech Rep 56-308, 1956, Wright Air Development Center.

18. Roger G. Peterson, *Design and Analysis of Experiments*, Marcel Dekker, New York, 1985.

Other References, Journal Articles

1. Benjamin A. Barnes, Elinor Pearson, and Eric Reiss, "The Analysis of Variance: A Graphical Representation of a Statistical Concept," *Journal of the American Statistical Association*, *50* (1955), 1064–1072.

2. David B. Duncan, "Bayes Rules for a Common Multiple Comparisons Problem and Related Student-*t* Problems," *Annals of Mathematical Statistics*, *32* (1961), 1013–1033.

3. David B. Duncan, "A Bayesian Approach to Multiple Comparisons," *Technometrics*, *7* (1965), 171–222.

4. Alva R. Feinstein, "Clinical Biostatistics. II. Statistics Versus Science in the Design of Experiments," *Clinical Pharmacology and Therapeutics*, *11* (1970), 282–292.

5. B. G. Greenberg, "Why Randomize?" *Biometrics*, *7* (1951), 309–322.

6. M. Harris, D. G. Horvitz, and A. M. Mood, "On the Determination of Sample Sizes in Designing Experiments," *Journal of the American Statistical Association*, *43* (1948), 391–402.

7. H. Leon Harter, "Multiple Comparison Procedures for Interactions," *The American Statistician*, *24* (December 1970), 30–32.

8. Carl E. Hopkins and Alan J. Gross, "Significance Levels in Multiple Comparison Tests," *Health Services Research*, *5* (Summer 1970), 132–140.

9. Richard J. Light and Barry H. Margolin, "An Analysis of Variance for Categorical Data," *Journal of the American Statistical Association*, *66* (1971), 534–544.

10. Stuart J. Pocock, "Current Issues in the Design and Interpretation of Clinical Trials," *British Medical Journal*, *290* (1985), 39–42.

11. K. L. Q. Read, "ANOVA Problems with Simple Numbers," *The American Statistician*, *39* (1985), 107–111.

12. Ken Sirotnik, "On the Meaning of the Mean in ANOVA (or the Case of the Missing Degree of Freedom)," *The American Statistician*, *25* (October 1971), 36–37.

13. David M. Steinberg and William G. Hunter, "Experimental Design: Review and Comment," (with discussion) *Technometrics*, *26* (1986), 71–130.

14. Ray A. Waller and David B. Duncan, "A Bayes Rule for the Symmetric Multiple Comparisons Problem," *Journal of the American Statistical Association*, *64* (1969), 1484–1503.

Other References, Other Publications

1. Hea Sook Kim, *A Practical Guide to the Multiple Comparison Procedures*, Master's Thesis, Georgia State University, Atlanta, 1985.

Applications References

A-1. Virginia M. Miller and Paul M. Vanhoutte, "Progesterone and Modulation of Endothelium-Dependent Responses in Canine Coronary Arteries," *American Journal of Physiology*, (*Regulatory Integrative Comp. Physiol. 30*), *261* (1991), R1022–R1027.

A-2. Vijendra K. Singh, Reed P. Warren, J. Dennis Odell, and Phyllis Cole, "Changes of Soluble Interleukin-2, Interleukin-2 Receptor, T8 Antigen, and Interleukin-1 in the Serum of Autistic Children," *Clinical Immunology and Immunopathology*, *61* (1991), 448–455.

A-3. David A. Schwartz, Robert K. Merchant, Richard A. Helmers, Steven R. Gilbert, Charles S. Dayton, and Gary W. Hunninghake, "The Influence of Cigarette Smoking on Lung Function in Patients with Idiopathic Pulmonary Fibrosis," *American Review of Respiratory Disease*, *144* (1991), 504–506.

A-4. Erika Szádóczky, Annamária Falus, Attila Németh, György Teszéri, and Erzsébet Moussong-Kovács, "Effect of Phototherapy on ^{3}H-imipramine Binding Sites in Patients with SAD, Non-SAD and in Healthy Controls," *Journal of Affective Disorders*, *22* (1991), 179–184.

A-5. Meg Gulanick, "Is Phase 2 Cardiac Rehabilitation Necessary for Early Recovery of Patients with Cardiac Disease? A Randomized, Controlled Study," *Heart & Lung, 20* (1991), 9–15.

A-6. E. Azoulay-Dupuis, J. B. Bedos, E. Vallée, D. J. Hardy, R. N. Swanson, and J. J. Pocidalo, "Antipneumococcal Activity of Ciprofloxacin, Ofloxacin, and Temafloxacin in an Experimental Mouse Pneumonia Model at Various Stages of the Disease," *Journal of Infectious Diseases, 163* (1991), 319–324.

A-7. Robert D. Budd, "Cocaine Abuse and Violent Death," *American Journal of Drug and Alcohol Abuse, 15* (1989), 375–382.

A-8. Jules Rosen, Charles F. Reynolds III, Amy L. Yeager, Patricia R. Houck, and Linda F. Hurwitz, "Sleep Disturbances in Survivors of the Nazi Holocaust," *American Journal of Psychiatry, 148* (1991), 62–66.

A-9. A. C. Regenstein, J. Belluomini, and M. Katz, "Terbutaline Tocolysis and Glucose Intolerance," *Obstetrics and Gynecology, 81* (May 1993), 739–741.

A-10. P. O. Jessee and C. E. Cecil, "Evaluation of Social Problem-Solving Abilities in Rural Home Health Visitors and Visiting Nurses," *Maternal-Child Nursing Journal, 20* (Summer 1992), 53–64.

A-11. Wilfred Druml, Georg Grimm, Anton N. Laggner, Kurt Lenz, and Bruno Schneeweiß, "Lactic Acid Kinetics in Respiratory Alkalosis," *Critical Care Medicine, 19* (1991), 1120–1124.

A-12. Brian J. McConville, M. Harold Fogelson, Andrew B. Norman, William M. Klykylo, Pat Z. Manderscheid, Karen W. Parker, and Paul R. Sanberg, "Nicotine Potentiation of Haloperidol in Reducing Tic Frequency in Tourette's Disorder," *American Journal of Psychiatry, 148* (1991), 793–794.

A-13. M. E. Valencia, G. McNeill, J. M. Brockway, and J. S. Smith, "The Effect of Environmental Temperature and Humidity on 24h Energy Expenditure in Men," *British Journal of Nutrition, 68* (September 1992), 319–27.

A-14. D. S. Hodgson, C. I. Dunlop, P. L. Chapman, and J. L. Grandy, "Cardiopulmonary Responses to Experimentally Induced Gastric Dilatation in Isoflurane-Anesthetized Dogs," *American Journal of Veterinary Research, 53* (June 1992), 938–943.

A-15. James O. Hill, John C. Peters, George W. Reed, David G. Schlundt, Teresa Sharp, and Harry L. Greene, "Nutrient Balance in Humans: Effect of Diet Composition," *American Journal of Clinical Nutrition, 54* (1991), 10–17.

A-16. Robert A. Blum, John H. Wilton, Donald M. Hilligoss, Mark J. Gardner, Eugenia B. Henry, Nedra J. Harrison, and Jerome J. Schentag, "Effect of Fluconazole on the Disposition of Phenytoin," *Clinical Pharmacology and Therapeutics, 49* (1991), 420–425.

A-17. Peter H. Abbrecht, Krishnan R. Rajagopal, and Richard R. Kyle, "Expiratory Muscle Recruitment During Inspiratory Flow-Resistive Loading and Exercise," *American Review of Respiratory Disease, 144* (1991), 113–120.

A-18. Jon Kabat-Zinn, Ann O. Massion, Jean Kristeller, Linda Gay Peterson, Kenneth E. Fletcher, Lori Pbert, William R. Lenderking, and Saki F. Santorelli, "Effectiveness of a Mediation-Based Stress Reduction Program in the Treatment of Anxiety Disorders,' *American Journal of Psychiatry, 149* (1992), 936–943.

A-19. M. Speechley, G. L. Dickie, W. W. Weston, and V. Orr, "Changes in Residents' Self-Assessed Competence During a Two-Year Family Practice Program," *Academic Medicine, 68* (February 1993), 163–165.

A-20. A. Barnett and R. J. Maughan, "Response of Unacclimatized Males to Repeated Weekly Bouts of Exercise in the Heat," *British Journal of Sports Medicine, 27* (March 1993), 39–44.

A-21. Michael W. Orth, Yisheng Bai, Ibrahim H. Zeytun, and Mark E. Cook, "Excess Levels of Cysteine and Homocysteine Induce Tibial Dyschondroplasia in Broiler Chicks," *Journal of Nutrition, 122* (1992), 482–487.

A-22. Carole Wood Gorenflo and Daniel W. Gorenflo, "The Effects of Information and Augmentative Communication Technique on Attitudes Toward Nonspeaking Individuals," *Journal of Speech and Hearing Research, 34* (February 1991), 19–26.

A-23. D. Ouerghi, S. Rivest, and D. Richard, "Adrenalectomy Attenuates the Effect of Chemical Castration on Energy Balance in Rats," *Journal of Nutrition*, *122* (1992), 369–373.

A-24. R. Niaura, D. B. Abrams, M. Pedraza, P. M. Monti, and D. J. Rohsenow, "Smokers' Reactions to Interpersonal Interaction and Presentation of Smoking Cues," *Addictive Behaviors*, *17* (November–December 1992), 557–566.

A-25. M. B. Max, D. Zeigler, S. E. Shoaf, E. Craig, J. Benjamin, S. H. Li, C. Buzzanell, M. Perez, and B. C. Ghosh, "Effects of a Single Oral Dose of Desipramine on Postoperative Morphine Analgesia," *Journal of Pain and Symptom Management*, *7* (November 1992), 454–462.

A-26. M. Maes, E. Bosmans, E. Suy, C. Vandervorst, C. Dejonckheere, and J. Raus, "Antiphospholipid, Antinuclear, Epstein-Barr and Cytomegalovirus Antibodies, and Soluble Interleukin-2 Receptors in Depressive Patients," *Journal of Affective Disorders*, *21* (1991), 133–140.

A-27. Elaine A. Graveley and John H. Littlefield, "A Cost-effectiveness Analysis of Three Staffing Models for the Delivery of Low-Risk Prenatal Care," *American Journal of Public Health*, *82* (1992), 180–184.

A-28. Tarun K. Das, Jean-Marie Moutquin, and Jean-Guy Parent, "Effect of Cigarette Smoking on Maternal Airway Function During Pregnancy," *American Journal of Obstetrics and Gynecology*, *165* (1991), 675–679.

A-29. Reed E. Pyeritz, Elliot K. Fishman, Barbara A. Bernhardt, and Stanley S. Siegelman, "Dural Ectasia Is a Common Feature of the Marfan Syndrome," *American Journal of Human Genetics*, *43* (1988), 726–732.

A-30. Sandra L. Nehlsen-Cannarella, David C. Nieman, Anne J. Balk-Lamberton, Patricia A. Markoff, Douglas B. W. Chritton, Gary Gusewitch, and Jerry W. Lee, "The Effects of Moderate Exercise Training on Immune Response," *Medicine and Science in Sports and Exercise*, *23* (1991), 64–70.

A-31. P. J. Roodenburg, J. W. Wladimiroff, A. van Es, and H. F. R. Prechtl, "Classification and Quantitative Aspects of Fetal Movements During the Second Half of Normal Pregnancy," *Early Human Development*, *25* (1991), 19–35.

A-32. J. Vasterling, R. A. Jenkins, D. M. Tope, and T. G. Burish, "Cognitive Distraction and Relaxation Training for the Control of Side Effects Due to Cancer Chemotherapy," *Journal of Behavioral Medicine*, *16* (February 1993), 65–80.

A-33. M. Huber, B. Kittner, C. Hojer, G. R. Fink, M. Neveling, and W. D. Heiss, "Effect of Propentofylline on Regional Cerebral Glucose Metabolism in Acute Ischemic Stroke," *Journal of Cerebral Blood Flow and Metabolism*, *13* (May 1993), 526–530.

A-34. L. L. Smith, M. H. Brunetz, T. C. Chenier, M. R. McCammon, J. A. Houmard, M. E. Franklin, and R. G. Israel, "The Effects of Static and Ballistic Stretching on Delayed Onset Muscle Soreness and Creatine Kinase," *Research Quarterly for Exercise and Sport*, *64* (March 1993), 103–107.

A-35. B. Cimprich, "Development of an Intervention to Restore Attention in Cancer Patients," *Cancer Nursing*, *16* (April 1993), 83–92.

A-36. D. Paradis, F. Vallee, S. Allard, C. Bisson, N. Daviau, C. Drapeau, F. Auger, and M. LeBel, "Comparative Study of Pharmacokinetics and Serum Bactericidal Activities of Cefpirome, Ceftazidime, Ceftriaxone, Imipenem, and Ciprofloxacin," *Antimicrobial Agents and Chemotherapy*, *36* (October 1992), 2085–2092.

Simple Linear Regression and Correlation

· ·

CONTENTS

9.1
Introduction

In analyzing data for the health sciences disciplines, we find that it is frequently desirable to learn something about the relationship between two variables. We may, for example, be interested in studying the relationship between blood pressure and age, height and weight, the concentration of an injected drug and heart rate, the consumption level of some nutrient and weight gain, the intensity of a stimulus and reaction time, or total family income and medical care expenditures. The nature and strength of the relationships between variables such as these may be examined by *regression* and *correlation* analysis, two statistical techniques that, although related, serve different purposes.

Regression   Regression analysis is helpful in ascertaining the probable form of the relationship between variables, and the ultimate objective when this method of analysis is employed usually is to *predict* or *estimate* the value of one variable corresponding to a given value of another variable. The ideas of regression were first elucidated by the English scientist Sir Francis Galton (1822–1911) in reports of his research on heredity—first in sweet peas and later in human stature (1–3). He described a tendency of adult offspring, having either short or tall parents, to revert back toward the average height of the general population. He first used the word *reversion*, and later *regression*, to refer to this phenomenon.

Correlation   Correlation analysis, on the other hand, is concerned with measuring the strength of the relationship between variables. When we compute measures of correlation from a set of data, we are interested in the degree of the *correlation* between variables. Again, the concepts and terminology of correlation analysis originated with Galton, who first used the word *correlation* in 1888 (4).

In this chapter our discussion is limited to the exploration of the relationship between two variables. The concepts and methods of regression are covered first, beginning in the next section. In Section 9.6 the ideas and techniques of correlation are introduced. In the next chapter we consider the case where there is an interest in the relationships among three or more variables.

Regression and correlation analysis are areas in which the speed and accuracy of a computer are most appreciated. The data for the exercises of this chapter, therefore, are presented in a way that makes them suitable for computer processing. As is always the case, the input requirements and output features of the particular programs and software packages to be used should be studied carefully.

9.2
The Regression Model

In the typical regression problem, as in most problems in applied statistics, researchers have available for analysis a sample of observations from some real or hypothetical population. Based on the results of their analysis of the sample data, they are interested in reaching decisions about the population from which the sample is presumed to have been drawn. It is important, therefore, that the researchers understand the nature of the population in which they are interested. They should know enough about the population to be able either to construct a mathematical model for its representation or to determine if it reasonably fits some established model. A researcher about to analyze a set of data by the methods of simple linear regression, for example, should be secure in the knowledge that the simple linear regression model is, at least, an approximate representation of the population. It is unlikely that the model will be a perfect portrait of the real situation, since this characteristic is seldom found in models of practical value. A model constructed so that it corresponds precisely with the details of the situation is usually too complicated to yield any information of value. On the other hand, the results obtained from the analysis of data that have been forced into a model that does not fit are also worthless. Fortunately, however, a perfectly fitting model is not a requirement for obtaining useful results. Researchers, then, should be able to distinguish between the occasion when their chosen models and the data are sufficiently compatible for them to proceed and the case where their chosen model must be abandoned.

Assumptions Underlying Simple Linear Regression   In the simple linear regression model two variables, X and Y, are of interest. The variable X is usually referred to as the *independent variable*, since frequently it is controlled by the investigator; that is, values of X may be selected by the investigator and, corresponding to each preselected value of X, one or more values of Y are obtained. The other variable, Y, accordingly, is called the *dependent variable*, and we speak of the regression of Y on X. The following are the assumptions underlying the simple linear regression model.

1. Values of the independent variable X are said to be "fixed." This means that the values of X are preselected by the investigator so that in the collection of the data they are not allowed to vary from these preselected values. In this model, X is referred to by some writers as a *nonrandom* variable and by others as a *mathematical* variable. It should be pointed out at this time that the statement of this assumption classifies our model as the *classical regression model*. Regression analysis also can be carried out on data in which X is a random variable.

2. The variable X is measured without error. Since no measuring procedure is perfect, this means that the magnitude of the measurement error in X is negligible.

3. For each value of X there is a subpopulation of Y values. For the usual inferential procedures of estimation and hypothesis testing to be valid, these subpopulations must be normally distributed. In order that these procedures may be presented it will be assumed that the Y values are normally distributed in the examples and exercises that follow.

4. The variances of the subpopulations of Y are all equal.

5. The means of the subpopulations of Y all lie on the same straight line. This is known as the *assumption of linearity*. This assumption may be expressed symbolically as

$$\mu_{y|x} = \alpha + \beta x \qquad (9.2.1)$$

.where $\mu_{y|x}$ is the mean of the subpopulation of Y values for a particular value of X, and α and β are called population regression coefficients. Geometrically, α and β represent the y-intercept and slope, respectively, of the line on which all the means are assumed to lie.

6. The Y values are statistically independent. In other words, in drawing the sample, it is assumed that the values of Y chosen at one value of X in no way depend on the values of Y chosen at another value of X.

These assumptions may be summarized by means of the following equation, which is called the regression model:

$$y = \alpha + \beta x + e \tag{9.2.2}$$

where y is a typical value from one of the subpopulations of Y, α and β are as defined for Equation 9.2.1, and e is called the error term. If we solve 9.2.2 for e, we have

$$e = y - (\alpha + \beta x)$$
$$= y - \mu_{y|x} \tag{9.2.3}$$

and we see that e shows the amount by which y deviates from the mean of the subpopulation of Y values from which it is drawn. As a consequence of the assumption that the subpopulations of Y values are normally distributed with equal variances, the e's for each subpopulation are normally distributed with a variance equal to the common variance of the subpopulations of Y values.

The following acronym will help the reader remember most of the assumptions necessary for inference in linear regression analysis:

LINE [Linear (assumption 5), Independent (assumption 6),

Normal (assumption 3), Equal variances (assumption 4)]

A graphical representation of the regression model is given in Figure 9.2.1.

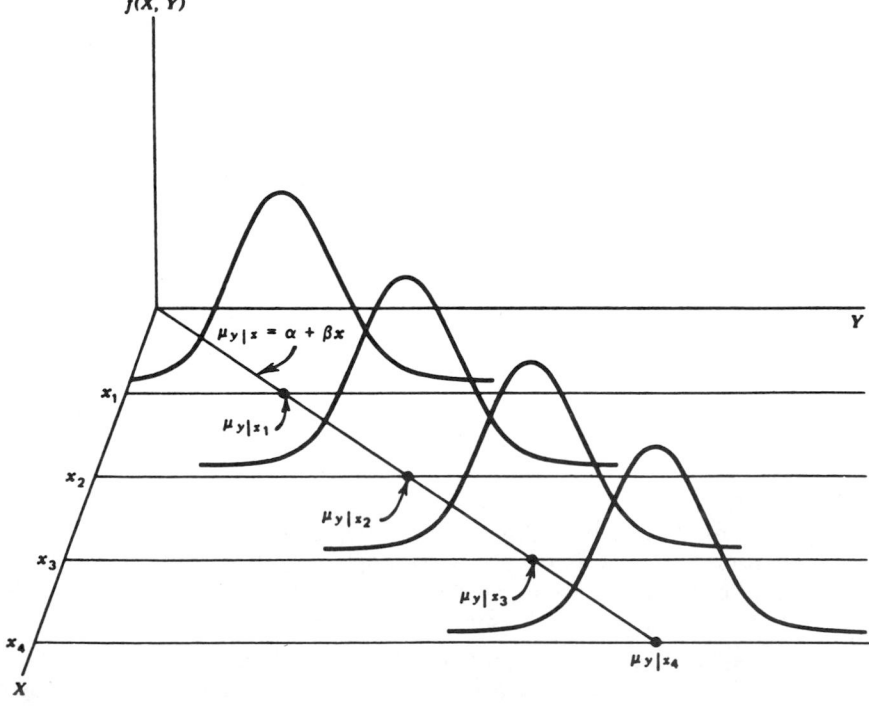

Figure 9.2.1   Representation of the simple linear regression model.

9.3
The Sample Regression Equation

In simple linear regression the object of the researcher's interest is the population regression equation—the equation that describes the true relationship between the dependent variable Y and the independent variable X.

In an effort to reach a decision regarding the likely form of this relationship, the researcher draws a sample from the population of interest and, using the resulting data, computes a sample regression equation that forms the basis for reaching conclusions regarding the unknown population regression equation.

Steps in Regression Analysis In the absence of extensive information regarding the nature of the variables of interest, a frequently employed strategy is to assume initially that they are linearly related. Subsequent analysis, then, involves the following steps.

1. Determine whether or not the assumptions underlying a linear relationship are met in the data available for analysis.
2. Obtain the equation for the line that best fits the sample data.
3. Evaluate the equation to obtain some idea of the strength of the relationship and the usefulness of the equation for predicting and estimating.
4. If the data appear to conform satisfactorily to the linear model, use the equation obtained from the sample data to predict and to estimate.

When we use the regression equation to *predict*, we will be predicting the value Y is likely to have when X has a given value. When we use the equation to *estimate*, we will be estimating the mean of the subpopulation of Y values assumed to exist at a given value of X. Note that the sample data used to obtain the regression equation consist of known values of both X and Y. When the equation is used to predict and to estimate Y, only the corresponding values of X will be known. We illustrate the steps involved in simple linear regression analysis by means of the following example.

Example 9.3.1 Després et al. (A-1) point out that the topography of adipose tissue (AT) is associated with metabolic complications considered as risk factors for cardiovascular disease. It is important, they state, to measure the amount of intraabdominal AT as part of the evaluation of the cardiovascular-disease risk of an individual. Computed tomography (CT), the only available technique that precisely and reliably measures the amount of deep abdominal AT, however, is costly and requires irradiation of the subject. In addition, the technique is not available to many physicians. Després and his colleagues conducted a study to develop equations to predict the amount of deep abdominal AT from simple anthropometric measurements. Their subjects were men between the ages of 18 and 42 years who were free from metabolic disease that would require treatment. Among the

TABLE 9.3.1 Waist Circumference (cm), X, and Deep Abdominal AT, Y, of 109 Men

Subject	X	Y	Subject	X	Y	Subject	X	Y
1	74.75	25.72	38	103.00	129.00	75	108.00	217.00
2	72.60	25.89	39	80.00	74.02	76	100.00	140.00
3	81.80	42.60	40	79.00	55.48	77	103.00	109.00
4	83.95	42.80	41	83.50	73.13	78	104.00	127.00
5	74.65	29.84	42	76.00	50.50	79	106.00	112.00
6	71.85	21.68	43	80.50	50.88	80	109.00	192.00
7	80.90	29.08	44	86.50	140.00	81	103.50	132.00
8	83.40	32.98	45	83.00	96.54	82	110.00	126.00
9	63.50	11.44	46	107.10	118.00	83	110.00	153.00
10	73.20	32.22	47	94.30	107.00	84	112.00	158.00
11	71.90	28.32	48	94.50	123.00	85	108.50	183.00
12	75.00	43.86	49	79.70	65.92	86	104.00	184.00
13	73.10	38.21	50	79.30	81.29	87	111.00	121.00
14	79.00	42.48	51	89.80	111.00	88	108.50	159.00
15	77.00	30.96	52	83.80	90.73	89	121.00	245.00
16	68.85	55.78	53	85.20	133.00	90	109.00	137.00
17	75.95	43.78	54	75.50	41.90	91	97.50	165.00
18	74.15	33.41	55	78.40	41.71	92	105.50	152.00
19	73.80	43.35	56	78.60	58.16	93	98.00	181.00
20	75.90	29.31	57	87.80	88.85	94	94.50	80.95
21	76.85	36.60	58	86.30	155.00	95	97.00	137.00
22	80.90	40.25	59	85.50	70.77	96	105.00	125.00
23	79.90	35.43	60	83.70	75.08	97	106.00	241.00
24	89.20	60.09	61	77.60	57.05	98	99.00	134.00
25	82.00	45.84	62	84.90	99.73	99	91.00	150.00
26	92.00	70.40	63	79.80	27.96	100	102.50	198.00
27	86.60	83.45	64	108.30	123.00	101	106.00	151.00
28	80.50	84.30	65	119.60	90.41	102	109.10	229.00
29	86.00	78.89	66	119.90	106.00	103	115.00	253.00
30	82.50	64.75	67	96.50	144.00	104	101.00	188.00
31	83.50	72.56	68	105.50	121.00	105	100.10	124.00
32	88.10	89.31	69	105.00	97.13	106	93.30	62.20
33	90.80	78.94	70	107.00	166.00	107	101.80	133.00
34	89.40	83.55	71	107.00	87.99	108	107.90	208.00
35	102.00	127.00	72	101.00	154.00	109	108.50	208.00
36	94.50	121.00	73	97.00	100.00			
37	91.00	107.00	74	100.00	123.00			

SOURCE: Jean-Pierre Després, Ph.D. Used by permission.

measurements taken on each subject were deep abdominal AT obtained by CT and waist circumference as shown in Table 9.3.1. A question of interest is how well can one predict and estimate deep abdominal AT from a knowledge of waist circumference. This question is typical of those that can be answered by means of regression analysis. Since deep abdominal AT is the variable about which we wish to make predictions and estimations, it is the dependent variable. The variable waist measurement, knowledge of which will be used to make the predictions and estimations, is the independent variable.

The Scatter Diagram   A first step that is usually useful in studying the relationship between two variables is to prepare a *scatter diagram* of the data such as

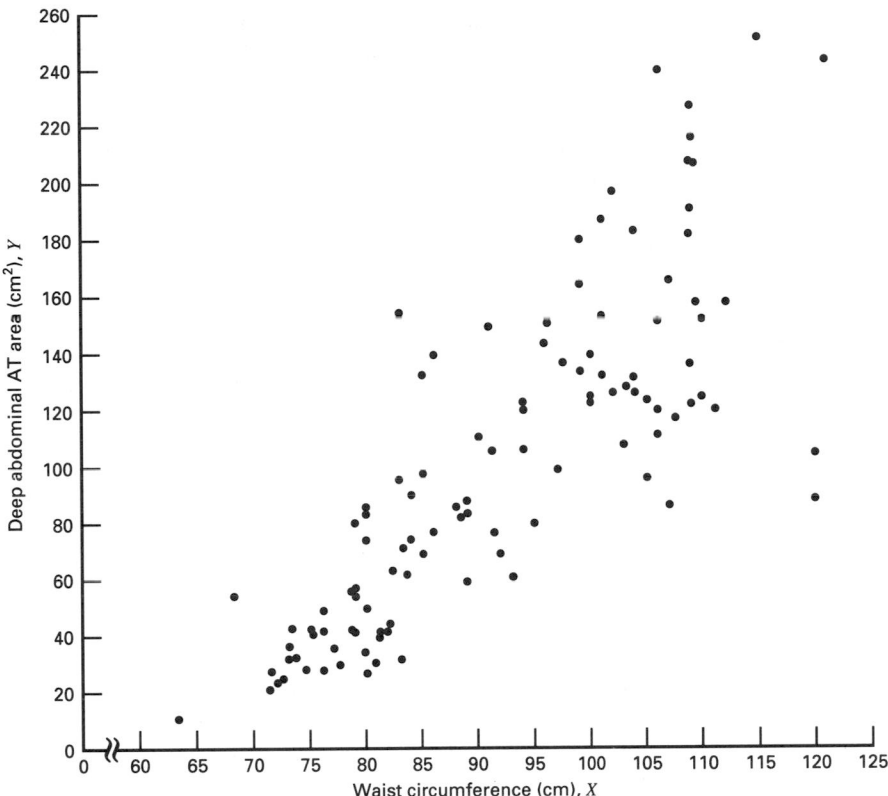

Figure 9.3.1 Scatter diagram of data shown in Table 9.3.1.

is shown in Figure 9.3.1. The points are plotted by assigning values of the independent variable X to the horizontal axis and values of the dependent variable Y to the vertical axis.

The pattern made by the points plotted on the scatter diagram usually suggests the basic nature and strength of the relationship between two variables. As we look at Figure 9.3.1, for example, the points seem to be scattered around an invisible straight line. The scatter diagram also shows that, in general, subjects with large waist circumferences also have larger amounts of deep abdominal AT. These impressions suggest that the relationship between the two variables may be described by a straight line crossing the Y-axis below the origin and making approximately a 45-degree angle with the X-axis. It looks as if it would be simple to draw, freehand, through the data points the line that describes the relationship between X and Y. It is highly unlikely, however, that the lines drawn by any two people would be exactly the same. In other words, for every person drawing such a line by eye, or freehand, we would expect a slightly different line. The question then arises as to which line best describes the relationship between the two variables. We cannot obtain an answer to this question by inspecting the lines. In fact, it is not likely that any freehand line drawn through the data will be the line that best describes the relationship between X and Y, since freehand lines will reflect any defects of vision or judgment of the person drawing the line. Similarly, when judging which of two lines best describes the relationship, subjective evaluation is liable to the same deficiencies.

What is needed for obtaining the desired line is some method that is not fraught with these difficulties.

The Least-Squares Line   The method usually employed for obtaining the desired line is known as the *method of least squares*, and the resulting line is called the *least-squares line*. The reason for calling the method by this name will be explained in the discussion that follows.

We recall from algebra that the general equation for a straight line may be written as

$$y = a + bx \tag{9.3.1}$$

where y is a value on the vertical axis, x is a value on the horizontal axis, a is the point where the line crosses the vertical axis, and b shows the amount by which y changes for each unit change in x. We refer to a as the y-intercept and b as the *slope* of the line. To draw a line based on Equation 9.3.1, we need the numerical values of the constants a and b. Given these constants, we may substitute various values of x into the equation to obtain corresponding values of y. The resulting points may be plotted. Since any two such coordinates determine a straight line, we may select any two, locate them on a graph, and connect them to obtain the line corresponding to the equation.

Normal Equations   It can be shown by mathematics beyond the scope of this book that a and b may be obtained by the simultaneous solution of the following two equations, which are known as the *normal equations* for a set of data:

$$\sum y_i = na + b \sum x_i \tag{9.3.2}$$

$$\sum x_i y_i = a \sum x_i + b \sum x_i^2 \tag{9.3.3}$$

In Table 9.3.2 we have the necessary values for substituting into the normal equations.

Substituting appropriate values from Table 9.3.2 into Equations 9.3.2 and 9.3.3 gives

$$11106.50 = 109a + 10017.30b$$

$$1089381.0 = 10017.30a + 940464.00b$$

We may solve these equations by any familiar method to obtain

$$a = -216.08 \quad \text{and} \quad b = 3.46$$

TABLE 9.3.2 Intermediate Computations for Normal Equations, Example 9.3.1

x	y	x^2	y^2	xy
74.75	25.72	5587.6	661.5	1922.6
72.60	25.89	5270.8	670.3	1879.6
81.80	42.60	6691.2	1814.8	3484.7
83.95	42.80	7047.6	1831.8	3593.1
74.65	29.84	5572.6	890.4	2227.6
71.85	21.68	5162.4	470.0	1557.7
80.90	29.08	6544.8	845.6	2352.6
83.40	32.98	6955.6	1087.7	2750.5
63.50	11.44	4032.2	130.9	726.4
73.20	32.22	5358.2	1038.1	2358.5
71.90	28.32	5169.6	802.0	2036.2
75.00	43.86	5625.0	1923.7	3289.5
73.10	38.21	5343.6	1460.0	2793.2
79.00	42.48	6241.0	1804.6	3355.9
77.00	30.96	5929.0	958.5	2383.9
68.85	55.78	4740.3	3111.4	3840.5
75.95	43.78	5768.4	1916.7	3325.1
74.15	33.41	5498.2	1116.2	2477.4
73.80	43.35	5446.4	1879.2	3199.2
75.90	29.31	5760.8	859.1	2224.6
76.85	36.60	5905.9	1339.6	2812.7
80.90	40.25	6544.8	1620.1	3256.2
79.90	35.43	6384.0	1255.3	2830.9
89.20	60.09	7956.6	3610.8	5360.0
82.00	45.84	6724.0	2101.3	3758.9
92.00	70.40	8464.0	4956.2	6476.8
86.60	83.45	7499.6	6963.9	7226.8
80.50	84.30	6480.2	7106.5	6786.2
86.00	78.89	7396.0	6223.6	6784.5
82.50	64.75	6806.2	4192.6	5341.9
83.50	72.56	6972.2	5265.0	6058.8
88.10	89.31	7761.6	7976.3	7868.2
90.80	78.94	8244.6	6231.5	7167.8
89.40	83.55	7992.4	6980.6	7469.4
102.00	127.00	10404.0	16129.0	12954.0
94.50	121.00	8930.3	14641.0	11434.5
91.00	107.00	8281.0	11449.0	9737.0
103.00	129.00	10609.0	16641.0	13287.0
80.00	74.02	6400.0	5479.0	5921.6
79.00	55.48	6241.0	3078.0	4382.9
83.50	73.13	6972.2	5348.0	6106.4
76.00	50.50	5776.0	2550.3	3838.0
80.50	50.88	6480.2	2588.8	4095.8
86.50	140.00	7482.2	19600.0	12110.0
83.00	96.54	6889.0	9320.0	8012.8
107.10	118.00	11470.4	13924.0	12637.8
94.30	107.00	8892.5	11449.0	10090.1
94.50	123.00	8930.3	15129.0	11623.5
79.70	65.92	6352.1	4345.4	5253.8
79.30	81.29	6288.5	6608.1	6446.3
89.80	111.00	8064.0	12321.0	9967.8
83.80	90.73	7022.4	8231.9	7603.2
85.20	133.00	7259.0	17689.0	11331.6
75.50	41.90	5700.3	1755.6	3163.5
78.40	41.71	6146.6	1739.7	3270.1

TABLE 9.3.2 (*Continued*)

x	y	x^2	y^2	xy
78.60	58.16	6178.0	3382.6	4571.4
87.80	88.85	7708.8	7894.3	7801.0
86.30	155.00	7447.7	24025.0	13376.5
85.50	70.77	7310.3	5008.4	6050.8
83.70	75.08	7005.7	5637.0	6284.2
77.60	57.05	6021.8	3254.7	4427.1
84.90	99.73	7208.0	9946.1	8467.1
79.80	27.96	6368.0	781.8	2231.2
108.30	123.00	11728.9	15129.0	13320.9
119.60	90.41	14304.2	8174.0	10813.0
119.90	106.00	14376.0	11236.0	12709.4
96.50	144.00	9312.3	20736.0	13896.0
105.50	121.00	11130.2	14641.0	12765.5
105.00	97.13	11025.0	9434.2	10198.6
107.00	166.00	11449.0	27556.0	17762.0
107.00	87.99	11449.0	7742.2	9414.9
101.00	154.00	10201.0	23716.0	15554.0
97.00	100.00	9409.0	10000.0	9700.0
100.00	123.00	10000.0	15129.0	12300.0
108.00	217.00	11664.0	47089.0	23436.0
100.00	140.00	10000.0	19600.0	14000.0
103.00	109.00	10609.0	11881.0	11227.0
104.00	127.00	10816.0	16129.0	13208.0
106.00	112.00	11236.0	12544.0	11872.0
109.00	192.00	11881.0	36864.0	20928.0
103.50	132.00	10712.2	17424.0	13662.0
110.00	126.00	12100.0	15876.0	13860.0
110.00	153.00	12100.0	23409.0	16830.0
112.00	158.00	12544.0	24964.0	17696.0
108.50	183.00	11772.2	33489.0	19855.5
104.00	184.00	10816.0	33856.0	19136.0
111.00	121.00	12321.0	14641.0	13431.0
108.50	159.00	11772.2	25281.0	17251.5
121.00	245.00	14641.0	60025.0	29645.0
109.00	137.00	11881.0	18769.0	14933.0
97.50	165.00	9506.3	27225.0	16087.5
105.50	152.00	11130.2	23104.0	16036.0
98.00	181.00	9604.0	32761.0	17738.0
94.50	80.95	8930.3	6552.9	7649.8
97.00	137.00	9409.0	18769.0	13289.0
105.00	125.00	11025.0	15625.0	13125.0
106.00	241.00	11236.0	58081.0	25546.0
99.00	134.00	9801.0	17956.0	13266.0
91.00	150.00	8281.0	22500.0	13650.0
102.50	198.00	10506.2	39204.0	20295.0
106.00	151.00	11236.0	22801.0	16006.0
109.10	229.00	11902.8	52441.0	24983.9
115.00	253.00	13225.0	64009.0	29095.0
101.00	188.00	10201.0	35344.0	18988.0
100.10	124.00	10020.0	15376.0	12412.4
93.30	62.20	8704.9	3868.8	5803.3
101.80	133.00	10363.2	17689.0	13539.4
107.90	208.00	11642.4	43264.0	22443.2
108.50	208.00	11772.2	43264.0	22568.0
Total 10017.30	11106.50	940464.0	1486212.0	1089381.0

The linear equation for the least-squares line that describes the relationship between waist circumference and deep abdominal AT may be written, then, as

$$\hat{y} = -216.08 + 3.46x \qquad (9.3.4)$$

This equation tells us that since a is negative, the line crosses the Y-axis below the origin, and that since b, the slope, is positive, the line extends from the lower left-hand corner of the graph to the upper right-hand corner. We see further that for each unit increase in x, y increases by an amount equal to 3.46. The symbol $\hat{y}$ denotes a value of y computed from the equation, rather than an observed value of Y.

By substituting two convenient values of X into Equation 9.3.4, we may obtain the necessary coordinates for drawing the line. Suppose, first, we let $X = 70$ and obtain

$$\hat{y} = -216.08 + 3.46(70) = 26.12$$

If we let $X = 110$ we obtain

$$\hat{y} = -216.08 + 3.46(110) = 164.52$$

The line, along with the original data, is shown in Figure 9.3.2.

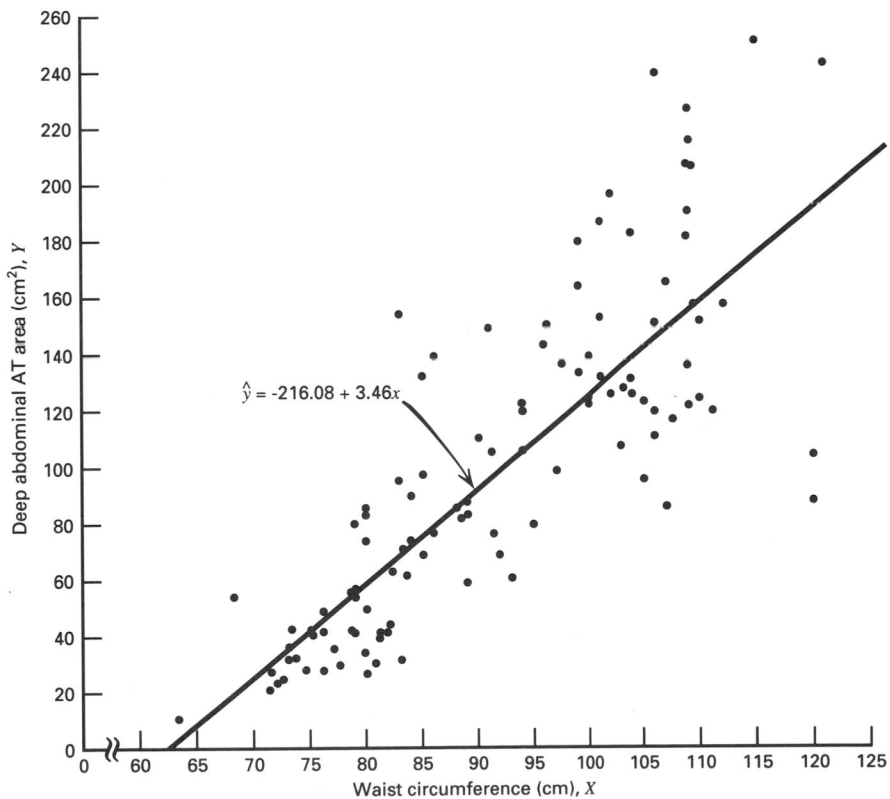

Figure 9.3.2 Original data and least-squares line for Example 9.3.1.

Alternative Formulas for *a* and *b*   Numerical values for *a* and *b* may be obtained by alternative formulas that do not directly involve the normal equations. The formulas are as follows:

$$b = \frac{n\sum xy - (\sum x)(\sum y)}{n\sum x^2 - (\sum x)^2} \tag{9.3.5}$$

$$a = \frac{\sum y - b\sum x}{n} \tag{9.3.6}$$

For the present example we have

$$b = \frac{109(1089381) - (10017.3)(11106.5)}{109(940464) - (10017.3)^2}$$

$$= 3.46$$

$$a = \frac{11106.5 - 3.46(10017.3)}{109}$$

$$= -216.08$$

Thus, we see that Equations 9.3.5 and 9.3.6 yield the same results as the normal equations.

The Least-Squares Criterion   Now that we have obtained what we call the "best" line for describing the relationship between our two variables, we need to determine by what criterion it is considered best. Before the criterion is stated, let us examine Figure 9.3.2. We note that generally the least-squares line does not pass through the observed points that are plotted on the scatter diagram. In other words, most of the observed points *deviate* from the line by varying amounts.

The line that we have drawn through the points is best in this sense:

The sum of the squared vertical deviations of the observed data points (y_i) from the least-squares line is smaller than the sum of the squared vertical deviations of the data points from any other line.

In other words, if we square the vertical distance from each observed point (y_i) to the least-squares line and add these squared values for all points, the resulting total will be smaller than the similarly computed total for any other line that can be drawn through the points. For this reason the line we have drawn is called the least-squares line.

EXERCISES

9.3.1 Plot each of the following regression equations on graph paper and state whether X and Y are directly or inversely related.
 (a) $\hat{y} = -3 + 2x$
 (b) $\hat{y} = 3 + 0.5x$
 (c) $\hat{y} = 10 - 0.75x$

9.3.2 The following scores represent a nurses' assessment (X) and a physicians' assessment (Y) of the condition of 10 patients at time of admission to a trauma center.

X:	18	13	18	15	10	12	8	4	7	3
Y:	23	20	18	16	14	11	10	7	6	4

 (a) Construct a scatter diagram for these data.
 (b) Plot the following regression equations on the scatter diagram and indicate which one you think best fits the data. State the reason for your choice.
   (1) $\hat{y} = 8 + 0.5x$
   (2) $\hat{y} = -10 + 2x$
   (3) $\hat{y} = 1 + 1x$

For each of the following exercises (a) draw a scatter diagram and (b) obtain the regression equation and plot it on the scatter diagram.

9.3.3 A research project by Phillips et al. (A-2) was motivated by the fact that there is wide variation in the clinical manifestations of sickle cell anemia (SCA). In an effort to explain this variability these investigators used a magneto-acoustic ball microrheometer developed in their laboratory to measure several rheologic parameters of suspensions of cells from individuals with SCA. They correlated their results with clinical events and end-organ failure in individuals with SCA. The following table shows scores for one of the rheologic measurements, viscous modulus (VI C) (X), and end organ failure score (Y). End-organ failure scores were based on the presence of nephropathy, avascular necrosis of bone, stroke, retinopathy, resting hypoxemia after acute chest syndrome(s), leg ulcer, and priapism with impotence.

X	Y	X	Y
.32	0	.57	2
.72	3	.63	5
.38	1	.37	1
.61	4	.45	1
.48	3	.85	4
.48	1	.80	4
.70	3	.36	1
.41	2	.69	4

SOURCE: George Phillips, Jr., Bruce Coffey, Roger Tran-Son-Tay, T. R. Kinney, Eugene P. Orringer, and R. M. Hochmuth, "Relationship of Clinical Severity to Packed Cell Rheology in Sickle Cell Anemia," *Blood*, **78** (1991), 2735–2739.

9.3.4 Habib and Lutchen (A-3) present a diagnostic technique that is of interest to respiratory disorder specialists. The following are the scores elicited by this technique, called AMDN, and the forced expiratory volume (FEV$_1$) scores (% predicted) for 22 subjects. The first seven subjects were healthy, subjects 8 through 17 had asthma, and the remaining subjects were cystic fibrosis patients.

Patient	AMDN	FEV_1
1	1.36	102
2	1.42	92
3	1.41	111
4	1.44	94
5	1.47	99
6	1.39	98
7	1.47	99
8	1.79	80
9	1.71	87
10	1.44	100
11	1.63	86
12	1.68	102
13	1.75	81
14	1.95	51
15	1.64	78
16	2.22	52
17	1.85	43
18	2.24	59
19	2.51	30
20	2.20	61
21	2.20	29
22	1.97	86

SOURCE: Robert H. Habib and Kenneth R. Lutchen, "Moment Analysis of a Multibreath Nitrogen Washout Based on an Alveolar Gas Dilution Number," *American Review of Respiratory Disease*, *144* (1991), 513–519.

9.3.5 In an article in the *American Journal of Clinical Pathology*, de Metz et al. (A-4) compare three methods for determining the percentage of dysmorphic erythrocytes in urine. The following are the results obtained when methods A (X) and B (Y) were used on 75 urine specimens.

X	Y	X	Y	X	Y	X	Y
0	0	20	16	65	55	89	81
0	1	16	18	66	71	90	80
0	11	17	30	67	70	91	90
2	0	19	30	69	71	90	97
5	0	20	29	74	60	92	89
6	3	18	35	75	59	93	98
7	3	25	32	73	70	93	97
9	5	30	40	75	69	94	98
8	6	32	45	76	70	95	89
9	7	39	49	78	80	95	95
10	15	40	50	78	82	95	97
10	17	48	41	77	90	95	98
13	13	47	43	82	73	97	85
15	8	57	42	85	74	98	95
18	7	50	60	85	80	99	95
19	9	60	65	86	75	100	96
20	9	60	70	88	74	100	100
16	13	59	69	88	83	100	99
19	16	62	70	88	91		

Source: Menno de Metz. Used by permission.

9.3.6 Height is frequently named as a good predictor variable for weight among people of the same age and gender. The following are the heights and weights of 14 males between the ages of 19 and 26 years who participated in a study conducted by Roberts et al. (A-5):

Weight	Height	Weight	Height
83.9	185	69.2	174
99.0	180	56.4	164
63.8	173	66.2	169
71.3	168	88.7	205
65.3	175	59.7	161
79.6	183	64.6	177
70.3	184	78.8	174

SOURCE: Susan B. Roberts. Used by permission.

9.3.7. Ogasawara (A-6) collected the following Full Scale IQ scores on 45 pairs of brothers with Duchenne progressive muscular dystrophy.

X	Y	X	Y
78	114	127	113
77	68	113	112
112	116	91	103
114	123	91	93
104	107	96	90
99	81	100	102
92	76	97	104
80	90	82	92
113	91	43	43
99	95	77	100
97	106	109	90
80	99	99	100
84	82	99	103
89	77	100	103
100	81	56	67
111	111	56	67
75	80	67	67
94	98	71	66
67	82	66	63
46	56	78	76
106	117	95	86
99	98	38	64
102	89		

SOURCE: Akihiko Ogasawara. Used by permission.

9.4
Evaluating the Regression Equation

Once the regression equation has been obtained it must be evaluated to determine whether it adequately describes the relationship between the two variables and whether it can be used effectively for prediction and estimation purposes.

When H_0: $\beta = 0$ Is Not Rejected   If in the population the relationship between X and Y is linear, β, the slope of the line that describes this relationship, will be either positive, negative, or zero. If β is zero, sample data drawn from the population will, in the long run, yield regression equations that are of little or no value for prediction and estimation purposes. Furthermore, even though we assume that the relationship between X and Y is linear, it may be that the relationship could be described better by some nonlinear model. When this is the case, sample data when fitted to a linear model will tend to yield results compatible with a population slope of zero. Thus, following a test in which the null hypothesis that β equals zero is not rejected, we may conclude (assuming that we have not made a type II error by accepting a false null hypothesis) either (1) that although the relationship between X and Y may be linear it is not strong enough for X to be of much value in predicting and estimating Y, or (2) that the relationship between X and Y is not linear; that is, some curvilinear model provides a better fit to the data. Figure 9.4.1 shows the kinds of relationships between X and Y in a population that may prevent rejection of the null hypothesis that $\beta = 0$.

When H_0: $\beta = 0$ Is Rejected   Now let us consider the situations in a population that may lead to rejection of the null hypothesis that $\beta = 0$. Assuming that we do not commit a type I error, rejection of the null hypothesis that $\beta = 0$ may be attributed to one of the following conditions in the population: (1) The relationship is linear and of sufficient strength to justify the use of sample regression equations to predict and estimate Y for given values of X. (2) There is a good fit of the data to a linear model, but some curvilinear model might provide an even better fit. Figure 9.4.2 illustrates the two population conditions that may lead to rejection of H_0: $\beta = 0$.

Thus we see that before using a sample regression equation to predict and estimate, it is desirable to test H_0: $\beta = 0$. We may do this either by using analysis of variance and the F statistic or by using the t statistic. We will illustrate both methods. Before we do this, however, let us see how we may investigate the strength of the relationship between X and Y.

The Coefficient of Determination   One way to evaluate the strength of the regression equation is to compare the scatter of the points about the regression line with the scatter about $\bar{y}$, the mean of the sample values of Y. If we take the scatter diagram for Example 9.3.1 and draw through the points a line that intersects the Y-axis at $\bar{y}$ and is parallel to the X-axis, we may obtain a visual impression of the relative magnitudes of the scatter of the points about this line and the regression line. This has been done in Figure 9.4.3.

It appears rather obvious from Figure 9.4.3 that the scatter of the points about the regression line is much less than the scatter about the $\bar{y}$ line. We would not wish, however, to decide on this basis alone that the equation is a useful one. The situation may not be always this clear-cut, so that an objective measure of some sort would be much more desirable. Such an objective measure, called the *coefficient of determination*, is available.

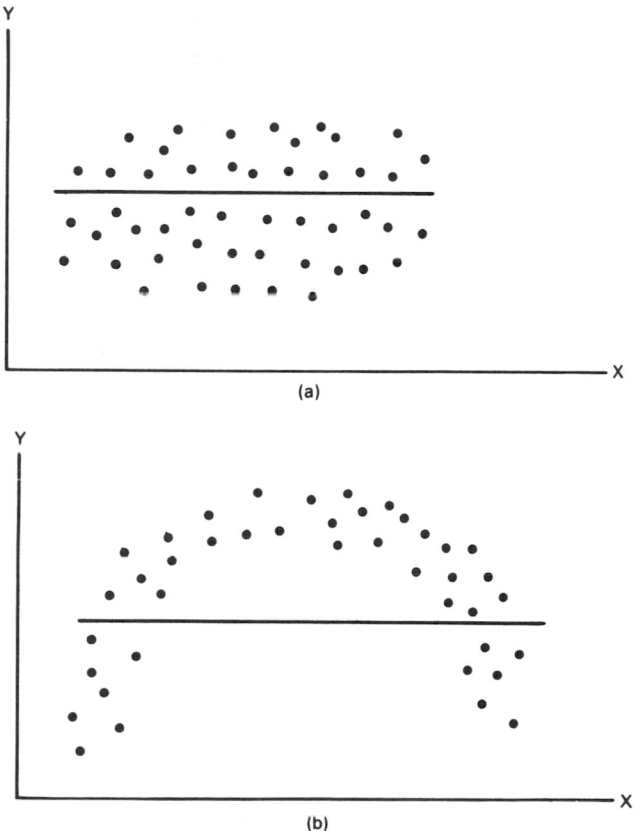

Figure 9.4.1 Conditions in a population that may prevent rejection of the null hypothesis that $\beta = 0$. (a) The relationship between X and Y is linear, but β is so close to zero that sample data are not likely to yield equations that are useful for predicting Y when X is given. (b) The relationship between X and Y is not linear; a curvilinear model provides a better fit to the data; sample data are not likely to yield equations that are useful for predicting Y when X is given.

The Total Deviation   Before defining the coefficient of determination, let us justify its use by examining the logic behind its computation. We begin by considering the point corresponding to any observed value, y_i, and by measuring its vertical distance from the $\bar{y}$ line. We call this the *total deviation* and designate it by $(y_i - \bar{y})$.

The Explained Deviation   If we measure the vertical distance from the regression line to the $\bar{y}$ line, we obtain $(\hat{y} - \bar{y})$, which is called the *explained deviation*, since it shows by how much the total deviation is reduced when the regression line is fitted to the points.

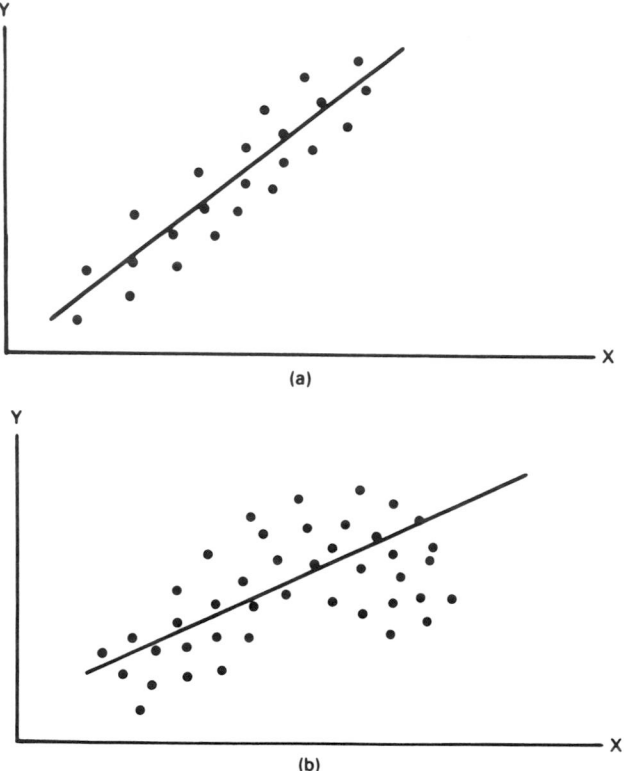

(a)

(b)

Figure 9.4.2 Population conditions relative to X and Y that may cause rejection of the null hypothesis that $\beta = 0$. (a) The relationship between X and Y is linear and of sufficient strength to justify the use of a sample regression equation to predict and estimate Y for given values of X. (b) A linear model provides a good fit to the data, but some curvilinear model would provide an even better fit.

Unexplained Deviation Finally, we measure the vertical distance of the observed point from the regression line to obtain $(y_i - \hat{y})$, which is called the *unexplained deviation*, since it represents the portion of the total deviation not "explained" or accounted for by the introduction of the regression line. These three quantities are shown for a typical value of Y in Figure 9.4.4.

It is seen, then, that the total deviation for a particular y_i is equal to the sum of the explained and unexplained deviations. We may write this symbolically as

$$(y_i - \bar{y}) = (\hat{y} - \bar{y}) - (y_i - \hat{y}) \tag{9.4.1}$$

$$\begin{array}{ccc} \text{total} & \text{explained} & \text{unexplained} \\ \text{deviation} & \text{deviation} & \text{deviation} \end{array}$$

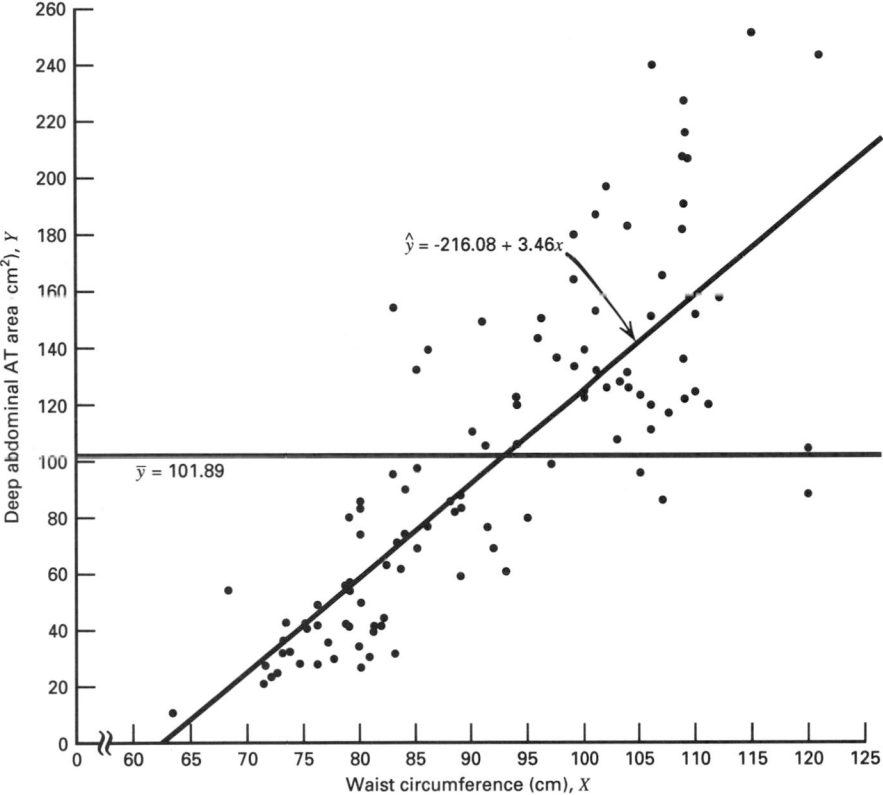

Figure 9.4.3 Scatter diagram, sample regression line, and y line for Example 9.3.1.

If we measure these deviations for each value of y_i and $\hat{y}$, square each deviation, and add up the squared deviations, we have

$$\sum (y_i - \bar{y})^2 = \sum (\hat{y} - \bar{y})^2 + \sum (y_i - \hat{y})^2 \qquad (9.4.2)$$

total	explained	unexplained
sum	sum	sum
of squares	of squares	of squares

These quantities may be considered measures of dispersion or variability.

Total Sum of Squares   The *total sum of squares* (*SST*), for example, is a measure of the dispersion of the observed values of Y about their mean $\bar{y}$; that is, this term is a measure of the total variation in the observed values of Y. The reader will recognize this term as the numerator of the familiar formula for the sample variance.

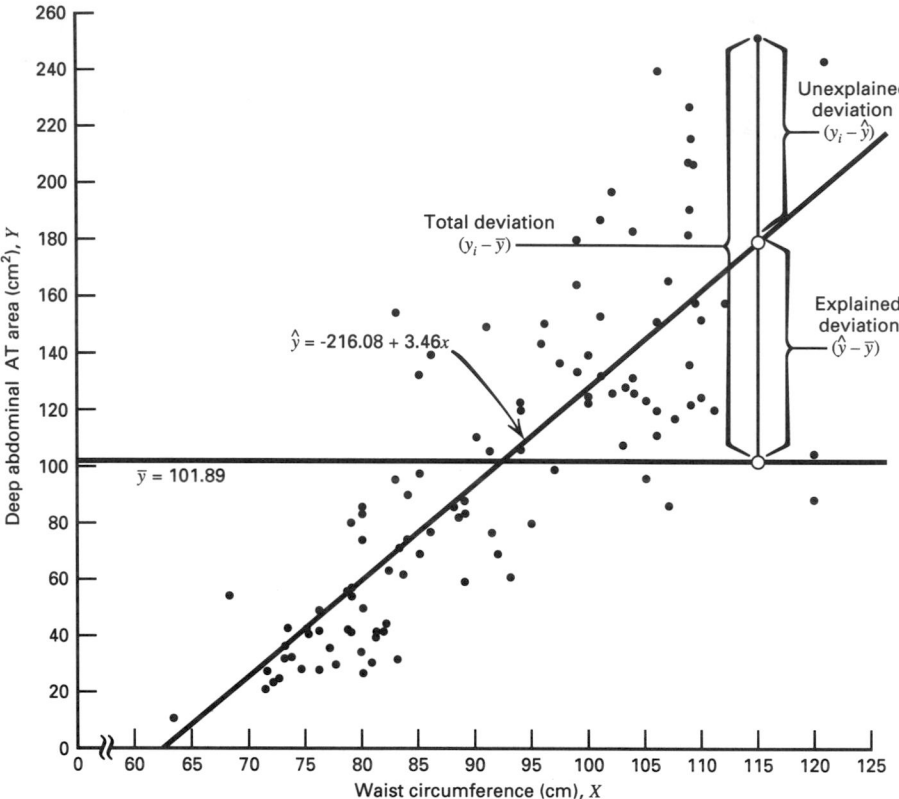

Figure 9.4.4 Scatter diagram showing the total, explained, and unexplained deviations for a selected value of Y, Example 9.3.1.

Explained Sum of Squares   The *explained sum of squares* measures the amount of the total variability in the observed values of Y that is accounted for by the linear relationship between the observed values of X and Y. This quantity is referred to also as the *sum of squares due to linear regression* (SSR).

Unexplained Sum of Squares   The *unexplained sum of squares* is a measure of the dispersion of the observed Y values about the regression line and is sometimes called the *error sum of squares*, or the *residual sum of squares* (SSE). It is this quantity that is minimized when the least-squares line is obtained.

We may express the relationship among the three sums of squares values as

$$SST = SSR + SSE$$

The necessary calculations for obtaining the total, the regression, and the error sums of squares for our illustrative example are displayed in Table 9.4.1.

TABLE 9.4.1 Calculation of Total, Explained, and Unexplained Sums of Squares

Subject	AT (y_i)	$\hat{y} = -216.08 + 3.46x$	$(y_i - \bar{y})$	$(y_i - \bar{y})^2$	$(y_i - \hat{y})$	$(y_i - \hat{y})^2$	$(\hat{y} - \bar{y})$	$(\hat{y} - \bar{y})^2$
1	25.72	43.42	−76.17	5801.8689	−17.70	313.2900	−58.47	3418.7409
2	25.89	36.50	−76.00	5776.0000	−10.61	112.5721	−65.39	4275.8521
3	42.60	67.64	−59.29	3515.3041	−25.04	627.0016	−34.25	1173.0625
⋮	⋮	⋮	⋮	⋮	⋮	⋮	⋮	⋮
109	208.00	159.33	106.11	11259.3321	48.67	2368.7689	57.44	3299.3536
Total	11106.50			$SST = 354531.0000$		$SSE = 116982.000$		$SSR = 237549.0000$
$\bar{y} = 101.89$								

For our illustrative example we have

$$SST = SSR + SSE$$

$$354531.0000 = 237549.0000 + 116982.0000$$

$$354531.0000 = 354531.0000$$

We may calculate the total sum of squares by the more convenient formula

$$\sum (y_i - \bar{y})^2 = \sum y_i^2 - \frac{\left(\sum y_i\right)^2}{n} \tag{9.4.3}$$

and the regression sum of squares may be computed by

$$\sum (\hat{y} - \bar{y})^2 = b^2 \sum (x_i - \bar{x})^2 = b^2 \left[\sum x_i^2 - \left(\sum x_i\right)^2 / n \right] \tag{9.4.4}$$

The error sum of squares is more conveniently obtained by subtraction. For our illustrative example we have

$$SST = 25.72^2 + 25.89^2 + \cdots + 208.00^2 - \frac{11106.50^2}{109} = 354531.0000$$

$$SSR = 3.46^2 \left[74.75^2 + 72.60^2 + \cdots + 108.50^2 - \frac{10017.30^2}{109} \right]$$

$$= 237549.0000$$

and

$$SSE = SST - SSR$$

$$= 354531.0000 - 237549.0000$$

$$= 116982.0000$$

The results using the computationally more convenient formulas are the same results as those shown in Table 9.4.1.

Calculating r^2 It is intuitively appealing to speculate that if a regression equation does a good job of describing the relationship between two variables, the explained or regression sum of squares should constitute a large proportion of the total sum of squares. It would be of interest, then, to determine the magnitude of this proportion by computing the ratio of the explained sum of squares to the total sum of squares. This is exactly what is done in evaluating a regression equation based on sample data, and the result is called the sample *coefficient of determination*, r^2. That is,

$$r^2 = \frac{\sum (\hat{y} - \bar{y})^2}{\sum (y_i - \bar{y})^2} = \frac{b^2 \left[\sum x_i^2 - \left(\sum x_i \right)^2 \big/ n \right]}{\sum y_i^2 - \dfrac{\left(\sum y_i \right)^2}{n}} = SSR/SST$$

In our present example we have, using the sums of squares values computed by Equations 9.4.3 and 9.4.4,

$$r^2 = \frac{237549.0000}{354531.0000} = .67$$

The sample coefficient of determination measures the closeness of fit of the sample regression equation to the observed values of Y. When the quantities $(y_i - \hat{y})$, the vertical distances of the observed values of Y from the equation, are small, the unexplained sum of squares is small. This leads to a large explained sum of squares that leads, in turn, to a large value of r^2. This is illustrated in Figure 9.4.5.

In Figure 9.4.5*a* we see that the observations all lie close to the regression line, and we would expect r^2 to be large. In fact, the computed r^2 for these data is .986, indicating that about 99 percent of the total variation in the y_i is explained by the regression.

In Figure 9.4.5*b* we illustrate a case where the y_i are widely scattered about the regression line, and there we suspect that r^2 is small. The computed r^2 for the data is .403, that is, less than 50 percent of the total variation in the y_i is explained by the regression.

The largest value that r^2 can assume is 1, a result that occurs when all the variation in the y_i is explained by the regression. When $r^2 = 1$ all the observations fall on the regression line. This situation is shown in Figure 9.4.5*c*.

The lower limit of r^2 is 0. This result is obtained when the regression line and the line drawn through $\bar{y}$ coincide. In this situation none of the variation in the y_i is explained by the regression. Figure 9.4.5*d* illustrates a situation in which r^2 is close to zero.

When r^2 is large, then, the regression has accounted for a large proportion of the total variability in the observed values of Y, and we look with favor on the regression equation. On the other hand, a small r^2, which indicates a failure of the regression to account for a large proportion of the total variation in the observed values of Y, tends to cast doubt on the usefulness of the regression equation for predicting and estimating purposes. We do not, however, pass final judgment on the equation until it has been subjected to an objective statistical test.

Testing H_0: $\beta = 0$ with the *F* Statistic   The following example illustrates one method for reaching a conclusion regarding the relationship between X and Y.

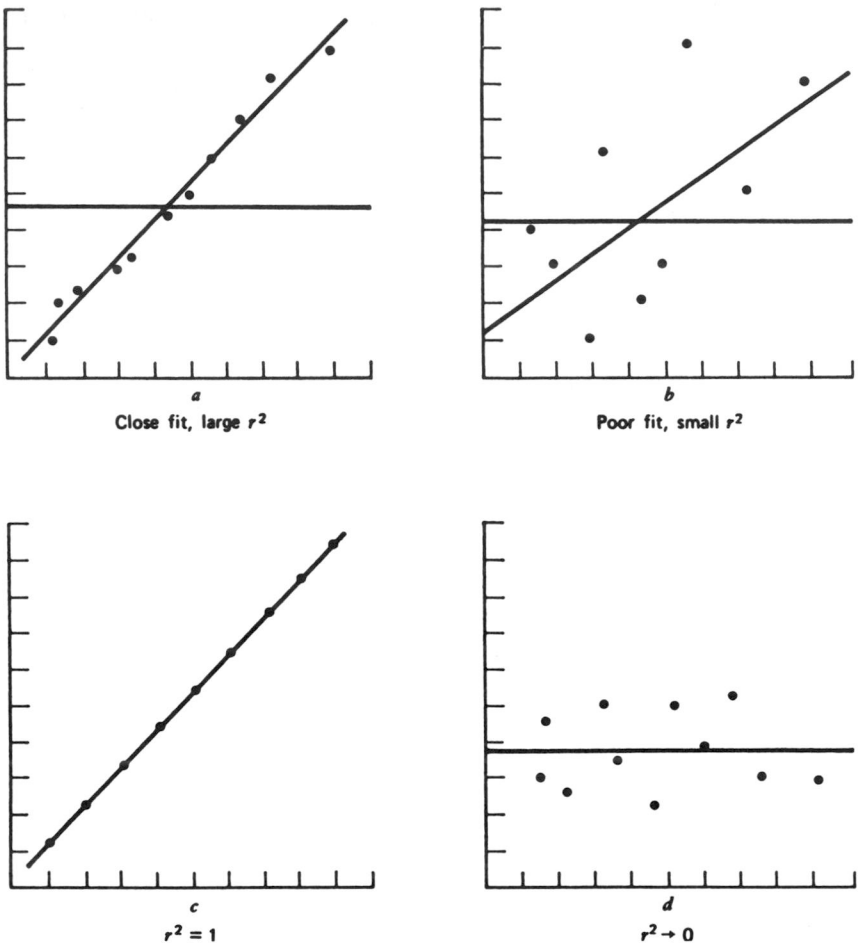

Figure 9.4.5 r^2 as a measure of closeness-of-fit of the sample regression line to the sample observations.

Example 9.4.1   Refer to Example 9.3.1. We wish to know if we can conclude that, in the population from which our sample was drawn, X and Y are linearly related.

Solution: The steps in the hypothesis testing procedure are as follows:

1. *Data*   The data were described in the opening statement of Example 9.3.1.

2. *Assumptions*   We presume that the simple linear regression model and its underlying assumptions as given in Section 9.2 are applicable.

3. *Hypotheses*

$$H_0: \beta = 0$$

$$H_A: \beta \neq 0$$

$$\alpha = .05$$

TABLE 9.4.2 ANOVA Table for Simple Linear Regression

Source of Variation	SS	d.f.	MS	V.R.
Linear regression	SSR	1	$SSR/1$	MSR/MSE
Residual	SSE	$n-2$	$SSE/(n-2)$	
Total	SST	$n-1$		

4. *Test Statistic* The test statistic is V.R. as explained in the discussion that follows.

From the three sum-of-squares terms and their associated degrees of freedom the analysis of variance table of Table 9.4.2 may be constructed.

In general, the degrees of freedom associated with the sum of squares due to regression is equal to the number of constants in the regression equation minus 1. In the simple linear case we have two constants, a and b, hence the degrees of freedom for regression are $2 - 1 = 1$.

5. *Distribution of Test Statistic* It can be shown that when the hypothesis of no linear relationship between X and Y is true, and when the assumptions underlying regression are met, the ratio obtained by dividing the regression mean square by the residual mean square is distributed as F with 1 and $n - 2$ degrees of freedom.

6. *Decision Rule* Reject H_0 if the computed value of V.R. is equal to or greater than the critical value of F.

7. *Calculation of the Test Statistic* Substituting appropriate numerical values into Table 9.4.2 gives Table 9.4.3.

8. *Statistical Decision* Since 217.279 is greater than 8.25, the critical value of F (obtained by interpolation) for 1 and 107 degrees of freedom, the null hypothesis is rejected.

9. *Conclusion* We conclude that the linear model provides a good fit to the data. For this test, since $217.279 > 13.61$, we have $p < .005$.

TABLE 9.4.3 ANOVA Table for Example 9.3.1

Source of Variation	SS	d.f	MS	V.R.
Linear regression	237549.0000	1	237549.0000	217.279
Residual	116982.0000	107	1093.2897	
Total	354531.0000	108		

Estimating the Population Coefficient of Determination The sample coefficient of determination provides a point estimate of ρ^2, the *population coefficient of determination*. The population coefficient of determination, ρ^2, has the same function relative to the population as r^2 has to the sample. It shows what proportion of the total population variation in Y is explained by the regression of Y on X. When the number of degrees of freedom are small, r^2 is positively biased. That is, r^2 tends to be large. An unbiased estimator of ρ^2 is provided by

$$\tilde{r}^2 = 1 - \frac{\sum(y_i - \hat{y})^2 / (n-2)}{\sum(y_i - \bar{y})^2 / (n-1)} \tag{9.4.5}$$

Observe that the numerator of the fraction in Equation 9.4.5 is the unexplained mean square and the denominator is the total mean square. These quantities appear in the analysis of variance table. For our illustrative example we have, using the data from Table 9.4.3,

$$\tilde{r}^2 = 1 - \frac{116982.0000 / 107}{354531.0000 / 108} = .66695$$

We see that this value is slightly less than

$$r^2 = 1 - \frac{116982.0000}{354531.0000} = .67004$$

We see that the difference in r^2 and $\tilde{r}^2$ is due to the factor $(n-1)/(n-2)$. When n is large, this factor will approach 1 and the difference between r^2 and $\tilde{r}^2$ will approach zero.

Testing H_0: $\beta = 0$ with the t Statistic When the assumptions stated in Section 9.2 are met, a and b are unbiased point estimators of the corresponding parameters α and β. Since, under these assumptions, the subpopulations of Y values are normally distributed, we may construct confidence intervals for and test hypotheses about α and β.

When the assumptions of Section 9.2 hold true, the sampling distributions of a and b are each normally distributed with means and variances as follows:

$$\mu_a = \alpha \tag{9.4.6}$$

$$\sigma_a^2 = \frac{\sigma_{y|x}^2 \sum x_i^2}{n \sum (x_i - \bar{x})^2} \tag{9.4.7}$$

$$\mu_b = \beta \tag{9.4.8}$$

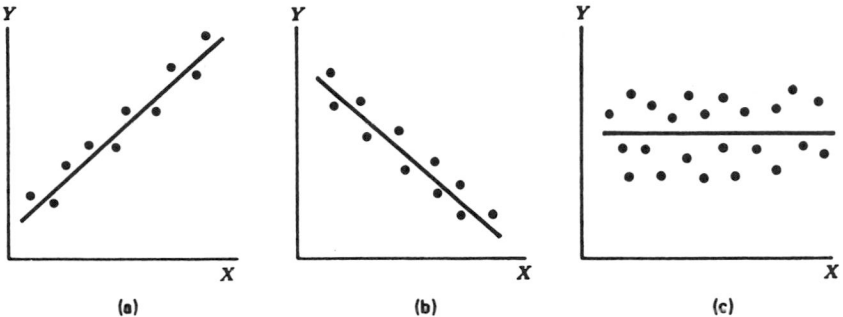

Figure 9.4.6 Scatter diagrams showing (a) direct linear relationship, (b) inverse linear relationship, and (c) no linear relationship between X and Y.

and

$$\sigma_b^2 = \frac{\sigma_{y|x}^2}{\sum (x_i - \bar{x})^2} \tag{9.4.9}$$

In Equations 9.4.7 and 9.4.9 $\sigma_{y|x}^2$ is the unexplained variance of the subpopulations of Y values.

With knowledge of the sampling distributions of a and b we may construct confidence intervals and test hypotheses relative to α and β in the usual manner. Inferences regarding α are usually not of interest. On the other hand, as we have seen, a great deal of interest centers on inferential procedures with respect to β. The reason for this is the fact that β tells us so much about the form of the relationship between X and Y. When X and Y are linearly related a positive β indicates that, in general, Y increases as X increases, and we say that there is a *direct linear relationship* between X and Y. A negative β indicates that values of Y tend to decrease as values of X increase, and we say that there is an *inverse linear relationship* between X and Y. When there is no linear relationship between X and Y, β is equal to zero. These three situations are illustrated in Figure 9.4.6.

The Test Statistic   For testing hypotheses about β the test statistic when $\sigma_{y|x}^2$ is known is

$$z = \frac{b - \beta_0}{\sigma_b} \tag{9.4.10}$$

where β_0 is the hypothesized value of β. The hypothesized value of β does not have to be zero, but in practice, more often than not, the null hypothesis of interest is that $\beta = 0$.

As a rule $\sigma_{y|x}^2$ is unknown. When this is the case, the test statistic is

$$t = \frac{b - \beta_0}{s_b} \tag{9.4.11}$$

where s_b is an estimate of σ_b, and t is distributed as Student's t with $n-2$ degrees of freedom. To obtain s_b, we must first estimate $\sigma_{y|x}^2$. An unbiased estimator of this parameter is provided by the unexplained variance computed from the sample data. That is,

$$s_{y|x}^2 = \frac{\sum (y_i - \hat{y})^2}{n-2} \qquad (9.4.12)$$

is an unbiased estimator of $\sigma_{y|x}^2$. This is the unexplained mean square that appears in the analysis of variance table.

The terms $(y_i - \hat{y})$ in Equation 9.4.12 are called the *residuals*. Some computer programs for regression analysis routinely give the residuals as part of the output. When this is the case one may obtain $s_{y|x}^2$ by squaring the residuals, adding the squared terms, and dividing the result by $n-2$. An alternative formula for $s_{y|x}^2$ is

$$s_{y|x}^2 = \frac{n-1}{n-2}\left(s_y^2 - b^2 s_x^2\right) \qquad (9.4.13)$$

where s_y^2 and s_x^2 are the variances of the y and x observations, respectively. For our illustrative example we have

$$s_y^2 = 3282.5999 \qquad \text{and} \qquad s_x^2 = 183.8495$$

so that

$$s_{y|x}^2 = \frac{108}{107}\left[3282.5999 - (3.46)^2(183.8495)\right] = 1091.73589$$

a result that agrees with the residual mean square in Table 9.4.3.

The square root of $s_{y|x}^2$, is $s_{y|x}$, the standard deviation of the observations about the fitted regression line, and measures the dispersion of these points about the line. The greater $s_{y|x}$, the poorer the fit of the line to the observed data.

When $s_{y|x}^2$ is used to estimate $\sigma_{y|x}^2$ we may obtain the desired and unbiased estimator of σ_b^2 by

$$s_b^2 = \frac{s_{y|x}^2}{\sum (x_i - \bar{x})^2} \qquad (9.4.14)$$

We may write Equation 9.4.14 in the following computationally more convenient form:

$$s_b^2 = \frac{s_{y|x}^2}{\sum x_i^2 - \left(\sum x_i\right)^2 / n} \qquad (9.4.15)$$

If the probability of observing a value as extreme as the value of the test statistic computed by Equation 9.4.11 when the null hypothesis is true is less than $\alpha/2$ (since we have a two-sided test), the null hypothesis is rejected.

Example 9.4.2

Refer to Example 9.3.1. We wish to know if we can conclude that the slope of the population regression line describing the relationship between X and Y is zero.

Solution:

1. *Data* See Example 9.3.1.

2. *Assumptions* We presume that the simple linear regression model and its underlying assumptions are applicable.

3. *Hypotheses*

$$H_0: \beta = 0$$

$$H_A: \beta \neq 0$$

$$\alpha = .05$$

4. *Test Statistic* The test statistic is given by Equation 9.4.11.

5. *Distribution of the Test Statistic* When the assumptions are met and H_0 is true, the test statistic is distributed as Student's t with $n - 2$ degrees of freedom.

6. *Decision Rule* Reject H_0 if the computed value of t is either greater than or equal to 1.2896 or less than or equal to -1.2896 (obtained by interpolation).

7. *Calculation of the Statistic* We first compute s_b^2. From Table 9.4.3 we have $s_{y|x}^2 = 1091.73589$, so that we may compute

$$s_b^2 = \frac{1091.73589}{940464 - (10017.3)^2/109} = .054983$$

We may compute our test statistic

$$t = \frac{3.46 - 0}{\sqrt{.054983}} = 14.7558$$

8. *Statistical Decision* Reject H_0 because $14.7558 > 1.2896$. The p value for this test is less than .01, since, when H_0 is true, the probability of getting a value of t as large as or larger than 2.6230 (obtained by interpolation) is .005 and the probability of getting a value of t as small as or smaller than -2.6230 is also .005. Since 14.7558 is greater than 2.6230, the probability of observing a value of t as large as or larger than 14.7558 when the null hypothesis is true, is less than .005. We double this value to obtain $2(.005) = .01$.

9. *Conclusion* We conclude that the slope of the true regression line is not zero. The practical implication is that we can expect to get better predictions and

estimates of Y if we use the sample regression equation than we would get if we ignore the relationship between X and Y. The fact that b is positive leads us to believe that β is positive and that the relationship between X and Y is a direct linear relationship.

As has already been pointed out, Equation 9.4.11 may be used to test the null hypothesis that β is equal to some value other than 0. The hypothesized value for β, β_0, is substituted into Equation 9.4.11 rather than 0. All other quantities, as well as the computations, are the same as in the illustrative example. The degrees of freedom and the method of determining significance are also the same.

A Confidence Interval for β   Once it has been determined that it is unlikely, in light of sample evidence, that β is zero, the researcher may be interested in obtaining an interval estimate of β. The general formula for a confidence interval,

$$\text{estimator} \pm (\text{reliability factor})(\text{standard error of the estimate})$$

may be used. When obtaining a confidence interval for β, the estimator is b, the reliability factor is some value of z or t (depending on whether or not $\sigma_{y|x}^2$ is known), and the standard error of the estimator is

$$\sigma_b = \sqrt{\frac{\sigma_{y|x}^2}{\sum (x_i - \bar{x})^2}}$$

When $\sigma_{y|x}^2$ is unknown, σ_b is estimated by

$$s_b = \sqrt{\frac{s_{y|x}^2}{\sum (x_i - \bar{x})^2}}$$

so that in most practical situations our $100(1 - \alpha)$ percent confidence interval for β is

$$b \pm t_{(1-\alpha/2)}\sqrt{\frac{s_{y|x}^2}{\sum (x_i - \bar{x})^2}} \qquad (9.4.16)$$

For our illustrative example we construct the following 95 percent confidence interval for β:

$$3.46 \pm 1.2896\sqrt{.054983}$$

$$3.16, 3.76$$

We interpret this interval in the usual manner. From the probabilistic point of view we say that in repeated sampling 95 percent of the intervals constructed in this way will include β. The practical interpretation is that we are 95 percent confident that the single interval constructed includes β.

Using the Confidence Interval To Test H_0: $\beta = 0$ It is instructive to note that the confidence interval we constructed does not include zero, so that zero is not a candidate for the parameter being estimated. We feel, then, that it is unlikely that $\beta = 0$. This is compatible with the results of our hypothesis test in which we rejected the null hypothesis that $\beta = 0$. Actually, we can always test H_0: $\beta = 0$ at the α significance level by constructing the $100(1 - \alpha)$ percent confidence interval for β, and we can reject or fail to reject the hypothesis on the basis of whether or not the interval includes zero. If the interval contains zero, the null hypothesis is not rejected; and if zero is not contained in the interval, we reject the null hypothesis.

Interpreting the Results It must be emphasized that failure to reject the null hypothesis that $\beta = 0$ does not mean that X and Y are not related. Not only is it possible that a type II error may have been committed but it may be true that X and Y are related in some nonlinear manner. On the other hand, when we reject the null hypothesis that $\beta = 0$, we cannot conclude that the *true* relationship between X and Y is linear. Again, it may be that although the data fit the linear regression model fairly well (as evidenced by the fact that the null hypothesis that $\beta = 0$ is rejected), some nonlinear model would provide an even better fit. Consequently, when we reject H_0 that $\beta = 0$, the best we can say is that more useful results (discussed below) may be obtained by taking into account the regression of Y on X than in ignoring it.

EXERCISES

9.4.1 to 9.4.5 Refer to Exercises 9.3.3 to 9.3.7 and for each one do the following:
  a. Compute the coefficient of determination.
  b. Prepare an ANOVA table and use the F statistic to test the null hypothesis that $\beta = 0$. Let $\alpha = .05$.
  c. Use the t statistic to test the null hypothesis that $\beta = 0$ at the .05 level of significance.
  d. Determine the p value for each hypothesis test.
  e. State your conclusions in terms of the problem.
  f. Construct the 95 percent confidence interval for β.

9.5
Using the Regression Equation

If the results of the evaluation of the sample regression equation indicate that there is a relationship between the two variables of interest, we can put the regression equation to practical use. There are two ways in which the equation can be used. It can be used to *predict* what value Y is likely to assume given a particular value of X. When the normality assumption of Section 9.2 is met, a *prediction interval* for this predicted value of Y may be constructed.

We may also use the regression equation to *estimate* the mean of the subpopulation of Y values assumed to exist at any particular value of X. Again, if the assumption of normally distributed populations holds, a confidence interval for this parameter may be constructed. The predicted value of Y and the point estimate of the mean of the subpopulation of Y will be numerically equivalent for any particular value of X but, as we will see, the prediction interval will be wider than the confidence interval.

Predicting *Y* for a Given *X*   Suppose, in our illustrative example, we have a subject whose waist measurement is 100 cm. We want to predict his deep abdominal adipose tissue. To obtain the predicted value, we substitute 100 for x in the sample regression equation to obtain

$$\hat{y} = -216.08 + 3.46(100) = 129.92$$

Since we have no confidence in this point prediction, we would prefer an interval with an associated level of confidence. If it is known, or if we are willing to assume that the assumptions of Section 9.2 are met, and when $\sigma^2_{y|x}$ is unknown, then the $100(1 - \alpha)$ percent prediction interval for Y is given by

$$\hat{y} \pm t_{(1-\alpha/2)} s_{y|x} \sqrt{1 + \frac{1}{n} + \frac{\left(x_p - \bar{x}\right)^2}{\sum \left(x_i - \bar{x}\right)^2}} \tag{9.5.1}$$

where x_p is the particular value of x at which we wish to obtain a prediction interval for Y and the degrees of freedom used in selecting t are $n - 2$. For our illustrative example we may construct the following 95 percent prediction interval:

$$129.92 \pm 1.2896\sqrt{1091.73589}\sqrt{1 + \frac{1}{109} + \frac{\left(100 - 91.9018\right)^2}{\left[940464 - \left(10017.3\right)^2/109\right]}}$$

$$87.04, \ 172.80$$

Our interpretation of a prediction interval is similar to the interpretation of a confidence interval. If we repeatedly draw samples, do a regression analysis, and construct prediction intervals for men who have a waist circumference of 100 cm, about 95 percent of them will include the man's deep abdominal AT value. This is the probabilistic interpretation. The practical interpretation is that we are 95 percent confident that a man who has a waist circumference of 100 cm will have a deep abdominal AT area of somewhere between 87.04 and 172.80 square centimeters.

Estimating the Mean of *Y* for a Given *X* If, in our illustrative example, we are interested in estimating the mean deep abdominal AT area for a subpopulation of men all of whom have a waist circumference of 100 cm, we would again calculate

$$\hat{y} = -216.08 + 3.46(100) = 129.92$$

The $100(1 - \alpha)$ percent confidence interval for $\mu_{y|x}$, when $\sigma^2_{y|x}$ is unknown, is given by

$$\hat{y} \pm t_{(1-\alpha/2)}s_{y|x}\sqrt{\frac{1}{n} + \frac{\left(x_p - \bar{x}\right)^2}{\sum\left(x_i - \bar{x}\right)^2}} \qquad (9.5.2)$$

We can obtain the following 95 percent confidence interval for $\mu_{y|x=100}$ of our present example by making proper substitutions:

$$129.92 \pm 1.2896\sqrt{1091.73589}\sqrt{\frac{1}{109} + \frac{(100 - 91.9018)^2}{\left[940464 - (10017.3)^2/109\right]}}$$

$$125.16, 134.68$$

If we repeatedly drew samples from our population of men, performed a regression analysis, and estimated $\mu_{y|x=100}$ with a similarly constructed confidence interval, about 95 percent of such intervals would include the mean amount of deep abdominal AT for the population. For this reason we are 95 percent confident that the single interval constructed contains the population mean.

Computer Analysis Now let us use MINITAB to obtain a computer analysis of the data of Example 9.3.1. We enter the *X* measurements into column 1 and the *Y* measurements into column 2. We issue the following command to label the column contents *X* and *Y*, respectively:

```
NAME C1 = 'X', C2 = 'Y'
```

The following commands produce the analysis and the accompanying printout. The command "BRIEF 3" is needed to obtain the full printout.

```
BRIEF 3
REGRESS 'Y' ON 1 PREDICTOR 'X'
```

Figure 9.5.1 shows a partial computer printout from the MINITAB simple linear regression program. We see that the printout contains information with which we are already familiar.

```
The regression equation is
Y = -216 + 3.46 X

Predictor        Coef       Stdev     t-ratio        p
Constant       -215.98      21.80      -9.91     0.0000
X               3.4569      0.2347     14.74     0.0000

s = 33.06        R-sq = 67.0%     R-sq(adj) = 66.7%

Analysis of Variance
SOURCE         DF         SS          MS         F          p
Regression      1       237549      237549     217.28     0.000
Error         107       116982       1093
Total         108       354531
```

Figure 9.5.1 Partial printout of the computer analysis of the data given in Example 9.3.1, using the MINITAB software package.

```
                     ANALYSIS OF VARIANCE
                     SUM OF            MEAN
SOURCE      DF       SQUARES          SQUARE      F VALUE      PROB > F
MODEL        1     237548.52       237548.52     217.279       0.0001
ERROR      107     116981.99      1093.28959
C TOTAL    108     354530.50
      ROOT MSE     33.06493        R-SQUARE       0.6700
      DEP MEAN       101.894       ADJ R-SQ       0.6670
      C.V.         32.45031
                     PARAMETER ESTIMATES
                  PARAMETER        STANDARD     T FOR HO:
VARIABLE    DF    ESTIMATE            ERROR   PARAMETER = 0    PROB > |T|
  INTERCEPT  1   -215.98149     21.79627076      -9.909         0.0001
  X          1    3.45885939     0.23465205      14.740         0.0001
```

Figure 9.5.2 Partial printout of the computer analysis of the data given in Example 9.3.1, using the SAS software package.

Figure 9.5.2 contains a partial printout of the SAS simple linear regression analysis of the data of Example 9.3.1. Differences occur in the numerical values of the output as a result of different rounding practices.

EXERCISES

In each exercise refer to the appropriate previous exercise and, for the value of X indicated (a) construct the 95 percent confidence interval for $\mu_{y|x}$ and (b) construct the 95 percent prediction interval for Y.

9.5.1 Refer to Exercise 9.3.3 and let $X = .75$.

9.5.2 Refer to Exercise 9.3.4 and let $X = 2.00$ (AMDN), 100 (FEV$_1$).

9.5.3 Refer to Exercise 9.3.5 and let $X = 60$.

9.5.4 Refer to Exercise 9.3.6 and let $X = 200$.

9.5.5 Refer to Exercise 9.3.7 and let $X = 100$.

9.6
The Correlation Model

In the classic regression model, which has been the underlying model in our discussion up to this point, only Y, which has been called the dependent variable, is required to be random. The variable X is defined as a fixed (nonrandom or mathematical) variable and is referred to as the independent variable. Recall, also, that under this model observations are frequently obtained by preselecting values of X and determining corresponding values of Y.

When both Y and X are random variables, we have what is called the *correlation model*. Typically, under the correlation model, sample observations are obtained by selecting a random sample of the *units of association* (which may be persons, places, animals, points in time, or any other element on which the two measurements are taken) and by taking on each a measurement of X and a measurement of Y. In this procedure, values of X are not preselected, but occur at random, depending on the unit of association selected in the sample.

Although correlation analysis cannot be carried out meaningfully under the classic regression model, regression analysis can be carried out under the correlation model. Correlation involving two variables implies a co-relationship between variables that puts them on an equal footing and does not distinguish between them by referring to one as the dependent and the other as the independent variable. In fact, in the basic computational procedures, which are the same as for the regression model, we may fit a straight line to the data either by minimizing $\Sigma(y_i - \hat{y})^2$ or by minimizing $\Sigma(x_i - \hat{x})^2$. In other words, we may do a regression of X on Y as well as a regression of Y on X. The fitted line in the two cases in general will be different, and a logical question arises as to which line to fit.

If the objective is solely to obtain a measure of the strength of the relationship between the two variables, it does not matter which line is fitted, since the measure usually computed will be the same in either case. If, however, it is desired to use the equation describing the relationship between the two variables for the purposes discussed in the preceding sections, it does matter which line is fitted. The variable for which we wish to estimate means or to make predictions should be treated as the dependent variable; that is, this variable should be regressed on the other variable.

The Bivariate Normal Distribution   Under the correlation model, X and Y are assumed to vary together in what is called a *joint distribution*. If this joint distribution is a normal distribution, it is referred to as a *bivariate normal distribution*. Inferences regarding this population may be made based on the results of samples properly drawn from it. If, on the other hand, the form of the joint distribution is known to be nonnormal, or if the form is unknown and there is no justification for assuming normality, inferential procedures are invalid, although descriptive measures may be computed.

Correlation Assumptions   The following assumptions must hold for inferences about the population to be valid when sampling is from a bivariate distribution.

1. For each value of X there is a normally distributed subpopulation of Y values.

2. For each value of Y there is a normally distributed subpopulation of X values.

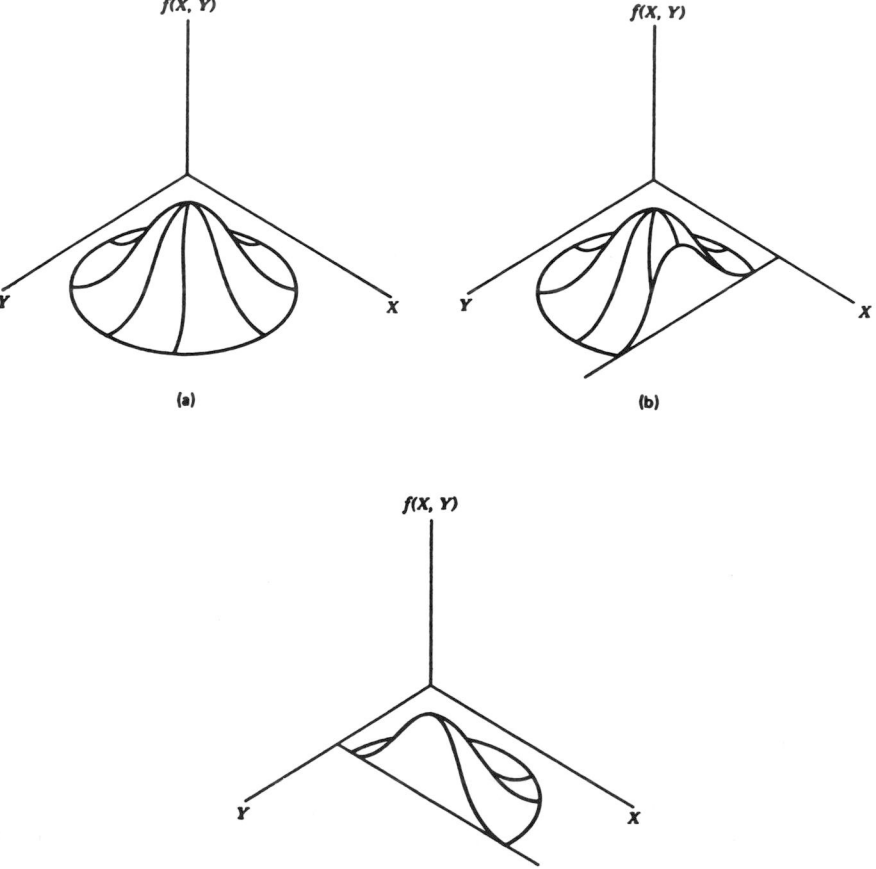

Figure 9.6.1   A bivariate normal distribution. (*a*) A bivariate normal distribution. (*b*) A cutaway showing normally distributed subpopulation of Y for given X. (*c*) A cutaway showing normally distributed subpopulation of X for given Y.

3. The joint distribution of X and Y is a normal distribution called the *bivariate normal distribution*.

4. The subpopulations of Y values all have the same variance.

5. The subpopulations of X values all have the same variance.

The bivariate distribution is represented graphically in Figure 9.6.1. In this illustration we see that if we slice the mound parallel to Y at some value of X, the cutaway reveals the corresponding normal distribution of Y. Similarly, a slice through the mound parallel to X at some value of Y reveals the corresponding normally distributed subpopulation of X.

9.7
The Correlation Coefficient

The bivariate normal distribution discussed in Section 9.6 has five parameters, σ_x, σ_y, μ_x, μ_y, and ρ. The first four are, respectively, the standard deviations and means associated with the individual distributions. The other parameter, ρ, is called the population *correlation coefficient* and measures the strength of the linear relationship between X and Y.

The population correlation coefficient is the positive or negative square root of ρ^2, the population coefficient or determination previously discussed, and since the coefficient of determination takes on values between 0 and 1 inclusive, ρ may assume any value between -1 and $+1$. If $\rho = 1$ there is a perfect direct linear correlation between the two variables, while $\rho = -1$ indicates perfect inverse linear correlation. If $\rho = 0$ the two variables are not linearly correlated. The sign of ρ will always be the same as the sign of β, the slope of the population regression line for X and Y.

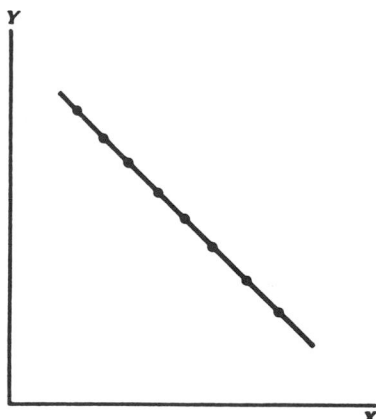

Figure 9.7.1 Scatter diagram for $r = -1$

The sample correlation coefficient, r, describes the linear relationship between the sample observations on two variables in the same way that ρ describes the relationship in a population.

Figures 9.4.5d and 9.4.5c, respectively, show typical scatter diagrams where $r \to 0$ ($r^2 \to 0$) and $r = +1$ ($r^2 = 1$). Figure 9.7.1 shows a typical scatter diagram where $r = -1$.

We are usually interested in knowing if we may conclude that $\rho \neq 0$, that is, that X and Y are linearly correlated. Since ρ is usually unknown, we draw a random sample from the population of interest, compute r, the estimate of ρ, and test H_0: $\rho = 0$ against the alternative $\rho \neq 0$. The procedure will be illustrated in the following example.

Example 9.7.1

Estellés et al. (A-7) studied the fibrinolytic parameters in normal pregnancy, in normotensive pregnancy with intrauterine fetal growth retardation (IUGR), and in patients with preeclampsia with and without IUGR. Table 9.7.1 shows the birth weights and plasminogen activator inhibitor Type 2 (PAI-2) levels in 26 cases

TABLE 9.7.1 Birth Weights (gm) and PAI-2 Levels (ng / ml) in Subjects Described in Example 9.7.1

Weight	PAI-2
2150	185
2050	200
1000	125
2300	25
900	25
2450	78
2350	290
2350	60
1900	65
2400	125
1700	122
1950	75
1250	25
1700	180
2000	170
920	12
1270	25
1550	25
1500	30
1900	24
2800	200
3600	300
3250	300
3000	200
3000	200
3050	230

Source: Justo Aznar, M.D., Ph.D. Used by permission.

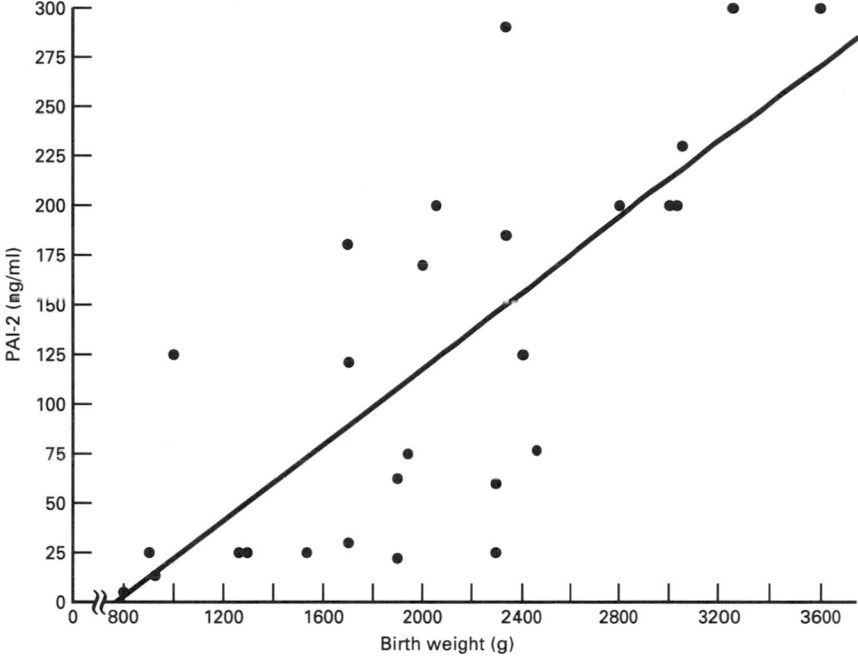

Figure 9.7.2 Birth weights and plasminogen activator inhibitor Type 2 (PAI-2) levels in subjects described in Example 9.7.1.

studied. We wish to assess the strength of the relationship between these two variables.

Solution: The scatter diagram and least-squares regression line are shown in Figure 9.7.2.

The preliminary calculations necessary for obtaining the least-squares regression line are shown in Table 9.7.2. Let us assume that the investigator wishes to obtain a regression equation to use for estimating and predicting purposes. In that case the sample correlation coefficient will be obtained by the methods discussed under the regression model.

The Regression Equation   Let us assume that we wish to be able to predict PAI-2 levels from a knowledge of birth weights. In that case we treat birth weight as the independent variable and PAI-2 level as the dependent variable and obtain the regression equation as follows.

By substituting from Table 9.7.2 into Equations 9.3.2 and 9.3.3, the following normal equations are obtained:

$$3296 = 26a + 54290b$$

$$8169390 = 54290a + 126874304b$$

TABLE 9.7.2 Preliminary Calculations for Obtaining Least-Squares Regression Line, Example 9.7.1

x Weight	y PAI-2	x^2	y^2	xy
2150	185	4622500	34225	397750
2050	200	4202500	40000	410000
1000	125	1000000	15625	125000
2300	25	5290000	625	57500
900	25	810000	625	22500
2450	78	6002500	6084	191100
2350	290	5522500	84100	681500
2350	60	5522500	3600	141000
1900	65	3610000	4225	123500
2400	125	5760000	15625	300000
1700	122	2890000	14884	207400
1950	75	3802500	5625	146250
1250	25	1562500	625	31250
1700	180	2890000	32400	306000
2000	170	4000000	28900	340000
920	12	846400	144	11040
1270	25	1612900	625	31750
1550	25	2402500	625	38750
1500	30	2250000	900	45000
1900	24	3610000	576	45600
2800	200	7840000	40000	560000
3600	300	12960000	90000	1080000
3250	300	10562500	90000	975000
3000	200	9000000	40000	600000
3000	200	9000000	40000	600000
3050	230	9302500	52900	701500
Total 54290	3296	126874304	642938	8169390

When these equations are solved we have

$$a = -72.1201$$

$$b = .09525$$

The least-squares equation is

$$\hat{y} = -72.1201 + .09525x$$

The coefficient of determination, which is equal to the explained sum of squares divided by the total sum of squares, is (using Equations 9.4.3 and 9.4.4)

$$r^2 = \frac{b^2\left[\sum x_i^2 - \left(\sum x_i\right)^2/n\right]}{\sum y_i^2 - \left(\sum y_i\right)^2/n} \tag{9.7.1}$$

Substituting values from Table 9.7.2 and the regression equation into Equation 9.7.1 gives

$$r^2 = \frac{(.09525)^2 \left[126874304 - (54290)^2/26 \right]}{642938 - (3296)^2/26}$$

$$= .5446$$

Finally, the correlation coefficient is

$$r = \sqrt{r^2} = \sqrt{.5446} = .7380$$

An alternative formula for computing r is given by

$$r = \frac{n \sum x_i y_i - \left(\sum x_i \right) \left(\sum y_i \right)}{\sqrt{n \sum x_i^2 - \left(\sum x_i \right)^2} \sqrt{n \sum y_i^2 - \left(\sum y_i \right)^2}} \tag{9.7.2}$$

An advantage of this formula is that r may be computed without first computing b. This is the desirable procedure when it is not anticipated that the regression equation will be used. Substituting from Table 9.7.2 in Equation 9.7.2 gives

$$r = \frac{26(8169390) - (54290)(3296)}{\sqrt{26(126874304) - (54290)^2} \sqrt{26(642938) - (3296)^2}}$$

$$= .7380$$

We know that r is positive because the slope of the regression line is positive.

Example 9.7.2

Refer to Example 9.7.1. We wish to see if the sample value of $r = .7380$ is of sufficient magnitude to indicate that in the population birth weight and PAI-2 levels are correlated.

Solution: We conduct a hypothesis test as follows.

1. *Data*   See the initial discussion of Example 9.7.1.
2. *Assumptions*   We presume that the assumptions given in Section 9.6 are applicable.
3. *Hypotheses*

$$H_0: \rho = 0$$

$$H_A: \rho \neq 0$$

4. *Test Statistic*   When $\rho = 0$, it can be shown that the appropriate test statistic is

$$t = r\sqrt{\frac{n-2}{1-r^2}} \tag{9.7.3}$$

5. *Distribution of Test Statistic*   When H_0 is true and the assumptions are met, the test statistic is distributed as Student's t distribution with $n - 2$ degrees of freedom.

6. *Decision Rule*   If we let $\alpha = .05$, the critical values of t in the present example are ± 2.0639. If, from our data, we compute a value of t that is either greater than or equal to $+2.0639$ or less than or equal to -2.0639, we will reject the null hypothesis.

7. *Calculation of Test Statistic*   Our calculated value of t is

$$t = .7380\sqrt{\frac{24}{1 - .5446}} = 5.3575$$

8. *Statistical Decision*   Since the computed value of the test statistic does exceed the critical value of t, we reject the null hypothesis.

9. *Conclusion*   We conclude that, in the population, birth weight and PAI-2 levels are linearly correlated. Since $5.3595 > 2.8039$, we have for this test, $p < .01$.

A Test for Use When the Hypothesized ρ is a Nonzero Value   The use of the t statistic computed in the above test is appropriate only for testing $H_0: \rho = 0$. If it is desired to test $H_0: \rho = \rho_0$, where ρ_0 is some value other than zero, we must use another approach. Fisher (5) suggests that r be transformed to z_r as follows:

$$z_r = \frac{1}{2}\ln\frac{1+r}{1-r} \tag{9.7.4}$$

where ln is a natural logarithm. It can be shown that z_r is approximately normally distributed with a mean of $z_\rho = \frac{1}{2}\ln\{(1 + \rho)/(1 - \rho)\}$ and estimated standard deviation of

$$\frac{1}{\sqrt{n-3}} \tag{9.7.5}$$

To test the null hypothesis that ρ is equal to some value other than zero the test statistic is

$$Z = \frac{z_r - z_\rho}{1/\sqrt{n-3}} \tag{9.7.6}$$

which follows approximately the standard normal distribution.

To determine z_r for an observed r and z_ρ for a hypothesized ρ, we consult Table I, thereby avoiding the direct use of natural logarithms.

Suppose in our present example we wish to test

$$H_0: \rho = .80$$

against the alternative

$$H_A: \rho \neq .80$$

at the .05 level of significance. By consulting Table I we find that for

$$r = .74 \qquad z_r = .95048$$

and for

$$\rho = .80 \qquad z_\rho = 1.09861$$

Our test statistic, then, is

$$Z = \frac{.95048 - 1.09861}{1/\sqrt{26 - 3}}$$

$$= -.71$$

Since $-.71$ is greater than the critical value of $z = -1.96$, we are unable to reject H_0 and conclude that the population correlation coefficient may be .80.

For sample sizes less than 25, Fisher's Z transformation should be used with caution, if at all. An alternative procedure from Hotelling (6) may be used for sample sizes equal to or greater than 10. In this procedure the following transformation of r is employed

$$z^* = z_r - \frac{3z_r + r}{4n} \tag{9.7.7}$$

The standard deviation of z^* is

$$\sigma_{z^*} = \frac{1}{\sqrt{n - 1}} \tag{9.7.8}$$

The test statistic is

$$Z^* = \frac{z^* - \zeta^*}{1/\sqrt{n - 1}} = (z^* - \zeta^*)\sqrt{n - 1} \tag{9.7.9}$$

where

$$\zeta^* \ (\text{pronounced zeta}) = z_p - \frac{(3z_p + \rho)}{4n}$$

Critical values for comparison purposes are obtained from the standard normal distribution.

In our present example, to test H_0: $\rho = .80$ against H_A: $\rho \neq .80$ using the Hotelling transformation and $\alpha = .05$, we have

$$z^* = .95048 - \frac{3(.95048) + .7380}{4(26)} = .915966$$

$$\zeta^* = 1.09861 - \frac{3(1.09861) + .80}{4(26)} = 1.059227$$

$$Z^* = (.915966 - 1.059227)\sqrt{26 - 1} = -.72$$

Since $-.72$ is greater than -1.96, the null hypothesis is not rejected, and the same conclusion is reached as when the Fisher transformation is used.

Alternatives   In some situations the data available for analysis do not meet the assumptions necessary for the valid use of the procedures discussed here for testing hypotheses about a population correlation coefficient. In such cases it may be more appropriate to use the Spearman rank correlation technique discussed in Chapter 13.

Confidence Interval for ρ   Fisher's transformation may be used to construct $100(1 - \alpha)$ percent confidence intervals for ρ. The general formula for a confidence interval

$$\text{estimator} \pm (\text{reliability factor})(\text{standard error})$$

is employed. We first convert our estimator, r, to z_r, construct a confidence interval about z_ρ, and then reconvert the limits to obtain a $100(1 - \alpha)$ percent confidence interval about ρ. The general formula then becomes

$$z_r \pm z\left(1/\sqrt{n - 3}\right) \tag{9.7.10}$$

For our present example the 95 percent confidence interval for z_ρ is given by

$$.95048 \pm 1.96\left(1/\sqrt{26-3}\right)$$

$$.54179, 1.35916$$

Converting these limits (by interpolation in Table I), which are values of z_r, into values of r gives

z_r	r
.54179	.494
1.35916	.876

We are 95 percent confident, then, that ρ is contained in the interval .494 to .876. Because of the limited entries in the table, these limits must be considered as only approximate.

An alternative method of constructing confidence intervals for ρ is to use the special charts prepared by David (7).

EXERCISES

In each of the following exercises:

a. Prepare a scatter diagram.
b. Compute the sample correlation coefficient.
c. Test H_0: $\rho = 0$ at the .05 level of significance and state your conclusions.
d. Determine the p value for the test.
e. Construct the 95 percent confidence interval for ρ.

9.7.1 The purpose of a study by Ruokonen et al. (A-8) was to evaluate the relationship between the mixed venous, hepatic, and femoral venous oxygen saturations before and during sympathomimetic drug infusions. The 24 subjects were all ICU patients who had had open-heart surgery (12 patients), had septic shock (8 patients), or had acute respiratory failure (4 patients). A measure of interest was the correlation between change in mixed venous (SvO_2), Y, and hepatic venous oxygen saturation (SvO_2), X, following vasoactive treatment. The following data, expressed as percents, were collected.

X	Y	X	Y
0.4	2.1	16.0	15.1
6.9	3.3	23.7	9.7
−0.1	4.4	15.1	6.8
12.4	4.9	25.1	12.2
−2.8	2.1	13.9	14.5
7.5	1.0	28.7	16.0
20.3	12.6	−8.5	2.9
2.5	0.8	11.6	8.8
12.4	9.7	32.4	9.4
10.1	9.1	18.2	11.6
−2.7	0.5	10.2	7.7
−3.8	−3.6	1.4	3.4

SOURCE: Jukka Takala, M.D. Used by permission.

9.7.2 Interest in the interactions between the brain, behavior, and immunity was the motivation for a study by Wodarz et al. (A-9). The subjects used in their study were 12 patients with severe unipolar major depressive disorder or bipolar depression (group 2) and 13 nonhospitalized healthy controls (group 1). A measure of interest was the correlation between subjects' cortisol and adrenocorticotropic hormone (ACTH) values. The following data were collected:

Group	Cortisol	ACTH
1	151.75	3.08
1	234.52	2.42
1	193.13	3.96
1	140.71	1.98
1	273.14	4.18
1	284.18	3.96
1	389.02	4.18
1	151.75	2.64
1	275.90	4.18
1	248.31	4.62
1	115.88	3.52
1	212.44	5.06
1	193.13	2.64
2	317.29	2.64
2	143.47	2.86
2	82.77	2.86
2	336.60	3.96
2	220.72	5.06
2	469.03	7.27
2	217.96	4.40
2	270.38	2.64
2	422.13	4.40
2	281.42	4.18
2	179.34	6.61
2	195.89	4.62

SOURCE: Dr. N. Wodarz. Used by permission.

9.7.3 A study by Kosten et al. (A-10) was concerned with the relationship between biological indications of addiction and the dependence syndrome. Subjects were 52 opiate addicts applying to a methadone maintenance program. Measures of concern to the investigators were the correlation between opiate withdrawal and opiate dependence and the correlation between opiate withdrawal and cocaine dependence. Opiate withdrawal was determined by the Naloxone Challenge Opiate Withdrawal

Test (NCTOT). The following data were obtained:

NCTOT	Opiate	Cocaine	NCTOT	Opiate	Cocaine
22	31	23	25	33	11
13	27	23	29	33	19
15	31	21	21	33	11
13	31	11	27	33	11
6	31	31	17	33	11
9	31	11	21	33	11
11	31	11	26	33	11
18	29	23	36	33	11
15	31	11	22	33	11
7	31	27	10	31	19
10	33	29	27	31	11
29	30	11	27	33	21
11	33	11	8	33	33
17	33	31	19	31	31
22	33	11	29	33	29
22	33	31	24	33	11
9	33	27	36	32	11
17	31	14	29	32	11
24	33	29	36	32	11
14	33	11	32	33	11
18	33	11	9	33	31
22	33	11	20	33	11
26	33	11	19	33	11
18	31	11	17	32	11
29	33	11	24	33	11
9	31	11	36	33	11

SOURCE: Therese A. Kosten, Ph.D. Used by permission.

9.7.4 The subjects in a study by Rondal et al. (A-11) were 21 children with Down's syndrome between the ages of 2 and 12 years. Among the variables on which the investigators collected data were mean length of utterance (MLU) and number of one-word utterances (OWU). MLU is computed by dividing the number of morphemes by the number of utterances in a sample of language. The number of OWU were computed on 100 utterances. The following values were collected:

MLU	OWU	MLU	OWU
.99	99	1.90	51
1.12	88	2.10	43
1.18	84	2.15	38
1.21	81	2.36	51
1.22	59	2.63	33
1.39	51	2.71	24
1.45	49	3.02	21
1.53	70	3.05	25
1.74	52	3.06	33
1.76	50	3.46	16
1.77	50		

SOURCE: J. A. Rondal, Ph.D. Used by permission.

9.7.5 Bryant and Eng⁻(A-12) conducted research to find a more precise, simpler, and less traumatic technique to study the relative maturation of the peripheral nerves in preterm and term infants. Subjects were 83 stable premature and full-term neonates from three nurseries in a metropolitan region. Among the measurements obtained were conceptional age in weeks (AGE) and soleus H-reflex latency (msec) per centimeter of infant leg length (MS/CM). The data were as follows:

Age	MS / CM	Age	MS / CM	Age	MS / CM
31.0	1.16129	38.0	.87368	32.0	1.16667
31.0	1.28750	39.0	.81000	37.0	.75897
34.0	1.18710	40.0	.78072	32.0	.97143
32.0	1.18621	41.0	.80941	42.0	.80909
35.0	1.07778	40.0	.84156	45.0	.59091
33.0	.88649	41.0	.98286	34.0	1.10000
33.0	1.01714	40.0	.73171	35.0	1.00000
32.0	1.25610	40.0	.81081	33.0	1.04242
32.0	1.04706	41.0	.76000	38.0	.87059
31.0	1.33333	42.0	.72821	38.0	.90000
34.0	.95385	42.0	.83902	34.0	.94194
33.0	1.11765	42.0	.84000	38.0	.69000
34.0	.93659	41.0	.85263	40.0	.74737
34.0	1.15000	40.0	.86667	37.0	1.01250
36.0	.85479	40.0	.90000	44.0	.69091
39.0	.83902	40.0	.81026	36.0	.85263
37.0	.87368	42.0	.83000	40.0	.72381
39.0	.86316	41.0	.81951	40.0	.75238
36.0	.94634	31.0	1.83077	32.0	1.28750
38.0	.95000	32.0	1.64615	32.0	1.22500
39.0	.83077	32.0	1.48571	34.0	1.37500
38.0	.90000	36.0	.91579	43.0	.60444
39.0	.89000	34.0	1.32000	40.0	.73043
39.0	.91282	34.0	1.05455	33.0	1.35714
39.0	.91000	40.0	.82353	33.0	1.17576
39.0	.81026	40.0	0.85263	38.5	.75122
39.0	.80000	31.0	1.76923	45.0	.56000
38.0	.77073	33.0	1.10000		

SOURCE: Gloria D. Eng, M.D. Used by permission.

9.7.6 A simple random sample of 15 apparently healthy children between the ages of 6 months and 15 years yielded the following data on age, X, and liver volume per unit of body weight (ml/kg), Y.

X	Y	X	Y
.5	41	10.0	26
.7	55	10.1	35
2.5	41	10.9	25
4.1	39	11.5	31
5.9	50	12.1	31
6.1	32	14.1	29
7.0	41	15.0	23
8.2	42		

9.8
Some Precautions

Regression and correlation analysis are powerful statistical tools when properly employed. Their inappropriate use, however, can lead only to meaningless results. To aid in the proper use of these techniques, we make the following suggestions:

1. The assumptions underlying regression and correlation analysis should be carefully reviewed before the data are collected. Although it is rare to find that assumptions are met to perfection, practitioners should have some idea about the magnitude of the gap that exists between the data to be analyzed and the assumptions of the proposed model, so that they may decide whether they should choose another model; proceed with the analysis, but use caution in the interpretation of the results; or use the chosen model with confidence.

2. In simple linear regression and correlation analysis, the two variables of interest are measured on the same entity, called the *unit of association*. If we are interested in the relationship between height and weight, for example, these two measurements are taken on the same individual. It usually does not make sense to speak of the correlation, say, between the heights of one group of individuals and the weights of another group.

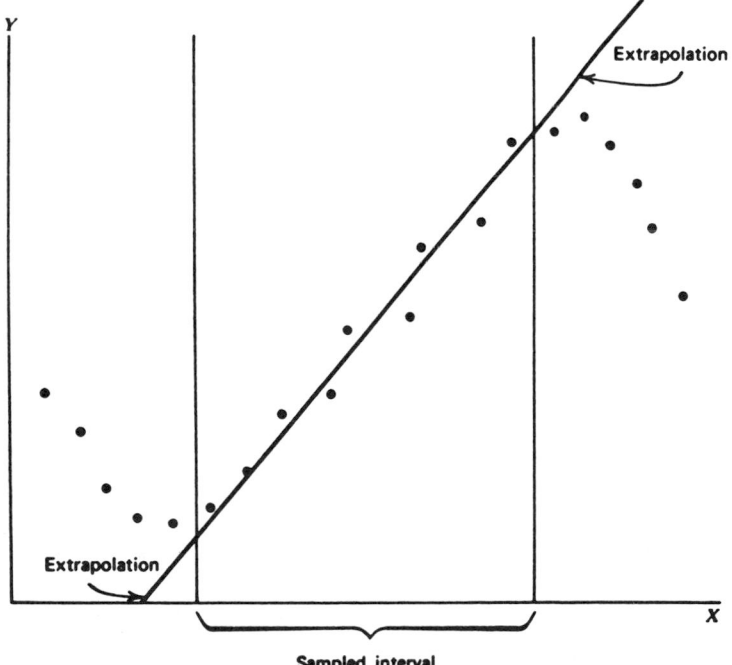

Figure 9.8.1 Example of extrapolation.

3. No matter how strong is the indication of a relationship between two variables, it should not be interpreted as one of cause and effect. If, for example, a significant sample correlation coefficient between two variables X and Y is observed, it can mean one of several things:

a. X causes Y.

b. Y causes X.

c. Some third factor, either directly or indirectly, causes both X and Y.

d. An unlikely event has occurred and a large sample correlation coefficient has been generated by chance from a population in which X and Y are, in fact, not correlated.

e. The correlation is purely nonsensical, a situation that may arise when measurement of X and Y are not taken on a common unit of association.

4. The sample regression equation should not be used to predict or estimate outside the range of values of the independent variable represented in the sample. This practice, called *extrapolation*, is risky. The true relationship between two variables, although linear over an interval of the independent variable, sometimes may be described at best as a curve outside this interval. If our sample by chance is drawn only from the interval where the relationship is linear, we have only a limited representation of the population, and to project the sample results beyond the interval represented by the sample may lead to false conclusions. Figure 9.8.1 illustrates the possible pitfalls of extrapolation.

9.9
Summary

In this chapter two important tools of statistical analysis, simple linear regression and correlation, are examined. The following outline for the application of these techniques has been suggested.

1. *Identify the Model*   Practitioners must know whether the regression model or the correlation model is the appropriate one for answering their questions.

2. *Review Assumptions*   It has been pointed out several times that the validity of the conclusions depends on how well the analyzed data fit the chosen model.

3. *Obtain the Regression Equation*   We have seen how the regression equation is obtained by the method of least squares. Although the computations, when done by hand, are rather lengthy, involved, and subject to error, this is not the problem today that it has been in the past. Computers are now in such widespread use that the researcher or statistician without access to one is the exception rather than the rule. No apology for lengthy computations is necessary to the researcher who has a computer available.

4. *Evaluate the Equation*   We have seen that the usefulness of the regression equation for estimating and predicting purposes is determined by means of the analysis of variance, which tests the significance of the regression mean square.

The strength of the relationship between two variables under the correlation model is assessed by testing the null hypothesis that there is no correlation in the population. If this hypothesis can be rejected we may conclude, at the chosen level of significance, that the two variables are correlated.

5. *Use the Equation*   Once it has been determined that it is likely that the regression equation provides a good description of the relationship between two variables, X and Y, it may be used for one of two purposes:

   a. To predict what value Y is likely to assume, given a particular value of X, or

   b. To estimate the mean of the subpopulation of Y values for a particular value of X.

This necessarily abridged treatment of simple linear regression and correlation may have raised more questions than it has answered. It may have occurred to the reader, for example, that a dependent variable can be more precisely predicted using two or more independent variables rather than one. Or, perhaps, he or she may feel that knowledge of the strength of the relationship among several variables might be of more interest than knowledge of the relationship between only two variables. The exploration of these possibilities is the subject of the next chapter, and the reader's curiosity along these lines should be at least partially relieved.

For those who would like to pursue the topic further, a number of excellent references, in addition to those already cited, follow at the end of this chapter.

REVIEW QUESTIONS AND EXERCISES

1. What are the assumptions underlying simple linear regression analysis when one of the objectives it to make inferences about the population from which the sample data were drawn?

2. Why is the regression equation called the least-squares equation?

3. Explain the meaning of a in the sample regression equation.

4. Explain the meaning of b in the sample regression equation.

5. Explain the following terms:
   a. Total sum of squares
   b. Explained sum of squares
   c. Unexplained sum of squares

6. Explain the meaning of and the method of computing the coefficient of determination.

7. What is the function of the analysis of variance in regression analysis?

8. Describe three ways in which one may test the null hypothesis that $\beta = 0$.

9. For what two purposes can a regression equation be used?

10. What are the assumptions underlying simple correlation analysis when inference is an objective?

11. What is meant by the unit of association in regression and correlation analysis?

12. What are the possible explanations for a significant sample correlation coefficient?

13. Explain why it is risky to use a sample regression equation to predict or to estimate outside the range of values of the independent variable represented in the sample.

14. Describe a situation in your particular area of interest where simple regression analysis would be useful. Use real or realistic data and do a complete regression analysis.

15. Describe a situation in your particular area of interest where simple correlation analysis would be useful. Use real or realistic data and do a complete correlation analysis.

In each of the following exercises carry out the required analysis and test hypotheses at the indicated significance levels. Compute the p value for each test.

16. A study by Scrogin et al. (A-13) was designed to assess the effects of concurrent manipulations of dietary NaCl and calcium on blood pressure as well as blood pressure and catecholamine responses to stress. Subjects were salt-sensitive male spontaneously hypertensive rats. Among the analyses performed by the investigators was a correlation between baseline blood pressure and plasma epinephrine concentration (E). The following data on these two variables were collected. Let $\alpha = .01$.

BP	PlasmaE	BP	PlasmaE
163.90	248.00	143.20	179.00
195.15	339.20	166.00	160.40
170.20	193.20	160.40	263.50
171.10	307.20	170.90	184.70
148.60	80.80	150.90	227.50
195.70	550.00	159.60	92.35
151.00	70.00	141.60	139.35
166.20	66.00	160.10	173.80
177.80	120.00	166.40	224.80
165.10	281.60	162.00	183.60
174.70	296.70	214.20	441.60
164.30	217.30	179.70	612.80
152.50	88.00	178.10	401.60
202.30	268.00	198.30	132.00
171.70	265.50		

SOURCE: Karie E. Scrogin. Used by permission.

17. Wada et al. (A-14) state that tumor necrosis factor (TNF) is an antitumoral cytokine that first attracted attention as a possible anticancer agent without side effects. TNF is also regarded as a possible mediator of disseminated intravascular coagulation (DIC) and multiple organ failure. Wada and colleagues evaluated the relationship between TNF and the pathology of DIC. Subjects were normal volunteers, DIC patients, pre-DIC patients, and non-DIC patients. The following data on plasma TNF levels (U/ml) and DIC score were collected for subjects without leukemia.

DIC	TNF	DIC	TNF
9	.48	5	.00
8	.46	7	.06
10	.00	8	.10
9	.20	7	.12
8	.10	9	.24
9	.18	9	.32
9	.14	6	.26
10	.16	10	.24
9	.20	8	.28
10	.72	7	.26
7	1.44	9	.12
7	.24	7	.14
11	.52	6	.24
6	.50	5	.14
8	.10	3	.12
5	.16	3	.00
4	.08	2	.00
3	.00	4	.00
6	.26	4	.14
5	.08	3	.00
3	.00	1	.00
6	.00	2	.00
4	.08	3	.20
4	.00		

SOURCE: Hideo Wada, M.D. Used by permission.

Perform a complete regression analysis with DIC score as the independent variable. Let $\alpha = .01$ for all tests.

18. Lipp-Ziff and Kawanishi (A-15) point out that, in certain situations, pulmonary artery diastolic pressure (PAD) is often used to estimate left ventricular end-diastolic pressure (LVEDP). These researchers used regression analysis to determine which point on the PAD waveform best estimates LVEDP. After correlating LVEDP with PAD measurements at three points on the waveform, they found the strongest relationship at .08 seconds after onset of the QRS complex (PAD .08). Their conclusion was based on an analysis of the following data:

PAD .08 (mm Hg)	LVEDP (mm Hg)	PAD .08 (mm Hg)	LVEDP (mm Hg)	PAD .08 (mm Hg)	LVEDP (mm Hg)
20	20	13	15	12	13
22	27	14	11	33	36
17	18	12	13	16	17
23	23	15	15	9	12
14	14	11	13	18	13
16	12	10	10	27	32
16	18	18	18	27	32
17	20	16	11	14	14
10	11	14	10	14	17
14	16	22	28	13	12
16	12	17	16	14	15
22	28	12	12	17	12
13	13	12	13	17	16

PAD .08 (mm Hg)	LVEDP (mm Hg)	PAD .08 (mm Hg)	LVEDP (mm Hg)	PAD .08 (mm Hg)	LVEDP (mm Hg)
23	31	13	17	14	12
26	32	16	20	16	21
18	18	18	24	14	13
17	20	11	15	13	14
18	18	13	14	12	13
26	28	11	16	18	20
11	8	16	17	22	25
22	27	11	10	19	36
30	43	16	19	27	28
18	18	23	25	17	18
22	16	10	11	17	20
30	30	23	29	17	19
42	37	11	14	25	30
26	29	31	35	10	12
11	15	14	19	16	15
10	12	13	14	24	24
12	11	22	30	9	12
20	21	11	10	11	7
15	14	13	16	10	10
21	13	24	26	11	15
13	18				

SOURCE: David T. Kawanishi, M.D., and Eileen L. Lipp-Ziff, R.N., M.S.N., C.C.R.N. Used by permission.

Perform a complete regression analysis of these data. Let $\alpha = .05$ for all tests.

19. Of concern to health scientists is mercury contamination of the terrestrial ecosystem. Crop plants provide a direct link for transportation of toxic metals such as mercury from soil to man. Panda et al. (A-16) studied the relationship between soil mercury and certain biological endpoints in barley. The source of mercury contamination was the solid waste of a chloralkali plant. Among the data analyzed were the following measures of concentration of mercury in the soil (mg/kg^{-1}) and percent of aberrant pollen mother cells (PMCs) based on meiotic analysis.

Hg	AbPMC(%)
.12	.50
21.87	.84
34.90	5.14
64.00	6.74
103.30	8.48

SOURCE: Kamal K. Panda, Ph.D. Used by permission.

Perform a complete regression analysis of these data. Let $\alpha = .05$ for all tests.

20. The following are the pulmonary blood flow (PBF) and pulmonary blood volume (PBV) values recorded for 16 infants and children with congenital heart disease.

Y PBV (ml / sqM)	X PBF (L / min / sqM)
168	4.31
280	3.40
391	6.20
420	17.30
303	12.30
429	13.99
605	8.73
522	8.90
224	5.87
291	5.00
233	3.51
370	4.24
531	19.41
516	16.61
211	7.21
439	11.60

Find the regression equation describing the linear relationship between the two variables, compute r^2, and test $H_0: \beta = 0$ by both the F test and the t test. Let $\alpha = .05$.

21. Fifteen specimens of human sera were tested comparatively for tuberculin antibody by two methods. The logarithms of the titers obtained by the two methods were as follows.

Method	
A (X)	B (Y)
3.31	4.09
2.41	3.84
2.72	3.65
2.41	3.20
2.11	2.97
2.11	3.22
3.01	3.96
2.13	2.76
2.41	3.42
2.10	3.38
2.41	3.28
2.09	2.93
3.00	3.54
2.08	3.14
2.11	2.76

Find the regression equation describing the relationship between the two variables, compute r^2, and test $H_0: \beta = 0$ by both the F test and the t test.

22. The following table shows the methyl mercury intake and whole blood mercury values in 12 subjects exposed to methyl mercury through consumption of contaminated fish.

X Methyl Mercury Intake (μg Hg / DAY)	Y Mercury in Whole Blood (ng / g)
180	90
200	120
230	125
410	290
600	310
550	290
275	170
580	375
105	70
250	105
460	205
650	480

Find the regression equation describing the linear relationship between the two variables, compute r^2, and test $H_0: \beta = 0$ by both the F and t tests.

23. The following are the weights (kg) and blood glucose levels (mg/100 ml) of 16 apparently healthy adult males.

Weight (X)	Glucose (Y)
64.0	108
75.3	109
73.0	104
82.1	102
76.2	105
95.7	121
59.4	79
93.4	107
82.1	101
78.9	85
76.7	99
82.1	100
83.9	108
73.0	104
64.4	102
77.6	87

Find the simple linear regression equation and test $H_0: \beta = 0$ using both ANOVA and the t test. Test $H_0: \rho = 0$ and construct a 95 percent confidence interval for ρ. What is the predicted glucose level for a man who weights 95 kg? Construct the 95 percent prediction interval for his weight. Let $\alpha = .05$ for all tests.

24. The following are the ages (years) and systolic blood pressures of 20 apparently healthy adults.

Age (X)	B.P. (Y)	Age (X)	B.P. (Y)
20	120	46	128
43	128	53	136
63	141	70	146
26	126	20	124
53	134	63	143
31	128	43	130
58	136	26	124
46	132	19	121
58	140	31	126
70	144	23	123

Find the simple linear regression equation and test H_0: $\beta = 0$ using both ANOVA and the t test. Test H_0: $\rho = 0$, and construct a 95 percent confidence interval for ρ. Find the 95 percent prediction interval for the systolic blood pressure of a person who is 25 years old. Let $\alpha = .05$ for all tests.

25. The following data were collected during an experiment in which laboratory animals were innoculated with a pathogen. The variables are time in hours after inoculation and temperature in degrees Celsius.

Time	Temperature	Time	Temperature
24	38.8	44	41.1
28	39.5	48	41.4
32	40.3	52	41.6
36	40.7	56	41.8
40	41.0	60	41.9

Find the simple linear regression equation and test H_0: $\beta = 0$ using both ANOVA and the t test. Test H_0: $\rho = 0$ and construct a 95 percent confidence interval for ρ. Construct the 95 percent prediction interval for the temperature at 50 hours after inoculation. Let $\alpha = .05$ for all tests.

For each of the studies described in Exercises 26 through 28, answer as many of the following questions as possible.

(a) Which is more relevant, regression analysis or correlation analysis, or are both techniques equally relevant?
(b) Which is the independent variable?
(c) Which is the dependent variable?
(d) What are the appropriate null and alternative hypotheses?
(e) Do you think the null hypothesis was rejected? Explain why or why not.
(f) Which is the more relevant objective, prediction or estimation, or are the two equally relevant?
(g) What is the sampled population?
(h) What is the target population?
(i) Are the variables directly or inversely related?

26. Tseng and Tai (A-17) report on a study to elucidate the presence of chronic hyperinsulinemia and its relation to clinical and biochemical variables. Subjects were 112 Chinese non-insulin-dependent diabetes mellitus patients under chlorpropamide therapy. Among other findings, the authors report that uric acid levels were correlated with insulin levels ($p < .05$).

27. To analyze their relative effects on premenopausal bone mass, Armamento-Villareal et al. (A-18) studied the impact of several variables on vertebral bone density (VBD).

Subjects were 63 premenopausal women between the ages of 19 and 40 years. Among the findings were a correlation between an estrogen score and VBD ($r = .44$, $p < .001$) and between age at menarche and VBD ($r = -.30$, $p = .03$).

28. Yamori et al. (A-19) investigated the epidemiological relationship of dietary factors to blood pressure (BP) and major cardiovascular diseases. Subjects were men and women aged 50 to 54 years randomly selected from 20 countries. Among the findings were relationships between body mass index and systolic blood pressure ($p < .01$) and between body mass index and diastolic blood pressure ($p < .01$) in men.

Exercises for Use With Large Data Sets Available on Computer Disk from the Publisher

1. Refer to the data for 1050 subjects with cerebral edema (CEREBRAL, Disk 2). Cerebral edema with consequent increased intracranial pressure frequently accompanies lesions resulting from head injury and other conditions that adversely affect the integrity of the brain. Available treatments for cerebral edema vary in effectiveness and undesirable side effects. One such treatment is glycerol, administered either orally or intravenously. Of interest to clinicians is the relationship between intracranial pressure and glycerol plasma concentration. Suppose you are a statistical consultant with a research team investigating the relationship between these two variables. Select a simple random sample from the population and perform the analysis that you think would be useful to the researchers. Present your findings and conclusions in narrative form and illustrate with graphs where appropriate. Compare your results with those of your classmates.

2. Refer to the data for 1050 subjects with essential hypertension (HYPERTEN, Disk 2). Suppose you are a statistical consultant to a medical research team interested in essential hypertension. Select a simple random sample from the population and perform the analyses that you think would be useful to the researchers. Present your findings and conclusions in narrative form and illustrate with graphs where appropriate. Compare your results with those of your classmates. Consult with your instructor regarding the size of sample you should select.

3. Refer to the data for 1200 patients with rheumatoid arthritis (CALCIUM, Disk 2). One hundred patients received the medicine at each dose level. Suppose you are a medical researcher wishing to gain insight into the nature of the relationship between dose level of prednisolone and total body calcium. Select a simple random sample of three patients from each dose level group and do the following.
   a. Use the total number of pairs of observations to obtain the least-squares equation describing the relationship between dose level (the independent variable) and total body calcium.
   b. Draw a scatter diagram of the data and plot the equation.
   c. Compute r and test for significance at the .05 level. Find the p value.
   d. Compare your results with those of your classmates.

REFERENCES

References Cited

1. Francis Galton, *Natural Inheritance*, Macmillan, London, 1899.
2. Francis Galton, *Memories of My Life*, Methuen, London, 1908.

3. Karl Pearson, *The Life, Letters and Labours of Francis Galton*, Volume III A, Cambridge at the University Press, 1930.

4. Francis Galton, "Co-relations and Their Measurement, Chiefly from Anthropometric Data," *Proceedings of the Royal Society*, *XLV* (1888), 135–145.

5. R. A. Fisher, "On the Probable Error of a Coefficient of Correlation Deduced from a Small Sample," *Metron*, 1 (1921), 3–21.

6. H. Hotelling, "New Light on the Correlation Coefficient and Its Transforms," *Journal of the Royal Statistical Society*, Ser B, *15* (1953), 193–232.

7. F. N. David, *Tables of the Ordinates and Probability Integral of the Distribution of the Correlation Coefficient in Small Samples*, Cambridge University Press, Cambridge, 1938.

Other References, Books

1. F. S. Acton, *Analysis of Straight Line Data*, Wiley, New York, 1959.

2. Andrew R. Baggaley, *Intermediate Correlational Methods*, Wiley, New York, 1964.

3. Cuthbert Daniel and Fred S. Wood, *Fitting Equations to Data*, Wiley-Interscience, New York, 1971.

4. N. R. Draper and H. Smith, *Applied Regression Analysis*, Second Edition, Wiley, New York, 1981.

5. Mordecai Ezekiel and Karl A. Fox, *Methods of Correlation and Regression Analysis*, Third Edition, Wiley, New York, 1959.

6. Arthur S. Goldberger, *Topics in Regression Analysis*, Macmillan, Toronto, 1968.

7. David G. Kleinbaum and Lawrence L. Kupper, *Applied Regression Analysis and Other Multivariable Methods*, Duxbury Press, North Scituate, Mass., 1978.

8. R. L. Plackett, *Principles of Regression Analysis*, Oxford University Press, London, 1960.

9. K. W. Smillie, *An Introduction to Regression and Correlation*, Academic Press, New York, 1966.

10. Peter Sprent, *Models in Regression*, Methuen, London, 1969.

11. E. J. Williams, *Regression Analysis*, Wiley, New York, 1959.

12. Stephen Wiseman, *Correlation Methods*, Manchester University Press, Manchester, 1966.

13. Dick R. Wittink, *The Application of Regression Analysis*, Allyn & Bacon, Boston, 1988.

14. Mary Sue Younger, *Handbook for Linear Regression*, Duxbury Press, North Scituate, Mass., 1979.

Other References, Journal Articles

1. R. G. D. Allen, "The Assumptions of Linear Regression," *Economica*, *6 N. S.* (1939), 191–204.

2. M. S. Bartlett, "The Fitting of Straight Lines If Both Variables Are Subject to Error," *Biometrics*, *5* (1949), 207–212.

3. J. Berkson, "Are There Two Regressions?" *Journal of the American Statistical Association*, *45* (1950), 164–180.

4. Dudley J. Cowden, "A Procedure for Computing Regression Coefficients," *Journal of the American Statistical Association*, *53* (1958), 144–150.

5. Lorraine Denby and Daryl Pregibon, "An Example of the Use of Graphics in Regression," *The American Statistician*, *41* (1987), 33–38.

6. A. S. C. Ehrenberg, "Bivariate Regression Is Useless," *Applied Statistics*, *12* (1963), 161–179.

7. M. G. Kendall, "Regression, Structure, and Functional Relationship, Part I," *Biometrika*, *28* (1951), 11–25.

8. M. G. Kendall, "Regression, Structure, and Functional Relationship II," *Biometrika*, *39* (1952), 96–108.

9 D. V. Lindley, "Regression Lines and the Linear Functional Relationship," *Journal of the Royal Statistical Society* (Supplement), *9* (1947), 218–244.

10. A. Madansky, "The Fitting of Straight Lines When Both Variables Are Subject to Error," *Journal of the American Statistical Association*, *54* (1959), 173–205.

11. A. Wald, "The Fitting of Straight Lines if Both Variables Are Subject to Error," *Annals of Mathematical Statistics*, *11* (1940), 284–300.

12. W. G. Warrn, "Correlation or Regression: Bias or Precision," *Applied Statistics*, *20* (1971), 148–164.

13. Charles P. Winsor, "Which Regression?" *Biometrics*, *2* (1946), 101–109.

Applications References

A-1. Jean-Pierre Després, Denis Prud'homme, Marie-Christine Pouliot, Angelo Tremblay, and Claude Bouchard, "Estimation of Deep Abdominal Adipose-Tissue Accumulation from Simple Anthropometric Measurements in Men," *American Journal of Clinical Nutrition*, *54* (1991), 471–477.

A-2. George Phillips, Jr., Bruce Coffey, Roger Tran-Son-Tay, T. R. Kinney, Eugene P. Orringer, and R. M. Hochmuth, "Relationship of Clinical Severity to Packed Cell Rheology in Sickle Cell Anemia," *Blood*, *78* (1991), 2735–2739.

A-3. Robert H. Habib and Kenneth R. Lutchen, "Moment Analysis of a Multibreath Nitrogen Washout Based on an Alveolar Gas Dilution Number," *American Review of Respiratory Disease*, *144* (1991), 513–519.

A-4. Menno de Metz, Pieter Paul Schiphorst, and Roy I. H. Go, "The Analysis of Erythrocyte Morphologic Characteristics in Urine Using a Hematologic Flow Cytometer and Microscopic Methods," *American Journal of Clinical Pathology*, *95* (1991), 257–261.

A-5. Susan B. Roberts, Melvin B. Heyman, William J. Evans, Paul Fuss, Rita Tsay, and Vernon R. Young, "Dietary Energy Requirements of Young Adult Men, Determined by Using the Doubly Labeled Water Method," *American Journal of Clinical Nutrition*, *54* (1991), 499–505.

A-6. Akihiko Ogasawara, "Similarity of IQs of Siblings with Duchenne Progressive Muscular Dystrophy," *American Journal on Mental Retardation*, *93* (1989), 548–550.

A-7. Amparo Estellés, Juan Gilabert, Francisco España, Justo Aznar, and Manuel Galbis, "Fibrinolytic Parameters in Normotensive Pregnancy with Intrauterine Fetal Growth Retardation and in Severe Preeclampsia," *American Journal of Obstetrics and Gynecology*, *165* (1991), 138–142.

A-8. Esko Ruokonen, Jukka Takala, and Ari Uusaro, "Effect of Vasoactive Treatment on the Relationship Between Mixed Venous and Regional Oxygen Saturation," *Critical Care Medicine*, *19* (1991), 1365–1369.

A-9. N. Wodarz, R. Rupprecht, J. Kornhuber, B. Schmitz, K. Wild, H. U. Braner, and P. Riederer, "Normal Lymphocyte Responsiveness to Lectins but Impaired Sensitivity to in Vitro Glucocorticoids in Major Depression," *Journal of Affective Disorders*, *22* (1991), 241–248.

A-10. Therese A. Kosten, Leslie K. Jacobsen, and Thomas R. Kosten, "Severity of Precipitated Opiate Withdrawal Predicts Drug Dependence by DSM-III-R Criteria," *American Journal of Drug and Alcohol Abuse*, *15* (1989), 237–250.

A-11. Jean A. Rondal, Martine Ghiotto, Serge Brédart, and Jean-François Bachelet, "Mean Length of Utterance of Children with Down Syndrome," *American Journal on Mental Retardation*, *93* (1988), 64–66.

A-12. Phillip R. Bryant and Gloria D. Eng, "Normal Values for the Soleus H-Reflex in Newborn Infants 31–45 Weeks Post Conceptional Age," *Archives of Physical Medicine and Rehabilitation*, *72* (1991), 28–30.

A-13. Karie E. Scrogin, Daniel C. Hatton, and David A. McCarron, "The Interactive Effects of Dietary Sodium Chloride and Calcium on Cardiovascular Stress Responses," *American Journal of Physiology* (*Regulatory Integrative Comp. Physiol. 30*), *261* (1991), R945–R949.

A-14. Hideo Wada, Michiaki Ohiwa, Toshihiro Kaneko, Shigehisa Tramaki, Motoaki Tanigawa, Mikio Takagi, Yoshitaka Mori, and Shigeru Shirakawa, "Plasma Level of Tumor Necrosis Factor in Disseminated Intravascular Coagulation," *American Journal of Hematology*, *37* (1991), 147–151.

A-15. Eileen L. Lipp-Ziff and David T. Kawanishi, "A Technique for Improving Accuracy of the Pulmonary Artery Diastolic Pressure as an Estimate of Left Ventricular End-diastolic Pressure," *Heart & Lung*, *20* (1991), 107–115.

A-16. Kamal K. Panda, Maheswar Lenka, and Brahma B. Panda, "Monitoring and Assessment of Mercury Pollution in the Vicinity of a Chloralkali Plant. II. Plant-Availability, Tissue-concentration and Genotoxicity of Mercury from Agricultural Soil Contaminated with Solid Waste Assessed in Barley (*Hordeum vulgare L.*)," *Environmental Pollution, 76* (1992), 33–42.

A-17. C. H. Tseng and T. Y. Tai, "Risk Factors for Hyperinsulinemia in Chlorpropamide-treated Diabetic Patients: A Three-year Follow-up," *Journal of the Formosan Medical Association, 91* (August 1992), 770–774.

A-18. R. Armamento-Villareal, D. T. Villareal, L. V. Avioli, and R. Civitelli, "Estrogen Status and Heredity Are Major Determinants of Premenopausal Bone Mass," *Journal of Clinical Investigation, 90* (December 1992), 2464–2471.

A-19. Y. Yamori, Y. Nara, S. Mizushima, M. Mano, M. Sawamura, M. Kihara, and R. Horie, "International Cooperative Study on the Relationship Between Dietary Factors and Blood Pressure: A Preliminary Report from the Cardiovascular Diseases and Alimentary Comparison (CARDIAC) Study. The CARDIAC Cooperative Study Research Group," *Nutrition and Health, 8* (2–3, 1992), 77–90.

CHAPTER **10**

Multiple Regression and Correlation

· ·

CONTENTS

10.1
Introduction

In Chapter 9 we explored the concepts and techniques for analyzing and making use of the linear relationship between two variables. We saw that this analysis may lead to an equation that can be used to predict the value of some dependent variable given the value of an associated independent variable.

Intuition tells us that, in general, we ought to be able to improve our predicting ability by including more independent variables in such an equation. For example, a researcher may find that intelligence scores of individuals may be predicted from physical factors such as birth order, birth weight, and length of gestation along with certain hereditary and external environmental factors. Length of stay in a chronic disease hospital may be related to the patient's age, marital status, sex, and income, not to mention the obvious factor of diagnosis. The response of an experimental animal to some drug may depend on the size of the dose and the age and weight of the animal. A nursing supervisor may be interested in the strength of the relationship between a nurse's performance on the job, score on the state board examination, scholastic record, and score on some achievement or aptitude test. Or a hospital administrator studying admissions from various communities served by the hospital may be interested in determining what factors seem to be responsible for differences in admission rates.

The concepts and techniques for analyzing the associations among several variables are natural extensions of those explored in the previous chapters. The computations, as one would expect, are more complex and tedious. However, as is pointed out in Chapter 9, this presents no real problem when a computer is available. It is not unusual to find researchers investigating the relationships among a dozen or more variables. For those who have access to a computer, the decision as to how many variables to include in an analysis is based not on the complexity and length of the computations but on such considerations as their meaningfulness, the cost of their inclusion, and the importance of their contribution.

In this chapter we follow closely the sequence of the previous chapter. The regression model is considered first, followed by a discussion of the correlation model. In considering the regression model, the following points are covered: a description of the model, methods for obtaining the regression equation, evaluation of the equation, and the uses that may be made of the equation. In both models the possible inferential procedures and their underlying assumptions are discussed.

10.2
The Multiple Linear Regression Model

In the multiple regression model we assume that a linear relationship exists between some variable Y, which we call the dependent variable, and k independent variables, $X_1, X_2, \ldots, X_k$. The independent variables are sometimes referred to as *explanatory variables*, because of their use in explaining the variation in Y. They are also called *predictor variables*, because of their use in predicting Y.

Assumptions   The assumptions underlying multiple regression analysis are as follows.

1. The X_i are nonrandom (fixed) variables. This assumption distinguishes the multiple regression model from the multiple correlation model, which will be presented in Section 10.6. This condition indicates that any inferences that are drawn from sample data apply only to the set of X values observed and not to some larger collection of X's. Under the regression model, correlation analysis is not meaningful. Under the correlation model to be presented later, the regression techniques that follow may be applied.

2. For each set of X_i values there is a subpopulation of Y values. To construct certain confidence intervals and test hypotheses it must be known, or the researcher must be willing to assume, that these subpopulations of Y values are normally distributed. Since we will want to demonstrate these inferential procedures, the assumption of normality will be made in the examples and exercises in this chapter.

3. The variances of the subpopulations of Y are all equal.

4. The Y values are independent. That is, the values of Y selected for one set of X values do not depend on the values of Y selected at another set of X values.

The Model Equation   The assumptions for multiple regression analysis may be stated in more compact fashion as

$$y_j = \beta_0 + \beta_1 x_{1j} + \beta_2 x_{2j} + \cdots + \beta_k x_{kj} + e_j \qquad (10.2.1)$$

where y_j is a typical value from one of the subpopulations of Y values, the β_i are called the regression coefficients, $x_{1j}, x_{2j}, \ldots, x_{kj}$ are, respectively, particular values of the independent variables $X_1, X_2, \ldots, X_k$, and e_j is a random variable with mean 0 and variance σ^2, the common variance of the subpopulations of Y values. To construct confidence interavls for and test hypotheses about the regression coefficients, we assume that the e_j are normally and independently distributed. The statements regarding e_j are a consequence of the assumptions regarding the distributions of Y values. We will refer to Equation 10.2.1 as the *multiple linear regression model*.

When Equation 10.2.1 consists of one dependent variable and two independent variables, that is, when the model is written

$$y_j = \beta_0 + \beta_1 x_{1j} + \beta_2 x_{2j} + e_j \qquad (10.2.2)$$

a *plane* in three-dimensional space may be fitted to the data points as illustrated in Figure 10.2.1. When the model contains more than two independent variables, it is described geometrically as a *hyperplane*.

In Figure 10.2.1 the observer should visualize some of the points as being located above the plane and some as being located below the plane. The deviation of a point from the plane is represented by

$$e_j = y_j - \beta_0 - \beta_1 x_{1j} - \beta_2 x_{2j} \qquad (10.2.3)$$

In Equation 10.2.2, β_0 represents the point where the plane cuts the Y-axis, that is, it represents the Y-intercept of the plane. β_1 measures the average change in Y for a unit change in X_1 when X_2 remains unchanged, and β_2 measures the average change in Y for a unit change in X_2 when X_1 remains unchanged. For this reason β_1 and β_2 are referred to as *partial regression coefficients*.

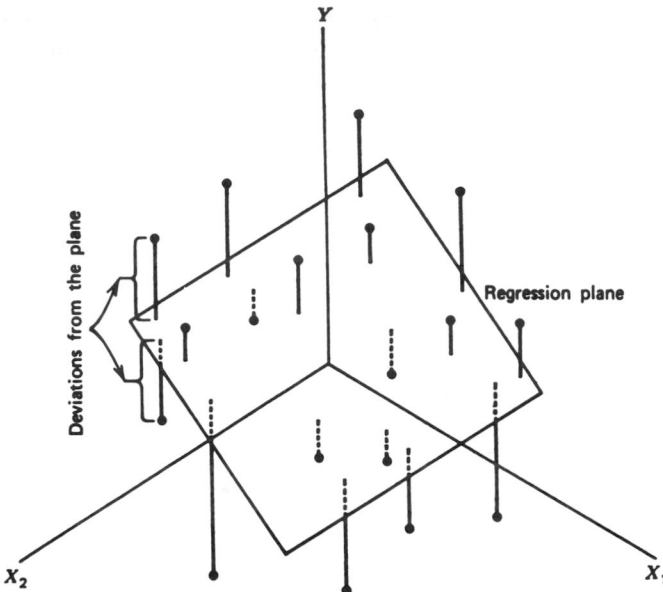

Figure 10.2.1 Multiple regression plane and scatter of points.

10.3
Obtaining the Multiple
Regression Equation

Unbiased estimates of the parameters $\beta_0, \beta_1, \ldots, \beta_k$ of the model specified in Equation 10.2.1 are obtained by the method of least squares. This means that the sum of the squared deviations of the observed values of Y from the resulting regression surface is minimized. In the three-variable case, as illustrated in Figure 10.2.1, the sum of the squared deviations of the observations from the plane are a minimum when β_0, β_1, and β_2 are estimated by the method of least squares. In other words, by the method of least squares, sample estimates of $\beta_0, \beta_1, \ldots, \beta_k$ are selected in such a way that the quantity

$$\sum e_j^2 = \sum \left(y_j - \beta_0 x_{1j} - \beta_1 x_{2j} - \cdots - \beta x_{kj} \right)^2$$

is minimized. This quantity, referred to as the sum of squares of the residuals, may also be written as

$$\sum \left(y_j - \hat{y} \right)^2 \tag{10.3.1}$$

indicating the fact that the sum of squares of deviations of the observed values of Y from the values of Y calculated from the estimated equation is minimized.

The Normal Equations Estimates, $b_0, b_1, b_2, \ldots, b_k$, of the regression coefficients are obtained by solving the following set of normal equations:

$$
\left.
\begin{aligned}
nb_0 + b_1 \sum x_{1j} + b_2 \sum x_{2j} + \cdots + b_k \sum x_{kj} &= \sum y_j \\
b_0 \sum x_{1j} + b_1 \sum x_{1j}^2 + b_2 \sum x_{1j}x_{2j} + \cdots + b_k \sum x_{1j}x_{kj} &= \sum x_{1j}y_j \\
b_0 \sum x_{2j} + b_1 \sum x_{2j}x_{1j} + b_2 \sum x_{2j}^2 + \cdots + b_k \sum x_{2j}x_{kj} &= \sum x_{2j}y_j \\
\cdots \quad \cdots \quad \cdots \quad \cdots \quad \cdots \quad \cdots \quad \cdots \quad \cdots \\
b_0 \sum x_{kj} + b_1 \sum x_{kj}x_{1j} + b_2 \sum x_{kj}x_{2j} + \cdots + b_k \sum x_{kj}^2 - \sum x_{kj}y_j
\end{aligned}
\right\} \quad (10.3.2)
$$

When the model contains only two independent variables, the sample regression equation is

$$
\hat{y}_j = b_0 + b_1 x_{1j} + b_2 x_{2j} \tag{10.3.3}
$$

The number of equations required to obtain estimates of the regression coefficients is equal to the number of parameters to be estimated. We may solve the equations as they stand or we may reduce them to a set of k equations by transforming each value into a deviation from its mean. For simplicity consider the case in which we have two independent variables.

To obtain the least-squares equation, the following normal equations must be solved for the sample regression coefficients:

$$
\left.
\begin{aligned}
nb_0 + b_1 \sum x_{1j} + b_2 \sum x_{2j} &= \sum y_j \\
b_0 \sum x_{1j} + b_1 \sum x_{1j}^2 + b_2 \sum x_{1j}x_{2j} &= \sum x_{1j}y_j \\
b_0 \sum x_{2j} + b_1 \sum x_{1j}x_{2j} + b_2 \sum x_{2j}^2 &= \sum x_{2j}y_j
\end{aligned}
\right\} \quad (10.3.4)
$$

If the calculations must be done with the aid of a desk calculator or a hand-held calculator the arithmetic can be formidable, as the discussion that follows well demonstrates. Those who have access to a computer, however, may, if they wish, skip most of the following explanation of computations.

If we designate these deviations of the measurements from their mean by y_j', x_{1j}', and x_{2j}', respectively, we have

$$
\left.
\begin{aligned}
y_j' &= y_j - \bar{y} \\
x_{1j}' &= x_{1j} - \bar{x}_1 \\
x_{2j}' &= x_{2j} - \bar{x}_2
\end{aligned}
\right\} \quad (10.3.5)
$$

If we restate the original sample regression equation (Equation 10.3.3) in terms of these transformations, we have

$$
\hat{y}_j' = b_0' + b_1' x_{1j}' + b_2' x_{2j}' \tag{10.3.6}
$$

where b_0', b_1', and b_2' are appropriate coefficients for the transformed variables. The relationship between the two sets of coefficients can be determined by substituting the deviations from the means of the original variables into Equation 10.3.6 and then simplifying. Thus,

$$\hat{y}_j - \bar{y} = b_0' + b_1'\left(x_{1j} - \bar{x}_1\right) + b_2'\left(x_{2j} - \bar{x}_2\right)$$

$$\hat{y}_j = \bar{y} + b_0' + b_1'x_{1j} - b_1'\bar{x}_1 + b_2'x_{2j} - b_2'\bar{x}_2 \qquad (10.3.7)$$

$$\hat{y}_j = b_0' + \bar{y} - b_1'\bar{x}_1 - b_2'\bar{x}_2 + b_1'x_{1j} + b_2'x_{2j}$$

When we set the coefficients of like terms in Equations 10.3.3 and 10.3.7 equal to each other, we obtain

$$b_1 = b_1'$$

$$b_2 = b_2'$$

and, therefore,

$$b_0 = b_0' + \bar{y} - b_1'\bar{x}_1 - b_2'\bar{x}_2 = b_0' + \bar{y} - b_1\bar{x}_1 - b_2\bar{x}_2 \qquad (10.3.8)$$

A new net of normal equations based on Equation 10.3.6 is

$$nb_0' + b_1'\sum x_{1j}' + b_2'\sum x_{2j}' = \sum y_j'$$

$$b_0'\sum x_{1j}' + b_1'\sum x_{1j}'^2 + b_2'\sum x_{1j}'x_{2j}' = \sum x_{1j}'y_j$$

$$b_0'\sum x_{2j}' + b_1'\sum x_{1j}'x_{2j}' + b_2'\sum x_{2j}'^2 = \sum x_{2j}'y_j$$

Using the transformations from Equation 10.3.5 and the property that $\sum(x_i - \bar{x}) = 0$, we obtain

$$nb_0' + b_1'(0) + b_2'(0) = 0$$

$$b_0'(0) + b_1'\sum\left(x_{1j} - \bar{x}_1\right)^2 + b_2'\sum\left(x_{1j} - \bar{x}_1\right)\left(x_{2j} - \bar{x}_2\right) = \sum\left(x_{1j} - \bar{x}_1\right)\left(y_j - \bar{y}\right)$$

$$b_0'(0) + b_1'\sum\left(x_{1j} - \bar{x}_1\right)\left(x_{2j} - \bar{x}_2\right) + b_2'\sum\left(x_{2j} - \bar{x}_2\right)^2 = \sum\left(x_{2j} - \bar{x}_2\right)\left(y_j - \bar{y}\right)$$

Note that $b_0' = 0$. Thus by Equation 10.3.8

$$b_0 = \bar{y} - b_1\bar{x}_1 - b_2\bar{x}_2$$

and when we substitute b_1 and b_2 for b'_1 and b'_2, respectively, our normal equations collapse to the following.

$$
\left.
\begin{aligned}
b_1 \sum x'^2_{1j} + b_2 \sum x'_{1j} x'_{2j} &= \sum x'_{1j} y'_j \\
b_1 \sum x'_{1j} x'_{2j} + b_2 \sum x'^2_{2j} &= \sum x'_{2j} y'_j
\end{aligned}
\right\}
\qquad (10.3.9)
$$

Example 10.3.1

Kalow and Tang (A-1) conducted a study to establish the variation of cytochrome P-450IA2 activities as determined by means of caffeine in a population of healthy volunteers. A second purpose of the study was to see how the variation in smokers compared with that of the nonsmoking majority of the population. Subjects responded to advertising posters displayed in a university medical sciences building. The variables on which the investigators collected data were (1) P-450IA2 index (IA2Index), (2) number of cigarettes smoked per day (Cig/Day), and (3) urinary cotinine level (Cot). The measurements on these three variables for 19 subjects are shown in Table 10.3.1. We wish to obtain the sample multiple regression equation.

Solution: Table 10.3.2 contains the sums of squares and cross products of the original values necessary for computing the sums of squares and cross products of y'_j, x'_{1j}, and x'_{2j}.

TABLE 10.3.1 Number of Cigarettes Smoked per Day, Urine Cotinine Level, and P-450IA2 Index for 19 Subjects Described in Example 10.3.1

Cig / Day	Cot	IA2Index
1	.0000	4.1648
1	.0000	3.7314
1	.0000	5.7481
1	.0000	4.4370
1	.0000	6.4687
3	.0000	3.8923
8	10.5950	5.2952
8	4.6154	4.6031
8	27.1902	5.8112
8	5.5319	3.6890
8	2.7778	3.3722
10	19.7856	8.0213
10	22.8045	10.8367
15	.0000	4.1148
15	14.5193	5.5429
15	36.7113	11.3531
20	21.2267	7.5637
20	21.1273	7.2158
24	63.2125	13.5000

SOURCE: Werner Kalow. Used by permission.

TABLE 10.3.2 Sums of Squares and Sums of Cross Products for Example 10.3.1

x_{1j} Cig / Day	x_{2j} Cot	y_j IA2Index	x_{1j}^2	x_{2j}^2	y_j^2	$x_{1j}x_{2j}$	$x_{1j}y_j$	$x_{2j}y_j$
1	.0000	4.1648	1	.00	17.346	.00	4.165	.000
1	.0000	3.7314	1	.00	13.923	.00	3.731	.000
1	.0000	5.7484	1	.00	33.044	.00	5.748	.000
1	.0000	4.4370	1	.00	19.687	.00	4.437	.000
1	.0000	6.4687	1	.00	41.844	.00	6.469	.000
3	.0000	3.8923	9	.00	15.150	.00	11.677	.000
8	10.5950	5.2952	64	112.26	28.039	84.76	42.361	56.103
8	4.6154	4.6031	64	21.30	21.189	36.92	36.825	21.245
8	27.1902	5.8112	64	739.31	33.770	217.52	46.489	158.007
8	5.5319	3.6890	64	30.60	13.609	44.26	29.512	20.408
8	2.7778	3.3722	64	7.72	11.372	22.22	26.978	9.367
10	19.7856	8.0213	100	391.47	64.341	197.86	80.213	158.705
10	22.8045	10.8367	100	520.05	117.435	228.05	108.367	247.126
15	.0000	4.1148	225	.00	16.931	.00	61.721	.000
15	14.5193	5.5429	225	210.81	30.724	217.79	83.144	80.479
15	36.7113	11.3531	225	1347.72	128.892	550.67	170.296	416.785
20	21.2267	7.5637	400	450.57	57.210	424.53	151.275	160.554
20	21.1273	7.2157	400	446.36	52.067	422.55	144.315	152.449
24	63.2125	13.5000	576	3995.82	182.250	1517.10	324.000	853.369
Totals 177	250.098	119.362	2585	8273.98	898.822	3964.22	1341.72	2334.60
Means 9.3158	13.1630	6.2822						

Using the data in Table 10.3.2, we compute

$$\sum x_{1j}'^2 = \sum (x_{1j} - \bar{x}_1)^2 = \sum x_{1j}^2 - \left(\sum x_{1j}\right)^2 \big/ n$$

$$= 2585 - (177)^2 / 19 = 936.105263$$

$$\sum x_{2j}'^2 = \sum (x_{2j} - \bar{x}_2)^2 = \sum x_{2j}^2 - \left(\sum x_{2j}\right)^2 \big/ n$$

$$= 8273.98 - (250.098)^2 / 19 = 4981.92686$$

$$\sum x_{1j}' x_{2j}' = \sum (x_{1j} - \bar{x}_1)(x_{2j} - \bar{x}_2) = \sum x_{1j}x_{2j} - \sum x_{1j} \sum x_{2j} \big/ n$$

$$= 3964.22 - (177.000)(250.098)/19 = 1634.35968$$

$$\sum x_{1j}' y_j' = \sum (x_{1j} - \bar{x}_1)(y_j - \bar{y}) = \sum x_{1j}y_j - \sum x_{1j} \sum y_j \big/ n$$

$$= 1341.72 - (177.000)(119.362)/19 = 229.76874$$

$$\sum x_{2j}' y_j' = \sum (x_{2j} - \bar{x}_2)(y_j - \bar{y}) = \sum x_{2j}y_j - \sum x_{2j} \sum y_j \big/ n$$

$$= 2334.60 - (250.098)(119.362)/19 = 763.43171$$

When we substitute these values into Equations 10.3.9, we have

$$\left.\begin{array}{l}936.105263b_1 + 1634.35968b_2 = 229.76874 \\ 1634.35968b_1 + 4981.92686b_2 = 763.43171\end{array}\right\} \quad (10.3.10)$$

These equations may be solved by any standard method to obtain

$$b_1 = -.05171$$

$$b_2 = .170204$$

We obtain b_0 from the relationship

$$b_0 = \bar{y} - b_1\bar{x}_1 - b_2\bar{x}_2 \quad (10.3.11)$$

For our example, we have

$$b_0 = 6.2822 - (-.05171)(9.3158) - (.170204)(13.1630) = 4.5235$$

Our sample multiple regression equation, then, is

$$\hat{y} = 4.5235 - .05171x_{1j} + .170204x_{2j} \quad (10.3.12)$$

Extension for Four or More Variables We have used an example containing only three variables for simplicity. As the number of variables increases, the algebraic manipulations and arithmetic calculations become more tedious and subject to error, although they are natural extensions of the procedures given in the present example.

Snedecor and Cochran (1) and Steel and Torrie (2) give numerical examples for four variables, and Anderson and Bancroft (3) illustrate the calculations involved when there are five variables. The techniques used by these authors are applicable for any number of variables.

After the multiple regression equation has been obtained, the next step involves its evaluation and interpretation. We cover this facet of the analysis in the next section.

EXERCISES

Obtain the regression equation for each of the following sets of data.

10.3.1 The subjects of a study by Malec et al. (A-2) were 16 graduates of a comprehensive, postacute brain injury rehabilitation program. The researchers examined the relationship among a number of variables, including work outcome (scaled from 1 for unemployed to 5, which represents competitive nonsheltered employment), score at time of initial evaluation on the Portland Adaptability Inventory (PAI), and length of stay (LOS) in days. The following measurements on these three variables were collected.

y Work Outcome	x_2 PAI PRE	x_1 Length of Stay (days)
5	19	67
4	17	157
2	23	242
4	14	255
1	27	227
4	22	140
1	23	179
4	18	258
4	16	85
5	22	52
3	15	296
1	30	256
4	21	198
1	22	224
4	19	126
4	8	156

SOURCE: James Malec, Ph.D. Used by permission.

10.3.2   David and Riley (A-3) examined the cognitive factors measured by the Allen Cognitive Level Test (ACL) as well as the test's relationship to level of psychopathology. Subjects were patients from a general hospital psychiatry unit. Among the variables on which the investigators collected data, in addition to ACL, were scores on the vocabulary (V) and abstraction (A) components of the Shipley Institute of Living Scale, and scores on the Symbol-Digit Modalities Test (SDMT). The following measures on 69 patients were recorded. The dependent variable is ACL.

Subject	ACL	SDMT	V	A	Subject	ACL	SDMT	V	A
1	6.0	70	28	36	17	5.9	42	30	32
2	5.4	49	34	32	18	4.7	52	17	26
3	4.7	28	19	8	19	4.7	35	26	26
4	4.8	47	32	28	20	3.8	41	18	28
5	4.9	29	22	4	21	6.0	58	32	26
6	4.5	23	24	24	22	5.6	41	19	16
7	6.3	40	24	12	23	4.8	13	14	10
8	5.9	50	18	14	24	5.8	62	27	36
9	4.1	32	31	20	25	4.5	46	21	20
10	4.8	27	14	8	26	4.8	52	26	28
11	4.0	33	24	8	27	4.7	63	22	14
12	4.5	40	34	36	28	4.5	42	22	26
13	5.8	66	29	20	29	6.0	66	30	26
14	6.0	46	27	34	30	5.6	55	26	26
15	4.5	26	15	10	31	6.3	55	22	28
16	4.7	42	31	24	32	5.2	43	22	28

Subject	ACL	SDMT	V	A	Subject	ACL	SDMT	V	A
33	4.8	48	16	10	52	4.5	44	29	24
34	5.8	47	32	36	53	4.9	51	28	36
35	4.8	50	26	30	54	4.2	37	20	8
36	3.7	29	11	16	55	4.5	56	32	36
37	4.5	17	18	8	56	4.8	37	33	36
38	4.9	39	14	2	57	6.0	76	26	20
39	5.0	31	30	32	58	4.0	42	26	8
40	3.9	61	30	36	59	4.5	20	13	10
41	3.7	45	31	18	60	4.0	48	27	16
42	5.6	56	23	18	61	4.7	54	40	40
43	4.8	53	28	20	62	6.0	53	25	32
44	5.6	29	17	8	63	4.5	39	20	8
45	6.6	63	31	30	64	4.8	35	26	10
46	4.3	19	12	6	65	6.6	63	26	30
47	4.0	23	18	6	66	4.1	17	16	16
48	4.2	40	23	8	67	4.5	44	31	24
49	5.6	20	22	6	68	6.6	47	30	36
50	3.4	2	13	8	69	4.9	35	10	19
51	4.0	41	30	22					

SOURCE: Sandra K. David, OTR/L. Used by permission.

10.3.3 In a study of factors thought to be related to admission patterns to a large general hospital, a hospital administrator obtained these data on 10 communities in the hospital's catchment area.

Community	Persons per 1000 Population Admitted During Study Period (Y)	Index of Availability of Other Health Services (X_1)	Index of Indigency (X_2)
1	61.6	6.0	6.3
2	53.2	4.4	5.5
3	65.5	9.1	3.6
4	64.9	8.1	5.8
5	72.7	9.7	6.8
6	52.2	4.8	7.9
7	50.2	7.6	4.2
8	44.0	4.4	6.0
9	53.8	9.1	2.8
10	53.5	6.7	6.7
Total	571.6	69.9	55.6

$$\sum x_{1j}^2 = 525.73 \qquad \sum x_{2j}^2 = 331.56 \qquad \sum y_j^2 = 33{,}349.92$$

$$\sum x_{1j}x_{2j} = 374.31 \qquad \sum x_{1j}y_j = 4104.32 \qquad \sum x_{2j}y_j = 3183.57$$

10.3.4 The administrator of a general hospital obtained the following data on 20 surgery patients during a study to determine what factors appear to be related to length of stay.

Postoperative Length of Stay in Days (Y)	Number of Current Medical Problems (X_1)	Preoperative Length of Stay in Days (X_2)
6	1	1
6	2	1
11	2	2
9	1	3
16	3	3
16	1	5
4	1	1
8	3	1
11	2	2
13	3	2
13	1	4
9	1	2
17	3	3
17	2	4
12	4	1
6	1	1
5	1	1
12	3	2
8	1	2
9	2	2
Total 208	38	43

$$\sum x_{1j}^2 = 90 \qquad \sum x_{2j}^2 = 119 \qquad \sum y_j^2 = 2478$$

$$\sum x_{1j}x_{2j} = 79 \qquad \sum x_{1j}y_j = 430 \qquad \sum x_{2j}y_j = 519$$

10.3.5 A random sample of 25 nurses selected from a state registry of nurses yielded the following information on each nurse's score on the state board examination and his or her final score in school. Both scores relate to the nurse's area of affiliation. Additional information on the score made by each nurse on an aptitude test, taken at the time of entering nursing school, was made available to the researcher. The complete data are as follows.

State Board Score (Y)	Final Score (X_1)	Aptitude Test Score (X_2)
440	87	92
480	87	79
535	87	99
460	88	91
525	88	84
480	89	71
510	89	78
530	89	78
545	89	71
600	89	76
495	90	89
545	90	90
575	90	73
525	91	71
575	91	81
600	91	84

State Board Score (Y)	Final Score (X_1)	Aptitude Test Score (X_2)
490	92	70
510	92	85
575	92	71
540	93	76
595	93	90
525	94	94
545	94	94
600	94	93
625	94	73
Total 13,425	2263	2053

$$\sum x_{1j}^2 = 204{,}977 \qquad \sum x_{2j}^2 = 170{,}569 \qquad \sum y_j^2 = 7{,}264{,}525$$

$$\sum x_{1j}x_{2j} = 185{,}838 \qquad \sum x_{1j}y_j = 1{,}216{,}685 \qquad \sum x_{2j}y_j = 1{,}101{,}220$$

10.3.6 The following data were collected on a simple random sample of 20 patients with hypertension. The variables are

$$Y = \text{mean arterial blood pressure (mm Hg)}$$

$$X_1 = \text{age (years)}$$

$$X_2 = \text{weight (kg)}$$

$$X_3 = \text{body surface area (sq m)}$$

$$X_4 = \text{duration of hypertension (years)}$$

$$X_5 = \text{basal pulse (beats/min)}$$

$$X_6 = \text{measure of stress}$$

PATIENT	Y	X_1	X_2	X_3	X_4	X_5	X_6
1	105	47	85.4	1.75	5.1	63	33
2	115	49	94.2	2.10	3.8	70	14
3	116	49	95.3	1.98	8.2	72	10
4	117	50	94.7	2.01	5.8	73	99
5	112	51	89.4	1.89	7.0	72	95
6	121	48	99.5	2.25	9.3	71	10
7	121	49	99.8	2.25	2.5	69	42
8	110	47	90.9	1.90	6.2	66	8
9	110	49	89.2	1.83	7.1	69	62
10	114	48	92.7	2.07	5.6	64	35
11	114	47	94.4	2.07	5.3	74	90
12	115	49	94.1	1.98	5.6	71	21
13	114	50	91.6	2.05	10.2	68	47
14	106	45	87.1	1.92	5.6	67	80
15	125	52	101.3	2.19	10.0	76	98
16	114	46	94.5	1.98	7.4	69	95
17	106	46	87.0	1.87	3.6	62	18
18	113	46	94.5	1.90	4.3	70	12
19	110	48	90.5	1.88	9.0	71	99
20	122	56	95.7	2.09	7.0	75	99

10.4
Evaluating the Multiple
Regression Equation

Before one uses a multiple regression equation to predict and estimate, it is desirable to determine first whether it is, in fact, worth using. In our study of simple linear regression we have learned that the usefulness of a regression equation may be evaluated by a consideration of the sample coefficient of determination and estimated slope. In evaluating a multiple regression equation we focus our attention on the *coefficient of multiple determination* and the partial regression coefficients.

The Coefficient of Multiple Determination   In Chapter 9 the coefficient of determination is discussed in considerable detail. The concept extends logically to the multiple regression case. The total variation present in the Y values may be partitioned into two components—the explained variation, which measures the amount of the total variation that is explained by the fitted regression surface, and the unexplained variation, which is that part of the total variation not explained by fitting the regression surface. The measure of variation in each case is a sum of squared deviations. The total variation is the sum of squared deviations of each observation of Y from the mean of the observations and is designated by $\Sigma(y_j - \hat{y})^2$ or SST. The explained variation, designated by $\Sigma(\hat{y} - \bar{y})^2$, is the sum of squared deviations of the calculated values from the mean of the observed Y values. This sum of squared deviations is called the *sum of squares due to regression* (SSR). The unexplained variation, written as $\Sigma(\hat{y}_j - \bar{y})^2$, is the sum of squared deviations of the original observations from the calculated values. This quantity is referred to as the *sum of squares about regression* or the *error sum of squares* (SSE). We may summarize the relationship among the three sums of squares with the following equation:

$$\Sigma\left(y_j - \bar{y}\right)^2 = \Sigma\left(\hat{y} - \bar{y}\right)^2 + \Sigma\left(y_j - \hat{y}\right)^2$$

$$SST = SSR + SSE \tag{10.4.1}$$

total sum of squares = explained (regression) sum of squares

+ unexplained (error) sum of squares

The total, explained, and unexplained sum of squares are computed as follows:

$$SST = \Sigma\left(y_j - \bar{y}\right)^2 = \Sigma y_j^2 - \left(\Sigma y_j\right)^2 / n \tag{10.4.2}$$

$$SSR = \Sigma\left(\hat{y} - \bar{y}\right)^2$$

$$= b_1 \Sigma x_{1j}' y_j' + b_2 \Sigma x_{2j}' y_j' + \cdots + b_k \Sigma x_{kj}' y_j' \tag{10.4.3}$$

$$SSE = SST - SSR \tag{10.4.4}$$

The coefficient of multiple determination, $R^2_{y.12\ldots k}$ is obtained by dividing the explained sum of squares by the total sum of squares. That is,

$$R^2_{y.12\ldots k} = \frac{\sum (\hat{y} - \bar{y})^2}{\sum (y_j - \bar{y})^2} \qquad (10.4.5)$$

The subscript $y.12\ldots k$ indicates that in the analysis Y is treated as the dependent variable and the X variables from X_1 through X_k are treated as the independent variables. The value of $R^2_{y.12\ldots k}$ indicates what proportion of the total variation in the observed Y values is explained by the regression of Y on $X_1, X_2, \ldots, X_k$. In other words, we may say that $R^2_{y.12\ldots k}$ is a measure of the goodness of fit of the regression surface. This quantity is analogous to r^2, which was computed in Chapter 9.

Example 10.4.1

Refer to Example 10.3.1. Compute $R^2_{y.12}$.

Solution: For our illustrative example we have (using the data from Table 10.3.2 and some previous calculations)

$$SST = 898.822 - (119.362)^2 / 19 = 148.9648$$

$$SSR = (-.05171)(229.76874) + (.170204)(763.43171) = 118.0578$$

$$SSE = 148.9648 - 118.0578 = 30.907$$

$$R^2_{y.12} = \frac{118.0578}{148.9648} = .7925$$

We say that 79.25 percent of the total variation in the Y values is explained by the fitted regression plane; that is, by the linear relationship with X_1 and X_2.

Testing the Regression Hypothesis To determine whether the overall regression is significant (that is, to determine whether $R^2_{y.12}$ is significant), we may perform a hypothesis test as follows.

1. *Data* The research situation and the data generated by the research are examined to determine if multiple regression is an appropriate technique for analysis.

2. *Assumptions* We presume that the multiple regression model and its underlying assumptions as presented in Section 10.2 are applicable.

3. *Hypotheses* In general, the null hypothesis is H_0: $\beta_1 = \beta_2 = \beta_3 = \cdots = \beta_k = 0$ and the alternative is H_A: not all $\beta_i = 0$. In words, the null hypothesis states that all the independent variables are of no value in explaining the variation in the Y values.

TABLE 10.4.1 ANOVA Table for Multiple Regression

Source	SS	d.f.	MS	V.R.
Due to regression	SSR	k	$MSR = SSR/k$	MSR/MSE
About regression	SSE	$n - k - 1$	$MSE = SSE/(n - k - 1)$	
Total	SST	$n - 1$		

4. *Test Statistic*   The appropriate test statistic is V.R., which is computed as part of an analysis of variance. The general ANOVA table is shown as Table 10.4.1. In Table 10.4.1, *MSR* stands for mean square due to regression and *MSE* stands for mean square about regression or, as it is sometimes called, the error mean square.

5. *Distribution of the Test Statistic*   When H_0 is true and the assumptions are met, V.R. is distributed as F with k and $n - k - 1$ degrees of freedom.

6. *Decision Rule*   Reject H_0 if the computed value of V.R. is equal to or greater than the critical value of F.

7. *Calculation of Test Statistic*   See Table 10.4.1.

8. *Statistical Decision*   Reject or fail to reject H_0 in accordance with the decision rule.

9. *Conclusion*   If we reject H_0, we conclude that, in the population from which the sample was drawn, the dependent variable is linearly related to the independent variables as a group. If we fail to reject H_0, we conclude that, in the population from which our sample was drawn, there is no linear relationship between the dependent variable and the independent variables as a group.

We illustrate the hypothesis testing procedure by means of the following example.

Example 10.4.2

We wish to test the null hypothesis of no linear relationship among the three variables discussed in Example 10.3.1: I-450IA2 index, number of cigarettes smoked per day, and urinary cotinine level.

Solution:

1. *Data*   See the description of the data given in Example 10.3.1.

2. *Assumptions*   We presume that the assumptions discussed in Section 10.2 are met.

3. *Hypotheses*

$$H_0: = \beta_1 = \beta_2 = 0$$

$$H_A: = \text{not all } \beta_i = 0$$

TABLE 10.4.2 ANOVA Table, Example 10.3.1

Source	SS	d.f.	MS	V.R.
Due to regression	118.0578	2	59.0289	30.55
About regression	30.907	16	1.9317	
Total	148.9648	18		

4. *Test Statistic*   The test statistic is V.R.

5. *Distribution of the Test Statistic*   If H_0 is true and the assumptions are met, the test statistic is distributed as F with 2 numerator and 16 denominator degrees of freedom.

6. *Decision Rule*   Let us use a significance level of $\alpha = .01$. The decision rule, then, is reject H_0 if the computed value of V.R. is equal to or greater than 6.23.

7. *Calculation of Test Statistic*   The ANOVA for the example is shown in Table 10.4.2, where we see that the computed value of V.R. is 30.55.

8. *Statistical Decision*   Since 30.55 is greater than 6.23, we reject H_0.

9. *Conclusion*   We conclude that, in the population from which the sample came, there is a linear relationship among the three variables.

Since 30.55 is greater than 7.51, the *p* value for the test is less than .005.

Inferences Regarding Individual β's   Frequently we wish to evaluate the strength of the linear relationship between Y and the independent variables individually. That is, we may want to test the null hypothesis that $\beta_i = 0$ against the alternative $\beta_i \neq 0$ $(i = 1, 2, \ldots, k)$. The validity of this procedure rests on the assumptions stated earlier: that for each combination of X_i values there is a normally distributed subpopulation of Y values with variance σ^2. When these assumptions hold true, it can be shown that each of the sample estimates b_i is normally distributed with mean β_i and variance $c_{ii}\sigma^2$. Since σ^2 is unknown, it will have to be estimated. An estimate is provided by the mean square about regression that is shown in the ANOVA table. We may designate this quantity generally as $s^2_{y.12\ldots k}$. For our particular example we have, from Table 10.4.2, $s^2_{y.12} = 1.9317$, and $s_{y.12} = 1.3898$. We must digress briefly at this point, however, to explain the computation of c_{ii}.

Computation of c_{ii}   The c_{ii} values are called *Gauss multipliers*. For those familiar with matrix algebra it may be enlightening to point out that they may be obtained by inverting the matrix of sums of squares and cross products that can be constructed by using the left-hand terms of the normal equations given in Equation 10.3.5. The c's may be found without the use of matrix algebra by solving the following two sets of equations:

$$c_{11} \sum x_{1j}'^2 + c_{12} \sum x_{1j}' x_{2j}' = 1 \atop c_{11} \sum x_{1j}' x_{2j}' + c_{12} \sum x_{2j}'^2 = 0 \Bigg\} \qquad (10.4.6)$$

$$c_{21} \sum x_{1j}'^2 + c_{22} \sum x_{1j}' x_{2j}' = 0 \atop c_{21} \sum x_{1j}' x_{2j}' + c_{22} \sum x_{2j}'^2 = 1 \Bigg\} \qquad (10.4.7)$$

In these equations $c_{12} = c_{21}$. Note also that the sums of squares and cross products are the same as those in the normal equations (Equation 10.3.5).

When the analysis involves more than two independent variables, the c's are obtained by expanding Equations 10.4.6 and 10.4.7 so that there is one set of equations for each independent variable. Each set of equations also contains as many individual equations as there are independent variables. The 1 is placed to the right of the equal sign in all equations containing a term of the form $c_{ii} \sum x_i'^2$. For example, in Equation 10.4.6, a 1 is to the right of the equal sign in the equation containing $c_{11} \sum x_{1j}'^2$. Ezekiel and Fox (4) have written out the equations for the case of three independent variables, and they, as well as Snedecor and Cochran (1), Steel and Torrie (2), and Anderson and Bancroft (3), demonstrate the use of the abbreviated Doolittle method (5) of obtaining the c's as well as the regression coefficients. Anderson and Bancroft (3) give a numerical example for four independent variables.

When we substitute data from our illustrative example into Equations 10.4.6 and 10.4.7, we have

$$936.105263c_{11} + 1634.35968c_{12} = 1 \atop 1634.35968c_{11} + 4981.92686c_{12} = 0 \Bigg\}$$

$$936.105263c_{21} + 1634.35968c_{22} = 0 \atop 1634.35968c_{21} + 4981.92686c_{22} = 1 \Bigg\}$$

The solution of these equations yields

$$c_{11} = .002500367$$

$$c_{12} = c_{21} = -.000820265$$

$$c_{22} = .00046982$$

Hypothesis Tests for the β_i   We may now return to the problem of inference procedures regarding the individual partial regression coefficients. To test the null hypothesis that β_i is equal to some particular value, say β_{i0}, the following t

statistic may be computed:

$$t = \frac{b_i - \beta_{i0}}{s_{b_i}} \qquad (10.4.8)$$

where the degrees of freedom are equal to $n - k - 1$, and

$$s_{b_i} = s_{y.12\ldots k} \sqrt{c_{ii}} \qquad (10.4.9)$$

The standard error of the difference between two partial regression coefficients is given by

$$s_{(b_i - b_j)} = \sqrt{s^2_{y.12\ldots k}\left(c_{ii} + c_{jj} - 2c_{ij}\right)} \qquad (10.4.10)$$

so that we may test $H_0: \beta_i = \beta_j$ by computing

$$t = \frac{b_i - b_j}{s_{(b_i - b_j)}} \qquad (10.4.11)$$

which has $n - k - 1$ degrees of freedom.

Example 10.4.3   Let us refer to Example 10.3.1 and test the null hypothesis that number of cigarettes smoked per day (Cig/Day) is irrelevant in predicting the IA2Index.

Solution:

1. *Data*   See Example 10.3.1.
2. *Assumptions*   See Section 10.2.
3. *Hypotheses*

$$H_0: \beta_1 = 0$$

$$H_A: \beta_1 \neq 0$$

$$\text{Let } \alpha = .05$$

4. *Test Statistic*   See Equation 10.4.8.
5. *Distribution of the Test Statistic*   When H_0 is true and the assumptions are met, the test statistic is distributed as Student's t with 16 degrees of freedom.
6. *Decision Rule*   Reject H_0 if the computed t is either greater than or equal to 2.1199 or less than or equal to -2.1199.
7. *Calculation of the Test Statistic*   By Equation 10.4.8 we compute

$$t = \frac{b_1 - 0}{s_{b_1}} = \frac{-.0517}{1.3898\sqrt{.002500367}} = -.7439$$

8. *Statistical Decision* The null hypothesis is not rejected, since the computed value of t, $-.7439$, is between -2.1199 and $+2.1199$, the critical values of t for a two-sided test when $\alpha = .05$ and the degrees of freedom are 16.

9. *Conclusion* We conclude, then, that there may not be a significant linear relationship between IA2Index and number of cigarettes smoked per day in the presence of urinary cotinine level. At least these data do not provide evidence for such a relationship. In other words, the data of the present sample do not provide sufficient evidence to indicate that number of cigarettes smoked per day, when used in a regression equation along with urinary cotinine, is a useful variable in predicting the IA2Index. [For this test, $p > 2(.10) = .20$.]

Now, let us perform a similar test for the second partial regression coefficient, β_2:

$$H_0: \beta_2 = 0$$

$$H_A: \beta_2 \neq 0$$

$$\alpha = .05$$

$$t = \frac{b_2 - 0}{s_{b_2}} = \frac{.1702}{1.3898\sqrt{.00046982}} = 5.6499$$

In this case the null hypothesis is rejected, since 5.6499 is greater than 2.1199. We conclude that there is a linear relationship between urinary cotinine level and IA2 Index in the presence of number of cigarettes smoked per day, and that urinary cotinine level, used in this manner, is a useful variable for predicting IA2 Index. [For this test, $p < 2(.005) = .01$.]

Confidence Intervals for the β_i When the researcher has been led to conclude that a partial regression coefficient is not 0, he or she may be interested in obtaining a confidence interval for this β_i. Confidence intervals for the β_i may be constructed in the usual way by using a value from the t distribution for the reliability factor and standard errors given above.

A $100(1 - \alpha)$ percent confidence interval for β_i is given by

$$b_i \pm t_{1-(\alpha/2), n-k-1} s_{y.12\ldots k} \sqrt{c_{ii}}$$

For our illustrative example we may compute the following 95 percent confidence interval for β_2:

$$.1702 \pm (2.1199)(1.3898)\sqrt{.00046982}$$

$$.1702 \pm .063860664$$

$$.1063, .2341$$

We may give this interval the usual probabilistic and practical interpretations. We are 95 percent confident that β_2 is contained in the interval from .1036 to .2341 since, in repeated sampling, 95 percent of the intervals that may be constructed in this manner will include the true parameter.

Some Precautions   One should be aware of the problems involved in carrying out multiple hypothesis tests and constructing multiple confidence intervals from the same sample data. The effect on α of performing multiple hypothesis tests from the same data is discussed in Section 8.2. A similar problem arises when one wishes to construct confidence intervals for two or more partial regression coefficients. The intervals will not be independent, so that the tabulated confidence coefficient does not, in general, apply. In other words, all such intervals would not be $100(1 - \alpha)$ percent confidence intervals. Durand (6) gives a procedure that may be followed when confidence intervals for more than one partial regression coefficient are desired. See also the book by Neter et al. (7).

Another problem sometimes encountered in the application of multiple regression is an apparent incompatibility in the results of the various tests of significance that one may perform. In a given problem for a given level of significance, one or the other of the following situations may be observed.

1. R^2 and all b_i significant.
2. R^2 and some but not all b_i significant.
3. R^2 significant but none of the b_i significant.
4. All b_i significant but not R^2.
5. Some b_i significant, but not all nor R^2.
6. Neither R^2 nor any b_i significant.

Geary and Leser (8) identify these six situations and, after pointing out that situations 1 and 6 present no problem (since they both imply compatible results), discuss each of the other situations in some detail.

Notice that situation 2 exists in our illustrative example, where we have a significant R^2 but only one out of two significant regression coefficients. Geary and Leser (8) point out that this situation is very common, especially when a large number of independent variables have been included in the regression equation, and that the only problem is to decide whether or not to eliminate from the analysis one or more of the variables associated with nonsignificant coefficients.

EXERCISES

10.4.1 Refer to Exercise 10.3.1. (a) Calculate the coefficient of multiple determination; (b) perform an analysis of variance; (c) test the significance of each b_i ($i > 0$). Let $\alpha = .05$ for all tests of significance. Determine the p value for all tests.

10.4.2 Refer to Exercise 10.3.2. Do the analysis suggested in 10.4.1.

10.5
Using the Multiple
Regression Equation

As we learned in the previous chapter, a regression equation may be used to obtain a computed value of Y, $\hat{y}$, when a particular value of X is given. Similarly, we may use our multiple regression equation to obtain a $\hat{y}$ value when we are given particular values of the two or more X variables present in the equation.

Just as was the case in simple linear regression, we may, in multiple regression, interpret a $\hat{y}$ value in one of two ways. First we may interpret $\hat{y}$ as an estimate of the mean of the subpopulation of Y values assumed to exist for particular combinations of X_i values. Under this interpretation $\hat{y}$ is called an *estimate*, and when it is used for this purpose, the equation is thought of as an *estimating equation*. The second interpretation of $\hat{y}$ is that it is the value Y is most likely to assume for given values of the X_i. In this case $\hat{y}$ is called the *predicted value* of Y, and the equation is called a *prediction equation*. In both cases, intervals may be constructed about the $\hat{y}$ value when the normality assumption of Section 10.2 holds true. When $\hat{y}$ is interpreted as an estimate of a population mean, the interval is called a *confidence interval*, and when $\hat{y}$ is interpreted as a predicted value of Y, the interval is called a *prediction interval*. Now let us see how each of these intervals is constructed.

The Confidence Interval for the Mean of a Subpopulation of Y Values Given Particular Values of the X_i We have seen that a $100(1 - \alpha)$ percent confidence interval for a parameter may be constructed by the general procedure of adding to and subtracting from the estimator a quantity equal to the reliability factor corresponding to $1 - \alpha$ multiplied by the standard error of the estimator. We have also seen that in multiple regression the estimator is

$$\hat{y} = b_0 + b_1 x_{1j} + b_2 x_{2j} + \cdots + b_k x_{kj} \tag{10.5.1}$$

The standard error of this estimator for the case of two independent variables is given by

$$s_{y.12}\sqrt{\frac{1}{n} + c_{11}x_{1j}'^2 + c_{22}x_{2j}'^2 + 2c_{12}x_{1j}'x_{2j}'} \tag{10.5.2}$$

where x'_{ij} values are particular values of the X_i expressed as deviations from their mean. Expression 10.5.2 is easily generalized to any number of independent variables. See for example, Anderson and Bancroft (3). The $100(1 - \alpha)$ percent confidence interval for the three-variable case, then, is as follows:

$$\hat{y} \pm t_{1-(\alpha/2), n-k-1} s_{y.12} \sqrt{\frac{1}{n} + c_{11}x'^2_{1j} + c_{22}x'^2_{2j} + 2c_{12}x'_{1j}x'_{2j}} \qquad (10.5.3)$$

Example 10.5.1

To illustrate the construction of a confidence interval for a subpopulation of Y values for given values of the X_i we refer to Example 10.3.1. The regression equation is

$$\hat{y} = 4.5235 - .05171x_{1j} + .170204x_{2j}$$

We wish to construct a 95 percent confidence interval for the mean IA2Index (Y) in a population of subjects all of whom smoke 12 cigarettes a day (X_1) and whose urinary cotinine levels (X_2) are all 10.

Solution: The point estimate of the mean of IA2Index is

$$\hat{y} = 4.5235 - .05171(12) + .170204(10) = 5.60502$$

To compute the standard error of this estimate, we first obtain $x'_{1j} = (x_{1j} - \bar{x}_1) = (12 - 9.32) = 2.68$ and $x'_{2j} = (x_{2j} - \bar{x}_2) = (10 - 13.16) = -3.16$. Recall that $c_{11} = .002500367$, $c_{22} = .00046982$, and $c_{12} = -.000820265$. The reliability factor for 95 percent confidence and 16 degrees of freedom is $t = 2.1199$. Substituting these values into Expression 10.5.3 gives

$$5.60502 \pm 2.1199(1.3898)$$

$$\times \sqrt{(1/19) + (.002500367)(2.68)^2 + (.00046982)(-3.16)^2 + 2(-.000820265)(2.68)(-3.16)}$$

$$= 5.60502 \pm .879810555$$

$$= 4.7252, 6.4848.$$

We interpret this interval in the usual ways. We are 95 percent confident that the interval from 4.7252 to 6.4848 includes the mean of the subpopulation of Y values for the specified combination of X_i values, since this parameter would be included in about 95 percent of the intervals that can be constructed in the manner shown.

The Prediction Interval for a Particular Value of Y Given Particular Values of the X When we interpret $\hat{y}$ as the value Y is most likely to assume when particular values of the X_i are observed, we may construct a prediction interval in the same way in which the confidence interval was constructed. The only difference in the two is the standard error. The standard error of the prediction is slightly larger than the standard error of the estimate, which causes the prediction interval to be wider than the confidence interval.

The standard error of the prediction for the three-variable case is given by

$$s_{y.12}\sqrt{1 + \frac{1}{n} + c_{11}x'^2_{1j} + c_{22}x'^2_{2j} + 2c_{12}x'_{1j}x'_{2j}} \qquad (10.5.4)$$

so that the $100(1 - \alpha)$ percent prediction interval is

$$\hat{y} \pm t_{1-(\alpha/2),\,n-k-1}s_{y.12}\sqrt{1 + \frac{1}{n} + c_{11}x'^2_{1j} + c_{22}x'^2_{2j} + 2c_{12}x'_{1j}x'_{2j}} \qquad (10.5.5)$$

Example 10.5.2   Let us refer again to Example 10.3.1. Suppose we have a subject who smokes 12 cigarettes per day and has a urinary cotinine level of 10. What do we predict this subject's IA2Index to be?

Solution: The point prediction, which is the same as the point estimate obtained previously, is

$$\hat{y} = 4.5235 - .05171(12) + .170204(10) = 5.60502$$

The values needed for the construction of the prediction interval are the same as for the confidence interval. When we substitute these values into Expression 10.5.5 we have

$5.60502 \pm 2.1199(1.3898)$

$$\times \sqrt{1 + (1/19) + (.002500367)(2.68)^2 + (.00046982)(-3.16)^2 + 2(-.000820265)(2.68)(-3.16)}$$

$= 5.60502 \pm 3.068168195$

$= 2.5368, 8.6732.$

We are 95 percent confident that this subject would have an IA2Index somewhere between 2.5368 and 8.6732.

Computer Analysis   Figure 10.5.1 shows the results of a computer analysis of the data of Example 10.3.1 using the MINITAB multiple regression program. The data were entered into columns 1 through 3 and renamed by the following command

```
NAME C3 'Y', C2 'X2', C3 'X1'
```

The following commands were issued to obtain the analysis and accompanying

```
The regression equation is
Y = 4.52 - 0.0517 X1 + 0.170 X2
Predictor         Coef      Stdev       t-ratio        p
Constant        4.5234     0.5381          8.41     0.000
X1             -0.05170   0.06950         -0.74     0.468
X2              0.17020   0.03013          5.65     0.000

s = 1.390          R-sq = 79.2%      R-sq (adj) = 76.7%

Analysis of Variance

Source              DF         SS          MS          F         p
Regression           2    118.059      59.029      30.55     0.000
Error               16     30.912       1.932
Total               18    148.970

Source              DF      SEQ SS
X1                   1      56.401
X2                   1      61.658

Obs.      X1         Y       Fit   Stdev. Fit   Residual   St. Resid
  1      1.0     4.165     4.472        0.496     -0.307       -0.24
  2      1.0     3.731     4.472        0.496     -0.740       -0.57
  3      1.0     5.748     4.472        0.496      1.277        0.98
  4      1.0     4.437     4.472        0.496     -0.035       -0.03
  5      1.0     6.469     4.472        0.496      1.997        1.54
  6      3.0     3.892     4.368        0.434     -0.476       -0.36
  7      8.0     5.295     5.913        0.325     -0.618       -0.46
  8      8.0     4.603     4.895        0.375     -0.292       -0.22
  9      8.0     5.811     8.738        0.589     -2.926       -2.32R
 10      8.0     3.689     5.051        0.362     -1.362       -1.02
 11      8.0     3.372     4.583        0.406     -1.210       -0.91
 12     10.0     8.021     7.374        0.360      0.647        0.48
 13     10.0    10.837     7.888        0.409      2.949        2.22R
 14     15.0     4.115     3.748        0.808      0.367        0.32
 15     15.0     5.543     6.219        0.485     -0.676       -0.52
 16     15.0    11.353     9.996        0.580      1.357        1.07
 17     20.0     7.564     7.102        0.663      0.461        0.38
 18     20.0     7.216     7.085        0.664      0.130        0.11
 19     24.0    13.500    14.042        1.043     -0.542       -0.59X
R denotes an obs. with a large st. resid.
X denotes an obs. whose X value gives it large influence.
```

Figure 10.5.1 Partial printout of analysis of data of Example 10.3.1, using MINITAB regression analysis program.

printout:

```
BRIEF 3
REGRESS Y IN C3 ON 2 PREDICTORS IN C1 C2
```

```
                                    SAS
          DEP VARIABLE:    IA2INDEX
                              ANALYSIS OF VARIANCE
                              SUM OF         MEAN
          SOURCE      DF     SQUARES        SQUARE       F VALUE    PROB>F

          MODEL        2    118.06041   59.03020419       30.555    0.0001
          ERROR       16  30.91079933    1.93192496
          C TOTAL     18   148.97121

                 ROOT MSE        1.389937     R-SQUARE     0.7925
                 DEP MEAN        6.282174     ADJ R-SQ     0.7666
                      C.V.        22.1251
                              PARAMETER ESTIMATES

                           PARAMETER       STANDARD    T FOR HO:
          VARIABLE DF       ESTIMATE         ERROR   PARAMETER = 0   PROB>|T|
          INTERCEP  1     4.52338314    0.53806674        8.407      0.0001
          CIGDAY    1    -0.05169327    0.06950225       -0.744      0.4678
          COT       1     0.17020054    0.03012742        5.649      0.0001
```

Figure 10.5.2 Partial SAS regression printout for the data of Example 10.3.1.

Note that the column labeled Stdev.Fit contains, for each set of the observed X's, numerical values of the standard error obtained by Expression 10.5.2.

The entries under SEQ SS show how much of the regression sum of squares, 118.059 is attributable to each of the explanatory variables X_1 and X_2. The residuals are the differences between the observed Y values and the fitted or predicted Y values. The entries under St.Resid are the standardized residuals. Standardized residuals are frequently calculated by dividing the raw residuals by the standard deviation, s, that appears on the printout. The standardized residuals on the printout are the result of a different procedure that we will not go into. On the printout, unusual observations are marked with an X if the predictor is unusual, and by an R if the response is unusual. For further details on the interpretation of these codes consult your MINITAB manual.

Figure 10.5.2 shows the partial SAS regression printout for the data in Example 10.3.1.

EXERCISES

For each of the following exercises compute the $\hat{y}$ value and construct (a) 95 percent confidence and (b) 95 percent prediction intervals for the specified values of X_i.

10.5.1 Refer to Exercise 10.3.1 and let $x_{1j} = 200$ and $x_{2j} = 20$.

10.5.2 Refer to Exercise 10.3.2 and let $x_{1j} = 50$, $x_{2j} = 30$, and $x_{3j} = 25$.

10.5.3 Refer to Exercise 10.3.3 and let $x_{1j} = 5$ and $x_{2j} = 6$.

10.5.4 Refer to Exercise 10.3.4 and let $x_{1j} = 1$ and $x_{2j} = 2$.

10.5.5 Refer to Exercise 10.3.5 and let $x_{1j} = 90$ and $x_{2j} = 80$.

10.5.6 Refer to Exercise 10.3.6 and let $x_{1j} = 50$, $x_{2j} = 95.0$, $x_{3j} = 2.00$, $x_{4j} = 6.00$, $x_{5j} = 75$, and $x_{6j} = 70$.

10.6
The Multiple Correlation Model

We pointed out in the preceding chapter that while regression analysis is concerned with the form of the relationship between variables, the objective of correlation analysis is to gain insight into the strength of the relationship. This is also true in the multivariable case, and in this section we investigate methods for measuring the strength of the relationship among several variables. First, however, let us define the model and assumptions on which our analysis rests.

The Model Equation We may write the correlation model as

$$y_j = \beta_0 + \beta_1 x_{1j} + \beta_2 x_{2j} + \cdots + \beta_k x_{kj} + e_j \qquad (10.6.1)$$

where y_j is a typical value from the population of values of the variable Y, the β's are the regression coefficients defined in Section 10.2, the x_{ij} are particular (known) values of the random variables X_i. This model is similar to the multiple regression model, but there is one important distinction. In the multiple regression model, given in Equation 10.2.1, the X_i are nonrandom variables, but in the multiple correlation model the X_i are random variables. In other words, in the correlation model there is a joint distribution of Y and the X_i that we call a *multivariate distribution*. Under this model, the variables are no longer thought of as being dependent or independent, since logically they are interchangeable and either of the X_i may play the role of Y.

Typically random samples of units of association are drawn from a population of interest, and measurements of Y and the X_i are made.

A least-squares plane or hyperplane is fitted to the sample data by methods described in Section 10.3, and the same uses may be made of the resulting equation. Inferences may be made about the population from which the sample was drawn if it can be assumed that the underlying distribution is normal, that is, if it can be assumed that the joint distribution of Y and X_i is a *multivariate normal distribution*. In addition, sample measures of the degree of the relationship among the variables may be computed and, under the assumption that sampling is from a multivariate normal distribution, the corresponding parameters may be estimated by means of confidence intervals, and hypothesis tests may be carried out. Specifically, we may compute an estimate of the *multiple correlation coefficient* that measures the dependence between Y and the X_i. This is a straightforward extension of the concept of correlation between two variables that we discuss in Chapter 9. We may also compute *partial correlation coefficients* that measure the intensity of the relationship between any two variables when the influence of all other variables has been removed.

The Multiple Correlation Coefficient   As a first step in analyzing the relationships among the variables, we look at the multiple correlation coefficient.

The multiple correlation coefficient is the square root of the coefficient of multiple determination and, consequently, the sample value may be computed by taking the square root of Equation 10.4.5. That is,

$$R_{y.12\ldots k} = \sqrt{R_{y.12\ldots k}^2} = \sqrt{\frac{\sum(\hat{y}-\bar{y})^2}{\sum(y_j-\bar{y})^2}} \qquad (10.6.2)$$

The numerator of the term under the radical in Equation 10.6.2, which is the explained sum of squares, is given by Equation 10.4.3, which we recall contains b_1 and b_2, the sample partial regression coefficients. We compute these by the methods of Section 10.3.

To illustrate the concepts and techniques of multiple correlation analysis, let us consider an example.

Example
10.6.1   Benowitz et al. (A-4) note that an understanding of the disposition kinetics and bioavailability from different routes of exposure is central to an understanding of nicotine dependence and the rational use of nicotine as a medication. The researchers reported their investigation of these phenomena and reported the results in the journal *Clinical Pharmacology & Therapeutics*. Their subjects were healthy men, 24 to 48 years of age, who were regular cigarette smokers. Among the data collected on each subject were puffs per cigarette, total particulate matter per cigarette, and nicotine intake per cigarette. The data on nine subjects are shown in Table 10.6.1. We wish to analyze the nature and strength of the relationship among these three variables.

Solution: First, the various sums, sums of squares, and sums of cross products must be computed. They are as follows:

$$\sum x_{1j} = 95.5000 \qquad \sum x_{2j} = 360.700 \qquad \sum y_j = 22.4500$$
$$\sum x_{1j}^2 = 1061.75 \qquad \sum x_{2j}^2 = 15546.3 \qquad \sum y_j^2 = 60.8605$$
$$\sum x_{1j}x_{2j} = 3956.25 \qquad \sum x_{1j}y_j = 251.660 \qquad \sum x_{2j}y_j = 954.332$$

When we compute the sums of squares and cross products of

$$y_j' = (y_j - \bar{y})$$

$$x_{1j}' = (x_{1j} - \bar{x}_1) \qquad \text{and} \qquad x_{2j}' = (x_{2j} - \bar{x}_2)$$

TABLE 10.6.1 Smoking Data for 9 Subjects

X_1	X_2	Y
7.5	21.9	1.38
9.0	46.4	1.78
8.5	24.0	1.68
10.0	28.8	2.12
14.5	43.8	3.26
11.0	48.1	2.98
9.0	50.8	2.56
12.0	47.8	3.47
14.0	49.1	3.22

X_1 = puffs/cigarette, X_2 = total particulate matter (mg/cigarette), Y = nicotine intake/cigarette (mg)

SOURCE: Neal L. Benowitz, Peyton Jacob III, Charles Denaro, and Roger Jenkins, "Stable Isotope Studies of Nicotine Kinetics and Bioavailability," *Clinical Pharmacology & Therapeutics, 49* (1991), 270–277.

we have

$$\sum x_{1j}'^2 = 1061.75 - (95.5)^2/9 = 48.38889$$

$$\sum x_{2j}'^2 = 15546.3 - (360.7)^2/9 = 1090.24556$$

$$\sum y_j'^2 = 60.8605 - (22.45)^2/9 = 4.86022$$

$$\sum x_{1j}' x_{2j}' = 3956.25 - (95.5)(360.7)/9 = 128.82222$$

$$\sum x_{1j}' y_j' = 251.66 - (95.5)(22.45)/9 = 13.44056$$

$$\sum x_{2j}' y_j' = 954.332 - (360.7)(22.45)/9 = 54.58589$$

The normal equations, by Equations 10.3.9, are

$$48.38889b_1 + 128.82222b_2 = 13.44056$$
$$128.82222b_1 + 1090.24556b_2 = 54.58589$$

The simultaneous solution of these equations gives $b_1 = .21077$, $b_2 = .02516$. We obtain b_0 by substituting appropriate values into Equation 10.3.11:

$$b_0 = 2.494 - (.21077)(10.611) - (.02516)(40.08) = -.75089$$

The least-squares equation, then, is

$$\hat{y} = -.75089 + .21077x_{1j} + .02516x_{2j}$$

This equation may be used for estimation and prediction purposes and may be evaluated by the methods discussed in Section 10.4.

Calculation of $R^2_{y.12}$ We now have the necessary quantities for computing the multiple correlation coefficient. We first compute the explained sum of squares by Equation 10.4.3:

$$SSR = (.21077)(13.44056) + (.02516)(54.58589)$$

$$= 4.20625$$

The total sum of squares by Equation 10.4.2 is

$$SST = 60.8605 - (22.45)^2/9 = 4.86022$$

The coefficient of multiple determination, then, is

$$R^2_{y.12} = \frac{4.20625}{4.86022} = .865444$$

and the multiple correlation coefficient is

$$R_{y.12} = \sqrt{.865444} = .93029$$

Interpretation of $R^2_{y.12}$ We interpret $R_{y.12}$ as a measure of the correlation among the variables nicotine intake per cigarette, number of puffs per cigarette, and total particulate matter per cigarette in the sample of nine healthy men between the ages of 24 and 48. If our data constitute a random sample from the population of such persons we may use $R_{y.12}$ as an estimate of $\rho_{y.12}$, the true population multiple correlation coefficient. We may also interpret $R_{y.12}$ as the simple correlation coefficient between y_j and $\hat{y}$, the observed and calculated values, respectively, of the "dependent" variable. Perfect correspondence between the observed and calculated values of Y will result in a correlation coefficient of 1, while a complete lack of a linear relationship between observed and calculated values yields a correlation coefficient of 0. The multiple correlation coefficient is always given a positive sign. We may test the null hypothesis that $\rho_{y.12\ldots k} = 0$ by computing

$$F = \frac{R^2_{y.12\ldots k}}{1 - R^2_{y.12\ldots k}} \cdot \frac{n - k - 1}{k} \tag{10.6.3}$$

The numerical value obtained from Equation 10.6.3 is compared with the tabulated value of F with k and $n - k - 1$ degrees of freedom. The reader will recall that this is identical to the test of H_0: $\beta_1 = \beta_2 = \cdots = \beta_k = 0$ described in Section 10.4.

For our present example let us test the null hypothesis that $\rho_{y.12} = 0$ against the alternative that $\rho_{y.12} \neq 0$. We compute

$$F = \frac{.865444}{(1 - .865444)} \cdot \frac{9 - 2 - 1}{2} = 19.2955$$

Since 19.2955 is greater than 14.54, $p < .005$, so that we may reject the null hypothesis at the .005 level of significance and conclude that nicotine intake is linearly correlated with puffs per cigarette and total particulate matter per cigarette in the sampled population.

Further comments on the significance of observed multiple correlation coefficients may be found in Ezekiel and Fox (4), who discuss a paper on the subject by R. A. Fisher (9) and present graphs for constructing confidence intervals when the number of variables is eight or less. Kramer (10) presents tables for constructing confidence limits when the number of variables is greater than eight.

Partial Correlation The researcher may wish to have a measure of the strength of the linear relationship between two variables when the effect of the remaining variables has been removed. Such a measure is provided by the *partial correlation* coefficient. For example, the partial sample correlation coefficient $r_{y1.2}$ is a measure of the correlation between Y and X_1 when X_2 is held constant.

The partial correlation coefficients may be computed from the *simple correlation coefficients*. The simple correlation coefficients measure the correlation between two variables when no effort has been made to control other variables. In other words, they are the coefficients for any pair of variables that would be obtained by the methods of simple correlation discussed in Chapter 9.

Suppose we have three variables, Y, X_1, and X_2. The sample partial correlation coefficient measuring the correlation between Y and X_1 with X_2 held constant, for example, is written $r_{y1.2}$. In the subscript, the symbol to the right of the decimal point indicates which variable is held constant, while the two symbols to the left of the decimal point indicate which variables are being correlated. For the three-variable case, there are two other sample partial correlation coefficients that we may compute. They are $r_{y2.1}$ and $r_{12.y}$.

The Coefficient of Partial Determination The square of the partial correlation coefficient is called the coefficient of partial determination. It provides useful information about the interrelationships among variables. Consider $r_{y1.2}$, for example. Its square, $r_{y1.2}^2$, tells us what proportion of the remaining variability in Y is explained by X_1 after X_2 has explained as much of the total variability in Y as it can.

Calculating the Partial Correlation Coefficients   For three variables the following simple correlation coefficients are obtained first:

r_{y1}, the simple correlation between Y and X_1

r_{y2}, the simple correlation between Y and X_2

r_{12}, the simple correlation between X_1 and X_2

These simple correlation coefficients may be computed as follows:

$$r_{y1} = \sum x'_{1j}y'_j \Big/ \sqrt{\sum x'^2_{1j}\sum y'^2_j} \qquad (10.6.4)$$

$$r_{y2} = \sum x'_{2j}y'_j \Big/ \sqrt{\sum x'^2_{2j}\sum y'^2_j} \qquad (10.6.5)$$

$$r_{12} = \sum x'_{1j}x'_{2j} \Big/ \sqrt{\sum x'^2_{1j}\sum x'^2_{2j}} \qquad (10.6.6)$$

The sample partial correlation coefficients that may be computed in the three-variable case are

1. The partial correlation between Y and X_1 when X_2 is held constant:

$$r_{y1.2} = \left(r_{y1} - r_{y2}r_{12}\right) \Big/ \sqrt{\left(1 - r^2_{y2}\right)\left(1 - r^2_{12}\right)} \qquad (10.6.7)$$

2. The partial correlation between Y and X_2 when X_1 is held constant:

$$r_{y2.1} = \left(r_{y2} - r_{y1}r_{12}\right) \Big/ \sqrt{\left(1 - r^2_{y1}\right)\left(1 - r^2_{12}\right)} \qquad (10.6.8)$$

3. The partial correlation between X_1 and X_2 when Y is held constant:

$$r_{12.y} = \left(r_{12} - r_{y1}r_{y2}\right) \Big/ \sqrt{\left(1 - r^2_{y1}\right)\left(1 - r^2_{y2}\right)} \qquad (10.6.9)$$

Example 10.6.2   To illustrate the calculation of sample partial correlation coefficients, let us refer to Example 10.6.1, and calculate the partial correlation coefficients among the variables nicotine intake (Y), puffs per cigarette (X_1), and total particulate matter (X_2).

Solution: First, we calculate the simple correlation coefficients for each pair of variables as follows:

$$r_{y1} = 13.44056\Big/\sqrt{(48.38889)(4.86022)} = .8764$$

$$r_{y2} = 54.58589\Big/\sqrt{(1090.24556)(4.86022)} = .7499$$

$$r_{12} = 128.82222\Big/\sqrt{(48.38889)(1090.24556)} = .5609$$

We use the simple correlation coefficients to obtain the following partial correlation coefficients:

$$r_{y1.2} = \big[.8764 - (.7499)(.5609)\big]\Big/\sqrt{(1 - .7499^2)(1 - .5609^2)} = .8322$$

$$r_{y2.1} = \big[.7499 - (.8764)(.5609)\big]\Big/\sqrt{(1 - .8764^2)(1 - .5609^2)} = .6479$$

$$r_{12.y} = \big[.5609 - (.8764)(.7499)\big]\Big/\sqrt{(1 - .8764^2)(1 - .7499^2)} = -.3023$$

Testing Hypotheses About Partial Correlation Coefficients We may test the null hypothesis that any one of the population partial correlation coefficients is 0 by means of the t test. For example, to test H_0: $\rho_{y1.2\ldots k} = 0$, we compute

$$t = r_{y1.2\ldots k}\sqrt{\frac{n - k - 1}{1 - r_{y1.2\ldots k}^2}} \qquad (10.6.10)$$

which is distributed as Student's t with $n - k - 1$ degrees of freedom.

Let us illustrate the procedure for our current example by testing H_0: $\rho_{y1.2} = 0$ against the alternative, H_A: $\rho_{y1.2} \neq 0$. The computed t is

$$t = .8322\sqrt{\frac{9 - 2 - 1}{1 - .8322^2}} = 3.6764$$

Since the computed t of 3.6764 is larger than the tabulated t of 2.4469 for 6 degrees of freedom and $\alpha = .05$, (two-sided test), we may reject H_0 at the .05 level of significance and conclude that there is a significant correlation between nicotine intake and puff per cigarette when total particulate matter is held constant. Significance tests for the other two partial correlation coefficients will be left as an exercise for the reader.

Although our illustration of correlation analysis is limited to the three-variable case, the concepts and techniques extend logically to the case of four or more variables. The number and complexity of the calculations increase rapidly as the number of variables increases.

EXERCISES

10.6.1 The objective of a study by Steinhorn and Green (A-5) was to determine whether the metabolic response to illness in children as measured by direct means is correlated with the estimated severity of illness. Subjects were 12 patients between the ages of two and 120 months with a variety of illnesses including sepsis, bacterial meningitis, and respiratory failure. Severity of illness was assessed by means of the Physiologic Stability Index (PSI) and the Pediatric Risk of Mortality scoring system (PRISM). Scores were also obtained on the Therapeutic Intervention Scoring System (TISS) and the Nursing Utilization Management Intervention System (NUMIS) instruments. Measurements were obtained on the following variables commonly used as biochemical markers of physiologic stress: total urinary nitrogen (TUN), minute oxygen consumption ($\dot{V}o_2$), and branch chain to aromatic amino acid ratio (BC : AA). The resulting measurements on these variables were as follows:

PRISM	PSI	TISS	NUMIS	$\dot{V}o_2$	TUN	BC : AA
15.0	14.0	10.0	8.0	146.0	3.1	1.8
27.0	18.0	52.0	10.0	171.0	4.3	1.4
5.0	4.0	15.0	8.0	121.0	2.4	2.2
23.0	18.0	22.0	8.0	185.0	4.1	1.4
4.0	12.0	27.0	8.0	130.0	2.2	1.7
6.0	4.0	8.0	8.0	101.0	2.0	2.4
18.0	17.0	42.0	8.0	127.0	4.6	1.7
15.0	14.0	47.0	9.0	161.0	3.7	1.6
12.0	11.0	51.0	9.0	145.0	6.4	1.3
1.0	4.0	15.0	7.0	116.0	2.5	2.3
50.0	63.0	64.0	10.0	190.0	7.8	1.6
9.0	10.0	42.0	8.0	135.0	3.7	1.8

SOURCE: David M. Steinhorn and Thomas P. Green, "Severity of Illness Correlates With Alterations in Energy Metabolism in the Pediatric Intensive Care Unit," *Critical Care Medicine*, *19* (1991), 1503–1509. © by Williams & Wilkins, 1991.

a. Compute the simple correlation coefficients between all possible pairs of variables.

b. Compute the multiple correlation coefficient among the variables NUMIS, TUN, $\dot{V}o_2$, and BC : AA. Test the overall correlation for significance.

c. Calculate the partial correlations between NUMIS and each one of the other variables specified in part b while the other two are held constant. (These are called second-order partial correlation coefficients.) You will want to use a software package such as SAS© to perform these calculations.

d. Repeat c above with the variable PRISM instead of NUMIS.

e. Repeat c above with the variable PSI instead of NUMIS.

f. Repeat c above with the variable TISS instead of NUMIS.

10.6.2 The following data were obtained on 12 males between the ages of 12 and 18 years (all measurements are in centimeters).

Height (Y)	Radius Length (X_1)	Femur Length (X_2)
149.0	21.00	42.50
152.0	21.79	43.70
155.7	22.40	44.75
159.0	23.00	46.00
163.3	23.70	47.00
166.0	24.30	47.90
169.0	24.92	48.95
172.0	25.50	49.90
174.5	25.80	50.30
176.1	26.01	50.90
176.5	26.15	50.85
179.0	26.30	51.10
Total 1992.1	290.87	573.85

$$\sum x_{1j}^2 = 7087.6731 \qquad \sum x_{2j}^2 = 27541.8575 \qquad \sum y_j^2 = 331851.09$$

$$\sum x_{1j}x_{2j} = 13970.5835 \qquad \sum x_{1j}y_j = 48492.886 \qquad \sum x_{2j}y_j = 95601.09$$

a. Find the sample multiple correlation coefficient and test the null hypothesis that $\rho_{y.12} = 0$

b. Find each of the partial correlation coefficients and test each for significance. Let $\alpha = .05$ for all tests.

c. Determine the p value for each test.

d. State your conclusions.

10.6.3 The following data were collected on 15 obese girls.

Weight in Kilograms (Y)	Lean Body Weight (X_1)	Mean Daily Caloric Intake (X_2)
79.2	54.3	2670
64.0	44.3	820
67.0	47.8	1210
78.4	53.9	2678
66.0	47.5	1205
63.0	43.0	815
65.9	47.1	1200
63.1	44.0	1180
73.2	44.1	1850
66.5	48.3	1260
61.9	43.5	1170
72.5	43.3	1852
101.1	66.4	1790
66.2	47.5	1250
99.9	66.1	1789
Total 1087.9	741.1	22739

$$\sum x_{1j}^2 = 37,439.95 \qquad \sum x_{2j}^2 = 39,161,759 \qquad \sum y_j^2 = 81,105.63$$

$$\sum x_{1j}x_{2j} = 1,154,225.2 \qquad \sum x_{1j}y_j = 55,021.31 \qquad \sum x_{2j}y_j = 1,707,725.3$$

a. Find the multiple correlation coefficient and test it for significance.
b. Find each of the partial correlation coefficients and test each for significance. Let $\alpha = .05$ for all tests.
c. Determine the p value for each test.
d. State your conclusions.

10.6.4 A research project was conducted to study the relationships among intelligence, aphasia, and apraxia. The subjects were patients with focal left hemisphere damage. Scores on the following variables were obtained through application of standard tests.

$$Y = \text{intelligence}$$

$$X_1 = \text{ideomotor apraxia}$$

$$X_2 = \text{constructive apraxia}$$

$$X_3 = \text{lesion volume (pixels)}$$

$$X_4 = \text{severity of aphasia}$$

The results are shown in the following table. Find the multiple correlation coefficient and test for significance. Let $a = .05$ and find the p value.

Subject	Y	X_1	X_2	X_3	X_4
1	66	7.6	7.4	2296.87	2
2	78	13.2	11.9	2975.82	8
3	79	13.0	12.4	2839.38	11
4	84	14.2	13.3	3136.58	15
5	77	11.4	11.2	2470.50	5
6	82	14.4	13.1	3136.58	9
7	82	13.3	12.8	2799.55	8
8	75	12.4	11.9	2565.50	6
9	81	10.7	11.5	2429.49	11
10	71	7.6	7.8	2369.37	6
11	77	11.2	10.8	2644.62	7
12	74	9.7	9.7	2647.45	9
13	77	10.2	10.0	2672.92	7
14	74	10.1	9.7	2640.25	8
15	68	6.1	7.2	1926.60	5

10.7
Summary

In this chapter we examine how the concepts and techniques of simple linear regression and correlation analysis are extended to the multiple-variable case. The least-squares method of obtaining the regression equation is presented and illustrated. This chapter also is concerned with the calculation of descriptive measures, tests of significance, and the uses to be made of the multiple regression equation. In addition, the methods and concepts of correlation analysis, including partial correlation, are discussed. For those who wish to extend their knowledge of multiple regression and correlation analysis the references at the end of the chapter provide a good beginning.

When the assumptions underlying the methods of regression and correlation presented in this and the previous chapter are not met, the researcher must resort to alternative techniques. One alternative is to use a nonparametric procedure such as the ones discussed by Daniel (11, 12).

REVIEW QUESTIONS AND EXERCISES

1. What are the assumptions underlying multiple regression analysis when one wishes to infer about the population from which the sample data have been drawn?

2. What are the assumptions underlying the correlation model when inference is an objective?

3. Explain fully the following terms:
   a. Coefficient of multiple determination
   b. Multiple correlation coefficient
   c. Simple correlation coefficient
   d. Partial correlation coefficient

4. Describe a situation in your particular area of interest where multiple regression analysis would be useful. Use real or realistic data and do a complete regression analysis.

5. Describe a situation in your particular area of interest where multiple correlation analysis would be useful. Use real or realistic data and do a complete correlation analysis.

   In the exercises that follow carry out the indicated analysis and test hypotheses at the indicated significance levels. Compute the p-value for each test.

6. The following table shows certain pulmonary function values observed in 10 hospitalized patients.

X_1 Vital Capacity (Liters)	X_2 Total Lung Capacity (Liters)	Y Forced Expiratory Volume (Liters) per Second
2.2	2.5	1.6
1.5	3.2	1.0
1.6	5.0	1.4
3.4	4.4	2.6
2.0	4.4	1.2
1.9	3.3	1.5
2.2	3.2	1.6
3.3	3.3	2.3
2.4	3.7	2.1
.9	3.6	.7

Compute the multiple correlation coefficient and test for significance at the .05 level.

7. The following table shows the weight and total cholesterol and triglyceride levels in 15 patients with primary type II hyperlipoproteinemia just prior to initiation of treatment.

Y Weight (kg)	X_1 Total Cholesterol (mg / 100 ml)	X_2 Triglyceride (mg / 100 ml)
76	302	139
97	336	101
83	220	57
52	300	56
70	382	113
67	379	42
75	331	84
78	332	186
70	426	164
99	399	205
75	279	230
78	332	186
70	410	160
77	389	153
76	302	139

Compute the multiple correlation coefficient and test for significance at the .05 level.

8. In a study of the relationship between creatinine excretion, height, and weight the data shown in the following table were collected on 20 infant males.

Infant	Creatinine Excretion (mg / day) Y	Weight (kg) X_1	Height (cm) X_2
1	100	9	72
2	115	10	76
3	52	6	59
4	85	8	68
5	135	10	60
6	58	5	58
7	90	8	70
8	60	7	65
9	45	4	54
10	125	11	83
11	86	7	64
12	80	7	66
13	65	6	61
14	95	8	66
15	25	5	57
16	125	11	81
17	40	5	59
18	95	9	71
19	70	6	62
20	120	10	75

a. Find the multiple regression equation describing the relationship among these variables.
b. Compute R^2 and do an analysis of variance.
c. Let $X_1 = 10$ and $X_2 = 60$ and find the predicted value of Y.

9. A study was conducted to examine those variables throught to be related to the job satisfaction of nonprofessional hospital employees. A random sample of 15 employees gave the following results:

Score on Job Satisfaction Test (Y)	Coded Intelligence Score (X_1)	Index of Personal Adjustment (X_2)
54	15	8
37	13	1
30	15	1
48	15	7
37	10	4
37	14	2
31	8	3
49	12	7
43	1	9
12	3	1
30	15	1
37	14	2
61	14	10
31	9	1
31	4	5

a. Find the multiple regression equation describing the relationship among these variables.
b. Compute the coefficient of multiple determination and do an analysis of variance.
c. Let $X_1 = 10$ and $X_2 = 5$ and find the predicted value of Y.

10. A medical research team obtained the index of adiposity, basal insulin, and basal glucose values on 21 normal subjects. The results are shown in the following table. The researchers wished to investigate the strength of the association among these variables.

Index of Adiposity Y	Basal Insulin ($\mu U / ml$) X_1	Basal Glucose ($mg / 100\,ml$) X_2
90	12	98
112	10	103
127	14	101
137	11	102
103	10	90
140	38	108
105	9	100
92	6	101
92	8	92
96	6	91
114	9	95
108	9	95
160	41	117
91	7	101
115	9	86
167	40	106
108	9	84
156	43	117
167	17	99
165	40	104
168	22	85

Compute the multiple correlation coefficient and test for significance at the .05 level.

11. As part of a study to investigate the relationship between stress and certain other variables the following data were collected on a simple random sample of 15 corporate executives.
   a. Find the least-squares regression equation for these data.
   b. Construct the analysis of variance table and test the null hypothesis of no relationship among the five variables.
   c. Test the null hypothesis that each slope in the regression model is equal to zero.
   d. Find the multiple coefficient of determination and the multiple correlation coefficient. Let $\alpha = .05$ and find the p value for each test.

Measure of Stress (Y)	Measure of Firm Size (X_1)	Number of Years in Present Position (X_2)	Annual Salary $(\times 1000)$ (X_3)	Age (X_4)
101	812	15	$30	38
60	334	8	20	52
10	377	5	20	27
27	303	10	54	36
89	505	13	52	34
60	401	4	27	45
16	177	6	26	50
184	598	9	52	60
34	412	16	34	44
17	127	2	28	39
78	601	8	42	41
141	297	11	84	58
11	205	4	31	51
104	603	5	38	63
76	484	8	41	30

For each of the studies described in Exercises 12 through 16, answer as many of the following questions as possible:
   (a) Which is more relevant, regression analysis or correlation analysis, or are both techniques equally relevant?
   (b) Which is the dependent variable?
   (c) What are the independent variables?
   (d) What are the appropriate null and alternative hypotheses?
   (e) Which null hypotheses do you think were rejected? Why?
   (f) Which is the more relevant objective, prediction or estimation, or are the two equally relevant? Explain your answer.
   (g) What is the sampled population?
   (h) What is the target population?
   (i) Which variables are related to which other variables? Are the relationships direct or inverse?
   (j) Write out the regression equation using appropriate numbers for parameter estimates.
   (k) What is the numerical value of the coefficient of multiple determination?
   (l) Give numerical values for any correlation coefficients that you can.

12. Hursting et al. (A-6) evaluated the effects of certain demographic variables on prothrombin fragment 1.2 (F1.2) concentrations in a healthy population. Data were ob-

tained from 357 healthy individuals. In a multiple linear regression model, the logarithms of F1.2 concentrations were regressed on age, race, sex, and smoking status. The significant explanatory variables were age, sex, and smoking.

13. The relations between mechanical parameters and myosin heavy chain isoforms were studied in ovariectomized rats and estrogen-treated, ovariectomized rats by Hewett et al. (A-7). The researchers found that both maximum velocity of shortening (V_{max}) and maximum isometric force (P_{max}) correlated significantly with myosin heavy chain isoform (SM1) as a percentage of the total isoform species. The investigators used a multiple regression analysis with a model in which V_{max} is to be predicted from a knowledge of percent SM1 and P_{max} in that order. The model intercept is $-.246$, the regression coefficient associated with percent SM1 is .005, and the regression coefficient associated with P_{max} is .00005. Student t tests of the significance of the regression coefficients yielded p values of $p < .0002$ for percent SM1 and $p < .61$ for P_{max}.

14. Maier et al. (A-8) conducted a study to investigate the relationship between erythropoietin concentration in umbilical venous blood and clinical signs of fetal hypoxia. Subjects were 200 consecutively born neonates. Using a multiple regression analysis the investigators found that the erythropoietin concentration correlated significantly ($p < .01$) with fetal growth retardation and umbilical acidosis but not with gestational age, meconium-stained amniotic fluid, abnormal fetal heart rate pattern, or Apgar score at 5 minutes.

15. In a study by Sinha et al. (A-9) the correlation between dietary vitamin C and plasma ascorbic acid (AA) was examined in 68 nonsmoking male volunteers aged 30–59 years. The determinants of plasma AA were examined by a multiple regression model containing dietary vitamin C, calories, body weight, and amount of beverages consumed. A calculation of the relationship between vitamin C intake and plasma AA yielded $r = .43$ ($p < .0003$).

16. Carr et al. (A-10) investigated the relation between serum lipids, membrane fluidity, insulin, and the activity of the sodium–hydrogen exchanger in human lymphocytes from 83 subjects with no current disease. As part of a multiple regression analysis, tests were conducted of the strength of the relationship between the maximal proton efflux rate and age ($p = .005$), systolic blood pressure ($p = .04$), membrane anisotropy ($p = .03$), and serum cholesterol ($p = .03$).

Exercises for Use With the Large Data Sets Available on Computer Disk from the Publisher

1. Refer to the data on 500 patients who have sought treatment for the relief of respiratory disease symptoms (RESPDIS, Disk 2). A medical research team is conducting a study to determine what factors may be related to respiratory disease. The dependent variable Y is a measure of the severity of the disease. A larger value indicates a more serious condition. The independent variables are as follows.

X_1 = education (highest grade completed)

X_2 = measure of crowding of living quarters

X_3 = measure of air quality at place of residence

(a larger number indicates poorer quality)

X_4 = nutritional status (a large number indicates a higher level of nutrition)

X_5 = smoking status (0 = smoker, 1 = nonsmoker)

Select a simple random sample of subjects from this population and conduct a statistical analysis that you think would be of value to the research team. Prepare a narrative report of your results and conclusions. Use graphic illustrations where appropriate. Compare your results with those of your classmates. Consult your instructor regarding the size of sample you should select.

2. Refer to the data on cardiovascular risk factors (RISKFACT, Disk 3). The subjects are 1000 males engaged in sedentary occupations. You wish to study the relationships among risk factors in this population. The variables are

$$Y = \text{oxygen consumption}$$

$$X_1 = \text{systolic blood pressure (mm Hg)}$$

$$X_2 = \text{total cholesterol (mg/DL)}$$

$$X_3 = \text{HDL cholesterol (mg/DL)}$$

$$X_4 = \text{triglycerides (mg/DL)}$$

Select a simple random sample from this population and carry out an appropriate statistical analysis. Prepare a narrative report of your findings and compare them with those of your classmates. Consult with your instructor regarding the size of the sample.

REFERENCES

References Cited

1. George W. Snedecor and William G. Cochran, *Statistical Methods*, Sixth Edition, The Iowa State University Press, Ames, 1967.

2. Robert G. D. Steel and James H. Torrie, *Principles and Procedures of Statistics*, McGraw-Hill, New York, 1960.

3. R. L. Anderson and T. A. Bancroft, *Statistical Theory in Research*, McGraw-Hill, New York, 1952.

4. Mordecai Ezekiel and Karl A. Fox, *Methods of Correlation and Regression Analysis*, Third Edition, Wiley, New York, 1963.

5. M. H. Doolittle, "Method Employed in the Solution of Normal Equation and the Adjustment of a Triangulation," *U.S. Coast and Geodetic Survey Report*, 1878.

6. David Durand, "Joint Confidence Region for Multiple Regression Coefficients," *Journal of the American Statistical Association*, *49* (1954), 130–146.

7. John Neter, William Wasserman, and Michael H. Kutner, *Applied Linear Regression Models*, Second Edition, Irwin, Homewood, Ill., 1989.

8. R. C. Geary and C. E. V. Leser, "Significance Tests in Multiple Regression" *The American Statistician*, *22* (February 1968), 20–21.

9. R. A. Fisher, "The General Sampling Distribution of the Multiple Correlation Coefficient," *Proceedings of the Royal Society A*, *121* (1928), 654–673.

10. K. H. Kramer, "Tables for Constructing Confidence Limits on the Multiple Correlation Coefficient," *Journal of the American Statistical Association*, *58* (1963), 1082–1085.

11. Wayne W. Daniel, *Applied Nonparametric Statistics*, Second Edition, PWS-Kent, Boston, 1989.
12. Wayne W. Daniel, *Nonparametric, Distribution-Free, and Robust Procedures in Regression Analysis: A Selected Bibliography*, Vance Bibliographies, Monticello, Ill., June 1980.

Other References, Books

1. T. W. Anderson, *Introduction to Multivariate Statistical Analysis*, Wiley, New York, 1958.
2. Frank Andrews, James Morgan and John Sonquist, *Multiple Classification Analysis*, Survey Research Center, Ann Arbor, Mich., 1967.
3. William D. Berry and Stanley Feldman, *Multiple Regression in Practice*, Sage, Beverly Hills, Calif., 1985.
4. Cuthbert Daniel and Fred S. Wood, *Fitting Equations to Data*, Second Edition, Wiley-Interscience, New York, 1979.
5. Alan E. Treloar, *Correlation Analysis*, Burgess, Minneapolis, 1949.

Other References, Journal Articles

1. G. Heitmann and K. Ord, "An Interpretation of the Least Squares Regression Surface," *The American Statistician*, *39* (1985), 120–123.
2. R. G. Newton and D. J. Spurrell, "A Development of Multiple Regression for the Analysis of Routine Data," *Applied Statistic*, *16* (1967), 51–64.
3. Potluri Rao, "Some Notes on Misspecification in Multiple Regression," *The American Statistician*, *25* (*December* 1971), 37–39.
4. Neil S. Weiss, "A Graphical Representation of the Relationships Between Multiple Regression and Multiple Correlation," *The American Statistician*, *24* (April 1970), 25–29.
5. E. J. Williams, "The Analysis of Association Among Many Variates," *Journal of the Royal Statistical Society*, *29* (1967), 199–242.

Other References, Other Publications

1. R. L. Bottenberg and Y. H. Ward, Jr., *Applied Multiple Linear Regression*, U.S. Department of Commerce, Office of Technical Services, AD 413128, 1963.
2. Wayne W. Daniel, *Ridge Regression: A Selected Bibliography*, Vance Bibliographies, Monticello, Ill., October 1980.
3. Wayne W. Daniel, *Outliers in Research Data: A Selected Bibliography*, Vance Bibliographies, Monticello, Ill., July 1980.
4. Jean Draper, *Interpretation of Multiple Regression Analysis Part I, Problems of Interpreting Large Samples of Data*, The University of Arizona, College of Business and Public Administration, Division of Economics and Business Research, 1968.

Applications References

A-1. Werner Kalow and Bing-Kou Tang, "Caffeine as a Metabolic Probe: Exploration of the Enzyme-Inducing Effect of Cigarette Smoking," *Clinical Pharmacology & Threapeutics*, *49* (1991), 44–48.
A-2. James F. Malec, Jeffrey S. Smigielski, and Robert W. DePompolo, "Goal Attainment Scaling and Outcome Measurement in Postacute Brain Injury Rehabilitation," *Archives of Physical Medicine and Rehabilitation*, *72* (1991), 138–143.
A-3. Sandra K. David and William T. Riley, "The Relationship of the Allen Cognitive Level Test to Cognitive Abilities and Psychopathology," *American Journal of Occupational Therapy*, *44* (1990), 493–497.
A-4. Neal L. Benowitz, Peyton Jacob, III, Charles Denaro, and Roger Jenkins, "Stable Isotope Studies of Nicotine Kinetics and Bioavailability," *Clinical Pharmacology & Therapeutics*, *49* (1991), 270–277.

A-5. David M. Steinhorn and Thomas P. Green, "Severity of Illness Correlates With Alterations in Energy Metabolism in the Pediatric Intensive Care Unit," *Critical Care Medicine*, *19* (1991), 1503–1509.

A-6. M. J. Hursting, A. G. Stead, F. V. Crout, B. Z. Horvath, and B. M. Moore, "Effects of Age, Race, Sex, and Smoking on Prothrombin Fragment 1.2 in a Healthy Population," *Clinical Chemistry*, *39* (April 1993), 683–686.

A-7. T. E. Hewett, A. F. Martin, and R. J. Paul, "Correlations Between Myosin Heavy Chain Isoforms and Mechanical Parameters in Rat Myometrium," *Journal of Physiology (Cambridge)*, *460* (January 1993), 351–364.

A-8. R. F. Maier, K. Bohme, J. W. Dudenhausen, and M. Obladen, "Cord Erythropoietin in Relation to Different Markers of Fetal Hypoxia," *Obstetrics and Gynecology*, *81* (1993), 575–580.

A-9. R. Sinha, G. Block, and P. R. Taylor, "Determinants of Plasma Ascorbic Acid in a Healthy Male Population," *Cancer Epidemiology, Biomarkers and Prevention*, *1* (May–June 1992), 297–302.

A-10. P. Carr, N. A. Taub, G. F. Watts, and L. Poston, "Human Lymphocyte Sodium–Hydrogen Exchange. The Influences of Lipids, Membrane Fluidity, and Insulin," *Hypertension*, *21* (March 1993), 344–352.

CHAPTER **11**

Regression Analysis — Some Additional Techniques

· · · · · · · · · · · · · · · · · ·

CONTENTS

11.1 Introduction
11.2 Qualitative Independent Variables
11.3 Variable Selection Procedures
11.4 Logistic Regression
11.5 Summary

11.1
Introduction

The basic concepts and methodology of regression analysis are covered in Chapters 9 and 10. In Chapter 9 we discuss the situation in which the objective is to obtain an equation that can be used to make predictions and estimates about some dependent variable from a knowledge of some other single variable that we call the independent, predictor, or explanatory variable. In Chapter 10 the ideas and techniques learned in Chapter 9 are expanded to cover the situation in which it is believed that the inclusion of information on two or more independent variables will yield a better equation for use in making predictions and estimations. Regression analysis is a complex and powerful statistical tool that is widely employed in health sciences research. To do the subject justice requires more space than is available in an introductory statistics textbook. However, for the benefit of those

459

who wish additional coverage of regression analysis we present in this chapter some additional topics that should prove helpful to the student and practitioner of statistics.

11.2
Qualitative Independent Variables

The independent variables considered in the discussion in Chapter 10 were all quantitative; that is, they yielded numerical values that either were counts or were measurements in the usual sense of the word. For example, some of the independent variables used in our examples and exercises were age, urinary cotinine level, number of cigarettes smoked per day, and minute oxygen consumption, aptitude test scores, and number of current medical problems. Frequently, however, it is desirable to use one or more qualitative variables as independent variables in the regression model. Qualitative variables, it will be recalled, are those variables whose "values" are categories and convey the concept of attribute rather than amount or quantity. The variable marital status, for example, is a qualitative variable whose categories are "single," "married," "widowed," and "divorced." Other examples of qualitative variables include sex (male or female), diagnosis, race, occupation, and immunity status to some disease. In certain situations an investigator may suspect that including one or more variables such as these in the regression equation would contribute significantly to the reduction of the error sum of squares and thereby provide more precise estimates of the parameters of interest.

Suppose, for example, that we are studying the relationship between the dependent variable systolic blood pressure and the independent variables weight and age. We might also want to include the qualitative variable sex as one of the independent variables. Or suppose we wish to gain insight into the nature of the relationship between lung capacity and other relevant variables. Candidates for inclusion in the model might consist of such quantitative variables as height, weight, and age, as well as qualitative variables like sex, area of residence (urban, suburban, rural), and smoking status (current smoker, ex-smoker, never smoked).

Dummy Variables   In order to incorporate a qualitative independent variable in the multiple regression model it must be quantified in some manner. This may be accomplished through the use of what are known as *dummy variables*.

A dummy variable is a variable that assumes only a finite number of values (such as 0 or 1) for the purpose of identifying the different categories of a qualitative variable.

The term "dummy" is used to indicate the fact that the numerical values (such as 0 and 1) assumed by the variable have no quantitative meaning but are used merely to identify different categories of the qualitative variable under consideration.

The following are some examples of qualitative variables and the dummy variables used to quantify them.

Qualitative Variable	Dummy Variable
Sex (male, female):	$x_1 = \begin{cases} 1 \text{ for male} \\ 0 \text{ for female} \end{cases}$
Place of residence (urban, rural, suburban):	$x_1 = \begin{cases} 1 \text{ for urban} \\ 0 \text{ for rural and suburban} \end{cases}$ $x_2 = \begin{cases} 1 \text{ for rural} \\ 0 \text{ for urban and suburban} \end{cases}$
Smoking status [current smoker, ex-smoker (has not smoked for 5 years or less), ex-smoker (has not smoked for more than 5 years), never smoked]:	$x_1 = \begin{cases} 1 \text{ for current smoker} \\ 0 \text{ otherwise} \end{cases}$ $x_2 = \begin{cases} 1 \text{ for ex-smoker } (\leq 5 \text{ years}) \\ 0 \text{ otherwise} \end{cases}$ $x_3 = \begin{cases} 1 \text{ for ex-smoker } (> 5 \text{ years}) \\ 0 \text{ otherwise} \end{cases}$

Note in these examples that when the qualitative variable has k categories, $k - 1$ dummy variables must be defined for all the categories to be properly coded. This rule is applicable for any multiple regression containing an intercept constant. The variable sex, with two categories, can be quantified by the use of only one dummy variable, while three dummy variables are required to quantify the variable smoking status, which has four categories.

The following examples illustrate some of the uses of qualitative variable in multiple regression. In the first example we assume that there is no interaction between the independent variables. Since the assumption of no interaction is not realistic in many instances, we illustrate, in the second example, the analysis that is appropriate when interaction between variables is accounted for.

Example 11.2.1

In a study of factors thought to be associated with birth weight, data from a simple random sample of 32 birth records were examined. Table 11.2.1 shows part of the data that were extracted from each record. There we see that we have two independent variables: length of gestation in weeks, which is quantitative; and smoking status of mother, a qualitative variable.

Solution: For the analysis of the data we will quantify smoking status by means of a dummy variable that is coded 1 if the mother is a smoker and 0 if she is a nonsmoker. The data in Table 11.2.1 are plotted as a scatter diagram in Figure 11.2.1. The scatter diagram suggests that, in general, longer periods of gestation are associated with larger birth weights.

TABLE 11.2.1 Data Collected on a Simple Random Sample of 32 Births, Example 11.2.1

Case	Y Birth Weight (Grams)	X_1 Gestation (Weeks)	X_2 Smoking Status of Mother
1	2940	38	Smoker (S)
2	3130	38	Nonsmoker (N)
3	2420	36	S
4	2450	34	N
5	2760	39	S
6	2440	35	S
7	3226	40	N
8	3301	42	S
9	2729	37	N
10	3410	40	N
11	2715	36	S
12	3095	39	N
13	3130	39	S
14	3244	39	N
15	2520	35	N
16	2928	39	S
17	3523	41	N
18	3446	42	S
19	2920	38	N
20	2957	39	S
21	3530	42	N
22	2580	38	S
23	3040	37	N
24	3500	42	S
25	3200	41	S
26	3322	39	N
27	3459	40	N
28	3346	42	S
29	2619	35	N
30	3175	41	S
31	2740	38	S
32	2841	36	N

To obtain additional insight into the nature of these data we may enter them into a computer and employ an appropriate program to perform further analyses. For example, we enter the observations $y_1 = 2940$, $x_{11} = 38$, $x_{21} = 1$, for the first case, $y_2 = 3130$, $x_{12} = 38$, $x_{22} = 0$ for the second case, and so on. Figure 11.2.2 shows the computer output obtained with the use of the MINITAB multiple regression program.

We see in the printout that the multiple regression equation is

$$\hat{y}_j = b_0 + b_1 x_{1j} + b_2 x_{2j}$$

$$\hat{y}_j = -2390 + 143 x_{1j} - 245 x_{2j} \tag{11.2.1}$$

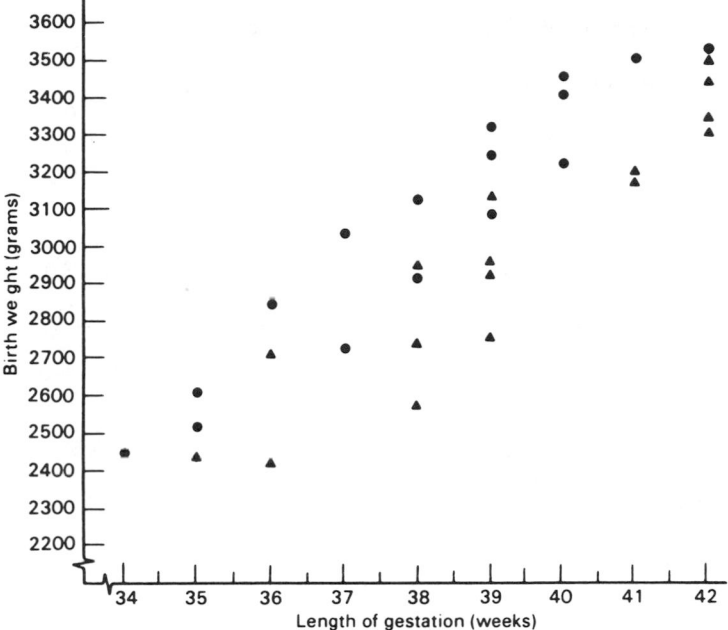

Figure 11.2.1 Birth weights and lengths of gestation for 32 births: (▲) smoking and (●) nonsmoking mothers.

To observe the effect on this equation when we wish to consider only the births to smoking mothers, we let $x_{2j} = 1$. The equation then becomes

$$\hat{y}_j = -2390 + 143x_{1j} - 245(1)$$

$$= -2635 + 143x_{1j} \qquad (11.2.2)$$

which has a y-intercept of -2635 and a slope of 143. Note that the y-intercept for the new equation is equal to $(b_0 + b_1) = [-2390 + (-245)] = -2635$.

Now let us consider only births to nonsmoking mothers. When we let $x_2 = 0$, our regression equation reduces to

$$\hat{y}_j = -2390 + 143x_{1j} - 245(0)$$

$$= -2390 + 143x_{1j} \qquad (11.2.3)$$

The slope of this equation is the same as the slope of the equation for smoking mothers, but the y-intercepts are different. The y-intercept for the equation associated with nonsmoking mothers is larger than the one for the smoking mothers. These results show that for this sample babies born to mothers who do not smoke weighed, on the average, more than babies born to mothers who do

```
The regression equation is

y = - 2390 + 143 x1 + -245 x2

 Predictor  Coef      Stdev    t-ratio   p
 Constant   -2389.6   349.2    -6.84     0.000
 x1         143.100   9.128    15.68     0.000
 x2         -244.54   41.98    -5.83     0.000


 s = 115.5   R-sq = 89.6%   R-sq(adj) = 88.9%

Analysis of Variance


 SOURCE       DF   SS        MS        F        p
 Regression   2    3348720   1674360   125.45   0.000
 Error        29   387070    13347
 Total        31   3735789


 SOURCE       DF   SEQ SS
 x1           1    2895839
 x2           1    452881
```

Figure 11.2.2 Partial computer printout, MINITAB multiple regression analysis, Example 11.2.1.

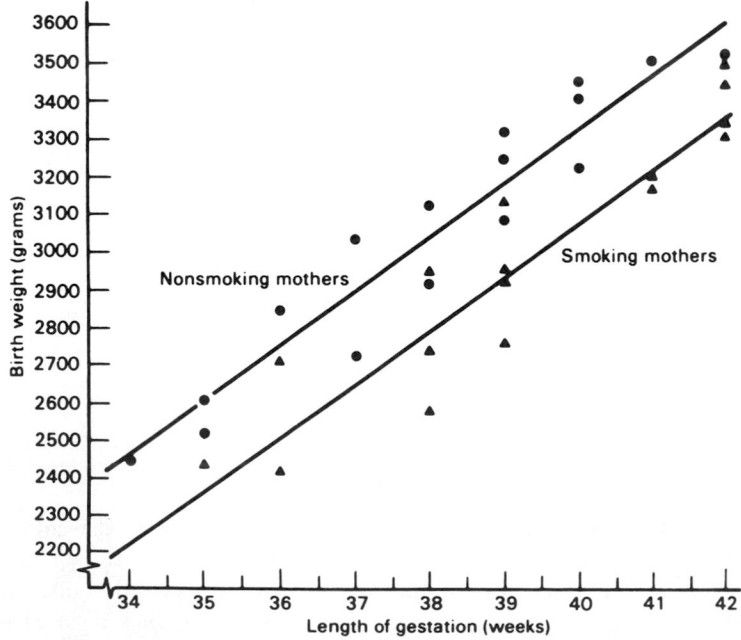

Figure 11.2.3 Birth weights and length of gestation for 32 births and the fitted regression lines: (▲) smoking and (●) nonsmoking mothers.

smoke, when length of gestation is taken into account. The amount of the difference, on the average, is 245 grams. Stated another way, we can say that for this sample babies born to mothers who smoke weighed, on the average, 245 grams less than the babies born to mothers who do not smoke, when length of gestation is taken into account. Figure 11.2.3 shows the scatter diagram of the original data along with a plot of the two regression lines (Equations 11.2.2 and 11.2.3).

**Example
11.2.2**

At this point a question arises regarding what inferences we can make about the sampled population on the basis of the sample results obtained in Example 11.2.1. First of all, we wish to know if the sample difference of 245 grams is significant. In other words, does smoking have an effect on birth weight? We may answer this question through the following hypothesis testing procedure.

Solution:

1. *Data*   The data are as given in Example 11.2.1.

2. *Assumptions*   We presume that the assumptions underlying multiple regression analysis are met.

3. *Hypotheses* H_0: $\beta_2 = 0$; H_A: $\beta_2 \neq 0$. Suppose we let $\alpha = .05$.

4. *Test Statistic*   The test statistic is $t = (b_2 - 0)/s_{b_2}$.

5. *Distribution of Test Statistic*   When the assumptions are met and H_0 is true the test statistic is distributed as Student's t with 29 degrees of freedom.

6. *Decision Rule*   We reject H_0 if the computed t is either greater than or equal to 2.0452 or less than or equal to -2.0452.

7. *Calculation of Test Statistic*   The calculated value of the test statistic appears in Figure 11.2.2 as the t ratio for the coefficient associated with the variable appearing in column 3 of Table 11.2.1. This coefficient, of course, is b_2. We see that the computed t is -5.83.

8. *Statistical Decision*   Since $-5.83 < -2.0452$, we reject H_0.

9. *Conclusion*   We conclude that, in the sampled population, whether or not the mothers smoke does have an effect on the birth weights of their babies.

   For this test we have $p < 2(.005)$ since -5.83 is less than -2.7564.

A Confidence Interval for β_2   Given that we are able to conclude that in the sampled population the smoking status of the mothers does have an effect on the birth weights of their babies, we may now inquire as to the magnitude of the effect. Our best point estimate of the average difference in birth weights, when length of gestation is taken into account, is 245 grams in favor of babies born to mothers who do not smoke. We may obtain an interval estimate of the mean amount of the difference by using information from the computer printout by means of the following expression:

$$b_2 \pm t s_{b_2}$$

For a 95 percent confidence interval we have

$$-244.54 \pm 2.0452(41.98)$$

$$-330.3975, \; -158.6825$$

Thus we are 95 percent confident that the difference is somewhere between about 159 grams and 331 grams.

Advantages of Dummy Variables   The reader may have correctly surmised that an alternative analysis of the data of Example 11.2.1 would consist of fitting two separate regression equations: one to the subsample of mothers who smoke and another to the subsample of those who do not. Such an approach, however, lacks some of the advantages of the dummy variable technique and is a less desirable procedure when the latter procedure is valid. If we can justify the assumption that the two separate regression lines have the same slope, we can get a better estimate of this common slope through the use of dummy variables, which entails pooling of the data from the two subsamples. In Example 11.2.1 the estimate using a dummy variable is based on a total sample size of 32 observations, whereas separate estimates would each be based on a sample of only 16 observations. The dummy variable approach also yields more precise inferences regarding other parameters since more degrees of freedom are available for the calculation of the error mean square.

Use of Dummy Variables — Interaction Present   Now let us consider the situation in which interaction between the variables is assumed to be present. Suppose, for example, that we have two independent variables: one quantitative variable x_1 and one qualitative variable with three response levels yielding the two dummy variables X_2 and X_3. The model, then, would be

$$y_j = \beta_0 + \beta_1 X_{1j} + \beta_2 X_{2j} + \beta_3 X_{3j} + \beta_4 X_{1j} X_{2j} + \beta_5 X_{1j} X_{3j} + e_j \qquad (11.2.4)$$

in which $\beta_4 X_{1j} X_{2j}$ and $\beta_5 X_{1j} X_{3j}$ are called *interaction terms* and represent the interaction between the quantitative and the qualitative independent variables. Note that there is no need to include in the model the term containing $X_{2j} X_{3j}$; it will always be zero because when $X_2 = 1$, $X_3 = 0$ and when $X_3 = 1$, $X_2 = 0$. The model of Equation 11.2.4 allows for a different slope and Y-intercept for each level of the qualitative variable.

Suppose we use dummy variable coding to quantify the qualitative variable as follows:

$$X_3 = \begin{cases} 1 \text{ for level 1} \\ 0 \text{ otherwise} \end{cases}$$

$$X_2 = \begin{cases} 1 \text{ for level 2} \\ 0 \text{ otherwise} \end{cases}$$

The three sample regression equations for the three levels of the qualitative variable, then, are as follows:

Level 1 ($X_2 = 1$, $X_3 = 0$):

$$\hat{y}_j = b_0 + b_1 x_{1j} + b_2(1) + b_3(0) + b_4 x_{1j}(1) + b_5 x_{1j}(0)$$

$$= b_0 + b_1 x_{1j} + b_2 + b_4 x_{1j}$$

$$= (b_0 + b_2) + (b_1 + b_4)x_{1j} \qquad (11.2.5)$$

Level 2 ($X_2 = 0$, $X_3 = 1$):

$$\hat{y}_j = b_0 + b_1 x_{1j} + b_2(0) + b_3(1) + b_4 x_{1j}(0) + b_5 x_{1j}(1)$$

$$= b_0 + b_1 x_{1j} + b_3 + b_5 x_{1j}$$

$$= (b_0 + b_3) + (b_1 + b_5)x_{1j} \qquad (11.2.6)$$

Level 3 ($X_2 = 0$, $X_3 = 0$):

$$\hat{y} = b_0 + b_1 x_{1j} + b_2(0) + b_3(0) + b_4 x_{1j}(0) + b_5 x_{1j}(0)$$

$$\hat{y}_j = b_0 + b_1 x_{1j} \qquad (11.2.7)$$

Let us illustrate these results by means of an example.

Example 11.2.3

A team of mental health researchers wishes to compare three methods (A, B, and C) of treating severe depression. They would also like to study the relationship between age and treatment effectiveness as well as the interaction (if any) between age and treatment. Each member of a simple random sample of 36 patients, comparable with respect to diagnosis and severity of depression, was randomly assigned to receive treatment A, B, or C. The results are shown in Table 11.2.2. The dependent variable Y is treatment effectiveness, the quantitative independent variable X_1 is patient's age at nearest birthday, and the independent variable type of treatment is a qualitative variable that occurs at three levels. The following dummy variable coding is used to quantify the qualitative variable:

$$X_2 = \begin{cases} 1 \text{ if treatment A} \\ 0 \text{ otherwise} \end{cases}$$

$$X_3 = \begin{cases} 1 \text{ if treatment B} \\ 0 \text{ otherwise} \end{cases}$$

The scatter diagram for these data is shown in Figure 11.2.4. Table 11.2.3 shows the data as they were entered into a computer for analysis, and Figure 11.2.5

TABLE 11.2.2 Data for Example 11.2.3

Measure of Effectiveness	Age	Method of Treatment
56	21	A
41	23	B
40	30	B
28	19	C
55	28	A
25	23	C
46	33	B
71	67	C
48	42	B
63	33	A
52	33	A
62	56	C
50	45	C
45	43	B
58	38	A
46	37	C
58	43	B
34	27	C
65	43	A
55	45	B
57	48	B
59	47	C
64	48	A
61	53	A
62	58	B
36	29	C
69	53	A
47	29	B
73	58	A
64	66	B
60	67	B
62	63	A
71	59	C
62	51	C
70	67	A
71	63	C

contains the printout of the analysis using the MINITAB multiple regression program.

Solution: Now let us examine the printout to see what it provides in the way of insight into the nature of the relationships among the variables. The least-squares equation is

$$\hat{y}_j = 6.21 + 1.03x_{1j} + 41.3x_{2j} + 22.7x_{3j} - .703x_{1j}x_{2j} - .510x_{1j}x_{3j}$$

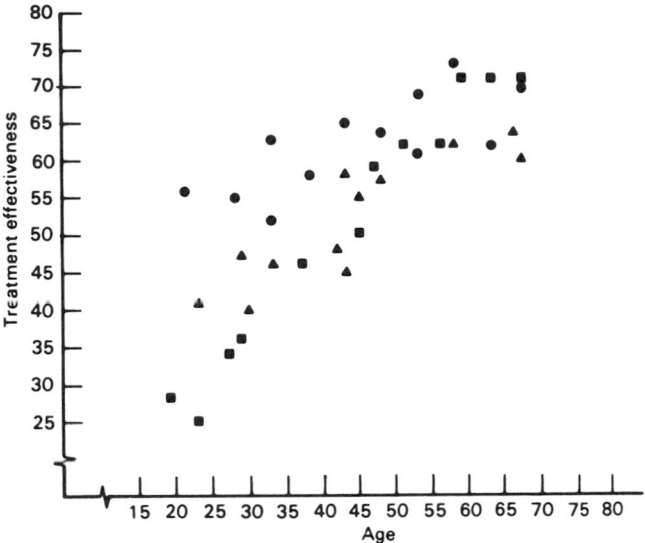

Figure 11.2.4 Scatter diagram of data for Example 11.2.3 (●) treatment A, (▲) treatment B, (■) treatment C.

The three regression equations for the three treatments are as follows:

Treatment A (Equation 11.2.5):

$$\hat{y}_j = (6.21 + 41.3) + (1.03 - .703)x_{1j}$$

$$= 47.51 + .327x_{1j}$$

Treatment B (Equation 11.2.6):

$$\hat{y}_j = (6.21 + 22.7) + (1.03 - .510)x_{1j}$$

$$= 28.91 + .520x_{1j}$$

Treatment C (Equation 11.2.7):

$$\hat{y}_j = 6.21 + 1.03x_{1j}$$

Figure 11.2.6 contains the scatter diagram of the original data along with the regression equations for the three treatments. Visual inspection of Figure 11.2.6 suggests that treatments A and B do not differ greatly with respect to their slopes, but their y-intercepts are considerably different. The graph suggests that treatment A is better than treatment B for younger patients, but the difference is less dramatic with older patients. Treatment C appears to be decidedly less desirable than both treatments A and B for younger patients, but is about as effective as

TABLE 11.2.3 Data for Example 11.2.3 Coded for Computer Analysis

Y	X_1	X_2	X_3	X_1X_2	X_1X_3
56	21	1	0	21	0
55	28	1	0	28	0
63	33	1	0	33	0
52	33	1	0	33	0
58	38	1	0	38	0
65	43	1	0	43	0
64	48	1	0	48	0
61	53	1	0	53	0
69	53	1	0	53	0
73	58	1	0	58	0
62	63	1	0	63	0
70	67	1	0	67	0
41	23	0	1	0	23
40	30	0	1	0	30
46	33	0	1	0	33
48	42	0	1	0	42
45	43	0	1	0	43
58	43	0	1	0	43
55	45	0	1	0	45
57	48	0	1	0	48
62	58	0	1	0	58
47	29	0	1	0	29
64	66	0	1	0	66
60	67	0	1	0	67
28	19	0	0	0	0
25	23	0	0	0	0
71	67	0	0	0	0
62	56	0	0	0	0
50	45	0	0	0	0
46	37	0	0	0	0
34	27	0	0	0	0
59	47	0	0	0	0
36	29	0	0	0	0
71	59	0	0	0	0
62	51	0	0	0	0
71	63	0	0	0	0

treatment B for older patients. These subjective impressions are compatible with the contention that there is interaction between treatments and age.

Inference Procedures   The relationships we see in Figure 11.2.6, however, are sample results. What can we conclude about the population from which the sample was drawn?

For an answer let us look at the t ratios on the computer printout in Figure 11.2.5. Each of these is the test statistic

$$t = \frac{b_i - 0}{s_{b_i}}$$

```
The regression equation is
y = 6.21 + 1.03 x1 + 41.3 x2 + 22.7 x3 - 0.703 x4
  - 0.510 x5


Predictor   Coef      Stdev     t-ratio   p
Constant    6.211     3.350     1.85      0.074
x1          1.03339   0.07233   14.29     0.000
x2          41.304    5.085     8.12      0.000
x3          22.707    5.091     4.46      0.000
x4         -0.7029    0.1090   -6.45      0.000
x5         -0.5097    0.1104   -4.62      0.000


s = 3.925   R-sq = 91.4%   R-sq(adj) = 90.0%

Analysis of Variance


SOURCE        DF    SS        MS       F       p
Regression    5     4932.85   986.57   64.04   0.000
Error         30     462.15    15.40
Total         35    5395.00

SOURCE        DF    SEQ SS
x1            1     3424.43
x2            1      803.80
x3            1        1.19
x4            1      375.00
x5            1      328.42
```

Figure 11.2.5 Computer printout, MINITAB multiple regression analysis, Example 11.2.3.

for testing H_0: $\beta_i = 0$. We see by Equation 11.2.5 that the y-intercept of the regression line for treatment A is equal to $b_0 + b_2$. Since the t ratio of 8.12 for testing H_0: $\beta_2 = 0$ is greater than the critical t of 2.0423 (for $\alpha = .05$), we can reject H_0 that $\beta_2 = 0$ and conclude that the y-intercept of the population regression line for treatment A is different from the y-intercept of the population regression line for treatment C, which has a y-intercept of β_0. Similarly, since the t ratio of 4.46 for testing H_0: $\beta_3 = 0$ is also greater than the critical t of 2.0423, we can conclude (at the .05 level of significance) that the y-intercept of the population regression line for treatment B is also different from the y-intercept of the population regression line for treatment C. (See the y-intercept of Equation 11.2.6.)

Now let us consider the slopes. We see by Equation 11.2.5 that the slope of the regression line for treatment A is equal to b_1 (the slope of the line for treatment

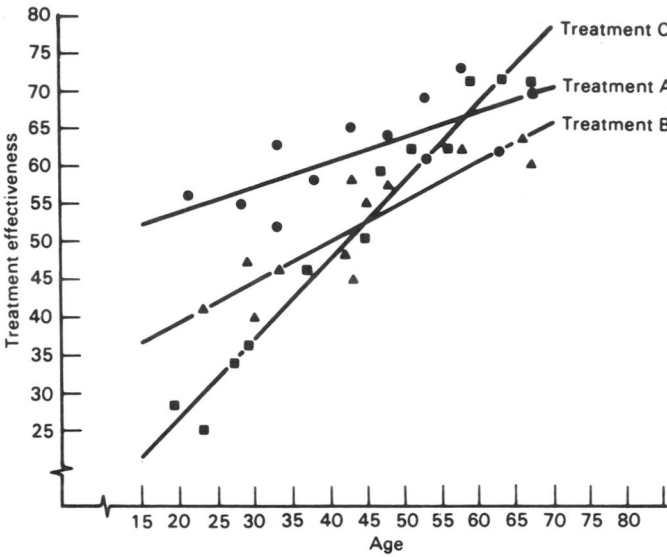

Figure 11.2.6 Scatter diagram of data for Example 11.2.3 with the fitted regression lines: (●) treatment A, (▲) treatment B, (■) treatment C.

C) $+ b_4$. Since the t ratio of -6.45 for testing H_0: $\beta_4 = 0$ is less than the critical t of -2.0423, we can conclude (for $\alpha = .05$) that the slopes of the population regression lines for treatments A and C are different. Similarly, since the computed t ratio for testing H_0: $\beta_5 = 0$ is also less than -2.0423, we conclude (for $\alpha = .05$) that the population regression lines for treatments B and C have different slopes (see the slope of Equation 11.2.6). Thus we conclude that there is interaction between age and type of treatment. This is reflected by a lack of parallelism among the regression lines in Figure 11.2.6.

Another question of interest is this: Is the slope of the population regression line for treatment A different from the slope of the population regression line for treatment B? To answer this question requires computational techniques beyond the scope of this text. The interested reader is referred to the books by Neter et al. (1) and Kleinbaum et al. (2) for help with this problem.

In Section 10.4 the reader was warned that there are problems involved in making multiple inferences from the same sample data. The references cited in that section may be consulted for procedures to be followed when multiple inferences, such as those discussed in this section, are desired.

We have discussed only two situations in which the use of dummy variables is appropriate. More complex models involving the use of one or more qualitative independent variables in the presence of two or more quantitative variables may be appropriate in certain circumstances. More complex models are discussed by

Mendenhall and McClave (3), Kleinbaum et al. (2), Draper and Smith (4), and Neter et al. (1).

EXERCISES

For each exercise do the following:

(a) Draw a scatter diagram of the data using different symbols for the different categorical variables.

(b) Use dummy variable coding and regression to analyze the data.

(c) Perform appropriate hypothesis tests and construct appropriate confidence intervals using your choice of significance and confidence levels

(d) Find the p value for each test that you perform.

11.2.1 Woo et al. (A-1) point out that current methods of measuring cardiac output require the invasive insertion of a thermodilution catheter, a procedure accompanied by risks and complications. These researchers examined the noninvasive method of transthoracic electrical bioimpedance (TEB) in comparison with the invasive procedure (Td). Their subjects were critically ill patients with poor left ventricular function and with either ischemic or idiopathic dilated cardiomyopathy. Resulting pairs of cardiac outputs measured by the two methods were divided into two categories, those in which the difference between outputs for the two methods was less than .5 l/min and those in which the difference was greater than .5 l/min. The results were as follows:

Less than .5 l / min. Difference		More than .5 l / min. Difference			
Td	**TEB**	**Td**	**TEB**	**Td**	**TEB**
4.88	5.03	3.64	2.8	3.97	2.9
2.8	3.23	7.41	8.1	3.64	4.18
4.82	4.37	3.98	2.57	5.48	4.08
5.7	5.6	8.57	5.5	7.73	3.57
3.7	3.4	2.18	3.3	4.74	5.3
2.86	3.13	3.38	2.73	4.64	2.9
2.36	2.83	2.49	5.8	3.49	4.23
4.04	4.03	3.1	7	2.57	3.47
4.33	4.4	2.69	5.9	4.3	6.33
4.51	4.8	2.64	3.4	3.1	4.1
7.36	7.2	4.16	5.6	5.82	6.9
2.38	2.37	1.9	3.73	3.28	5.33
3.29	3.13	3.4	4.3	6.58	7.93
5.2	5.35	7.5	6.6	4.79	3.4
3.49	3.13	4.41	3.25	8.05	5.7
4.08	4.5	5.06	3.13	2.92	5.13
3.89	3.4	6.5	10.03		
3.41	3.9	5.59	3.03		
4.38	4	4.48	2.17		
2.8	2.73	2.63	5.7		
3.5	3.15	6.03	7		

Table (*continued*)

Less than .5 l / min. Difference		More than .5 l / min. Difference			
Td	**TEB**	**Td**	**TEB**	**Td**	**TEB**
3.45	3.47	2.92	4.2		
4.17	4.1	5.75	4.53		
2.49	2.77	3.43	6.17		
4.89	4.63	4.36	6.17		
		2.18	3.03		
		4.95	2.9		
		3.91	4.58		
		6.23	3.63		
		4.76	3.77		
		3.66	2.85		
		4.95	6.17		
		2.7	3.53		
		3.58	2.23		
		3.13	2.05		
		2.9	4.9		
		6.19	5.63		
		6.1	7.4		
		7.15	5.1		

SOURCE: Mary A. Woo, DNSc., R.N. Used by permission.

11.2.2 According to Schwartz et al. (A-2) investigators have demonstrated that in patients with obstructive sleep apnea weight reduction results in a decrease in apnea severity. The mechanism involved is unclear, but Schwartz and his colleagues hypothesize that decreases in upper airway collapsibility account for decreases in apnea severity with weight loss. To determine whether weight loss causes decreases in collapsibility, they measured the upper airway critical pressure before and after reduction in body mass index in 13 patients with obstructive sleep apnea. Thirteen weight-stable control subjects matched for age, body mass index, gender (all men), and nonrapid eye movement disordered breathing rate were studied before and after usual care intervention. The following are the changes in upper airway critical pressure (CPCRIT) (cm H_2O) and body mass index (CBMI) (kg/m^2) following intervention and group membership (0 = weight-loss group, 1 = usual-care group) of the subjects.

Subject	CPCRIT	CBMI	Group
1	−4.0	−7.4420	0
2	−5.2	−6.2894	0
3	−9.2	−8.9897	0
4	−5.9	−4.2663	0
5	−7.2	−8.0755	0
6	−6.3	−10.5133	0
7	−4.7	−3.1076	0
8	−9.3	−6.6595	0
9	−4.9	−5.7514	0
10	.4	−5.3274	0
11	−2.7	−10.5106	0
12	−10.4	−14.9994	0
13	−1.7	−2.5526	0

Subject	CPCRIT	CBMI	Group
14	.2	−.9783	1
15	−2.7	.0000	1
16	−2.8	.0000	1
17	−1.8	.4440	1
18	−2.2	1.3548	1
19	−.3	−.9278	1
20	−.9	−.7464	1
21	−.4	1.9881	1
22	−1.7	−.9783	1
23	2.7	1.3591	1
24	1.3	.9031	1
25	1.0	−1.4125	1
26	.3	−.1430	1

SOURCE: Alan R. Schwartz, M.D. Used by permission.

11.2.3 The purpose of a study by Loi et al. (A-3) was to investigate the effect of mexiletine on theophylline metabolism in young, healthy male and female nonsmokers. Theophylline is a bronchodilator used in the treatment of asthma and chronic obstructive pulmonary disease. Mexiletine is an effective type I antiarrhythmic agent used in the treatment of ventricular arrhythmias. The following table shows the percent change in plasma clearance of theophylline (Y), the mean steady-state plasma concentration of mexiletine (μg/ml) (X), and gender of the 15 subjects who participated in the study.

Subject	Y	X	Gender[a]
1	41.0	1.05	1
2	46.2	.46	1
3	44.3	.58	1
4	53.1	.70	1
5	57.8	1.07	1
6	48.4	.68	1
7	31.3	.71	1
8	39.6	.87	1
9	21.8	.73	0
10	49.1	.72	0
11	47.4	.82	0
12	27.3	.54	0
13	39.7	.58	0
14	48.5	1.53	0
15	39.7	.57	0

[a] 1 = female, 0 = male.
SOURCE: Robert E. Vestal, M.D. Used by permission.

11.2.4 Researchers wished to study the effect of biofeedback and manual dexterity on the ability of patients to perform a complicated task accurately. Twenty-eight patients were randomly selected from those referred for physical therapy. The 28 were then randomly assigned to either receive or not receive biofeedback. The dependent variable is the number of consecutive repetitions of the task completed before an error was made. The following are the results.

Biofeedback	Manual Dexterity Score	Number of Repetitions (Y)
Yes	225	88
Yes	88	102
No	162	73
Yes	90	105
No	245	51
Yes	150	52
Yes	87	106
Yes	212	76
Yes	112	100
Yes	77	112
No	137	89
No	171	52
No	199	49
Yes	137	75
No	149	50
Yes	251	75
No	102	75
Yes	90	112
No	180	55
Yes	25	115
No	142	50
No	88	87
No	87	106
No	101	91
Yes	211	75
Yes	136	70
No	100	100
Yes	100	100

11.3
Variable Selection Procedures

Health sciences researchers contemplating the use of multiple regression analysis to solve problems usually find that they have a large number of variables from which to select the independent variables to be employed as predictors of the dependent variable. Such investigators will want to include in their model as many variables as possible in order to maximize the model's predictive ability. The investigator must realize, however, that adding another independent variable to a set of independent variables always increases the coefficient of determination R^2. Therefore, independent variables should not be added to the model indiscriminately, but only for good reason. In most situations, for example, some potential predictor variables are more expensive than others in terms of data-collection costs. The cost-conscious investigator, therefore, will not want to include an expensive variable in a model unless there is evidence that it makes a worthwhile contribution to the predictive ability of the model.

The investigator who wishes to use multiple regression analysis most effectively must be able to employ some strategy for making intelligent selections from among those potential predictor variables that are available. Many such strategies are in current use, and each has its proponents. The strategies vary in terms of complexity and the tedium involved in their employment. Unfortunately, the strategies do not always lead to the same solution when applied to the same problem.

Stepwise Regression Perhaps the most widely used strategy for selecting independent variables for a multiple regression model is the stepwise procedure. The procedure consists of a series of steps. At each step of the procedure each variable then in the model is evaluated to see if, according to specified criteria, it should remain in the model.

Suppose, for example, that we wish to perform stepwise regression for a model containing k predictor variables. The criterion measure is computed for each variable. Of all the variables that do not satisfy the criterion for inclusion in the model, the one that least satisfies the criterion is removed from the model. If a variable is removed in this step, the regression equation for the smaller model is calculated and the criterion measure is computed for each variable now in the model. If any of these variables fail to satisfy the criterion for inclusion in the model, the one that least satisfies the criterion is removed. If a variable is removed at this step, the variable that was removed in the first step is reentered into the model, and the evaluation procedure is continued. This process continues until no more variables can be entered or removed.

The nature of the stepwise procedure is such that, although a variable may be deleted from the model in one step, it is evaluated for possible reentry into the model in subsequent steps.

MINITAB'S STEPWISE procedure, for example, uses the associated F statistic as the evaluative criterion for deciding whether a variable should be deleted or added to the model. Unless otherwise specified, the cutoff value is $F = 4$. The printout of the STEPWISE results contains t statistics (the square root of F) rather than F statistics. At each step MINITAB calculates an F statistic for each variable then in the model. If the F statistic for any of these variables is less than the specified cutoff value (4 if some other value is not specified), the variable with the smallest F is removed from the model. The regression equation is refitted for the reduced model, the results are printed, and the procedure goes to the next step. If no variable can be removed, the procedure tries to add a variable. An F statistic is calculated for each variable not then in the model. Of these variables, the one with the largest associated F statistic is added, provided its F statistic is larger than the specified cutoff value (4 if some other value is not specified). The regression equation is refitted for the new model, the results are printed, and the procedure goes on to the next step. The procedure stops when no variable can be added or deleted.

To change the criterion for allowing a variable to enter the model from 4 to some other value K, we use the subcommand FENTER $= K$. The new criterion F statistic, then, is K rather than 4. To change the criterion for deleting a variable from the model, from 4 to some other value K, we use the subcommand FREMOVE $= K$. We must choose FENTER to be greater than or equal to FREMOVE. The following example illustrates the use of the stepwise procedure for selecting variables for a multiple regression model.

Example 11.3.1

A nursing director would like to use nurses' personal characteristics to develop a regression model for predicting the job performance (JOBPER). The following variables are available from which to choose the independent variables to include in the model:

$$X_1 = \text{assertiveness (ASRV)}$$

$$X_2 = \text{enthusiasm (ENTH)}$$

$$X_3 = \text{ambition (AMB)}$$

$$X_4 = \text{communication skills (COMM)}$$

$$X_5 = \text{problem solving skills (PROB)}$$

$$X_6 = \text{initiative (INIT)}$$

We wish to use the stepwise procedure for selecting independent variables from those available in the table to construct a multiple regression model for predicting job performance.

Solution: Table 11.3.1 shows the measurements taken on the dependent variable, JOBPER, and each of the six independent variables for a sample of 30 nurses.

We use MINITAB to obtain a useful model by the stepwise procedure. Observations on the dependent variable job performance (JOBPER) and the six candidate independent variables are stored, as before, in MINITAB columns 1 through 7, respectively. Figure 11.3.1 shows the appropriate MINITAB command and the printout of the results.

To obtain the results in Figure 11.3.1, the values of FENTER and FREMOVE both were set automatically at 4. In step 1 there are no variables to be considered for deletion from the model. The variable AMB (column 4) has the largest associated F statistic which is $F = (9.74)^2 = 94.8676$. Since 94.8676 is greater than 4, AMB is added to the model. In step 2 the variable INIT (column 7) qualifies for addition to the model since its associated F of $(-2.2)^2 = 4.84$ is greater than 4 and it is the variable with the largest associated F statistic. It is added to the model. After step 2 no other variable could be added or deleted, and the procedure stopped. We see, then, that the model chosen by the stepwise procedure is a two-independent-variable model with AMB and INIT as the independent variables. The estimated regression equation is:

$$\hat{y} = 31.96 + .787x_3 - .45x_6$$

TABLE 11.3.1 Measurements on Seven Variables for Example 11.3.1

Y	X_1	X_2	X_3	X_4	X_5	X_6
45	74	29	40	66	93	47
65	65	50	64	68	74	49
73	71	67	79	81	87	33
63	64	44	57	59	85	37
83	79	55	76	76	84	33
45	56	48	54	59	50	42
60	68	41	66	71	69	37
73	76	49	65	75	67	43
71	83	71	77	76	81	33
69	62	44	57	67	81	43
66	54	52	67	63	68	36
69	61	46	66	64	75	43
71	63	56	67	60	64	35
70	84	82	68	64	78	37
79	78	53	82	84	78	39
83	65	49	82	65	55	38
75	86	63	79	84	80	41
67	61	64	75	60	81	45
67	71	45	67	80	86	48
52	59	67	64	69	79	54
52	71	32	44	48	65	43
66	62	51	72	71	81	43
55	67	51	60	68	81	39
42	65	41	45	55	58	51
65	55	41	58	71	76	35
68	78	65	73	93	77	42
80	76	57	84	85	79	35
50	58	43	55	56	84	40
87	86	70	81	82	75	30
84	83	38	83	69	79	41

```
STEPWISE REGRESSION OF    y     ON  6 PREDICTORS, WITH N =    30
      STEP        1       2
CONSTANT      7.226   31.955

C4            0.888    0.787
T-RATIO        9.74     8.13

C7                     -0.45
T-RATIO                -2.20

S              5.90     5.53
R-SQ          77.21    80.68
```

Figure 11.3.1 MINITAB printout of stepwise procedure for the data of Table 11.3.1.

EXERCISES

11.3.1 One of the objectives of a study by Brower et al. (A-4) was to determine if there are particular demographic, pharmacologic, or psychological correlates of dependence on anabolic-androgenic steroids (AASs). The subjects were male weight lifters, all users of AASs, who completed an anonymous, self-administered questionnaire. Variables on which data were collected included number of dependency symptoms (COUNT), number of different steroid drugs tried (DRUGNO), maximum dosage expressed as a z-score (MAXDOSE), difference in body weight in pounds before and after using steroids (NETWGT), number of aggressive symptoms reported (SIDEAGG), feeling not big enough before using steroids (on a scale of 1–5, with 1 signifying never feeling not big enough and 5 signifying feeling not big enough all the time) (NOTBIG), feeling not big enough after using steroids (same scale as for NOTBIG) (NOTBIG2), score on screening test for alcoholism (CAGE), and difference in the amount of weight in pounds lifted by the bench press method before and after using steroids (NETBENCH). The results for 31 subjects were as follows. Do a stepwise regression analysis of these data with COUNT as the dependent variable.

COUNT	DRUGNO	MAXDOSE	CAGE	SIDEAGG	NOTBIG	NOTBIG2	NETWGT	NETBENCH
3	5	2.41501	0	4	3	2	53	205
7	7	1.56525	1	4	4	4	40	130
3	2	1.42402	1	4	3	3	34	90
3	0	.81220	0	4	3	3	20	75
3	2	−1.22474	2	4	3	4	20	−15
3	7	1.61385	0	2	3	3	34	125
1	1	−1.02328	0	2	4	3	25	40
2	4	−.47416	0	4	4	5	44	85
4	2	1.24212	2	0	4	3	25	50
3	6	2.41501	0	4	3	3	55	125
0	2	.00000	0	2	1	1	17	65
2	1	2.94491	0	2	2	2	20	75
1	0	−1.08538	0	4	3	3	−60	100
0	2	−.56689	3	4	3	3	5	50
1	1	−.84476	2	1	5	3	13	40
1	3	−.29054	2	4	3	2	15	30
4	7	.20792	0	4	4	5	17	70
6	0	−.54549	3	4	4	4	16	15
3	3	1.42402	0	4	4	4	52	195
3	5	1.46032	0	4	4	5	35	90
4	1	.41846	4	4	4	3	15	50
3	2	.81220	1	4	1	1	20	30
2	8	1.61385	0	2	3	2	43	125
3	1	−.42369	4	1	1	4	0	20
2	4	1.89222	1	2	2	3	15	75
4	5	1.14967	2	3	3	3	49	130
6	3	−.41145	0	4	5	3	27	70
0	1	−.63423	0	0	3	3	15	25
3	1	2.39759	1	2	4	4	20	50
2	3	−.43849	2	2	3	3	13	65
7	8	2.03585	0	2	4	4	55	155

SOURCE: Kirk J. Brower, M.D. Used by permission.

11.3.2 Erickson and Yount (A-5) point out that an unintended fall in body temperature is commonly associated with surgery. They compared the effect of three combinations of aluminum-coated plastic covers (head cover, body covers, and both) and a control condition on tympanic temperature in 60 adults having major abdominal surgery under general anesthesia. Covers were applied from the time of transport to the operating room until exit from the postanesthesia care unit (PACU). The variables on which the investigators obtained measurements were pretransport temperature (TTEMP1), temperature at PACU admission (TTEMP4), age (AGE), body mass index (BMI), surgery time (SURGTM), body covers (BODY), head covers (HEAD), and cover with warmed blanket at operating room entry (BODYCOV). The results were as follows. Do a stepwise regression analysis of these data. The dependent variable is TTEMP4.

AGE	BMI	SURGTM	BODY	HEAD	BODYCOV	TTEMP1	TTEMPT4
59	19.2	1.2	1	1	1	99.8	97.5
39	26.6	1.3	0	0	0	99.0	96.2
75	23.7	1.7	1	0	0	98.5	96.6
34	24.0	.8	0	1	1	100.4	99.6
71	18.2	1.3	1	1	0	98.9	94.8
65	22.0	1.3	0	1	1	99.8	97.3
41	25.3	.6	1	0	1	99.7	99.3
46	20.5	1.0	1	0	0	100.7	98.1
56	28.8	1.7	0	0	1	98.8	97.2
42	27.2	2.6	0	1	0	99.6	95.8
51	37.7	1.8	0	0	1	100.3	98.7
38	22.7	1.0	1	0	1	100.0	98.6
68	28.3	2.0	1	1	0	99.7	95.9
37	29.8	1.0	0	0	1	100.6	99.5
35	36.2	2.2	0	1	1	100.4	99.0
65	34.9	1.6	1	1	0	100.3	97.6
71	31.4	3.7	1	0	0	99.1	97.2
65	27.5	.8	1	1	0	98.3	96.8
60	31.2	1.1	0	0	1	98.9	98.0
48	20.9	1.2	0	0	1	99.9	97.4
37	25.9	1.6	1	1	1	99.4	100.1
66	30.1	1.3	1	0	0	99.3	97.8
71	26.7	1.4	0	1	1	100.4	98.5
30	21.1	1.6	1	0	0	100.2	98.6
69	28.9	2.0	1	1	0	99.9	99.2
47	31.2	2.7	0	1	0	100.3	96.8
30	28.3	1.6	0	0	1	99.8	97.6
42	39.6	2.5	0	0	0	99.9	99.0
39	26.6	1.7	1	1	0	100.0	99.0
42	29.6	1.4	0	0	1	99.8	98.2
34	35.3	1.4	0	1	1	99.7	98.1
57	31.4	1.3	0	1	1	99.1	97.9
54	42.1	2.3	1	0	0	98.9	98.2
40	23.8	.9	1	1	0	99.1	97.1
45	29.9	1.7	1	1	1	100.5	99.3
50	28.7	2.0	1	0	0	99.4	96.9
46	33.4	1.3	0	1	1	99.2	97.4

Table (*continued*)

AGE	BMI	SURGTM	BODY	HEAD	BODYCOV	TTEMP1	TTEMPT4
33	25.3	1.4	0	0	1	99.0	98.6
45	32.1	1.8	0	1	1	99.2	97.8
63	33.4	.7	1	0	0	100.2	100.3
57	27.1	.7	1	1	0	98.5	97.5
43	21.7	1.2	0	0	0	100.6	98.7
75	25.6	1.1	1	1	0	99.1	97.2
45	48.6	2.4	0	1	1	100.4	98.7
41	21.5	1.5	0	0	0	100.0	96.7
75	25.7	1.6	0	1	0	99.6	97.2
40	28.4	2.6	1	0	0	100.6	97.8
71	19.4	2.2	0	0	1	99.6	96.2
76	29.1	3.5	1	1	0	99.9	96.6
61	29.3	1.6	0	1	0	99.1	97.1
38	30.4	1.7	1	1	1	99.8	98.8
25	21.6	2.8	0	0	1	99.2	96.9
80	24.6	4.2	1	0	0	100.5	96.0
62	26.6	1.9	1	0	0	99.2	97.6
34	20.4	1.5	0	1	1	100.1	96.6
70	27.5	1.3	1	0	1	98.9	98.4
41	27.4	1.3	0	0	1	99.0	96.3
43	24.6	1.3	1	1	1	99.5	97.3
65	24.8	2.1	1	0	0	100.0	99.1
45	21.5	1.9	0	1	1	100.4	95.6

SOURCE: Roberta S. Erickson, Ph.D., R.N. Used by permission.

11.3.3 Infant growth and the factors influencing it are considered in a study by Kusin et al. (A-6). Subjects were infants born in two villages in Madura, East Java. The researchers wished to assess the relation between infant feeding and growth through a longitudinal study in which growth and the intake of breast milk and additional foods were measured simultaneously. The variables on which measurements were obtained were birthweight in kilograms (GG), weight in kilograms at a specified age (GEW), calories from breastmilk (BMKC2), protein from breastmilk (BMPR2), sex (0 = girl, 1 = boy) (SX), breast feeding pattern (1 = mixed, 2, 3 = exclusively breastfed) (EB), calories from additional food (OTHER2), and protein from additional food (OTHPR2). The following data are for 28 subjects at 30 weeks of age. Perform a stepwise regression analysis of these data.

GG	SX	GEW	EB	BMKC2	OTHER2	BMPR2	OTHPR2
2.50	1	5.8	1	300.33	153.00	5.86	2.89
3.10	1	6.7	1	366.60	450.00	7.15	8.50
2.90	1	6.4	1	344.04	153.00	6.71	2.89
3.30	1	5.4	1	28.20	500.80	.55	11.90
3.30	1	7.1	1	383.52	342.00	7.48	6.46
2.80	2	6.0	1	389.16	63.00	7.59	1.19
3.00	2	6.5	1	407.49	.00	7.95	.00
3.00	1	6.9	1	415.95	208.40	8.11	3.73
3.40	1	8.3	1	396.21	126.00	7.73	2.38
3.00	1	6.6	3	455.43	.00	8.88	.00
3.00	2	6.0	1	353.91	126.00	6.90	2.38

GG	SX	GEW	EB	BMKC2	OTHER2	BMPR2	OTHPR2
3.00	1	7.5	1	382.11	318.40	7.45	5.24
2.80	2	6.6	1	417.36	104.40	8.14	1.97
3.10	1	6.9	1	322.89	243.00	6.30	4.59
3.20	1	7.1	1	338.40	228.70	6.60	3.64
2.75	1	7.0	1	365.19	198.00	7.12	3.74
2.70	2	8.7	3	482.22	.00	9.40	.00
3.50	1	8.5	1	366.60	270.00	7.15	5.10
2.80	2	4.9	1	280.59	144.00	5.47	2.72
3.10	1	6.9	3	296.10	.00	5.78	.00
3.00	1	8.0	1	363.78	166.00	7.10	2.92
3.25	1	8.7	1	399.88	99.00	7.80	1.87
3.30	1	7.6	2	305.97	.00	5.97	.00
3.00	1	6.9	1	372.24	288.00	7.26	5.44
3.30	2	6.3	2	358.14	.00	6.99	.00
3.20	1	8.9	2	441.33	.00	8.61	.00
3.00	2	6.7	1	473.76	185.40	9.24	3.50
3.60	2	7.5	1	432.87	126.00	8.44	2.38

Source: Ulla Renqvist. Used by permission.

11.4
Logistic Regression

Up to now our discussion of regression analysis has been limited to those situations in which the dependent variable is a continuous variable such as weight, blood pressure, or plasma levels of some hormone. Much research in the health sciences field is motivated by a desire to describe, understand, and make use of the relationship between independent variables and a dependent (or outcome) variable that is discrete. Particularly plentiful are circumstances in which the outcome variable is dichotomous. A dichotomous variable, we recall, is a variable that can assume only one of two mutually exclusive values. These values are usually coded $Y = 1$ for a success and $Y = 0$ for a nonsuccess, or failure. Dichotomous variables include those whose two possible values are such categories as died, did not die; cured, not cured; disease occurred, disease did not occur; and smoker, nonsmoker. The health sciences professional who either engages in research or needs to understand the results of research conducted by others will find it advantageous to have, at least, a basic understanding of *logistic regression*, the type of regression analysis that is usually employed when the dependent variable is dichotomous. The purpose of the present discussion is to provide the reader with this level of understanding. We shall limit our presentation to the case in which there is only one independent variable that may be either continuous or dichotomous.

The Logistic Regression Model   We recall that in Chapter 9 we referred to regression analysis involving only two variables as simple linear regression analysis.

The simple linear regression model was expressed by the equation

$$y = \alpha + \beta x + e \tag{11.4.1}$$

in which y is an arbitrary observed value of the continuous dependent variable. When the observed value of Y is $\mu_{y|x}$, the mean of a subpopulation of Y values for a given value of X, the quantity e, the difference between the observed Y and the regression line (see Figure 9.2.1) is zero, and we may write Equation 11.4.1 as

$$\mu_{y|x} = \alpha + \beta x \tag{11.4.2}$$

which may also be written as

$$E(y|x) = \alpha + \beta x \tag{11.4.3}$$

Generally the right-hand side of Equations 11.4.1 through 11.4.3 may assume any value between minus infinity and plus infinity.

Even though only two variables are involved, the simple linear regression model is not appropriate when Y is a dichotomous variable because the expected value (or mean) of Y is the probability that $Y = 1$ and, therefore, is limited to the range 0 through 1, inclusive. Equations 11.4.1 through 11.4.3, then, are incompatible with the reality of the situation.

If we let $p = P(Y = 1)$, then the ratio $p/(1 - p)$ can take on values between 0 and plus infinity. Furthermore, the natural logarithm (ln) of $p/(1 - p)$ can take on values between minus infinity and plus infinity just as can the right-hand side of Equations 11.4.1 through 11.4.3. Therefore, we may write

$$\ln\left[\frac{p}{1 - p}\right] = \alpha + \beta x \tag{11.4.4}$$

Equation 11.4.4 is called the *logistic regression model* because the transformation of $\mu_{y|x}$ (that is, p) to $\ln[p/(1 - p)]$ is called the *logit transformation*. Equation 11.4.4 may also be written as

$$p = \frac{\exp(\alpha + \beta x)}{1 + \exp(\alpha + \beta x)} \tag{11.4.5}$$

in which exp is the inverse of the natural logarithm.

The logistic regression model is widely used in health sciences research. For example, the model is frequently used by epidemiologists as a model for the probability (interpreted as the risk) that an individual will acquire a disease during some specified time period during which he/she is exposed to a condition (called a risk factor) known to be or suspected of being associated with the disease.

TABLE 11.4.1 Two Cross-Classified Dichotomous Variables Whose Values Are Coded 1 and 0

Dependent Variable (Y)	Independent Variable (X)	
	1	0
1	$n_{1,1}$	$n_{1,0}$
2	$n_{0,1}$	$n_{0,0}$

Logistic Regression — Dichotomous Independent Variable   The simplest situation in which logistic regression is applicable is one in which both the dependent and the independent variable are dichotomous. The values of the dependent (or outcome) variable usually indicate whether or not a subject acquired a disease or whether or not the subject died. The values of the independent variable indicate the status of the subject relative to the presence or absence of some risk factor. In the discussion that follows we assume that the dichotomies of the two variables are coded 0 and 1. When this is the case the variables may be cross-classified in a table, such as Table 11.4.1, that contains two rows and two columns. The cells of the table contain the frequencies of occurrence of all possible pairs of values of the two variables: $(1, 1)$, $(1, 0)$, $(0, 1)$ and $(0, 0)$.

An objective of the analysis of data that meet these criteria is a statistic known as the *odds ratio*. To understand the concept of the odds ratio, we must understand the term *odds*, which is frequently used by those who place bets on the outcomes of sporting events or participate in other types of gambling activities. Using probability terminology, Freund (5) defines odds as follows.

DEFINITION

The odds for success are the ratio of the probability of success to the probability of failure.

The odds ratio is a measure of how much greater (or less) the odds are for subjects possessing the risk factor to experience a particular outcome. This conclusion assumes that the outcome is a rare event. For example, when the outcome is the contracting of a disease, the interpretation of the odds ratio assumes that the disease is rare.

Suppose, for example, that the outcome variable is the acquisition or nonacquisition of skin cancer and the independent variable (or risk factor) is high levels of exposure to the sun. Analysis of such data collected on a sample of subjects might yield an odds ratio of 2, indicating that the odds of skin cancer are two times higher among subjects with high levels of exposure to the sun than among subjects without high levels of exposure.

Computer software packages that perform logistic regression frequently provide as part of their output estimates of α and β and the numerical value of the odds ratio. As it turns out the odds ratio is equal to $\exp(\beta)$.

TABLE 11.4.2 Cases of Acute Pelvic Inflammatory Disease and Control Subjects Classified by Smoking Status

Ever Smoked?	Cases	Controls	Total
Yes	77	123	200
No	54	171	225
Total	131	294	425

SOURCE: Delia Scholes, Janet R. Daling, and Andy S. Stergachis, "Current Cigarette Smoking and Risk of Acute Pelvic Inflammatory Disease," *American Journal of Public Health*, *82* (1992), 1352–1355. Used by permission of the American Public Health Association, the copyright holder.

Example 11.4.1   In a study of cigarette smoking and risk of acute pelvic inflammatory disease, Scholes et al. (A-7) reported the data shown in Table 11.4.2. We wish to use logistic regression analysis to determine how greater the odds are of finding cases of the disease among subjects who have ever smoked than among those who have never smoked.

Solution: We may use the SAS software package to analyze these data. The independent variable is smoking status (SMOKE), and the dependent variable is status relative to the presence of acute pelvic inflammatory disease. Use of the SAS command PROC LOGIST yields, as part of the resulting output, the statistics shown in Figure 11.4.1.

We see that the estimate of α is -1.1527 and the estimate of β is .6843. The estimated odds ratio, then, is $\widehat{OR} = \exp(.6843) = 1.98$. Thus we estimate that the odds of finding a case of pelvic inflammatory disease to be almost two times as high among subjects who have ever smoked as among subjects who have never smoked.

Logistic Regression — Continuous Independent Variable   Now let us consider the situation in which we have a dichotomous dependent variable and a continuous independent variable. We shall assume that a computer is available to perform the calculations. Our discussion, consequently, will focus on an evaluation

```
                  Parameter    Standard
     Variable      Estimate       Error

     INTERCPT       -1.1527      0.1561
     SMOKE           0.6843      0.2133
```

Figure 11.4.1 Partial output from use of SAS command PROC LOGIST with the data of Table 11.4.2.

TABLE 11.4.3 Hispanic Americans with Total Serum Cholesterol (TC) Levels Greater Than or Equal to 240 Milligrams per Deciliter by Age Group

Age Group (Years)	Number Examined (n_i)	Number with TC $\geq$ 240 (n_{i1})[a]
25–34	522	41
35–44	330	51
45–54	344	81
55–64	219	81
65–74	114	50

SOURCE: M. Carroll, C. Sempos, R. Fulwood, et al. *Serum Lipids and Lipoproteins of Hispanics, 1982–84.* National Center for Health Statistics. *Vital Health Statistics, 11*(240), (1990).
[a]The original publication reported percentages rather than frequencies. The frequencies appearing here were obtained by multiplying the percentages for each age group by the appropriate sample size.

of the adequacy of the model as a representation of the data at hand, interpretation of key elements of the computer printout, and the use of the results to answer relevant questions about the relationship between the two variables.

Example 11.4.2

In a survey of Hispanic Americans conducted by the National Center for Health Statistics the data on total serum cholesterol (TC) levels and age shown in Table 11.4.3 were collected (A-8). We wish to use these data to obtain information regarding the relationship between age and the presence or absence of TC values greater than or equal to 240. We wish also to know if we may use the results of our analysis to predict the likelihood of a Hispanic American's having a TC value $\geq$ 240 if we know that person's age.

Solution: The independent variable is the continuous variable age (AGE) and the dependent or response variable is status with respect to TC level. The dependent variable is a dichotomous variable that can assume one of two values: TC $\geq$ 240 or TC < 240. Since individual ages are not available we must base our analysis on the reported grouped data. We use the SAS software package. The computer input for the independent variable consists of the midpoints of the age groups: 29.5, 39.5, and so on. The SAS command is PROC CATMOD. A partial printout of the analysis is shown in Figure 11.4.2.

Effect	Parameter	Estimate	Standard Error	Chi-Square	Prob
INTERCEPT	1	-4.0388	0.2623	237.01	0.0000
AGE	2	0.0573	0.00521	121.06	0.0000

Figure 11.4.2 Partial SAS printout of the logistic regression analysis of the data in Table 11.4.3.

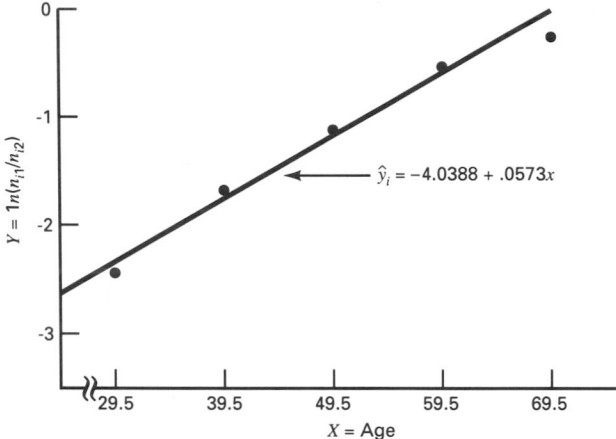

Figure 11.4.3 Fitted logistic regression line for Example 11.4.2.

The slope of our regression is .0573 and the intercept is −4.0388. The regression, then, is given by

$$\hat{y}_i = -4.0388 + .0573x$$

where $\hat{y}_i = \ln(n_{i1}/n_{i2})$, n_{i1} is the number of subjects in the ith age category who have TC values greater than or equal to 240, and $n_{i1} + n_{i2} = n_i$, the total number of subjects in the ith category who were examined.

Test of H_0 that $\beta = 0$ We search a conclusion about the adequacy of the logistic model by testing the null hypothesis that the slope of the regression line is zero. The test statistic is $z = b/s_b$, where z is the standard normal statistic, b is the sample slope (.0573), and s_b is its standard error (.00521) as shown in Figure 11.4.2. From these numbers we compute $z = .0573/.00521 = 10.99808$, which has an associated p value of less than .0001. We conclude, therefore, that the logistic model is adequate. The square of z is chi-square with 1 degree of freedom, a statistic that is shown in Figure 11.4.2.

To obtain a visual impression of how well the model fits the data we plot the midpoints of the age categories against $\ln(n_{i1}/n_{i2})$ and superimpose the fitted regression line on the graph. The results are shown in Figure 11.4.3.

Using the logistic regression to estimate p   We may use Equation 11.4.5 and the results of our analysis to estimate p, the probability that a Hispanic American of a given age (within the range of ages represented by the data) will have a TC

MAXIMUM-LIKELIHOOD PREDICTED VALUES FOR RESPONSE FUNCTIONS AND PROBABILITIES

Sample	AGE	EXM	Function Number	Observed Function	Observed Standard Error	Predicted Function	Predicted Standard Error	Residual
1	29.5		1	-2.4622952	0.16269372	-2.3493245	0.12050719	-0.1129707
		0	P1	0.07854406	0.01177494	0.08711948	0.0095339	-0.0085754
		1	P2	0.92145594	0.01177494	0.91288052	0.0095339	0.00857541
2	39.5		1	-1.6993861	0.15228944	-1.7766203	0.08256409	0.07723419
		0	P1	0.15454545	0.01989831	0.14472096	0.01021952	0.0098245
		1	P2	0.84545455	0.01989831	0.85527904	0.01021952	-0.0098245
3	49.5		1	-1.1777049	0.12707463	-1.2039161	0.06720744	0.02621126
		0	P1	0.23546512	0.02287614	0.23077929	0.01194343	0.00468583
		1	P2	0.76453488	0.02287614	0.76922071	0.01194343	-0.0046858
4	59.5		1	-0.5328045	0.13997163	-0.6312119	0.08753496	0.0984074
		0	P1	0.36986301	0.0326224	0.34723579	0.01984095	0.02262723
		1	P2	0.63013699	0.0326224	0.65276421	0.01984095	-0.0226272
5	69.5		1	-0.2468601	0.18874586	-0.0585077	0.12733053	-0.1883524
		0	P1	0.43859649	0.04647482	0.48537724	0.03180541	-0.0467807
		1	P2	0.56140351	0.04647482	0.51462276	0.03180541	0.04678075

Figure 11.4.4 Additional SAS printout of the logistic regression analysis of the data from Example 11.4.2.

489

value ≥ 240. Suppose, for example, that we wish to estimate the probability that a Hispanic American who is 29.5 years of age will have a TC value ≥ 240. Substituting 29.5 and the results shown in Figure 11.4.2 into Equation 11.4.5 gives

$$p = \frac{\exp[-4.0388 + (.0573)(29.5)]}{1 + \exp[-4.0388 + (.0573)(29.5)]} = .08719$$

SAS calculates the estimated probabilities for the given values of X. Those for the midpoints of our five age groups are shown in Figure 11.4.4. We note that because of rounding the values on the SAS printout differ from those we obtain by Equation 11.4.5. We see that the printout also contains the standard errors of the estimates, the observed proportions and their standard errors, the differences between observed and estimated values, and the values of $\hat{y}_i$ used to plot the regression line for Figure 11.4.3.

Further Reading   We have discussed only the basic concepts and applications of logistic regression. The technique has much wider application. For example, it may be used in situations in which there are two or more independent variables that may be continuous, dichotomous, or polytomous (discrete with more than two categories). Stepwise regression analysis may be used with logistic regression. There are also techniques available for constructing confidence intervals for odds ratios. The reader who wishes to learn more about logistic regression may consult the books by Fienberg (6), Hosmer and Lemeshow (7), Kahn and Sempos (8), Kleinbaum, Kupper, and Morgenstern (9), Schlesselman (10), and Woolson (11). Some of the references listed at the end of Chapters 9 and 10 also contain discussions of logistic regression.

EXERCISES

11.4.1 A sample of 500 elementary school children were cross-classified by nutritional status and academic performance as follows:

Nutritional Status and Academic
Performance of 500 Elementary School Children

Academic Performance	Nutritional Status		
	Poor	**Good**	**Total**
Poor	105	15	120
Satisfactory	80	300	380
Total	185	315	500

Use logistic regression analysis to find the regression coefficients and the estimate of the odds ratio. Write an interpretation of your results.

11.4.2 The following table shows, within each group, the number of patients admitted to a psychiatric treatment program and the number who were improved at the end of one year of treatment.

Age Group	Number Admitted	Number Improved
20–24	30	6
25–29	32	8
30–34	34	11
35–39	40	17
40–44	35	18
45–49	45	31
50–54	30	22
55–59	25	19
60–64	20	16

Use logistic regression to analyze these data as was done in Example 11.4.2. Write an interpretation of your results and a discussion of how they might be of use to a health professional.

11.5
Summary

This chapter is included for the benefit of those who wish to extend their understanding of regression analysis and their ability to apply techniques to models that are more complex than those covered in Chapters 9 and 10. In this chapter we present some additional topics from regression analysis. We discuss the analysis that is appropriate when one or more of the independent variables is dichotomous. In this discussion the concept of dummy variable coding is presented. A second topic that we discuss is how to select the most useful independent variables when we have a long list of potential candidates. The technique we illustrate for the purpose is stepwise regression analysis. Finally, we present the basic concepts and procedures that are involved in logistic regression analysis. We cover two situations, the case in which the independent variable is dichotomous and the case in which the independent variable is continuous.

Since the calculations involved in obtaining useful results from data that are appropriate for analysis by means of the techniques presented in this chapter are complicated and time-consuming when attempted by hand, it is recommended that a computer be used to work the exercises. For those who wish to pursue these topics further a list of references is presented at the end of the chapter.

REVIEW QUESTIONS AND EXERCISES

1. What is a qualitative variable?

2. What is a dummy variable?

3. Explain and illustrate the technique of dummy variable coding.

4. Why is a knowledge of variable selection techniques important to the health sciences researcher?

5. What is stepwise regression?

6. Explain the basic concept involved in stepwise regression.

7. When is logistic regression used?

8. Write out and explain the components of the logistic regression model.

9. Define the word *odds*.

10. What is an odds ratio?

11. Give an example in your field in which logistic regression analysis would be appropriate when the independent variable is dichotomous.

12. Give an example in your field in which logistic regression analysis would be appropriate when the independent variable is continuous.

13. Find a published article in the health sciences field in which each of the following techniques is employed:
    a. Dummy variable coding
    b. Stepwise regression
    c. Logistic regression

Write a report on the article in which you identify the variables involved, the reason for the choice of the technique, and the conclusions that the authors reach on the basis of their analysis.

14. The objective of a study by Porrini et al. (A-9) was to evaluate dietary intakes and their correlation to certain risk factors for coronary heart disease. The subjects were adults living in northern Italy. One of the risk factors for which data were collected was total cholesterol level (TC). Data on the following dietary variables were collected: energy (ENERGY), total fat (TOTFAT), saturated fat (SATFAT), polyunsaturated fat (POLY-FAT), vegetable fat (VEGFAT), animal fat (ANIMFAT), cholesterol (CHOL), fiber (FIBER), alcohol (ALCOHOL). In addition, measurements on body mass index (BMI) were taken. The measurement units are energy, mJ; cholesterol, mg; body mass index, kg/m^2; and grams (g) for all other variables. The following table shows the values for these variables for male subjects between the ages of 20 and 39 years. Use stepwise regression analysis to select the most useful variables to be in a model for predicting total cholesterol level.

TC	ENERGY	TOTFAT	SATFAT	POLYFAT	VEGFAT	ANIMFAT	CHOL	FIBER	ALCOHOL	BMI
223	2280.3	67.3	23.5	6.4	32.6	34.7	207.5	22.0	23.8	26.7
179	1718.9	68.0	29.0	7.5	29.6	38.3	332.5	15.2	.0	23.8
197	1644.8	58.9	20.4	10.7	28.1	30.8	272.9	12.5	26.3	21.8
187	2574.3	91.4	26.0	8.8	56.9	34.5	286.2	30.7	27.5	23.1
325	2891.7	97.3	37.0	10.4	35.9	61.4	309.5	23.2	63.6	28.3
281	2211.0	102.8	32.0	10.8	43.8	59.0	357.9	19.5	16.9	26.4
250	1853.4	69.9	27.7	10.0	24.1	45.8	346.0	14.2	2.3	23.6
183	2399.5	116.2	36.8	12.6	54.7	61.5	242.5	22.9	4.5	30.0
211	2028.9	62.6	22.3	7.5	30.6	32.0	213.5	19.9	63.6	27.7
248	2489.5	65.9	21.8	13.1	37.5	28.3	414.5	18.0	63.6	20.8
198	2242.8	85.9	28.8	6.1	42.1	43.7	239.9	21.3	.0	22.7
250	2754.5	53.9	17.4	5.0	22.4	31.5	159.0	24.3	91.5	21.9
178	2043.5	63.3	26.4	12.7	31.3	32.0	207.4	15.9	60.2	22.1
222	2077.6	70.6	29.0	8.1	22.4	48.2	302.3	22.1	16.7	26.6
205	2986.9	61.1	16.0	13.1	39.7	21.4	274.0	29.6	34.1	22.2
159	3229.2	92.1	34.7	10.2	31.4	60.8	258.2	24.6	84.8	21.9
215	1544.9	76.6	30.7	16.1	30.7	45.8	301.9	19.5	10.6	29.8
196	2700.8	93.7	33.6	9.1	40.8	52.9	372.5	32.8	.0	21.6
275	2646.6	105.9	32.4	12.4	59.2	46.7	414.2	30.1	5.3	27.3
269	2905.5	92.0	33.1	9.0	33.0	59.0	425.0	29.8	52.5	26.9
300	4259.5	133.9	38.0	21.2	82.4	51.5	519.1	40.9	39.8	28.7
220	3512.0	113.2	44.0	17.8	43.4	69.8	550.9	43.3	43.7	26.0
180	3130.6	123.6	37.6	14.1	65.7	57.8	342.0	26.3	.0	24.9
226	4358.6	167.5	54.4	34.3	91.2	76.3	437.5	38.5	31.8	23.1
202	3832.2	152.8	72.8	12.8	62.9	89.8	788.4	19.1	9.1	24.4
185	1782.5	67.9	20.7	8.0	19.8	48.0	295.1	16.2	9.6	18.8

Table (*continued*)

TC	ENERGY	TOTFAT	SATFAT	POLYFAT	VEGFAT	ANIMFAT	CHOL	FIBER	ALCOHOL	BMI
172	2041.3	78.8	31.5	5.8	42.0	36.8	487.5	17.1	31.8	21.0
285	4061.6	94.2	33.6	14.1	31.5	62.7	491.2	21.9	156.7	28.4
194	4280.2	142.5	51.5	7.3	56.0	86.5	747.0	46.9	31.8	23.5
257	2834.6	85.7	36.3	9.7	27.9	57.9	464.7	35.4	59.8	24.1
198	4032.4	143.6	52.3	16.9	67.3	76.3	446.9	62.2	31.8	23.1
180	3245.8	101.4	33.1	13.2	50.2	51.2	409.1	44.8	21.2	24.6
177	2379.4	74.3	24.3	7.8	35.3	39.0	257.4	20.9	63.5	27.3
183	2771.6	98.7	30.7	10.6	48.1	50.5	492.9	30.2	20.5	20.9
248	1888.4	71.7	21.9	14.6	33.0	38.7	215.4	20.9	.0	26.0
167	2387.1	32.3	11.0	2.5	22.4	9.9	234.2	43.3	.0	24.9
166	1474.0	60.2	20.5	12.6	22.8	37.4	222.5	11.9	6.0	25.2
197	2574.0	93.7	30.4	9.0	41.8	52.0	404.4	27.2	32.5	24.2
191	2999.0	110.1	38.5	12.2	43.3	66.8	421.3	24.8	36.1	23.8
183	2746.2	76.1	19.3	10.0	43.4	32.7	240.9	21.0	98.8	25.3
200	2959.8	91.7	30.5	10.2	42.6	49.1	403.2	40.0	65.0	29.0
206	4104.3	156.0	50.7	15.8	96.1	59.8	423.1	39.1	27.7	20.5
229	2731.9	122.2	38.9	26.3	77.0	45.2	365.2	27.0	.7	25.3
195	3440.6	132.1	42.1	12.4	65.6	66.4	526.1	45.1	41.7	23.2
202	3000.5	114.0	36.6	12.3	44.2	69.8	306.4	34.2	.0	27.8
273	2588.8	86.7	24.2	20.3	48.7	38.0	252.1	19.9	57.7	21.8
220	2144.1	91.0	23.3	10.4	52.6	38.3	310.2	23.3	43.9	24.6
155	2259.9	85.5	21.9	10.9	56.2	29.3	182.3	20.8	53.0	23.4
295	3694.9	121.8	43.7	21.7	47.9	73.8	418.5	16.1	88.6	25.4
211	3114.2	101.1	31.2	11.5	42.0	59.1	277.2	34.0	34.6	28.4
214	2183.0	85.9	31.6	7.4	33.5	52.4	372.9	21.7	37.0	23.8

SOURCE: Marisa Porrini. Used by permission.

15. In the following table are the cardiac output (l/min) and oxygen consumption (Vo_2) values for a sample of adults (A) and children (C), who particulated in a study designed to investigate the relationship among these variables.

Measurements were taken both at rest and during exercise. Treat cardiac output as the dependent variable and use dummy variable coding and analyze the data by regression techniques. Explain the results. Plot the original data and the fitted regression equations.

Cardiac Output (1 / min)	Vo_2 (1 / min)	Age Group
4.0	.21	A
7.5	.91	C
3.0	.22	C
8.9	.60	A
5.1	.59	C
5.8	.50	A
9.1	.99	A
3.5	.23	C
7.2	.51	A
5.1	.48	C
6.0	.74	C
5.7	.70	C
14.2	1.60	A
4.1	.30	C
4.0	.25	C
6.1	.22	A
6.2	.61	C
4.9	.45	C
14.0	1.55	A
12.9	1.11	A
11.3	1.45	A
5.7	.50	C
15.0	1.61	A
7.1	.83	C
8.0	.61	A
8.1	.82	A
9.0	1.15	C
6.1	.39	A

16. A simple random sample of normal subjects between the ages of 6 and 18 yielded the data on total body potassium (mEq) and total body water (liters) shown in the following table.

Let total potassium be the dependent variable and use dummy variable coding to quantify the qualitative variable. Analyze the data using regression techniques. Explain the results. Plot the original data and the fitted regression equations.

Total Body Potassium	Total Body Water	Sex
795	13	M
1590	16	F
1250	15	M
1680	21	M

Table (*continued*)

Total Body Potassium	Total Body Water	Sex
800	10	F
2100	26	M
1700	15	F
1260	16	M
1370	18	F
1000	11	F
1100	14	M
1500	20	F
1450	19	M
1100	14	M
950	12	F
2400	26	M
1600	24	F
2400	30	M
1695	26	F
1510	21	F
2000	27	F
3200	33	M
1050	14	F
2600	31	M
3000	37	M
1900	25	F
2200	30	F

17. The data shown in the following table were collected as part of a study in which the subjects were preterm infants with low birth weights born in three different hospitals.

Use dummy variable coding and multiple regression techniques to analyze these data. May we conclude that the three sample hospital populations differ with respect to mean birth weight when gestational age is taken into account? May we conclude that there is interaction between hospital of birth and gestational age? Plot the original data and the fitted regression equations.

Birth Weight (kg)	Gestation Age (weeks)	Hospital of Birth
1.4	30	A
.9	27	B
1.2	33	A
1.1	29	C
1.3	35	A
.8	27	B
1.0	32	A
.7	26	A
1.2	30	C
.8	28	A
1.5	32	B
1.3	31	A
1.4	32	C
1.5	33	B

Birth Weight (kg)	Gestation Age (weeks)	Hospital of Birth
1.0	27	A
1.8	35	B
1.4	36	C
1.2	34	A
1.1	28	B
1.2	30	B
1.0	29	C
1.4	33	C
.9	28	A
1.0	28	C
1.9	36	B
1.3	29	B
1.7	35	C
1.0	30	A
.9	28	A
1.0	31	A
1.6	31	B
1.6	33	B
1.7	34	B
1.6	35	C
1.2	28	A
1.5	30	B
1.8	34	B
1.5	34	C
1.2	30	A
1.2	32	C

18. Hertzman et al. (A-10) conducted a study to identify determinants of elevated blood lead levels in preschool children; to compare the current situation with past information; to determine historical trends in environmental lead contamination in a Canadian community; and to find a basis for identifying appropriate precautions and protection against future lead exposure. Subjects were children between the ages of two and five years inclusive who resided in a Canadian community that is the site of one of North America's largest lead-zinc smelters. Subjects were divided into two groups: (1) cases, consisting of children who had blood lead levels of 18 μg/ml or greater and (2) controls, consisting of subjects whose blood lead levels were 10 μg/dl or less. Lead levels were ascertained for samples of drinking water, paint, household dust, home-grown vegetables, and soil. Among the analyses performed by the investigators was a multiple logistic regression analysis with age, sex, and the logarithms of the lead levels of the environmental samples (covariates) as the independent variables. They found that soil lead level was the strongest risk factor for high blood lead levels. The analysis yielded an odds ratio of 14.25, which could be interpreted as "each ten-fold increase in soil lead level would increase the relative proportion of cases to controls by 14.25-fold." The following table shows the soil lead levels for the cases (coded 1) and the controls (coded 0). Use logistic regression to analyze these data. Obtain the odds ratio and compare it with the one obtained by the authors' analysis. Test for significance at the .05 level and find the p-value.

Subject Category	Soil Lead Level (ppm)	Subject Category	Soil Lead Level (ppm)	Subject Category	Soil Lead Level (ppm)
1 = case	1290	0	197	1	852
0 = control	90	1	916	0	137
1	894	1	755	0	137
0	193	1	59	0	125
1	1410	1	1720	1	562
1	410	1	574	0	325
1	1594	1	403	1	1317
0	321	1	61	1	2125
0	40	1	1290	1	2635
0	96	1	1409	1	2635
0	260	1	880	0	544
0	433	1	40	1	731
0	260	1	40	1	815
0	227	0	68	0	328
0	337	1	777	1	1455
1	867	1	1975	0	977
1	1694	1	1237	1	624
0	302	0	133	1	392
1	2860	0	269	1	427
1	2860	0	357	1	1000
1	4320	0	315	1	1009
1	859	0	315	0	1010
0	119	0	255	1	3053
1	115	0	422	0	1220
0	192	0	400	0	46
1	1345	0	400	0	181
0	55	0	229	0	87
0	55	1	229	0	131
1	606	0	768	0	131
1	1660	0	886	1	1890
0	82	1	58	1	221
0	1470	0	508	1	221
1	600	1	811	0	79
1	2120	1	527	1	1570
1	569	1	1753	1	909
0	105	0	57	1	1720
1	503	0	769	1	308
0	161	0	677	1	97
0	161	1	677	0	200
1	1670	1	424	0	1135
0	132	1	2230	0	320
1	974	0	421	1	5255
1	3795	1	628	0	176
0	548	1	1406	0	176
1	622	1	378	0	100
0	788	1	812		
1	2130	1	812		

SOURCE: Shona Kelly. Used by permission.

For each of the studies described in Exercises 19 through 21, answer as many of the following questions as possible.

(a) Which is the dependent variable?

(b) What are the independent variables?

(c) What are the appropriate null and alternative hypotheses?

(d) Which null hypotheses do you think were rejected? Why?

(e) Which is the more relevant objective, prediction or estimation, or are the two equally relevant? Explain your answer.

(f) What is the sampled population?

(g) What is the target population?

(h) Which variables are related to which other variables? Are the relationships direct or inverse?

(i) Write out the regression equation using appropriate numbers for parameter estimates.

(j) Give numerical values for any other statistics that you can.

(k) Identify each variable as to whether it is quantitative or qualitative.

(l) Explain the meaning of any statistics for which numerical values are given.

19. Brock and Brock (A-11) used a multiple regression model in a study of the influence of selected variables on plasma cholinesterase activity (ChE) in 650 males and 437 females with ChE–1 phenotype U or UA. With ChE measured on a logarithmic scale the researchers developed a linear model with an intercept term of 2.016 and regression coefficients and their associated variables as follows: ChE–1 phenotype $(-.308)$, sex $(-.104)$, weight $(.00765)$, height $(-.00723)$. The researchers reported $R = .535$, $p < .001$.

20. Ueshima et al. (A-12) report on a study designed to evaluate the response of patients with chronic atrial fibrillation (AF) to exercise. Seventy-nine male patients with AF underwent resting two-dimensional and M-mode echocardiography and symptom-limited treadmill testing with ventilatory gas exchange analysis. In a stepwise regression analysis to evaluate potential predictors of maximal oxygen uptake (Vo_2 max), the variables entering the procedure at steps 1 through 7, respectively, and the resulting R^2, and associated p values were as follows: maximal systolic blood pressure $(.35, < .01)$, maximal heart rate $(0.45, .03)$, left ventricular ejection fraction $(.47, .45)$, age $(.49, .51)$, left atrial dimension $(.50, .53)$, left ventricular diastolic dimension $(.50, .75)$, left ventricular systolic dimension $(.50, .84)$.

21. Ponticelli et al. (A-13) found arterial hypertension present at the end of one year in 81.6 percent of 212 cyclosporine-treated renal transplant recipients with stable graft function. Through logistic regression analysis the authors found that the presence of hypertension before transplantation ($p = .0001$; odds ratio 3.5), a plasma creatinine level higher than 2 mg/dl at one year ($p = .0001$, odds ratio 3.8), and a maintenance therapy with corticosteriods ($p = .008$, odds ratio 3.3) were positively associated with hypertension at one year after transplantation.

Exercise for Use With the Large Data Sets Available on Computer Disk from the Publisher

1. Refer to the weight loss data on 588 cancer patients and 600 healthy controls (WGTLOSS, Disk 2). Weight loss among cancer patients is a well-known phenomenon. Of interest to clinicians is the role played in the process by metabolic abnormalities. One investigation into the relationships among these variables yielded the following data on whole-body protein turnover (Y) and percentage of ideal body weight for height (X). Subjects were lung cancer patients and healthy controls of the same age. Select a simple random sample of size 15 from each group and do the following.

a. Draw a scatter diagram of the sample data using different symbols for each of the two groups.

b. Use dummy variable coding to analyze these data.

c. Plot the two regression lines on the scatter diagram. May one conclude that the two sampled populations differ with respect to mean protein turnover when percentage of ideal weight is taken into account?

May one conclude that there is interaction between health status and percentage of ideal body weight? Prepare a verbal interpretation of the results of your analysis and compare your results with those of your classmates.

REFERENCES

References Cited

1. John Neter, William Wasserman, and Michael H. Kutner, *Applied Linear Regression Models*, Second Edition, Irwin, Homewood, Ill., 1989.

2. David G. Kleinbaum, Lawrence L. Kupper, and Keith E. Muller, *Applied Regression Analysis and Other Multivariable Methods*, Second Edition, PWS-Kent, Boston, 1988.

3. William Mendenhall and James T. McClave, *A Second Course in Business Statistics: Regression Analysis*, Dellen Publishing Company, San Francisco, 1981.

4. N. R. Draper and H. Smith, *Applied Regression Analysis*, Second Edition, Wiley, New York, 1981.

5. John E. Freund, *Introduction to Probability*, Dickenson Publishing Company, *Encino, Calif.*, 1973.

6. Stephen E. Feinberg, *The Analysis of Cross-Classified Categorical Data*, Second Edition, The MIT Press, Cambridge, Mass., 1980.

7. David W. Hosmer and Stanley Lemeshow, *Applied Logistic Regression*, Wiley, New York, 1989.

8. Harold A. Kahn and Christopher T. Sempos, *Statistical Methods in Epidemiology*, Oxford University Press, New York, 1989.

9. David G. Kleinbaum, Lawrence L. Kupper, and Hal Morgenstern, *Epidemiologic Research: Principles and Quantitative Methods*, Lifetime Learning Publications, Belmont, Calif., 1982.

10. James J. Schlesselman, *Case-Control Studies: Design, Conduct, Analysis*, Oxford University Press, New York, 1982.

11. Robert F. Woolson, *Statistical Methods for the Analysis of Biomedical Data*, Wiley, New York, 1987.

Other References, Books

1. K. W. Smillie, *An Introduction to Regression and Correlation*, Academic Press, New York, 1966.

2. Peter Sprent, *Models in Regression*, Methuen, London, 1969.

Other References, Journal Articles

1. David M. Allen, "Mean Square-Error of Prediction as a Criterion for Selecting Variables," *Technometrics*, *13* (1971), 469–475.

2. E. M. L. Beale, M. G. Kendall, and D. W. Mann, "The Discarding of Variables in Multivariate Analysis," *Biometrika*, *54* (1967), 357–366.

3. M. J. Garside, "The Best Sub-Set in Multiple Regression Analysis," *Applied Statistics, 14* (1965), 196–200.

4. J. W. Gorman and R. J. Toman, "Selection of Variables for Fitting Equations to Data,"*Technometrics, 8* (1966), 27–52.

5. R. R. Hocking and R. N. Leslie, "Selection of the Best Sub-Set in Regression Analysis," *Technometrics, 9* (1967), 531–540.

6. H. J. Larson and T. A. Bancroft, "Sequential Model Building for Prediction in Regression Analysis I," *Annals of Mathematical Statistics, 34* (1963), 462–479.

7. D. V. Lindley, "The Choice of Variables in Multiple Regression," *Journal of the Royal Statistical Society B, 30* (1968), 31–66.

8. A. Summerfield and A. Lubin, "A Square Root Method of Selecting a Minimum Set of Variables in Multiple Regression: I, The Method," *Psychometrika, 16* (3): 271 (1951).

Other References, Other Publications

1. Wayne W. Daniel, *The Use of Dummy Variables in Regression Analysis: A Selected Bibliography With Annotations*, Vance Bibliographies, Monticello, Ill., November 1979.

2. E. F. Schultz, Jr. and J. F. Goggans, "A Systematic Procedure for Determining Potent Independent Variables in Multiple Regression nd Discriminant Analysis," Agri. Exp. Sta. Bull. 336, Auburn University, 1961.

Applications References

A-1. Mary A. Woo, Michele Hamilton, Lynne W. Stevenson, and Donna L. Vredevoe, "Comparison of Thermodilution and Transthoracic Electrical Bioimpedence Cardiac Outputs," *Heart & Lung, 20* (1991), 357–362.

A-2. Alan R. Schwartz, Avram R. Gold, Norman Schubert, Alexandra Stryzak, Robert A. Wise, Solbert Permutt, and Philip L. Smith, "Effect of Weight Loss on Upper Airway Collapsibility in Obstructive Sleep Apnea,' *American Review of Respiratory Disease, 144* (1991), 494–498.

A-3. Cho-Ming Loi, Xiaoxiong Wei, and Robert E. Vestal, "Inhibition of Theophylline Metabolism by Mexiletine in Young Male and Female Nonsmokers," *Clinical Pharmacology & Therapeutics, 49* (1991), 571–580.

A-4. Kirk J. Brower, Frederic C. Blow, James P. Young, and Elizabeth M. Hill, "Symptoms and Correlates of Anabolic–Androgenic Steroid Dependence," *British Journal of Addiction, 86* (1991), 759–768.

A-5. Roberta S. Erickson and Sue T. Yount, "Effect of Aluminized Covers on Body Temperature in Patients Having Abdominal Surgery," *Heart & Lung, 20* (1991), 255–264.

A-6. J. A. Kusin, Sri Kardjati, W. M. van Steenbergen, and U. H. Renqvist, "Nutritional Transition During Infancy in East Java, Indonesia: 2. A Longitudinal Study of Growth in Relation to the Intake of Breast Milk and Additional Foods," *European Journal of Clinical Nutrition, 45* (1991), 77–84.

A-7 Delia Scholes, Janet R. Daling, and Andy S. Stergachis, "Current Cigarette Smoking and Risk of Acute Pelvic Inflammatory Disease," *American Journal of Public Health, 82* (1992), 1352–1355.

A-8. M. Carroll, C. Sempos, R. Fulwood, et al. *Serum Lipids and Lipoproteins of Hispanics, 1982–84*. National Center for Health Statistics. *Vital and Health Statistics, 11*(240), (1990).

A-9. M. Porrini, P. Simonetti, G. Testolin, C. Roggi, M. S. Laddomada, and M. T. Tenconi, "Relation Between Diet Composition and Coronary Heart Disease Risk Factors," *Journal of Epidemiology and Community Health, 45* (1991), 148–151.

A-10. Clyde Hertzman, Helen Ward, Nelson Ames, Shona Kelly, and Cheryl Yates, "Childhood Lead Exposure in Trail Revisited," *Canadian Journal of Public Health, 82* (November/December 1991), 385–391.

A-11. A. Brock and V. Brock, "Factors Affecting Inter-Individual Variation in Human Plasma Cholinesterase Activity: Body Weight, Height, Sex, Genetic Polymorphism and Age," *Archives of Environmental Contamination and Toxicology*, *24* (January 1993), 93–99.

A-12. K. Ueshima, J. Myers, P. M. Ribisl., J. E. Atwood, C. K. Morris, T. Kawaguchi, J. Liu, and V. F. Froelicher, "Hemodyanmic Determinants of Exercise Capacity in Chronic Atrial Fibrillation," *American Heart Journal*, *125* (May 1993, No. 5, Part 1), 1301–1305.

A-13. C. Ponticelli, G. Montagnino, A. Aroldi, C. Angelini, M. Braga, and A. Tarantino, "Hypertension After Renal Transplantation," *American Journal of Kidney Diseases*, *21* (May 1993, No. 5 Supplement 2), 73–78.

The Chi-Square Distribution and the Analysis of Frequencies

· ·

CONTENTS

12.1
Introduction

In the chapters on estimation and hypothesis testing brief mention is made of the chi-square distribution in the construction of confidence intervals for and the testing of hypotheses concerning a population variance. This distribution, which is one of the most widely used distributions in statistical applications, has many other uses. Some of the more common ones are presented in this chapter along with a more complete description of the distribution itself, which follows in the next section.

The chi-square distribution is the most frequently employed statistical technique for the analysis of count or frequency data. For example, we may know for a sample of hospitalized patients how many are male and how many are female. For the same sample we may also know how many have private insurance coverage, how many have Medicare insurance, and how many are on Medicaid assistance. We may wish to know, for the population from which the sample was drawn, if the type of insurance coverage differs according to gender. For another sample of patients we may have frequencies for each diagnostic category represented and for each geographic area represented. We might want to know if, in the population from which the sample was drawn, there is a relationship between area of residence and diagnosis. We will learn how to use chi-square analysis to answer these types of questions.

There are other statistical techniques that may be used to analyze frequency data in an effort to answer other types of questions. In this chapter we will also learn about these techniques.

12.2
The Mathematical Properties
of the Chi-Square Distribution

The chi-square distribution may be derived from normal distributions. Suppose that from a normally distributed random variable Y with mean μ and variance σ^2 we randomly and independently select samples of size $n = 1$. Each value selected may be transformed to the standard normal variable z by the familiar formula

$$z = \frac{y_i - \mu}{\sigma} \qquad (12.2.1)$$

Each value of z may be squared to obtain z^2. When we investigate the sampling distribution of z^2, we find that it follows a chi-square distribution with 1 degree of freedom. That is,

$$\chi^2_{(1)} = \left(\frac{y - \mu}{\sigma}\right)^2 = z^2$$

Now suppose that we randomly and independently select samples of size $n = 2$ from the normally distributed population of Y values. Within each sample we may transform each value of y to the standard normal variable z and square as before.

If the resulting values of z^2 for each sample are added, we may designate this sum by

$$\chi^2_{(2)} = \left(\frac{y_1 - \mu}{\sigma}\right)^2 + \left(\frac{y_2 - \mu}{\sigma}\right)^2 = z_1^2 + z_2^2$$

since it follows the chi-square distribution with 2 degrees of freedom, the number of independent squared terms that are added together.

The procedure may be repeated for any sample size n. The sum of the resulting z^2 values in each case will be distributed as chi-square with n degrees of freedom. In general, then,

$$\chi^2_{(n)} = z_1^2 + z_2^2 + \cdots + z_n^2 \qquad (12.2.2)$$

follows the chi-square distribution with n degrees of freedom. The mathematical form of the chi-square distribution is as follows:

$$f(u) = \frac{1}{\left(\frac{k}{2} - 1\right)!} \frac{1}{2^{k/2}} u^{(k/2)-1} e^{-(u/2)}, \qquad u > 0 \qquad (12.2.3)$$

where e is the irrational number $2.71828\ldots$ and k is the number of degrees of freedom. The variate u is usually designated by the Greek letter chi (χ) and, hence, the distribution is called the chi-square distribution. As we pointed out in Chapter 6, the chi-square distribution has been tabulated in Table F. Further use of the table is demonstrated as the need arises in succeeding sections.

The mean and variance of the chi-square distribution are k and $2k$, respectively. The modal value of the distribution is $k - 2$ for values of k greater than or equal to 2 and is zero for $k = 1$.

The shapes of the chi-square distributions for several values of k are shown in Figure 6.9.1. We observe in this figure that the shapes for $k = 1$ and $k = 2$ are quite different from the general shape of the distribution for $k > 2$. We also see from this figure that chi-square assumes values between 0 and infinity. It cannot take on negative values, since it is the sum of values that have been squared. A final characteristic of the chi-square distribution worth noting is that the sum of two or more independent chi-square variables also follows a chi-square distribution.

Types of Chi-Square Tests   As already noted, we make use of the chi-square distribution in this chapter in testing hypotheses where the data available for analysis are in the form of frequencies. These hypothesis testing procedures are discussed under the topics of *tests of goodness-of-fit*, *tests of independence*, and *tests of homogeneity*. We will discover that, in a sense, all of the chi-square tests that we employ may be thought of as goodness-of-fit tests, in that they test the goodness-of-fit of observed frequencies to frequencies that one would expect if the data were generated under some particular theory or hypothesis. We, however, reserve the phrase "goodness-of-fit" for use in a more restricted sense. We use the term "goodness-of-fit" to refer to a comparison of a sample distribution to some theoretical distribution that it is assumed describes the population from which the sample came. The justification of our use of the distribution in these situations is due to Karl Pearson (1), who showed that the chi-square distribution may be used as a test of the agreement between observation and hypothesis whenever the data are in the form of frequencies. An extensive treatment of the chi-square distribution is to be found in the book by Lancaster (2).

Observed Versus Expected Frequencies   The chi-square statistic is most appropriate for use with categorical variables, such as marital status, whose values are categories like married, single, widowed, and divorced. The quantitative data used in the computation of the test statistic are the frequencies associated with each category of the one or more variables under study. There are two sets of frequencies with which we are concerned, *observed frequencies* and *expected frequencies*. The observed frequencies are the number of subjects or objects in our sample that fall into the various categories of the variable of interest. For example, if we have a sample of 100 hospital patients we may observe that 50 are married, 30 are single, 15 are widowed, and 5 are divorced. Expected frequencies are the number of subjects or objects in our sample that we would expect to observe if some null hypothesis about the variable is true. For example, our null hypothesis might be that the four categories of marital status are equally represented in the population from which we drew our sample. In that case we would expect our sample to contain 25 married, 25 single, 25 widowed, and 25 divorced patients.

The Chi-Square Test Statistic   The test statistic for the chi-square tests we discuss in this chapter is

$$X^2 = \sum \left[\frac{(O_i - E_i)^2}{E_i} \right] \tag{12.2.4}$$

When the null hypothesis is true, X^2 is distributed approximately as χ^2 with $k - r$ degrees of freedom. In determining the degrees of freedom, k is equal to the number of groups for which observed and expected frequencies are available, and r is the number of restrictions or constraints imposed on the given comparison. A restriction is imposed when we force the sum of the expected frequencies to equal the sum of the observed frequencies, and an additional restriction is imposed for each parameter that is estimated from the sample. For a full discussion of the theoretical justification for subtracting one degree of freedom for each estimated parameter, see Cramer (3).

In Equation 12.2.4, O_i is the observed frequency for the ith category of the variable of interest, and E_i is the expected frequency (given that H_0 is true) for the ith category.

The quantity X^2 is a measure of the extent to which, in a given situation, pairs of observed and expected frequencies agree. As we will see, the nature of X^2 is such that when there is close agreement between observed and expected frequencies it is small, and when the agreement is poor it is large. Consequently only a sufficiently large value of X^2 will cause rejection of the null hypothesis.

If there is perfect agreement between the observed frequencies and the frequencies that one would expect, given that H_0 is true, the term $O_i - E_i$ in Equation 12.2.4 will be equal to zero for each pair of observed and expected frequencies. Such a result would yield a value of X^2 equal to zero, and we would be unable to reject H_0.

When there is disagreement between observed frequencies and the frequencies one would expect given that H_0 is true, at least one of the $O_i - E_i$ terms in Equation 12.2.4 will be a nonzero number. In general, the poorer the agreement between the O_i and the E_i, the greater and/or the more frequent will be these nonzero values. As noted previously, if the agreement between the O_i and the E_i is sufficiently poor (resulting in a sufficiently large X^2 value) we will be able to reject H_0.

When there is disagreement between a pair of observed and expected frequencies, the difference may be either positive or negative, depending on which of the two frequencies is the larger. Since the measure of agreement, X^2, is a sum of component quantities whose magnitudes depend on the difference $O_i - E_i$, positive and negative differences must be given equal weight. This is achieved by squaring each $O_i - E_i$ difference. Dividing the squared differences by the appropriate expected frequency converts the quantity to a term that is measured in original units. Adding these individual $(O_i - E_i)^2/E_i$ terms yields X^2, a summary statistic that reflects the extent of the overall agreement between observed and expected frequencies.

The Decision Rule The quantity $\Sigma[(O_i - E_i)^2/E_i]$ will be small if the observed and expected frequencies are close together and will be large if the differences are large.

The computed value of X^2 is compared with the tabulated value of χ^2 with $k - r$ degrees of freedom. The decision rule, then, is: Reject H_0 if X^2 is greater than or equal to the tabulated χ^2 for the chosen value of α.

12.3
Tests of Goodness-of-Fit

As we have pointed out, a goodness-of-fit test is appropriate when one wishes to decide if an observed distribution of frequencies is incompatible with some preconceived or hypothesized distribution.

We may, for example, wish to determine whether or not a sample of observed values of some random variable is compatible with the hypothesis that it was drawn from a population of values that is normally distributed. The procedure for reaching a decision consists of placing the values into mutually exclusive categories or class intervals and noting the frequency of occurrence of values in each category.

We then make use of our knowledge of normal distributions to determine the frequencies for each category that one could expect if the sample had come from a normal distribution. If the discrepancy is of such magnitude that it could have come about due to chance, we conclude that the sample may have come from a normal distribution. In a similar manner, tests of goodness-of-fit may be carried out in cases where the hypothesized distribution is the binomial, the Poisson, or any other distribution. Let us illustrate in more detail with some examples of tests of hypotheses of goodness-of-fit.

Example 12.3.1

The Normal Distribution

A research team making a study of hospitals in the United States collects data on a sample of 250 hospitals. The team computes for each hospital the inpatient occupancy ratio, a variable that shows, for a 12-month period, the ratio of average daily census to the average number of beds maintained. The sample yielded the distribution of ratios (expressed as percents), shown in Table 12.3.1.

We wish to know whether these data provide sufficient evidence to indicate that the sample did not come from a normally distributed population.

Solution:

1. *Data*   See Table 12.3.1.

2. *Assumptions*   We assume that the sample available for analysis is a simple random sample.

3. *Hypotheses*

   H_0: In the population from which the sample was drawn, inpatient occupancy ratios are normally distributed.

   H_A: The sampled population is not normally distributed.

4. *Test Statistic*   The test statistic is

$$X^2 = \sum_{i=1}^{k} \left[\frac{(O_i - E_i)^2}{E_i} \right]$$

TABLE 12.3.1 Results of Study Described in Example 12.3.1

Inpatient Occupancy Ratio	Number of Hospitals
0.0 to 39.9	16
40.0 to 49.9	18
50.0 to 59.9	22
60.0 to 69.9	51
70.0 to 79.9	62
80.0 to 89.9	55
90.0 to 99.9	22
100.0 to 109.9	4
Total	250

5. *Distribution of the Test Statistic* If H_0 is true the test statistic is distributed approximately as chi-square with $k - r$ degrees of freedom. The values of k and r will be determined later.

6. *Decision Rule* We will reject H_0 if the computed value of X^2 is equal to or greater than the critical value of chi-square.

7. *Calculation of Test Statistic* Since the mean and variance of the hypothesized distribution are not specified, the sample data must be used to estimate them. These parameters, or their estimates, will be needed to compute the frequency that would be expected in each class interval when the null hypothesis is true. The mean and standard deviation computed from the grouped data of Table 12.3.1 by the methods of Sections 2.6 and 2.7 are

$$\bar{x} = 69.91$$

$$x = 19.02$$

As the next step in the analysis we must obtain for each class interval the frequency of occurrence of values that we would expect when the null hypothesis is true, that is, if the sample were, in fact, drawn from a normally distributed population of values. To do this, we first determine the expected relative frequency of occurrence of values for each class interval and then multiply these expected relative frequencies by the total number of values to obtain the expected number of values for each interval.

The Expected Relative Frequencies It will be recalled from our study of the normal distribution that the relative frequency of occurrence of values equal to or less than some specified value, say x_0, of the normally distributed random variable X is equivalent to the area under the curve and to the left of x_0 as represented by the shaded area in Figure 12.3.1. We obtain the numerical value of this area by converting x_0 to a standard normal deviation by the formula $z_0 = (x_0 - \mu)/\sigma$ and

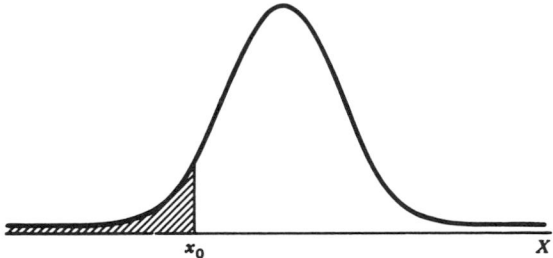

Figure 12.3.1 A normal distribution showing the relative frequency of occurrence of values less than or equal to x_0. The shaded area represents the relative frequency of occurrence of values equal to or less than x_0.

finding the appropriate value in Table D. We use this procedure to obtain the expected relative frequencies corresponding to each of the class intervals in Table 12.3.1. We estimate μ and σ with $\bar{x}$ and s as computed from the grouped sample data. The first step consists of obtaining z values corresponding to the lower limit of each class interval. The area between two successive z values will give the expected relative frequency of occurrence of values for the corresponding class interval.

For example, to obtain the expected relative frequency of occurrence of values in the interval 40.0 to 49.9 we proceed as follows:

$$\text{The } z \text{ value corresponding to } X = 40.0 \text{ is } z = \frac{40.0 - 69.91}{19.02} = -1.57$$

$$\text{The } z \text{ value corresponding to } X = 50.0 \text{ is } z = \frac{50.0 - 69.91}{19.02} = -1.05$$

In Table D we find that the area to the left of -1.05 is .1469, and the area to the left of -1.57 is .0582. The area between -1.05 and -1.57 is equal to .1469 − .0582 = .0887, which is equal to the expected relative frequency of occurrence of values of occupancy ratios within the interval 40.0 to 49.9. This tells us that if the null hypothesis is true, that is, if the occupancy ratio values are normally distributed, we should expect 8.87 percent of the values in our sample to be between 40.0 and 49.9. When we multiply our total sample size, 250, by .0887 we find the expected frequency for the interval to be 22.18. Similar calculations will give the expected frequencies for the other intervals as shown in Table 12.3.2.

Comparing Observed and Expected Frequencies   We are now interested in examining the magnitudes of the discrepancies between the observed frequencies and the expected frequencies, since we note that the two sets of frequencies do not agree. We know that even if our sample were drawn from a normal distribution of values,

TABLE 12.3.2 Class Intervals and Expected Frequencies for Example 12.3.1

Class Interval	$z = (x_i - \bar{x})/s$ At Lower Limit of Interval	Expected Relative Frequency	Expected Frequency
< 40.0		.0582	14.55
40.0 to 49.9	−1.57	.0887	22.18
50.0 to 59.9	−1.05	.1546	38.65
60.0 to 69.9	−.52	.1985	49.62
70.0 to 79.9	.00	.2019	50.48
80.0 to 89.9	.53	.1535	38.38
90.0 to 99.9	1.06	.0875	21.88
100.0 to 109.9	1.58	.0397	9.92
110.0 and greater	2.11	.0174	4.35
Total		1.0000	250.00

TABLE 12.3.3 Observed and Expected Frequencies and $(O_i - E_i)^2/E_i$ For Example 12.3.1

Class Interval	Observed Frequency (O_i)	Expected Frequency (E_i)	$(O_i - E_i)^2/E_i$
< 40.0	16	14.55	.145
40.0 to 49.9	18	22.18	.788
50.0 to 59.9	22	38.65	7.173
60.0 to 69.9	51	49.62	.038
70.0 to 79.9	62	50.48	2.629
80.0 to 89.9	55	38.38	7.197
90.0 to 99.9	22	21.88	.001
100.0 to 109.9	4	9.92	3.533
110.0 and greater	0	4.35	4.350
Total	250	250.00	25.854

sampling variability alone would make it highly unlikely that the observed and expected frequencies would agree perfectly. We wonder, then, if the discrepancies between the observed and expected frequencies are small enough that we feel it reasonable that they could have occurred by chance alone, when the null hypothesis is true. If they are of this magnitude, we will be unwilling to reject the null hypothesis that the sample came from a normally distributed population.

If the discrepancies are so large that it does not seem reasonable that they could have occurred by chance alone when the null hypothesis is true, we will want to reject the null hypothesis. The criterion against which we judge whether the discrepancies are "large" or "small" is provided by the chi-square distribution.

The observed and expected frequencies along with each value of $(O_i - E_i)^2/E_i$ are shown in Table 12.3.3. The first entry in the last column, for example, is computed from $(16 - 14.55)^2/14.55 = .145$. The other values of $(O_i - E_i)^2/E_i$ are computed in a similar manner.

From Table 12.3.3 we see that $X^2 = \Sigma[(O_i - E_i)^2/E_i] = 25.854$. The appropriate degrees of freedom are 9 (the number of groups or class intervals) − 3 (for the three restrictions: making $\Sigma E_i = \Sigma O_i$, and estimating μ and σ from the sample data) = 6.

8. *Statistical Decision* When we compare $X^2 = 25.854$ with values of χ^2 in Table F, we see that it is larger than $\chi^2_{.995} = 18.548$, so that we can reject the null hypothesis that the sample came from a normally distributed population at the .005 level of significance. In other words, the probability of obtaining a value of X^2 as large as 25.854, when the null hypothesis is true, is less than 5 in 1000 ($p < .005$). We say that such a rare event did not occur due to chance alone (when H_0 is true), so we look for another explanation. The other explanation is that the null hypothesis is false.

9. *Conclusion* We conclude that in the sampled population, inpatient occupancy ratios are not normally distributed.

Sometimes the parameters are specified in the null hypothesis. It should be noted that had the mean and variance of the population been specified as part of the null hypothesis in Example 12.3.1, we would not have had to estimate them from the sample and our degrees of freedom would have been $9 - 1 = 8$.

If parameters are estimated from ungrouped sample data rather than from grouped data as in our example, the distribution of X^2 may not be sufficiently approximated by the chi-square distribution to give satisfactory results. The problem is discussed by Dahiya and Gurland (4) and Watson (5–7). The same problem is encountered when parameters are estimated independently of the sample, as discussed by Chase (8).

Small Expected Frequencies Frequently in applications of the chi-square test the expected frequency for one or more categories will be small, perhaps much less than 1. In the literature the point is frequently made that the approximation of X^2 to χ^2 is not strictly valid when some of the expected frequencies are small. There is disagreement among writers, however, over what size expected frequencies are allowable before making some adjustment or abandoning χ^2 in favor of some alternative test. Some writers, especially the earlier ones, suggest lower limits of 10, whereas others suggest that all expected frequencies should be no less than 5. Cochran (9, 10), writing in the early 1950s, suggested that for goodness-of-fit tests of unimodal distributions (such as the normal) the minimum expected frequency can be as low as 1. If, in practice, one encounters one or more expected frequencies less than 1, adjacent categories may be combined to achieve the suggested minimum. Combining reduces the number of categories and, therefore, the number of degrees of freedom. Cochran's suggestions appear to have been followed extensively by practitioners in recent years. More recent research on the subject of small expected frequencies includes that of Roscoe and Byars (11), Yarnold (12), Tate and Hyer (13), Slakter (14, 15), and Lewontin and Felsenstein (16).

Alternatives Although one frequently encounters in the literature the use of chi-square to test for normality, it is not the most appropriate test to use when the hypothesized distribution is continuous. The Kolmogorov–Smirnov test, described in Chapter 13, was especially designed for goodness-of-fit tests involving continuous distributions.

Example 12.3.2 The Binomial Distribution In a study designed to determine patient acceptance of a new pain reliever, 100 physicians each selected a sample of 25 patients to participate in the study. Each patient, after trying the new pain relief for a specified period of time, was asked whether it was preferable to the pain reliever used regularly in the past.

The results of the study are shown in Table 12.3.4.

We are interested in determining whether or not these data are compatible with the hypothesis that they were drawn from a population that follows a binomial distribution. Again, we employ a chi-square goodness-of-fit test.

TABLE 12.3.4 Results of Study Described in Example 12.3.2

Number of Patients Out of 25 Preferring New Pain Reliever	Number of Doctors Reporting This Number	Total Number of Patients Preferring New Pain Reliever By Doctor
0	5	0
1	6	6
2	8	16
3	10	30
4	10	40
5	15	75
6	17	102
7	10	70
8	10	80
9	9	81
10 or more	0	0
Total	100	500

Solution: Since the binomial parameter, p, is not specified, it must be estimated from the sample data. A total of 500 patients out of the 2500 patients participating in the study said they preferred the new pain reliever, so that our point estimate of p is $\hat{p} = 500/2500 = .20$. The expected relative frequencies can be obtained by evaluating the binomial function

$$f(x) = \binom{25}{x}.2^x.8^{25-x}$$

for $x = 0, 1, \ldots, 25$. For example, to find the probability that out of a sample of 25 patients none would prefer the new pain reliever, when in the total population the true proportion preferring the new pain reliever is .2, we would evaluate

$$f(0) = \binom{25}{0}.2^0.8^{25-0}$$

This can be done most easily by consulting Table B, where we see that $P(X = 0) = .0038$. The relative frequency of occurrence of samples of size 25 in which no patients prefer the new pain reliever is .0038. To obtain the corresponding expected frequency, we multiply .0038 by 100 to get .38. Similar calculations yield the remaining expected frequencies which, along with the observed frequencies, are shown in Table 12.3.5. We see in this table that the first expected frequency is less than 1, so that we follow Cochran's suggestion and combine this group with the second group. When we do this, all the expected frequencies are greater than 1.

TABLE 12.3.5 Calculations for Example 12.3.2

Number of Patients Out of 25 Preferring New Pain Reliever	Number of Doctors Reporting This Number (Observed Frequency, O_i)	Expected Relative Frequency	Expected Frequency E_i
0	5 ⎱ 11	.0038	.38 ⎱ 2.74
1	6 ⎰	.0236	2.36 ⎰
2	8	.0708	7.08
3	10	.1358	13.58
4	10	.1867	18.67
5	15	.1960	19.60
6	17	.1633	16.33
7	10	.1109	11.09
8	10	.0623	6.23
9	9	.0295	2.95
10 or more	0	.0173	1.73
Total	100	1.0000	100.00

From the data we compute

$$X^2 = \frac{(11 - 2.74)^2}{2.74} + \frac{(8 - 7.08)^2}{7.08} + \cdots + \frac{(0 - 1.73)^2}{1.73} = 47.624$$

The appropriate degrees of freedom are 10 (the number of groups left after combining the first two) less 2, or 8. One degree of freedom is lost because we force the total of the expected frequencies to equal the total observed frequencies, and one degree of freedom is sacrificed because we estimate p from the sample data.

We compare our computed X^2 with the tabulated χ^2 with 8 degrees of freedom and find that it is significant at the .005 level of significance; that is, $p < .005$. We reject the null hypothesis that the data came from a binomial distribution.

Example 12.3.3 The Poisson Distribution   A hospital administrator wishes to test the null hypothesis that emergency admissions follow a Poisson distribution with $\lambda = 3$. Suppose that over a period of 90 days the numbers of emergency admissions were as shown in Table 12.3.6.

The data of Table 12.3.6 are summarized in Table 12.3.7.

Solution: To obtain the expected frequencies we first obtain the expected relative frequencies by evaluating the Poisson function given by Equation 4.4.1 for each entry in the left-hand column of Table 12.3.7. For example, the first expected relative frequency is obtained by evaluating

$$f(0) = \frac{e^{-3}3^0}{0!}$$

TABLE 12.3.6 Number of Emergency Admissions to a Hospital During a 90-Day Period

Day	Emergency Admissions	Day	Emergency Admissions	Day	Emergency Admissions	Day	Emergency Admissions
1	2	24	5	47	4	70	3
2	3	25	3	48	2	71	5
3	4	26	2	49	2	72	4
4	5	27	4	50	3	73	1
5	3	28	4	51	4	74	1
6	2	29	3	52	2	75	6
7	3	30	5	53	3	76	3
8	0	31	1	54	1	77	3
9	1	32	3	55	2	78	5
10	0	33	2	56	3	79	2
11	1	34	4	57	2	80	1
12	0	35	2	58	5	81	7
13	6	36	5	59	2	82	7
14	4	37	0	60	7	83	1
15	4	38	6	61	8	84	5
16	4	39	4	62	3	85	1
17	3	40	4	63	1	86	4
18	4	41	5	64	3	87	4
19	3	42	1	65	1	88	9
20	3	43	3	66	0	89	2
21	3	44	1	67	3	90	3
22	4	45	2	68	2		
23	3	46	3	69	1		

TABLE 12.3.7 Summary of Data Presented in Table 12.3.6

Number of Emergency Admissions in a Day	Number of Days This Number of Emergency Admissions of Occurred
0	5
1	14
2	15
3	23
4	16
5	9
6	3
7	3
8	1
9	1
10 or more	0
Total	90

TABLE 12.3.8 Observed and Expected Frequencies and Components of X^2 For Example 12.3.3

Number of Emergency Admissions	Number of Days This Number Occurred, O_i	Expected Relative Frequency	Expected Frequency	$\dfrac{(O_i - E_i)^2}{E_i}$
0	5	.050	4.50	.056
1	14	.149	13.41	.026
2	15	.224	20.16	1.321
3	23	.224	20.16	.400
4	16	.168	15.12	.051
5	9	.101	9.09	.001
6	3	.050	4.50	.500
7	3	.022	1.98	.525
8	1 ⎫	.008	.72 ⎫	
9	1 ⎬ 2	.003	.27 ⎬ .108	.784
10 or more	0 ⎭	.001	.09 ⎭	
Total	90	1.000	90.00	3.664

We may use Table C of Appendix II to find this and all the other expected relative frequencies that we need. Each of the expected relative frequencies is multiplied by 90 to obtain the corresponding expected frequencies. These values along with the observed and expected frequencies and the components of X^2, $(O_i - E_i)^2/E_i$, are displayed in Table 12.3.8. In Table 12.3.8 we see that

$$X^2 = \sum \left[\frac{(O_i - E_i)^2}{E_i} \right] = \frac{(5 - 4.50)^2}{4.50} + \cdots + \frac{(2 - 1.08)^2}{1.08} = 3.664$$

We also note that the last three expected frequencies are less than 1, so that they must be combined to avoid having any expected frequencies less than 1. This means that we have only nine effective categories for computing degrees of freedom. Since the parameter, λ, was specified in the null hypothesis, we do not lose a degree of freedom for reasons of estimation, so that the appropriate degrees of freedom are $9 - 1 = 8$. By consulting Table F of Appendix II, we find that the critical value of χ^2 for 8 degrees of freedom and $\alpha = .05$ is 15.507, so that we cannot reject the null hypothesis at the .05, or for that matter any reasonable level of significance ($p > .10$). We conclude, therefore, that emergency admissions at this hospital may follow a Poisson distribution with $\lambda = 3$. At least the observed data do not cast any doubt on that hypothesis.

If the parameter λ has to be estimated from sample data, the estimate is obtained by multiplying each value x by its frequency, summing these products, and dividing the total by the sum of the frequencies.

Example 12.3.4

A certain human trait is thought to be inherited according to the ratio $1:2:1$ for homozygous dominant, heterozygous, and homozygous recessive. An examination of a simple random sample of 200 individuals yielded the following distribution of the trait: dominant, 43; heterozygous, 125, and recessive, 32. We wish to know if these data provide sufficient evidence to cast doubt on the belief about the distribution of the trait.

Solution:

1. *Data* See statement of the example.
2. *Assumptions* We assume that the data meet the requirements for the application of the chi-square goodness-of-fit test.
3. *Hypotheses*

   H_0: The trait is distributed according to the ratio $1:2:1$ for homozygous dominant, heterozygous, and homozygous recessive.

   H_A: The trait is not distributed according to the ratio $1:2:1$.

4. *Test Statistic* The test statistic is

$$X^2 = \sum \left[\frac{(O - E)^2}{E} \right]$$

5. *Distribution of the Test Statistic* If H_0 is true, X^2 is distributed as chi-square with 2 degrees of freedom.
6. *Decision Rule* Suppose we let the probability of committing a type I error be .05. Reject H_0 if the computed value of X^2 is equal to or greater than 5.991.
7. *Calculation of the Test Statistic* If H_0 is true, the expected frequencies for the three manifestations of the trait are 50, 100, and 50 for dominant, heterozygous, and recessive, respectively. Consequently

$$X^2 = (43 - 50)^2/50 + (125 - 100)^2/100 + (32 - 50)^2/50 = 13.71$$

8. *Statistical Decision* Since $13.71 > 5.991$, we reject H_0.
9. *Conclusion* We conclude that the trait is not distributed according to the ratio $1:2:1$. Since $13.71 > 10.597$, the p value for the test is $p < .005$.

EXERCISES

12.3.1 The following table shows the distribution of uric acid determinations taken on 250 patients. Test the goodness-of-fit of these data to a normal distribution with $\mu = 5.74$ and $\sigma = 2.01$. Let $\alpha = .01$.

Uric Acid Determination	Observed Frequency
< 1	1
1 to 1.99	5
2 to 2.99	15
3 to 3.99	24
4 to 4.99	43
5 to 5.99	50
6 to 6.99	45
7 to 7.99	30
8 to 8.99	22
9 to 9.99	10
10 or higher	5
Total	250

12.3.2 The following data were collected on 300 eight-year-old girls. Test, at the .05 level of significance, the null hypothesis that the data are drawn from a normally distributed population. Use the methods of Chapter 1 to compute the sample mean and standard deviation from grouped data.

Height in Centimeters	Observed Frequency
114 to 115.9	5
116 to 117.9	10
118 to 119.9	14
120 to 121.9	21
122 to 123.9	30
124 to 125.9	40
126 to 127.9	45
128 to 129.9	43
130 to 131.9	42
132 to 133.9	30
134 to 135.9	11
136 to 137.9	5
138 to 139.9	4
Total	300

12.3.3 The face sheet of patients' records maintained in a local health department contains 10 entries. A sample of 100 records revealed the following distribution of erroneous entries.

Number of Erroneous Entries Out of 10	Number of Records
0	8
1	25
2	32
3	24
4	10
5 or more	1
Total	100

Test the goodness-of-fit of these data to the binomial distribution with $p = .20$. Find the p value for this test.

12.3.4 Jordan et al. (A-1) state that fragile sites are nonrandom, heritable sites on chromosomes that can be induced to form gaps, breaks, and rearrangements under specific conditions. They point out that one researcher has made the assumption that the distribution of events, X, pooled across individuals, follows a Poisson distribution, with the expected number of events per site as the mean and variance. To test this assumption, Jordan and her colleagues collected the following data on three pairs of like-sexed twins.

X	Observed Frequency of X	Expected Frequency
0	2070	1884.14
1	224	455.96
2	70	55.17
3	22	4.45
4	3	.27
5	2	.01
6	0	.00
7	0	.00
8	1	.00
9	1	.00
10	2	.00
11	1	.00
12	0	.00
13	0	.00
14	0	.00
15	3	.00
37	1	.00

SOURCE: Diane K. Jordan, Trudy L. Burns, James E. Divelbiss, Robert F. Woolson, and Shivanand R. Patil, "Variability in Expression of Common Fragile Sites: In Search of a New Criterion," *Human Genetics*, *85* (1990), 462–466.

Can we conclude on the basis of these data that the previously stated assumption is valid? Let $\alpha = .01$.

12.3.5 The following are the numbers of a particular organism found in 100 samples of water from a pond.

Number of Organisms Per Sample	Frequency
0	15
1	30
2	25
3	20
4	5
5	4
6	1
7	0
Total	100

Test the null hypothesis that these data were drawn from a Poisson distribution. Determine the p value for this test.

12.3.6 A research team conducted a survey in which the subjects were adult smokers. Each subject in a sample of 200 was asked to indicate the extent to which he/she agreed with the statement: "I would like to quit smoking." The results were as follows:

Response: Number Responding:	Strongly agree	Agree	Disagree	Strongly disagree
	102	30	60	8

Can one conclude on the basis of these data that, in the sampled population, opinions are not equally distributed over the four levels of agreement? Let the probability of committing a type I error be .05 and find the p value.

12.4
Tests of Independence

Another, and perhaps the most frequent, use of the chi-square distribution is to test the null hypothesis that two criteria of classification, when applied to the same set of entities, are independent. We say that two criteria of classification are independent if the distribution of one criterion is the same no matter what the distribution of the other criterion. For example, if socioeconomic status and area of residence of the inhabitants of a certain city are independent, we would expect to find the same proportion of families in the low, medium, and high socioeconomic groups in all areas of the city.

The Contingency Table   The classification, according to two criteria, of a set of entities, say people, can be shown by a table in which the r rows represent the various levels of one criterion of classification and the c columns represent the various levels of the second criterion. Such a table is generally called a *contingency table*. The classification according to two criteria of a finite population of entities is shown in Table 12.4.1.

We will be interested in testing the null hypothesis that in the population the two criteria of classification are independent. If the hypothesis is rejected, we will conclude that the two criteria of classification are not independent. A sample of size n will be drawn from the population of entities, and the frequency of occurrence of entities in the sample corresponding to the cells formed by the intersections of the rows and columns of Table 12.4.1 along with the marginal totals will be displayed in a table such as Table 12.4.2.

Calculating the Expected Frequencies   The expected frequencies, under the null hypothesis that the two criteria of classification are independent, are calculated for each cell.

We learned in Chapter 3 (see Equation 3.4.4) that if two events are independent, the probability of their joint occurrence is equal to the product of their individual probabilities. Under the assumption of independence, for example, we

TABLE 12.4.1 Two-Way Classification of a Finite Population of Entities

Second Criterion of Classification Level	First Criterion of Classification Level					Total
	1	**2**	**3**	$\cdots$	**c**	
1	N_{11}	N_{12}	N_{13}	$\cdots$	N_{1c}	$N_{1.}$
2	N_{21}	N_{22}	N_{23}	$\cdots$	N_{2c}	$N_{2.}$
3	N_{31}	N_{32}	N_{33}	$\cdots$	N_{3c}	$N_{3.}$
$\vdots$	$\vdots$	$\vdots$	$\vdots$	$\vdots$	$\vdots$	$\vdots$
r	N_{r1}	N_{r2}	N_{r3}	$\cdots$	N_{nc}	$N_{r.}$
Total	$N_{.1}$	$N_{.2}$	$N_{.3}$	$\cdots$	$N_{.c}$	N

TABLE 12.4.2 Two-Way Classification of a Sample of Entities

Second Criterion of Classification Level	First Criterion of Classification Level					Total
	1	**2**	**3**	$\cdots$	**c**	
1	n_{11}	n_{12}	n_{13}	$\cdots$	n_{1c}	$n_{1.}$
2	n_{21}	n_{22}	n_{23}	$\cdots$	n_{2c}	$n_{2.}$
3	n_{31}	n_{32}	n_{33}	$\cdots$	n_{3c}	$n_{3.}$
$\vdots$	$\vdots$	$\vdots$	$\vdots$		$\vdots$	$\vdots$
r	n_{r1}	n_{r2}	n_{r3}	$\cdots$	n_{rc}	$n_{r.}$
Total	$n_{.1}$	$n_{.2}$	$n_{.3}$	$\cdots$	$n_{.c}$	n

compute the probability that one of the n subjects represented in Table 12.4.2 will be counted in row 1 and column 1 of the table (that is, in cell 11) by multiplying the probability that the subject will be counted in row 1 by the probability that the subject will be counted in column 1. In the notation of the table, the desired calculation is

$$\left(\frac{n_{1.}}{n}\right)\left(\frac{n_{.1}}{n}\right)$$

To obtain the expected frequency for cell 11 we multiply this probability by the total number of subjects, n. That is, the expected frequency for cell 11 is given by

$$\left(\frac{n_{1.}}{n}\right)\left(\frac{n_{.1}}{n}\right)(n)$$

Since the n in one of the denominators cancels into numerator n, this expression reduces to

$$\frac{(n_{1.})(n_{.1})}{n}$$

In general, then, we see that to obtain the expected frequency for a given cell, we multiply the total of the row in which the cell is located by the total of the column in which the cell is located and divide the product by the grand total.

Observed Versus Expected Frequencies   The expected frequencies and observed frequencies are compared. If the discrepancy is sufficiently small, the null hypothesis is tenable. If the discrepancy is sufficiently large, the null hypothesis is rejected, and we conclude that the two criteria of classification are not independent. The decision as to whether the discrepancy between observed and expected frequencies is sufficiently large to cause rejection of H_0 will be made on the basis of the size of the quantity computed when we use Equation 12.3.1, where O_i and E_i refer, respectively, to the observed and expected frequencies in the cells of Table 12.4.2. It would be more logical to designate the observed and expected frequencies in these cells by O_{ij} and E_{ij}, but to keep the notation simple and to avoid the introduction of another formula, we have elected to use the simpler notation. It will be helpful to think of the cells as being numbered from 1 to k, where 1 refers to cell 11 and k refers to cell rc. It can be shown that X^2 as defined in this manner is distributed approximately as χ^2 with $(r - 1)(c - 1)$ degrees of freedom when the null hypothesis is true. If the computed value of X^2 is equal to or larger than the tabulated value of χ^2 for some α, the null hypothesis is rejected at the α level of significance. The hypothesis testing procedure is illustrated with the following example.

Example 12.4.1   The purpose of a study by Vermund et al. (A-2) was to investigate the hypothesis that HIV-infected women who are also infected with human papillomavirus (HPV), detected by molecular hybridization, are more likely to have cervical cytologic abnormalities than are women with only one or neither virus. The data shown in Table 12.4.3 were reported by the investigators. We wish to know if we may conclude that there is a relationship between HPV status and stage of HIV infection.

TABLE 12.4.3 HPV Status and Stage of HIV Infection Among 96 Women

HPV	HIV Seropositive, Symptomatic	Seropositive, Asymptomatic	Seronegative	Total
Positive	23	4	10	37
Negative	10	14	35	59
Total	33	18	45	96

SOURCE: Sten H. Vermund, Karen F. Kelley, Robert S. Klein, Anat R. Feingold, Klaus Schreiber, Gary Munk, and Robert D. Burk, "High Risk of Human Papillomavirus Infection and Cervical Squamous Intraepithelial Lesions Among Women with Symptomatic Human Immunodeficiency Virus Infection," *American Journal of Obstetrics and Gynecology*, *165* (1991), 392–400.

Solution:

1. *Data*   See Table 12.4.3.

2. *Assumptions*   We assume that the sample available for analysis is equivalent to a simple random sample drawn from the population of interest.

3. *Hypotheses*

   H_0:   HPV status and stage of HIV infection are independent.

   H_A: The two variables are not independent.

   Let $\alpha = .05$.

4. *Test Statistic*   The test statistic is

$$X^2 = \sum_{i=1}^{k} \left[\frac{(O_i - E_i)^2}{E_i} \right]$$

5. *Distribution of the Test Statistic*   When H_0 is true X^2 is distributed approximately as χ^2 with $(r - 1)(c - 1) = (2 - 1)(3 - 1) = (1)(2) = 2$ degrees of freedom.

6. *Decision Rule*   Reject H_0 if the computed value of X^2 is equal to or greater than 5.991.

7. *Calculation of Test Statistic*   The expected frequency for the first cell is $(33 \times 37)/96 = 12.72$. The other expected frequencies are calculated in a similar manner. Observed and expected frequencies are displayed together in Table 12.4.4. From the observed and expected frequencies we may compute

$$X^2 = \sum \left[\frac{(O_i - E_i)^2}{E_i} \right]$$

$$= \frac{(23 - 12.72)^2}{12.72} + \frac{(4 - 6.94)^2}{6.94} + \cdots + \frac{(35 - 27.66)^2}{27.66}$$

$$= 8.30805 + 1.24548 + \cdots + 1.94778 = 20.60081$$

TABLE 12.4.4 Observed and Expected Frequencies for Example 12.4.1

HPV	HIV Seropositive, Symptomatic	Seropositive, Asymptomatic	Seronegative	Total
Positive	23 (12.72)	4 (6.94)	10 (17.34)	37
Negative	10 (20.28)	14 (11.06)	35 (27.66)	59
Total	33	18	45	96

8. *Statistical Decision*   We reject H_0 since 20.60081 is > 5.991.

9. *Conclusion*   We conclude that H_0 is false, and that there is a relationship between HPV status and stage of HIV infection. Since 20.60081 is greater than 10.597, $p < .005$.

Small Expected Frequencies   The problem of small expected frequencies discussed in the previous section may be encountered when analyzing the data of contingency tables. Although there is a lack of consensus on how to handle this problem, many authors currently follow the rule given by Cochran (10). He suggests that for contingency tables with more than 1 degree of freedom a minimum expectation of 1 is allowable if no more than 20 percent of the cells have expected frequencies of less than 5. To meet this rule, adjacent rows and/or adjacent columns may be combined when to do so is logical in light of other considerations. If X^2 is based on less than 30 degrees of freedom, expected frequencies as small as 2 can be tolerated. We did not experience the problem of small expected frequencies in Example 12.4.1, since they were all greater than 5.

The 2 × 2 Contingency Table   Sometimes each of two criteria of classification may be broken down into only two categories, or levels. When data are cross-classified in this manner, the result is a contingency table consisting of two rows and two columns. Such a table is commonly referred to as a 2 × 2 table. The value of X^2 may be computed by first calculating the expected cell frequencies in the manner discussed above. In the case of a 2 × 2 contingency table, however, X^2 may be calculated by the following shortcut formula:

$$X^2 = \frac{n(ad - bc)^2}{(a + c)(b + d)(a + b)(c + d)} \tag{12.4.1}$$

where a, b, c, and d are the observed cell frequencies as shown in Table 12.4.5. When we apply the $(r - 1)(c - 1)$ rule for finding degrees of freedom to a 2 × 2 table, the result is 1 degree of freedom. Let us illustrate this with an example.

TABLE 12.4.5 A 2 × 2 Contingency Table

Second Criterion of Classification	First Criterion of Classification		
	1	2	Total
1	a	b	$a + b$
2	c	d	$c + d$
Total	$a + c$	$b + d$	n

Example 12.4.2

According to Chow et al. (A-3) *Enterobacter* species are a major cause of nosocomial gram-negative bacteremia. Of interest is the ability of the organism to develop resistance to the antibiotic administered. Chow and his colleagues conducted a study of *Enterobacter* bacteremia to determine the clinical setting in which the condition occurs, the effect of previously received antibiotics on the antibiotic susceptibility profile of the *Enterobacter* isolated, the effect of antibiotic susceptibility and other factors on mortality, the incidence and mechanisms of emergence of resistance to antibiotic therapy, and the efficacy of combination therapy compared with monotherapy on the emergence of resistance. The subjects were 129 patients with *Enterobacter* bacteremia. The *Enterobacter* sp. were found to be multiresistant in 37 of the 129 initial blood isolates. Multiresistant *Enterobacter* was found in blood isolates of the 103 patients who had received an antibiotic within two weeks prior to the initial positive blood culture. We wish to know if we can conclude that there is a relationship between multiresistant *Enterobacter* status and status with regard to previous use of antibiotics.

Solution:

1. *Data* From the information given we may construct the 2 × 2 contingency table displayed as Table 12.4.6.

2. *Assumptions* We assume that the sample is equivalent to a simple random sample.

3. *Hypotheses*

H_0: Status with regard to multiresistant *Enterobacter* and status with regard to previous use of antibiotics are independent.

H_A: The two variables are not independent.

Let $\alpha = .05$.

TABLE 12.4.6 Contingency Table for the Data of Example 12.4.2

| Antibiotic in Past 2 Weeks | Multiresistant *Enterobacter* Isolate | | |
	Yes	No	Total
Yes	36	67	103
No	1	25	26
Total	37	92	129

SOURCE: Reproduced with permission, from Joseph W. Chow, Michael J. Fine, David M. Shlaes, John P. Quinn, David C. Hooper, Michael P. Johnson, Rueben Ramphal, Marilyn M. Wagener, Deborah K. Miyashiro, and Victor L. Yu, "*Enterobacter* Bacteremia: Clinical Features and Emergence of Antibiotic Resistance During Therapy," *Annals of Internal Medicine*, *115* (1991), 585–590.

4. *Test Statistic*   The test statistic is

$$X^2 = \sum_{k=1}^{i} \left[\frac{(O_i - E_i)^2}{E_i} \right]$$

5. *Distribution of the Test Statistic*   When H_0 is true X^2 is distributed approximately as χ^2 with $(2-1)(2-1) = (1)(1) = 1$ degree of freedom.

6. *Decision Rule*   Reject H_0 if the computed value of X^2 is equal to or greater than 3.841.

7. *Calculation of the Test Statistic*   By Equation 12.4.1 we compute

$$X^2 = \frac{129\big[(36)(25) - (67)(1)\big]^2}{(37)(92)(103)(26)}$$

$$= 9.8193$$

8. *Statistical Decision*   Since $9.8193 > 3.841$, we reject H_0. For this test, $p < .005$.

9. *Conclusion*   The researcher may conclude that there is a relationship between the two variables under study.

Small Expected Frequencies   The problems of how to handle small expected frequencies and small total sample sizes may arise in the analysis of 2×2 contingency tables. Cochran (10) suggests that the χ^2 test should not be used if $n < 20$ or if $20 < n < 40$ and any expected frequency is less than 5. When $n \geq 40$ an expected cell frequency as small as 1 can be tolerated.

Yates' Correction   The observed frequencies in a contingency table are discrete and thereby give rise to a discrete statistic, X^2, which is approximated by the χ^2 distribution, which is continuous. Yates (17) in 1934 proposed a procedure for correcting for this in the case of 2×2 tables. The correction, as shown in Equation 12.4.2, consists of subtracting half the total number of observations from the absolute value of the quantity $ad - bc$ before squaring. That is,

$$X^2_{\text{corrected}} = \frac{n\big(|ad - bc| - .5n\big)^2}{(a + c)(b + d)(a + b)(c + d)} \tag{12.4.2}$$

It is generally agreed that no correction is necessary for larger contingency tables. Although Yates' correction for 2×2 tables has been used extensively in the past, recent investigators, for example, Grizzle (18), Lancaster (19), Pearson (20), and Plackett (21), have questioned its use. The work of Grizzle, in particular, has strengthened the case against the use of the correction on the basis that it too often results in an overly conservative test; that is, the use of the correction too often leads to nonrejection of the null hypothesis. As a result some practitioners are recommending against its use. This seems to be a reasonable recommendation to follow.

We may, as a matter of interest, apply the correction to our current example. Using Equation 12.4.2 and the data from Table 12.4.6, we may compute

$$X^2_{corrected} = \frac{129\left[|(36)(25) - (67)(1)| - .5(129)\right]^2}{(37)(92)(103)(26)}$$

$$= 8.3575$$

As might be expected, with a sample this large, the difference in the two results is not dramatic.

Tests of Independence-Characteristics   The characteristics of a chi-square test of independence that distinguish it from other chi-square tests are as follows:

1. A single sample is selected from a population of interest and the subjects or objects are cross-classified on the basis of the two variables of interest.

2. The rationale for calculating expected cell frequencies is based on the probability law, which states that if two events (here the two criteria of classification) are independent, the probability of their joint occurrence is equal to the product of their individual probabilities.

3. The hypotheses and conclusions are stated in terms of the independence (or lack of independence) of two variables.

EXERCISES

In the exercises that follow perform the test at the indicated level of significance and determine the p value.

12.4.1   The object of a research project by de Figueiredo et al. (A-4) was to identify and measure the differences among the following three groups of psychiatric outpatients: (1) those with family problems but without mental disorders, (2) those with both family problems and mental disorders, and (3) those with a mental disorder but without family problems. The following table shows the study subjects cross-classified by group membership and source of referral.

Source of Referral	Type of Problem		
	1	**2**	**3**
Self	15	37	16
Family	25	25	17
Mental health agency	14	40	27
Court	11	4	1
Other health agency	9	23	14
Other	3	8	1

SOURCE: John M. de Figueiredo, Heidi Boerstler, and Lisa O'Connell, "Conditions Not Attributable to a Mental Disorder: An Epidemiological Study of Family Problems," *American Journal of Psychiatry, 148* (1991), 780–783.

Do these data provide sufficient evidence to warrant the conclusion that problem category and source of referral are related? Let $\alpha = .01$.

12.4.2 The sharing of injecting equipment among drug users was investigated by Klee et al. (A-5). As part of their research they collected the following information regarding use of needle exchanges of injecting drug users who were located either through treatment agency files or through outreach work designed to involve those not receiving counselling treatment.

	Use of Needle Exchange			
	Regular	**Occasional**	**Never**	**Not known**
Agency	56	15	20	24
Non-agency	19	6	16	53

SOURCE: Hilary Klee, Jean Faugier, Cath Hayes, and Julie Morris, "The Sharing of Injecting Equipment Among Drug Users Attending Prescribing Clinics and Those Using Needle-Exchanges," *British Journal of Addiction*, *86* (1991), 217–223. © 1993, Society for the Study of Addiction to Alcohol and Other Drugs.

May we conclude from these data that use of needle exchange and agency status are related? Let $\alpha = .01$.

12.4.3 Concern about acquired immunodeficiency syndrome (AIDS) was the motivation for a survey conducted by Professor Patty J. Hale (A-6) of the University of Virginia. She used a mailed questionnaire to survey businesses. Among the information she collected were size of business and whether or not the employer had provided AIDS education for employees. The results were reported:

	AIDS Education Provided?	
Number of Employees	**Yes**	**No**
0–50	2	20
50–500	5	11
More than 500	11	5

SOURCE: Adapted from Patty J. Hale, "Employer Response to AIDS in a Low-Prevalence Area," *Family & Community Health*, *13* (No. 2, 1990), 38–45, with permission of Aspen Publishers, Inc., © 1990.

May we conclude on the basis of these data that whether or not a business provides AIDS education is independent of the size of the business? Let $\alpha = .05$.

12.4.4 Noting that *Chlamydia trachomatis* is the most prevalent sexually transmitted pathogen in many obstetric populations, Alger and Lovchik (A-7) conducted a study to determine the comparative efficacy of clindamycin and erythromycin in eradication of the pathogen from the lower genital tract in pregnant women and whether clindamycin is better tolerated. Out of 118 women treated, there were 70 whose compliance was good, and 8 of them experienced side effects. Thirty-nine maintained moderate compliance with 4 experiencing side effects, and of the 9 whose compliance was poor, 4 experienced side effects. May we conclude on the basis of these data that level of compliance and the experiencing of side effects are independent? Let $\alpha = .05$.

12.4.5 A sample of 500 college students participated in a study designed to evaluate the level of college students' knowledge of a certain group of common diseases. The following table shows the students classified by major field of study and level of knowledge of the group of diseases.

	Knowledge of Diseases		
Major	Good	Poor	Total
Premedical	31	91	122
Other	19	359	378
Total	50	450	500

Do these data suggest that there is a relationship between knowledge of the group of diseases and major field of study of the college students from which the present sample was drawn? Let $\alpha = .05$.

12.4.6 The following table shows the results of a survey in which the subjects were a sample of 300 adults residing in a certain metropolitan area. Each subject was asked to indicate which of three policies they favored with respect to smoking in public places.

	Policy Favored				
Highest Education Level	No Restrictions on Smoking	Smoking Allowed in Designated Areas Only	No Smoking at All	No Opinion	Total
College graduate	5	44	23	3	75
High school graduate	15	100	30	5	150
Grade school graduate	15	40	10	10	75
Total	35	184	63	18	300

Can one conclude from these data that, in the sampled population, there is a relationship between level of education and attitude toward smoking in public places? Let $\alpha = .05$.

12.5
Tests of Homogeneity

A characteristic of the examples and exercises presented in the last section is that, in each case, the total sample was assumed to have been drawn before the entities were classified according to the two criteria of classification. That is, the observed number of entities falling into each cell was determined after the sample was drawn. As a result, the row and column totals are chance quantities not under the control of the investigator. We think of the sample drawn under these conditions as a single sample drawn from a single population. On occasion, however, either row or column totals may be under the control of the investigator; that is, the investigator may specify that independent samples be drawn from each of several populations. In this case one set of marginal totals is said to be *fixed*, while the other set, corresponding to the criterion of classification applied to the samples, is *random*. The former procedure, as we have seen, leads to a chi-square test of independence. The latter situation leads to a chi-square *test of homogeneity*. The two situations not only involve different sampling procedures; they lead to different questions and null hypotheses. The test of independence is concerned with the question: Are the two criteria of classification independent? The homogeneity test is concerned with the question: Are the samples drawn from populations that are homogeneous with respect to some criterion of classification? In the latter case the null hypothesis states that the samples are drawn from the same population. Despite these differences in concept and sampling procedure, the two tests are mathematically identical, as we see when we consider the following example.

Calculating Expected Frequencies   Either the row categories or the column categories may represent the different populations from which the samples are drawn. If, for example, three populations are sampled, they may be designated as population 1, 2, and 3, in which case these labels may serve as either row or column headings. If the variable of interest has three categories, say A, B, and C, these labels may serve as headings for rows or columns, whichever is not used for the populations. If we use notation similar to that adopted for Table 12.4.2, the contingency table for this situation, with columns used to represent the populations, is shown as Table 12.5.1. Before computing our test statistic we need expected frequencies for each of the cells in Table 12.5.1. If the populations are indeed homogeneous, or, equivalently, if the samples are all drawn from the same population, with respect to the categories A, B, and C, our best estimate of the proportion in the combined population who belong to category A is $n_{A.}/n$. By the same token, if the three populations are homogeneous, we interpret this probability as applying to each of the populations individually. For example, under the null hypothesis, $n_{A.}$ is our best estimate of the probability that a subject picked at random from the combined population will belong to category A. We would expect, then, to find $n_{.1}(n_{A.}/n)$ of those in the sample from population 1 to belong to category A, $n_{.2}(n_{A.}/n)$ of those in the sample from Population 2 to belong to category A, and $n_{.3}(n_{A.}/n)$ of those in the sample from population 3 to belong to category A. These calculations yield the expected frequencies for the first row of

TABLE 12.5.1 A Contingency Table for Data for a Chi-Square Test of Homogeneity

Variable Category	Population			Total
	1	2	3	
A	n_{A1}	n_{A2}	n_{A3}	$n_{A.}$
B	n_{B1}	n_{B2}	n_{B3}	$n_{B.}$
C	n_{C1}	n_{C2}	n_{C3}	$n_{C.}$
Total	$n_{.1}$	$n_{.2}$	$n_{.3}$	n

TABLE 12.5.2 Frequency of Histologic Cell Type by Age Group

Age Group (years)	Number of Patients	Cell Type		
		Large Cell Nonkeratinizing Cell Type	Keratinizing Cell Type	Small Cell Nonkeratinizing Cell Type
30–39	34	18	7	9
40–49	97	56	29	12
50–59	144	83	38	23
60–69	105	62	25	18
Total	380	219	99	62

SOURCE: Shoji Kodama, Koji Kanazawa, Shigeru Honma, and Kenichi Tanaka, "Age as a Prognostic Factor in Patients With Squamous Cell Carcinoma of the Uterine Cervix," *Cancer*, *68* (1991), 2481–2485.

Table 12.5.1. Similar reasoning and calculations yield the expected frequencies for the other two rows.

We see again that the shortcut procedure of multiplying appropriate marginal totals and dividing by the grand total yields the expected frequencies for the cells. From the data in Table 12.5.1 we compute the following test statistic:

$$X^2 = \sum_{i=1}^{k} \left[\frac{(O_i - E_i)^2}{E_i} \right]$$

Example 12.5.1

Kodama et al. (A-8) studied the relationship between age and several prognostic factors in squamous cell carcinoma of the cervix. Among the data collected were the frequencies of histologic cell types in four age groups. The results are shown in Table 12.5.2. We wish to know if we may conclude that the populations represented by the four age-group samples are not homogeneous with respect to cell type.

Solution:

1. *Data* See Table 12.5.2.

2. *Assumptions* We assume that we have a simple random sample from each one of the four populations of interest.

3. *Hypotheses*

   H_0: The four populations are homogeneous with respect to cell type.

   H_A: The four populations are not homogeneous with respect to cell type.

   Let $\alpha = .05$.

4. *Test Statistic* The test statistic is $X^2 = \Sigma[(O_i - E_i)^2/E_i]$.

5. *Distribution of Test Statistic* If H_0 is true X^2 is distributed approximately as χ^2 with $(4 - 1)(3 - 1) = (3)(2) = 6$ degrees of freedom.

6. *Decision Rule* Reject H_0 if the computed value of X^2 is equal to or greater than 12.592.

TABLE 12.5.3 Observed and Expected Frequencies for Example 12.5.1

Age Group (years)	Number of Patients	Large Cell Nonkeratinizing Cell Type	Keratinizing Cell Type	Small Cell Nonkeratinizing Cell Type
		Cell Type		
30–39	34	18 (19.59)	7 (8.86)	9 (5.55)
40–49	97	56 (55.90)	29 (25.27)	12 (15.83)
50–59	144	83 (82.99)	38 (37.52)	23 (23.49)
60–69	105	62 (60.51)	25 (27.36)	18 (17.13)
Total	380	219	99	62

7. *Calculation of Test Statistic*   The observed and expected frequencies are shown in Table 12.5.3. From these data we compute the following value of the test statistic:

$$X^2 = \frac{(18 - 19.59)^2}{19.59} + \frac{(7 - 8.86)^2}{8.86} + \cdots + \frac{(18 - 17.13)^2}{17.13}$$

$$= 4.444$$

8. *Statistical Decision*   Since 4.444 is less than the critical value of 12.592, we are unable to reject the null hypothesis.

9. *Conclusion*   We conclude that the four populations may be homogeneous with respect to cell type.
Since 4.444 is less than 10.645, $p > .10$.

Small Expected Frequencies   The rules for small expected frequencies given in the previous section are applicable when carrying out a test of homogeneity.

When the chi-square test of homogeneity is used to test the null hypothesis that two populations are homogeneous, and when there are only two levels of the criterion of classification, the data may be displayed in a 2 × 2 contingency table. The analysis is identical to the analysis of 2 × 2 tables given in Section 12.4.

In summary, the chi-square test of homogeneity has the following characteristics:

1. Two or more populations are identified in advance and an independent sample is drawn from each.

2. Sample subjects or objects are placed in appropriate categories of the variable of interest.

3. The calculation of expected cell frequencies is based on the rationale that if the populations are homogeneous as stated in the null hypothesis, the best estimate of the probability that a subject or object will fall into a particular category of the variable of interest can be obtained by pooling the sample data.

4. The hypotheseses and conclusions are stated in terms of homogeneity (with respect to the variable of interest) of populations.

Test of Homogeneity and H_0: $p_1 = p_2$ The chi-square test of homogeneity for the two-sample case provides an alternative method for testing the null hypothesis that two population proportions are equal. In Section 7.6, it will be recalled, we learned to test H_0: $p_1 = p_2$ against H_A: $p_1 \neq p_2$ by means of the statistic

$$z = \frac{(\hat{p}_1 - \hat{p}_2) - (p_1 - p_2)_0}{\sqrt{\dfrac{\bar{p}(1 - \bar{p})}{n_1} + \dfrac{\bar{p}(1 - \bar{p})}{n_2}}}$$

where $\bar{p}$ is obtained by pooling the data of the two independent samples available for analysis.

Suppose, for example, that in a test of H_0: $p_1 = p_2$ against H_A: $p_1 \neq p_2$, the sample data were as follows: $n_1 = 100$, $\hat{p}_1 = .60$, $n_2 = 120$, $\hat{p}_2 = .40$. When we pool the sample data we have

$$\bar{p} = \frac{.60(100) + .40(120)}{100 + 120} = \frac{108}{220} = .4909$$

and

$$z = \frac{.60 - .40}{\sqrt{\dfrac{(.4909)(.5091)}{100} + \dfrac{(.4909)(.5091)}{120}}} = 2.95469$$

which is significant at the .05 level since it is greater than the critical value of 1.96.

If we wish to test the same hypothesis using the chi-square approach, our contingency table would be

	Characteristic Present		
Sample	Yes	No	Total
1	60	40	100
2	48	72	120
Total	108	112	220

By Equation 12.4.1 we compute

$$X^2 = \frac{220[(60)(72) - (40)(48)]^2}{(108)(112)(100)(120)} = 8.7302$$

which is significant at the .05 level since it is greater than the critical value of

```
Expected counts are printed below observed counts
              C1        C2        C3      Total
     1        23         4        10        37
            12.72      6.94     17.34

     2        10        14        35        59
            20.28     11.06     27.66


Total        33        18        45        96


ChiSq = 8.311 + 1.244 + 3.110 +
        5.212 + 0.780 + 1.950 = 20.606
df = 2
```

Figure 12.5.1 Printout of computer analysis of Example 12.4.1 using MINITAB.

3.841. We see, therefore, that we reach the same conclusion by both methods. This is not surprising since, as explained in Section 12.2, $\chi^2_{(1)} = z^2$. We note that $8.7302 = (2.95469)^2$ and that $3.841 = (1.96)^2$.

Computer Analysis The computer may be used to advantage in calculating X^2 for tests of independence and tests of homogeneity. Figure 12.5.1 shows the computer printout for Example 12.5.1 when the MINITAB program for computing X^2 from contingency tables is used. To obtain the analysis and accompanying

```
TABLE OF HPV BY HIV
HPV              HIV
FREQUENCY
EXPECTED      SERO POS     SERO POS     SERO NEG
              SYMPTOMA     ASYMPTOM                      TOTAL
POSITIVE           23            4           10            37
             -------------------------------------------
                 12.7          6.9         17.3
NEGATIVE           10           14           35            59
             -------------------------------------------
                 20.3         11.1         27.7
TOTAL              33           18           45            96
             -------------------------------------------

        STATISTICS FOR TABLE OF HPV BY HIV
        STATISTIC      DF      VALUE      PROB
        -----------------------------------------
        CHI- SQUARE     2     20.606     0.000
```

Figure 12.5.2 SAS® printout for the chi-square analysis of the data from Example 12.4.1

printout we enter the data into columns 1, 2, and 3 as follows

```
MTB  > read c1- c3
DATA > 23 4 10
DATA > 10 14 35
DATA > end
```

We then issue the command

```
MTB > chisquare c1- c3
```

We may use SAS to obtain an analysis and printout of contingency table data by using the PROC FREQ statement. Figure 12.5.2 shows a partial SAS® printout reflecting the analysis of the data of Example 12.4.1.

EXERCISES

In the exercises that follow perform the test at the indicated level of significance and determine the p value.

12.5.1 In a telephone survey conducted by Professor Bikram Garcha (A-9) respondents were asked to indicate their level of agreement with the statement "Cigarette smoking should be banned in public places." The results were as follows.

	Level of Agreement				
Gender	Strongly Agree	Agree	Neutral	Disagree	Strongly Disagree
Female	40	38	16	37	5
Male	16	25	11	25	11

SOURCE: Bikram Garcha, Ph.D. Used by permission.

Can we conclude on the basis of these data that males and females differ with respect to their levels of agreement on the banning of cigarette smoking in public places? Let $\alpha = .05$.

12.5.2 Dr. Lowell C. Wise (A-10) notes the impact on an organization's operation of what are called employee withdrawal behaviors: absenteeism, turnover, and systematic reduction in participation (SRP). He is especially interested in these phenomena as they occur in the nursing profession. He conducted research to investigate the interrelationships among different forms of withdrawal and the process by which employees choose among them and to learn more about SRP in particular. Subjects were 404 nurses hired during a two-year period in five hospitals. Among the data collected were the following, which show the subjects classified by type of withdrawal behavior and hospital:

Hospital	Withdrawal Behavior				
	Turnover Only	SRP Only	Both	Neither	Total
1	35	41	24	26	126
2	14	8	10	5	37
3	13	4	1	17	35
4	29	16	19	19	83
5	54	9	29	31	123
Total	145	78	83	98	404

SOURCE: Lowell C. Wise, "The Erosion of Nursing Resources: Employee Withdrawal Behaviors," *Research in Nursing & Health, 16* (1993), 67–75. Copyright © 1993. Reprinted by permission of John Wiley & Sons, Inc.

We wish to know if the five hospitals are homogeneous with respect to type of withdrawal behavior exhibited by its nurses. Let $\alpha = .05$.

12.5.3   The objective of s study by Sutker et al. (A-11) was to describe the long-term psychological and psychiatric sequelae of prisoner of war (POW) confinement against the backdrop of psychiatric evaluations of Korean conflict repatriates more than 35 years in the past. Subjects were 22 POWs and 22 combat veteran survivors of the Korean conflict. They were compared on measures of problem solving, personality characteristics, mood states, and psychiatric clinical diagnoses. Nineteen of the POWs reported problems with depression. The number of combat veterans reporting problems with depression was 9. Do these data provide sufficient evidence for us to conclude that the two populations are not homogeneous with respect to the incidence of problems of depression? Let $\alpha = .05$.

12.5.4   In an air pollution study, a random sample of 200 households was selected from each of two communities. A respondent in each household was asked whether or not anyone in the household was bothered by air pollution. The responses were as follows.

Community	Any Member of Household Bothered by Air Pollution?		
	Yes	No	Total
I	43	157	200
II	81	119	200
Total	124	276	400

Can the researchers conclude that the two communities differ with respect to the variable of interest? Let $\alpha = .05$.

12.5.5   In a simple random sample of 250 industrial workers with cancer, researchers found that 102 had worked at jobs classified as "high exposure" with respect to suspected cancer-causing agents. Of the remainder, 84 had worked at "moderate exposure" jobs, and 64 had experienced no known exposure because of their jobs. In an independent simple random sample of 250 industrial workers from the same area who had no history of cancer, 31 worked in "high exposure" jobs, 60 worked in "moderate exposure" jobs, and 1590 worked in jobs involving no known exposure to suspected cancer-causing agents. Does it appear from these data that persons working in jobs that expose them to suspected cancer-causing agents have an increased risk of contracting cancer? Let $\alpha = .05$.

12.6
The Fisher Exact Test

Sometimes we have data that can be summarized in a 2×2 contingency table, but these data are derived from very small samples. The chi-square test is not an appropriate method of analysis if minimum expected frequency requirements are not met. If, for example, n is less than 20 or if n is between 20 and 40 and one of the expected frequencies is less than 5, the chi-square test should be avoided.

A test that may be used when the size requirements of the chi-square test are not met was proposed in the mid-1930s almost simultaneously by Fisher (22, 23), Irwin (24), and Yates (25). The test has come to be known as the *Fisher exact test*. It is called exact because, if desired, it permits us to calculate the exact probability of obtaining the observed results or results that are more extreme.

Data Arrangement When we use the Fisher exact test, we arrange the data in the form of a 2×2 contingency table like Table 12.6.1. We arrange the frequencies in such a way that $A > B$ and choose the characteristic of interest so that $a/A > b/B$.

Some theorists believe that Fisher's exact test is appropriate only when both marginal totals of Table 12.6.1 are fixed by the experiment. This specific model does not appear to arise very frequently in practice. Many experimenters, therefore, use the test when both marginal totals are not fixed.

Assumptions The following are the assumptions for the Fisher exact test.

1. The data consist of A sample observations from population 1 and B sample observations from population 2.
2. The samples are random and independent.
3. Each observation can be categorized as one of two mutually exclusive types.

TABLE 12.6.1 A 2×2 Contingency Table for the Fisher Exact Test

Sample	With Characteristic	Without Characteristic	Total
1	a	$A - a$	A
2	b	$B - b$	B
Total	$a + b$	$A + B - a - b$	$A + B$

Hypotheses   The following are the null hypotheses that may be tested and their alternatives.

1. (Two-sided)

   H_0: The proportion with the characteristic of interest is the same in both populations; that is, $p_1 = p_2$

   H_A: The proportion with the characteristic of interest is not the same in both populations; $p_1 \neq p_2$

2. (One-sided)

   H_0: The proportion with the characteristic of interest in population 1 is less than or the same as the proportion in population 2; $p_1 \leq p_2$

   H_A: The proportion with the characteristic of interest is greater in population 1 than in population 2; $p_1 > p_2$

Test Statistic   The test statistic is b, the number in sample 2 with the characteristic of interest.

Decision Rule   Finney (26) has prepared critical values of b for $A \leq 15$. Latscha (27) has extended Finney's tables to accommodate values of A up to 20. Appendix Table J gives these critical values of b for A between 3 and 20, inclusive. Significance levels of 0.05, 0.025, 0.01, and 0.005 are included. The specific decision rules are as follows:

1. *Two-Sided Test*   Enter Table J with A, B, and a. If the observed value of b is equal to or less than the integer in a given column, reject H_0 at a level of significance equal to twice the significance level shown at the top of that column. For example, suppose $A = 8$, $B = 7$, $a = 7$, and the observed value of b is 1. We can reject the null hypothesis at the $2(0.05) = 0.10$, the $2(0.025) = 0.05$, and the $2(0.01) = 0.02$ levels of significance, but not at the $2(0.005) = 0.01$ level.

2. *One-Sided Test*   Enter Table J with A, B, and a. If the observed value of b is less than or equal to the integer in a given column, reject H_0 at the level of significance shown at the top of that column. For example, suppose that $A = 16$, $B = 8$, $a = 4$, and the observed value of b is 3. We can reject the null hypothesis at the 0.05 and 0.025 levels of significance, but not at the 0.01 or 0.005 levels.

Large-Sample Approximation   For sufficiently large samples we can test the null hypothesis of the equality of two population proportions by using the normal approximation. Compute

$$z = \frac{(a/A) - (b/B)}{\sqrt{\hat{p}(1 - \hat{p})(1/A + 1/B)}} \qquad (12.6.1)$$

where

$$\hat{p} = (a + b)/(A + B) \qquad (12.6.2)$$

and compare it for significance with appropriate critical values of the standard normal distribution. The use of the normal approximation is generally considered satisfactory if $a, b, A - a$, and $B - b$ are all greater than or equal to 5. Alternatively, when sample sizes are sufficiently large, we may test the null hypothesis by means of the chi-square test.

Further Reading The Fisher exact test has been the subject of some controversy among statisticians. Some feel that the assumption of fixed marginal totals is unrealistic in most practical applications. The controversy then centers around whether the test is appropriate when both marginal totals are not fixed. For further discussion of this and other points, see the articles by Barnard (28, 29, 30), Fisher (31), and Pearson (32).

Sweetland (33) compared the results of using the chi-square test with those obtained using the Fisher exact test for samples of size $A + B = 3$ to $A + B = 69$. He found close agreement when A and B were close in size and the test was one-sided.

Carr (34) presents an extension of the Fisher exact test to more than two samples of equal size and gives an example to demonstrate the calculations. Neave (35) presents the Fisher exact test in a new format; the test is treated as one of independence rather than of homogeneity. He has prepared extensive tables for use with his approach.

The sensitivity of Fisher's exact test to minor perturbations in 2×2 contingency tables is discussed by Dupont (36).

Example 12.6.1

The purpose of a study by Crozier et al. (A-12) was to document that patients with motor complete injury, but preserved pin appreciation, in addition to light touch, below the zone of injury have better prognoses with regard to ambulation than patients with only light touch preserved. Subjects were 27 patients with upper

TABLE 12.6.2 Ambulatory Status at Discharge of Group 1 and Group 2 Patients Described in Example 12.6.1

Group	Total	Ambulatory Status	
		Nonambulatory	Ambulatory
1	18	16	2
2	9	1	8
Total	27	17	10

SOURCE: Kelley S. Crozier, Virginia Graziani, John F. Ditunno, Jr., and Gerald J. Herbison, "Spinal Cord Injury: Prognosis for Ambulation Based on Sensory Examination in Patients Who Are Initially Motor Complete," *Archives of Physical Medicine and Rehabilitation, 72* (February 1991), 119–121.

TABLE 12.6.3 Data of Table 12.6.2 Rearranged to Conform to the Layout of Table 12.6.1

| | Ambulatory Status | | |
Group	Nonambulatory	Ambulatory	Total
1	$16 = a$	$2 = A - a$	$18 = A$
2	$1 = b$	$8 = B - b$	$9 = B$
Total	$17 = a + b$	$10 = A + B - a - b$	$27 = A + B$

motor neuron lesions admitted for treatment within 72 hours of injury. They were divided into two groups: Group 1 were patients who had touch sensation but no pin appreciation below the zone of injury. Group 2 were patients who had partial or complete pin appreciation and light touch sensation below the zone of injury. Table 12.6.2 shows the ambulatory status of these patients at time of discharge. We wish to know if we may conclude that patients classified as group 2 have a higher probability of ambulation at discharge than patients classified as group 1.

Solution:

1. *Data*   The data as reported are shown in Table 12.6.2. Table 12.6.3 shows the data rearranged to conform to the layout of Table 12.6.1. Nonambulation is the characteristic of interest.

2. *Assumptions*   We presume that the assumptions for application of the Fisher exact test are met.

3. *Hypotheses*

    H_0: The rate of ambulation at discharge in a population of patients classified as group 2 is the same as or less than the rate of ambulation at discharge in a population of patients classified as group 1.

    H_A: Group 2 patients have a higher rate of ambulation at discharge than group 1 patients.

4. *Test Statistic*   The test statistic is the observed value of b as shown in Table 12.6.3.

5. *Distribution of Test Statistic*   We determine the significance of b by consulting Table J.

6. *Decision Rule*   Suppose we let $\alpha = .01$. The decision rule, then, is to reject H_0 if the observed value of b is equal to or less than 3, the value of b in Table J for $A = 18$, $B = 9$, $a = 16$, and $\alpha = .01$.

7. *Calculation of Test Statistic*   The observed value of b, as shown in Table 12.6.3 is 1.

8. *Statistical Decision*   Since $1 < 3$, we reject H_0.

9. *Conclusion*   Since we reject H_0, we conclude that the alternative hypothesis is true. That is, we conclude that the probability of ambulation is higher in a population of group 2 patients than in a population of group 1 patients.

Finding the p Value We see in Table J that when $A = 18$, $B = 9$, and $a = 16$, the value of $b = 2$ has an exact probability of occurring by chance alone, when H_0 is true, of .001. Since the observed value of $b = 1$ is less than 2, its p value is less than .001.

EXERCISES

12.6.1 Levin et al. (A 13) studied the expression of class I histocompatibility antigens (HLA) in transitional cell carcinoma (TCC) of the urinary bladder by the immunoperoxidase technique and correlated the expression with tumor differentiation and survival. The investigators state that because β_2-microglobulin always is expressed on the cell surface with class I antigen, it has become a reliable marker for the presence of HLA class I antigens. Subjects were 33 patients with invasive TCC. The following table shows the subjects classified by expression of β_2-microglobulin on tumor cells in relation to tumor differentiation.

	Expression of β_2-Microglobulin	
Tumor Differentiation	**Positive**	**Negative**
Grade 1	5	1
Grade 2	8	5
Grade 3–4	6	8

SOURCE: I. Levin, T. Klein, J. Goldstein, O. Kuperman, J. Kanetti, and B. Klein, "Expression of Class I Histocompatibility Antigens in Transitional Cell Carcinoma of the Urinary Bladder in Relation to Survival," *Cancer*, *68* (1991), 2591–2594.

Combine grades 1 and 2 and test for a significant difference between grade 1–2 versus grade 3–4 with respect to the proportion of positive responses. Let $\alpha = .05$ and find the p value.

12.6.2 In a study by Schweizer et al. (A-14) patients with a history of difficulty discontinuing long-term, daily benzodiazepine therapy were randomly assigned, under double-blind conditions, to treatment with carbamazepine or placebo. A gradual taper off benzodiazepine therapy was then attempted. The following table shows the subjects' benzodiazepine status five weeks after taper.

	Benzodiazepine Use	
Treatment Group	**Yes**	**No**
Carbamazepine	1	18
Placebo	8	13

SOURCE: Modified from Edward Schweizer, Karl Rickels, Warren G. Case, and David J. Greenblatt, "Carbamazepine Treatment in Patients Discontinuing Long-term Benzodiazepine Therapy," *Archives of General Psychiatry*, *48* (1991), 448–452. Copyright 1991, American Medical Association.

May we conclude, on the basis of these data, that carbamazepine is effective in reducing dependence on benzodiazepine at the end of five weeks of treatment? Let $\alpha = .05$ and find the p value.

12.6.3 Robinson and Abraham (A-15) conducted an experiment in which 12 mice were subjected to cardiac puncture with resulting hemorrhage. A control group of 13 mice were subjected to cardiac puncture without blood withdrawal. After four days the mice were inoculated with *aeruginosa* organisms. Eight hemorrhaged mice died. None of the control mice died. On the basis of these data may we conclude that the chance of death is higher among mice exposed to *aeruginosa* organisms following hemorrhage than among those that do not hemorrhage? Let $\alpha = .01$ and find the p value.

12.7
Relative Risk, Odds Ratio, and the Mantel – Haenszel Statistic

In Chapter 8 we learned to use analysis of variance techniques to analyze data that arise from designed experiments, investigations in which at least one variable is manipulated in some way. Designed experiments, of course, are not the only sources of data that are of interest to clinicians and other health sciences professionals. Another important class of scientific investigation that is widely used is the *observational study*.

DEFINITION

An *observational study* is a scientific investigation in which neither the subjects under study nor any of the variables of interest are manipulated in any way.

An observational study, in other words, may be defined simply as an investigation that is not an experiment. The simplest form of observational study is one in which there are only two variables of interest. One of the variables is called the *risk factor*, or independent variable, and the other variable is referred to as the *outcome*, or dependent variable.

DEFINITION

The term *risk factor* is used to designate a variable that is thought to be related to some outcome variable. The risk factor may be a suspected cause of some specific state of the outcome variable.

In a particular investigation, for example, the outcome variable might be subjects' status relative to cancer and the risk factor might be their status with respect to cigarette smoking. The model is further simplified if the variables are categorical with only two categories per variable. For the outcome variable the categories might be cancer present and cancer absent. With respect to the risk factor subjects might be categorized as smokers and nonsmokers.

When the variables in observational studies are categorical the data pertaining to them may be displayed in a contingency table, and hence the inclusion of the topic in the present chapter. We shall limit our discussion to the situation in which the outcome variable and the risk factor are both dichotomous variables.

Types of Observational Studies There are two basic types of observational studies, *prospective studies* and *retrospective studies*.

DEFINITION

A *prospective study* is an observational study in which two random samples of subjects are selected: One sample consists of subjects possessing the risk factor and the other sample consists of subjects who do not possess the risk factor. The subjects are followed into the future (that is, they are followed prospectively) and a record is kept on the number of subjects in each sample who, at some point in time, are classifiable into each of the categories of the outcome variable.

The data resulting from a prospective study involving two dichotomous variables can be displayed in a 2×2 contingency table that usually provides information regarding the number of subjects with and without the risk factor and the number who did and did not succumb to the disease of interest as well as the frequencies for each combination of categories of the two variables.

DEFINITION

A *retrospective study* is the reverse of a prospective study. The samples are selected from those falling into the categories of the outcome variable. The investigator then looks back (that is, takes a retrospective look) at the subjects and determines which ones have (or had) and which ones do not have (or did not have) the risk factor.

From the data of a restrospective study we may construct a contingency table with frequencies similar to those that are possible for the data of a prospective study.

In general, the prospective study is more expensive to conduct than the retrospective study. The prospective study, however, more closely resembles an experiment.

Relative Risk The data resulting from a prospective study in which the dependent variable and the risk factor are both dichotomous may be displayed in a 2×2 contingency table such as Table 12.7.1. The risk of the development of the disease among the subjects with the risk factor is $a/(a + b)$. The risk of the

TABLE 12.7.1 Classification of a Sample of Subjects with Respect to Disease Status and Risk Factor

Risk Factor	Disease Status		Total at Risk
	Present	**Absent**	
Present	a	b	$a + b$
Absent	c	d	$c + d$
Total	$a + c$	$b + d$	n

development of the disease among the subjects without the risk factor is $c/(c + d)$. We define relative risk as follows.

DEFINITION

Relative risk is the ratio of the risk of developing a disease among subjects with the risk factor to the risk of developing the disease among subjects without the risk factor.

We represent the relative risk from a prospective study symbolically as

$$\widehat{RR} = \frac{a/(a + b)}{c/(c + d)} \tag{12.7.1}$$

where a, b, c, and d are as defined in Table 12.7.1, and $\widehat{RR}$ indicates that the relative risk is computed from a sample to be used as an estimate of the relative risk, RR, for the population from which the sample was drawn.

We may construct a confidence interval for RR by the following method proposed by Miettinen (37, 38)

$$100(1 - \alpha)\%\mathrm{CI} = \widehat{RR}^{1 \pm (z_\alpha/\sqrt{X^2})} \tag{12.7.2}$$

where z_α is the two-sided z value corresponding to the chosen confidence coefficient and X^2 is computed by Equation 12.4.1.

Interpretation of *RR* The value of RR may range anywhere between zero and infinity. A value of zero indicates that there is no association between the status of the risk factor and the status of the dependent variable. In most cases the two possible states of the dependent variable are disease present and disease absent. We interpret a RR of 1 to mean that the risk of acquiring the disease is the same for those subjects with the risk factor and those without the risk factor. A value of RR greater than 1 indicates that the risk of acquiring the disease is greater among subjects with the risk factor than among subjects without the risk factor. A RR value that is less than 1 indicates less risk of acquiring the disease among subjects with the risk factor than among subjects without the risk factor.

For example, a risk factor of 2 is taken to mean that those subjects with the risk factor are twice as likely to acquire the disease as compared to subjects without the risk factor.

We illustrate the calculation of relative risk by means of the following example.

Example 12.7.1

In a prospective study of postnatal depression in women, Boyce et al. (A-16) assessed women at four points in time, at baseline (during the second trimester of pregnancy), and at one, three, and six months postpartum. The subjects were primiparous women cohabiting in a married or de facto stable relationship. Among the data collected were those shown in Table 12.7.2 in which the risk factor is having a spouse characterized as being indifferent and lacking in warmth and affection. A case is a woman who became depressed according to an established criterion. From the sample of subjects in the study, we wish to estimate the relative risk of becoming a case of postnatal depression at one month postpartum when the risk factor is present.

Solution: By Equation 12.7.1 we compute

$$\widehat{RR} = \frac{5/26}{8/90} = \frac{.192308}{.088889} = 2.2$$

These data indicate that the risk of becoming a case of postnatal depression at one month postpartum when the spouse is indifferent and lacking in warmth and affection is 2.2 times as great as it is among women whose spouses do not exhibit these behaviors.

We compute the 95 percent confidence interval for RR as follows. By Equation 12.4.1. we compute from the data in Table 12.7.2

$$X^2 = \frac{116[(5)(82) - (21)(8)]^2}{(13)(103)(26)(90)} = 2.1682$$

By Equation 12.7.2, the lower and upper confidence limits are, respectively, $2.2^{1-1.96/\sqrt{2.1682}} = .77$ and $2.2^{1+1.96/\sqrt{2.1682}} = 6.28$. Since the interval includes 1, we conclude, at the .05 level of significance, that the population odds ratio may be 1. In other words, we conclude that in the population, there may not be an increased

TABLE 12.7.2 Subjects With and Without the Risk Factor who Became Cases of Postnatal Depression at 1 Month Postpartum

Risk Factor	Cases	Noncases	Total
Present	5	21	26
Absent	8	82	90
Total	13	103	116

SOURCE: Philip Boyce, Ian Hickie, and Gordon Parker, "Parents, Partners or Personality? Risk Factors for Post-natal Depression," *Journal of Affective Disorders, 21* (1991), 245–255.

risk of becoming a case of postnatal depression at one month postpartum when the spouse is indifferent and lacking in warmth and affection.

Odds Ratio   When the data to be analyzed come from a retrospective study, relative risk is not a meaningful measure for comparing two groups. As we have seen, a retrospective study is based on a sample of subjects with the disease (cases) and a separate sample of subjects without the disease (controls or noncases). We then retrospectively determine the distribution of the risk factor among the cases and controls. Given the results of a retrospective study involving two samples of subjects, cases and controls, we may display the data in a 2 × 2 table such as Table 12.7.3, in which subjects are dichotomized with respect to the presence and absence of the risk factor. Note that the column headings in Table 12.7.3 differ from those in Table 12.7.1 to emphasize the fact that the data are from a retrospective study and that the subjects were selected because they were either cases or controls. When the data from a retrospective study are displayed as in Table 12.7.3, the ratio $a/(a + b)$, for example, is not an estimate of the risk of disease for subjects with the risk factor. The appropriate measure for comparing cases and controls in a retrospective study is the *odds ratio*. As noted in Chapter 11, in order to understand the concept of the odds ratio, we must understand the term *odds*, which is frequently used by those who place bets on the outcomes of sporting events or participate in other types of gambling activities. Using probability terminology Freund (39) defines odds as follows.

DEFINITION

The odds for success are the ratio of the probability of success to the probability of failure

We use this definition of odds to define two odds that we can calculate from data displayed as in Table 12.7.3:

1. The odds of being a case (having the disease) to being a control (not having the disease) among subjects with the risk factor is $[a/(a + b)]/[b/(a + b)] = a/b$.

2. The odds of being a case (having the disease) to being a control (not having the disease) among subjects without the risk factor is $[c/(c + d)]/[d/(c + d)] = c/d$.

TABLE 12.7.3 Subjects of a Retrospective Study Classified According to Status Relative to a Risk Factor and Whether They Are Cases or Controls

Risk Factor	Sample		
	Cases	Controls	Total
Present	a	b	$a + b$
Absent	c	d	$c + d$
Total	$a + c$	$b + d$	n

We now define the odds ratio that we may compute from the data of a retrospective study. We use the symbol $\widehat{OR}$ to indicate that the measure is computed from sample data and used as an estimate of the population odds ratio, OR.

DEFINITION

The estimate of the population odds ratio is

$$\widehat{OR} = \frac{a/b}{c/d} = \frac{ad}{bc} \qquad (12.7.3)$$

where a, b, c, and d are as defined in Table 12.7.3.

We may construct a confidence interval for OR by the following method proposed by Miettinen (37, 38)

$$100(1 - \alpha)\%\text{CI} = \widehat{OR}^{1 \pm (z_\alpha/\sqrt{X^2})} \qquad (12.7.4)$$

where z_α is the two-sided z value corresponding to the chosen confidence coefficient and X^2 is computed by Equation 12.4.1.

Interpretation of the Odds Ratio   In the case of a rare disease the population odds ratio provides a good approximation to the population relative risk. Consequently, the sample odds ratio, being an estimate of the population odds ratio, provides an indirect estimate of the population relative risk in the case of a rare disease.

The odds ratio can assume values between zero and ∞. A value of zero indicates no association between the risk factor and disease status. A value less than 1 indicates reduced odds of the disease among subjects with the risk factor. A value greater than 1 indicates increased odds of having the disease among subjects in whom the risk factor is present.

Example 12.7.2

Cohen et al. (A-17) collected data on men who were booked through the Men's Central Jail, the main custody facility for men in Los Angeles County. Table 12.7.4 shows 158 subjects classified as cases or noncases of syphilis infection and according to number of sexual partners (the risk factor) in the preceding 90 days. We wish to compare the odds of syphilis infection among those with three or more sexual partners in the preceding 90 days with the odds of syphilis infection among those with no sexual partners during the preceding 90 days.

Solution: The odds ratio is the appropriate measure for answering the question posed. By Equation 12.7.3 we compute

$$\widehat{OR} = \frac{(41)(49)}{(58)(10)} = 3.46$$

TABLE 12.7.4 Subjects Classified According to Syphilis Infection Status and Number of Sexual Partners in the Preceding 90 Days

Number of Sexual Partners (in last 90 days)	Syphilis Infection Status		
	Cases	Noncases	Total
≥ 3	41	58	99
0	10	49	59
Total	51	107	158

SOURCE: Deborah Cohen, Richard Scribner, John Clark, and David Cory, "The Potential Role of Custody Facilities in Controlling Sexually Transmitted Diseases," *American Journal of Public Health, 82* (1992), 552–556.

We see that cases are 3.46 times as likely as noncases to have had three or more sexual partners in the preceding 90 days.

We compute the 95 percent confidence interval for *OR* as follows. By Equation 12.4.1 we compute from the data in Table 12.7.4

$$X^2 = \frac{158\left[(41)(49) - (58)(10)\right]^2}{(51)(107)(99)(59)} = 10.1223$$

The lower and upper confidence limits for the population *OR*, respectively, are $3.46^{1 - 1.96/\sqrt{10.1223}} = 1.61$ and $3.46^{1 + 1.96/\sqrt{10.1223}} = 7.43$. We conclude with 95 percent confidence that the population *OR* is somewhere between 1.61 and 7.43. Since the interval does not include 1, we conclude that, in the population, cases are more likely than noncases to have had three or more sexual partners in the preceding 90 days.

The Mantel–Haenszel Statistic   Frequently when we are studying the relationship between the status of some disease and the status of some risk factor, we are aware of another variable that may be associated either with the disease, with the risk factor, or with both in such a way that the true relationship between the disease status and the risk factor is masked. Such a variable is called a *confounding variable*. For example, experience might indicate the possibility that the relationship between some disease and a suspected risk factor differs among different ethnic groups. We would then treat ethnic membership as a confounding variable. When they can be identified, it is desirable to control for confounding variables so that an unambiguous measure of the relationship between disease status and risk factor may be calculated. A technique for accomplishing this objective is the Mantel–Haenszel (40) procedure, so called in recognition of the two men who developed it. The procedure allows us to test the null hypothesis that there is no association between status with respect to disease and risk factor status. Initially used only with data from retrospective studies, the Mantel–Haenszel procedure is also appropriate for use with data from prospective studies, as discussed by Mantel (41).

In the application of the Mantel–Haenszel procedure, case and control subjects are assigned to strata corresponding to different values of the confounding variable. The data are then analyzed within individual strata as well as across all strata. The discussion that follows assumes that the data under analysis are from a retrospective or a prospective study with case and noncase subjects classified according to whether they have or do not have the suspected risk factor. The confounding variable is categorical, with the different categories defining the strata. If the confounding variable is continuous it must be categorized. For example, if the suspected confounding variable is age, we might group subjects into mutually exclusive age categories. The data before stratification may be displayed as shown in Table 12.7.3.

Application of the Mantel–Haenszel procedure consists of the following steps.

1. Form k strata corresponding to the k categories of the confounding variable. Table 12.7.5 shows the data display for the ith stratum.

2. For each stratum compute the expected frequency e_i of the upper left-hand cell of Table 12.7.5 as follows:

$$e_i = \frac{(a_i + b_i)(a_i + c_i)}{n_i} \qquad (12.7.5)$$

3. For each stratum compute

$$v_i = \frac{(a_i + b_i)(c_i + d_i)(a_i + c_i)(b_i + d_i)}{n_i^2(n_i - 1)} \qquad (12.7.6)$$

4. Compute the Mantel–Haenszel test statistic, χ_{MH}^2, as follows:

$$\chi_{MH}^2 = \frac{\left[\sum_{i=1}^{k}(a_i - e_i)\right]^2}{\sum_{i=1}^{k} v_i} \qquad (12.7.7)$$

TABLE 12.7.5 Subjects in the ith Stratum of a Confounding Variable Classified According to Status Relative to a Risk Factor and Whether They Are Cases or Controls

Risk Factor	Sample		Total
	Cases	Controls	
Present	a_i	b_i	$a_i + b_i$
Absent	c_i	d_i	$c_i + d_i$
Total	$a_i + c_i$	$b_i + d_i$	n_i

5. Reject the null hypothesis of no association between disease status and suspected risk factor status in the population if the computed value of χ^2_{MH} is equal to or greater than the critical value of the test statistic, which is the tabulated chi-square value for 1 degree of freedom and the chosen level of significance.

Mantel–Haenszel Estimator of the Common Odds Ratio   When we have k strata of data, each of which may be displayed in a table like Table 12.7.5, we may compute the Mantel–Haenszel estimator of the common odds ratio, $\widehat{OR}_{\mathrm{MH}}$, as follows

$$\widehat{OR}_{MH} = \frac{\displaystyle\sum_{i=1}^{k} (a_i d_i / n_i)}{\displaystyle\sum_{i=1}^{k} (b_i c_i / n_i)} \tag{12.7.8}$$

When we use the Mantel–Haenszel estimator given by Equation 12.7.4, we assume that in the population, the odds ratio is the same for each stratum.

We illustrate the use of the Mantel–Haenszel statistics with the following examples.

Example 12.7.3   Platt et al. (A-18) assessed the efficacy of perioperative antibiotic prophylaxis for surgery in a randomized, double-blind study of patients undergoing herniorrhaphy or surgery involving the breast. The patients received either cefonicid (1 g) or an identical-appearing placebo. Among the data collected are those in Table 12.7.6, which shows the patients classified according to type of surgery, whether they

TABLE 12.7.6 Breast Surgery and Herniorrhaphy Patients Classified by Perioperative Antibiotic Prophylaxis and Need for Postoperative Antibiotic Treatment for any Reason

	Cefonicid	Placebo
Breast Surgery		
Number of patients	303	303
Number receiving postoperative treatment for any reason	26	43
Herniorrhaphy		
Number of patients	301	311
Number receiving postoperative treatment for any reason	14	25

SOURCE: R. Platt, D. F. Zaleznik, C. C. Hopkins, E. P. Dellinger, A. W. Karchmer, C. S. Bryan, J. F. Burke, M. A. Wikler, S. K. Marino, K. F. Holbrook, T. D. Tosteson, and M. R. Segal, "Perioperative Antibiotic Prophylaxis for Herniorrhaphy and Breast Surgery," *New England Journal of Medicine*, *322* (1990), 153–160. Reprinted by permission of *The New England Journal of Medicine*.

received cefonicid or the placebo, and whether they received postoperative antibiotic treatment for any reason. We wish to know if we may conclude, on the basis of these data, that there is an association between perioperative antibiotic prophylaxis and need for postoperative antibiotic treatment among patients undergoing breast surgery or herniorrhaphy. We wish to control for type of surgical procedure.

Solution:

1. *Data*   See Table 12.7.6.

2. *Assumptions*   We presume that the assumptions discussed earlier for the valid use of the Mantel–Haenszel statistic are met.

3. *Hypotheses*

   H_0: There is no association between perioperative antibiotic prophylaxis and need for postoperative antibiotic treatment among patients undergoing breast surgery or herniorrhaphy
   H_1: There is a relationship between the two variables.

4. *Test Statistic*

$$\chi^2_{MH} = \frac{\sum\limits_{i=1}^{k} (a_i - e_i)^2}{\sum\limits_{i=1}^{k} v_i}$$

   as given in Equation 12.7.7.

5. *Distribution of Test Statistic*   Chi-square with 1 degree of freedom.

6. *Decision Rule*   Suppose we let $\alpha = .05$. Reject H_0 if the computed value of the test statistic is greater than or equal to 3.841.

7. *Calculation of Test Statistic*   First we form two strata as shown in Table 12.7.7. By Equation 12.7.5 we compute the following expected frequencies:

$$e_1 = (43 + 260)(43 + 26)/606 = (303)(69)/606 = 34.50$$

$$e_2 = (25 + 286)(25 + 14)/612 = (311)(39)/606 = 19.82$$

By Equation 12.7.6 we compute

$$v_1 = (303)(303)(69)(537)/(606^2)(606 - 1) = 15.3112$$

$$v_2 = (311)(301)(39)(573)/(612^2)(612 - 1) = 9.1418$$

TABLE 12.7.7 Patients Undergoing Breast Surgery or Herniorrhaphy Stratified by Type of Surgery and Classified Case Status and Risk Factor Status

Stratum 1 (Breast Surgery)			
Risk Factor[a]	Cases[b]	Noncases	Total
Present	43	260	303
Absent	26	277	303
Total	69	537	606

Stratum 2 (Herniorrhaphy)			
Risk Factor[a]	Cases[b]	Noncases	Total
Present	25	286	311
Absent	14	287	301
Total	39	573	612

[a] The risk factor is not receiving perioperative antibiotic prophylaxis.
[b] A case is a patient who required postoperative antibiotic treatment for any reason.

Finally by Equation 12.7.7 we compute

$$\chi^2_{MH} = \frac{(43 - 34.50)^2 + (25 - 19.82)^2}{15.3112 + 9.1418} = 4.05$$

8. *Statistical Decision*   Since $4.05 > 3.841$, we reject H_0.

9. *Conclusion*   We conclude that there is a relationship between perioperative antibiotic prophylaxis and need for postoperative antibiotic treatment in patients undergoing breast surgery or herniorrhaphy.

Since $3.841 < 4.05 < 5.024$, the p value for this test is $.05 > p > .025$.

We now illustrate the calculation of the Mantel–Haenszel estimator of the common odds ratio.

Example 12.7.4   Let us refer to the data in Table 12.7.6 and compute the common odds ratio.

Solution: From the stratified data in Table 12.7.7 we compute the numerator of the ratio as follows:

$$(a_1 d_1/n_1) + (a_2 d_2/n_2) = [(43)(277)/606] + [(25)(287)/612]$$
$$= 31.378972$$

The denominator of the ratio is

$$(b_1 c_1/n_1) + (b_2 c_2/n_2) = [(260)(26)/606] + [(286)(14)/612]$$
$$= 17.697599$$

Now, by Equation 12.7.7, we compute the common odds ratio:

$$\widehat{OR}_{MH} = 31.378972/17.697599 = 1.77$$

From these results we estimate that patients undergoing breast surgery or herniorrhaphy who do not receive cefonicid are 1.77 times more likely to require postoperative antibiotic treatment for any reason than patients who do not receive cefonicid.

EXERCISES

12.7.1 Herrera et al. (A-19) reported the results of a study involving vitamin A supplementation among children aged 9 to 72 months in the Sudan. The investigators' objectives were to test the efficacy in reducing childhood mortality, morbidity, and malnutrition of large doses of vitamin A given every 6 months and to identify predictors for child death, including deficient dietary intake of vitamin A. Children in the study received every six months either vitamin A plus vitamin E (vitamin A group) or vitamin E alone (placebo group). The children were followed for 18 months. There were 120 deaths among the 14,343 children in the vitamin A group and 112 deaths among the 14,149 children in the placebo group. Compute the relative risk of death among subjects not receiving vitamin A. Does it appear from these data that vitamin A lowers child mortality?

12.7.2 The objective of a prospective study by Sepkowitz et al. (A-20) was to determine risk factors for the development of pneumothorax in patients with the acquired immunodeficiency syndrome (AIDS). Of 20 patients with pneumothorax, 18 had a history of aerosol pentamidine use. Among 1010 patients without pneumothorax, 336 had a history of aerosol pentamidine use. Compute the relative risk of aerosol pentamidine use in the development of pneumothorax in AIDS patients.

12.7.3 In a study of the familial occurrence of gastric cancer, Zanghieri et al. (A-21) wished to determine whether the occurrence of gastric cancer among relatives was related to the histotype. They reported the following data:

	Histologic Type		
	Diffuse	**Intestinal**	**Total**
Familiality +[a]	13	12	25
Familiality −	35	72	107
Total	48	84	132

[a]Number of patients with (familiality +) or without (familiality −) occurrence of gastric neoplasms among first-degree relatives.

SOURCE: Gianni Zanghieri, Carmela Di Gregorio, Carla Sacchetti, Rossella Fante, Romano Sassatelli, Giacomo Cannizzo, Alfonso Carriero, and Maurizio Ponz de Leon, "Familial Occurrence of Gastric Cancer in the 2-Year Experience of a Population-Based Registry," *Cancer*, *66* (1990), 1047–1051.

Compute the odds ratio that the investigators could use to answer their question. Use the chi-square test of independence to determine if one may conclude that there is an association between familiality and histologic type. Let $\alpha = .05$.

12.7.4 Childs et al. (A-22) described the prevalence of antibodies to leptospires in an inner-city population and examined risk factors associated with seropositivity. The subjects were persons visiting a sexually transmitted disease clinic. Among the data collected were those shown in the following table, in which the subjects are cross-classified according to age and status with regard to antibody titer to leptospires.

Age	Antibody Titers to Leptospires		
	≥ 200	< 200	Total
< 19	157	695	852
≥ 19	27	271	298
Total	184	966	1150

SOURCE: James E. Childs, ScD. Used by permission.

What is the estimated relative risk of antibody titers ≥ 200 among subjects under 19 years of age compared to those 19 or older? Compute the 95 percent confidence interval for the relative risk.

12.7.5 Telzak et al. (A-23) reported the following data for patients with diabetes who were exposed to *Salmonella enteritidis* through either a low-sodium diet (high exposure) or a regular-sodium diet (low exposure). Cases are those who became infected with the organism.

	High Exposure		Low Exposure	
	Cases ($n = 31$)	Controls ($n = 23$)	Cases ($n = 44$)	Controls ($n = 57$)
Number with diabetes	6	2	11	5

SOURCE: Edward E. Telzak, Michele S. Zweig Greenberg, Lawrence D. Budnick, Tejinder Singh, and Steve Blum, "Diabetes Mellitus—A Newly Described Risk Factor for Infection from *Salmonella enteritidis*," *The Journal of Infectious Diseases, 164* (1991), 538–541. Published by the University of Chicago. © 1991 by The University of Chicago. All rights reserved.

Compute the Mantel–Haenszel common odds ratio with stratification by exposure type. Use the Mantel–Haenszel test statistic to determine if we can conclude that there is an association between the risk factor and infection. Let $\alpha = .05$.

12.7.6 Noting that in studies of patients with benign prostatic hyperplasia (BPH), men undergoing transurethral resection of the prostate (TURP) had higher long-term mortality than men undergoing open prostatectomy, Concato et al. (A-24) speculated that increased mortality might be caused by older age and greater severity of comorbid disease at the time of surgery rather than by the transurethral procedure itself. To test their hypothesis, the investigators examined, in a retrospective study, the experiences and characteristics of men who underwent TURP or open prostatectomy over a three-year period. Subjects were categorized into three composite age-comorbidity stages according to baseline characteristics that cogently affect prognosis. Among the results reported were those regarding mortality and composite stage shown in the following table.

| Composite Stage | Treatment Group | | | |
| | TURP | | Open | |
	Deaths	No. of Subjects	Deaths	No. of Subjects
I	8	89	9	101
II	7	23	7	22
III	7	14	1	3
Total	22	126	17	126

SOURCE: Modified from John Concato, Ralph I. Horwitz, Alvan R. Feinstein, Joann G. Elmore, and Stephen F. Schiff, "Problems of Comorbidity in Mortality after Prostatectomy," *Journal of the American Medical Association*, *267* (1992), 1077–1082. Copyright 1992, American Medical Association.

Use the Mantel–Haenszel procedures to compute the common odds ratio and to test the null hypothesis of no relationship between treatment and mortality with stratification by composite stage. Let $\alpha = .05$.

12.8
Summary

In this chapter some uses of the versatile chi-square distribution are discussed. Chi-square goodness-of-fit tests applied to the normal, binomial, and Poisson distributions are presented. We see that the procedure consists of computing a statistic

$$X^2 = \sum \left[\frac{(O_i - E_i)^2}{E_i} \right]$$

that measures the discrepancy between the observed (O_i) and expected (E_i) frequencies of occurrence of values in certain discrete categories. When the appropriate null hypothesis is true, this quantity is distributed approximately as χ^2. When X^2 is greater than or equal to the tabulated value of χ^2 for some α, the null hypothesis is rejected at the α level of significance.

Tests of independence and tests of homogeneity are also discussed in this chapter. The tests are mathematically equivalent but conceptually different. Again, these tests essentially test the goodness-of-fit of observed data to expectation under hypotheses, respectively, of independence of two criteria of classifying the data and the homogeneity of proportions among two or more groups.

In addition, we discussed and illustrated in this chapter four other techniques for analyzing frequency data that can be presented in the form of a 2×2 contingency table: the Fisher exact test, the odds ratio, relative risk, and the Mantel–Haenszel procedure.

REVIEW QUESTIONS AND EXERCISES

1. Explain how the chi-square distribution may be derived.

2. What are the mean and variance of the chi-square distribution?

3. Explain how the degrees of freedom are computed for the chi-square goodness-of-fit tests.

4. State Cochran's rule for small expected frequencies in goodness-of-fit tests.

5. How does one adjust for small expected frequencies?

6. What is a contingency table?

7. How are the degrees of freedom computed when an X^2 value is computed from a contingency table?

8. Explain the rationale behind the method of computing the expected frequencies in a test of independence.

9. Explain the difference between a test of independence and a test of homogeneity.

10. Explain the rationale behind the method of computing the expected frequencies in a test of homogeneity.

11. When do researchers use the Fisher exact test rather than the chi-square test?

12. Define the following:
    a. Observational study
    b. Risk factor
    c. Outcome
    d. Retrospective study
    e. Prospective study
    f. Relative risk
    g. Odds
    h. Odds ratio
    i. Confounding variable

13. Under what conditions is the Mantel–Haenszel test appropriate?

14. Explain how researchers interpret the following measures:
    a. Relative risk
    b. Odds ratio
    c. Mantel–Haenszel common odds ratio

15. Sinton et al. (A-25) reported the following data regarding the incidence of antisperm antibodies in female infertility patients and their husbands.

| Antibody Status | Antibody Status of Wife | |
of Husband	Positive	Negative
Positive	17	34
Negative	10	64

SOURCE: Eleanor B. Sinton, D. C. Riemann, and Michael E. Ashton, "Antisperm Antibody Detection Using Concurrent Cytofluorometry and Indirect Immunofluorescence Microscopy," *American Journal of Clinical Pathology*, 95 (1991), 242–246.

Can we conclude on the basis of these data that antibody status in wives is independent of antibody status in their husbands? Let $\alpha = .05$.

16. Goodyer and Altham (A-26) compared the number of lifetime exit events occurring over the lives of children between the ages of 7 and 16 years who recently experienced new onset episodes of anxiety and depression (cases) with the incidence among community controls matched by age and social class. An exit event is defined as an event that results in a permanent removal of an individual from a person's social field. Among 100 cases 42 had experienced two or more exit events. The number with two or more exit events among the 100 controls was 25. May we conclude on the basis of these data that the two populations are not homogeneous with respect to exit event experience? Let $\alpha = .05$.

17. A sample of 150 chronic carriers of a certain antigen and a sample of 500 noncarriers revealed the following blood group distributions.

Blood Group	Carriers	Noncarriers	Total
0	72	230	302
A	54	192	246
B	16	63	79
AB	8	15	23
Total	150	500	650

Can one conclude from these data that the two populations from which the samples were drawn differ with respect to blood group distribution? Let $\alpha = .05$. What is the p value for this test?

18. The following table shows 200 males classified according to social class and headache status.

| Headache | Social Class | | | |
Group	A	B	C	Total
No headache (in previous year)	6	30	22	58
Simple headache	11	35	17	63
Unilateral headache (nonmigraine)	4	19	14	37
Migraine	5	25	12	42
Total	26	109	65	200

Do these data provide sufficient evidence to indicate that headache status and social class are related? Let $\alpha = .05$. What is the p value for this test?

19. The following is the frequency distribution of scores made on an aptitude test by 175 applicants to a physical therapy training facility.

Score	Number of Applicants
10–14	3
15–19	8
20–24	13
25–29	17
30–34	19
35–39	25
40–44	28
45–49	20
50–54	18
55–59	12
60–64	8
65–69	4
Total	175

Do these data provide sufficient evidence to indicate that the population of scores is not normally distributed? Let $\alpha = .05$. What is the p value for this test?

20. A local health department sponsored a venereal disease (VD) information program that was open to high school juniors and seniors who ranged in age from 16 through 19 years. The program director believed that each age level was equally interested in knowing more about VD. Since each age level was about equally represented in the area served, she felt that equal interest in VD would be reflected by equal age-level attendance at the program. The age breakdown of those attending was as follows:

Age	Number Attending
16	26
17	50
18	44
19	40

Are these data incompatible with the program director's belief that students in the four age levels are equally interested in VD? Let $\alpha = .05$. What is the p value for this test?

21. A survey of children under 15 years of age residing in the inner city area of a large city were classified according to ethnic group and hemoglobin level. The results were as follows:

| Ethnic Group | Hemoglobin Level (g / 100 ml) | | | |
	10.0 or greater	9.0–9.9	< 9.0	Total
A	80	100	20	200
B	99	190	96	385
C	70	30	10	110
Total	249	320	126	695

Do these data provide sufficient evidence to indicate, at the .05 level of significance, that the two variables are related? What is the p value for this test?

22. A sample of reported cases of mumps in preschool children showed the following distribution by age:

Age (Years)	Number of Cases
Under 1	6
1	20
2	35
3	41
4	48
Total	150

Test the hypothesis that cases occur with equal frequency in the five age categories. Let $\alpha = .05$. What is the p value for this test?

23. Each of a sample of 250 men drawn from a population of suspected joint disease victims was asked which of three symptoms bother him most. The same question was asked of a sample of 300 suspected women joint disease victims. The results were as follows:

Symptom by Which Bothered Most	Men	Women
Morning stiffness	111	102
Nocturnal pain	59	73
Joint swelling	80	125
Total	250	300

Do these data provide sufficient evidence to indicate that the two populations are not homogeneous with respect to major symptoms? Let $\alpha = .05$. What is the p value for this test?

For each of the following situations, indicate whether a null hypothesis of homogeneity or a null hypothesis of independence is appropriate.

24. A researcher wished to compare the status of three communities with respect to immunity against polio in preschool children. A sample of preschool children was drawn from each of the three communities.

25. In a study of the relationship between smoking and respiratory illness, a random sample of adults were classified according to consumption of tobacco and extent of respiratory symptoms.

26. A physician who wished to know more about the relationship between smoking and birth defects studies the health records of a sample of mothers and their children, including stillbirths and spontaneously aborted fetuses where possible.

27. A health research team believes that the incidence of depression is higher among people with hypoglycemia than among people who do not suffer from this condition.

28. In a simple random sample of 200 patients undergoing therapy at a drug abuse treatment center, 60 percent belonged to ethnic group I. The remainder belonged to ethnic group II. In ethnic group I, 60 were being treated for alcohol abuse (A), 25 for marijuana abuse (B), and 20 for abuse of heroin, illegal methadone, or some other opioid (C). The remainder had abused barbiturates, cocaine, amphetamines, hallucinogens, or some other nonopioid besides marijuana (D). In ethnic group II the abused drug category and the numbers involved were as follows:

A(28)   B(32)   C(13)   D(the remainder)

Can one conclude from these data that there is a relationship between ethnic group and choice of drug to abuse? Let $\alpha = .05$ and find the p value.

29. Volm and Mattern (A-27) analyzed human non-small cell lung carcinomas of previously untreated patients for expression of thymidylate synthase (TS) using immunohistochemistry. Thirteen patients were treated with combination chemotherapy. Seven of the 8 tumors that were TS-positive were clinically progressive, whereas 4 out of 5 tumors that were TS-negative showed clinical remission after chemotherapy. What statistical techniques studied in this chapter would be appropriate to analyze these data? What are the variables involved? Are the variables quantitative or qualitative? What null and alternative hypotheses are appropriate? If you think you have enough information to do so, carry out a complete hypothesis test. What are your conclusions?

30. The monthly pattern of distribution of endoscopically diagnosed duodenal ulcer disease was evaluated for the years 1975–1989 by Braverman et al. (A-28). Statistical analysis revealed differences for certain months. Slightly more of the 2020 patients with chronic duodenal bulb deformity presented in June and November, while more of the 1035 patients with acute duodenal ulcer presented in July, November, and December ($p <$ .001). What statistical technique studied in this chapter is appropriate for analyzing these data? What null and alternative hypotheses are appropriate? Describe the variables as to whether they are continuous, discrete, quantitative, or qualitative. What conclusions may be drawn from the given information?

31. Friedler et al. (A-29) conducted a prospective study on the incidence of intrauterine pathology diagnosed by hysteroscopy in 147 women who underwent dilatation and sharp curettage due to spontaneous first trimester abortion. Sixteen out of 98 subjects who had only one abortion were found to have intrauterine adhesions (IUA). The incidence of IUA after two abortions was 3 out of 21, and after three or more spontaneous abortions it was 9 out of 28. What statistical technique studied in this chapter would be appropriate for analyzing these data? Describe the variables involved as to whether they are continuous, discrete, quantitative, or qualitative. What null and alternative hypotheses are appropriate? If you think you have sufficient information conduct a complete hypothesis test. What are your conclusions?

32. Lehrer et al. (A-30) examined the relationship between pregnancy-induced hypertension and asthma. The subjects were 24,115 women without a history of chronic systemic hypertension who were delivered of live born and stillborn infants at a large medical center during a four-year period. The authors reported an upward trend in the incidence of asthma during pregnancy in women without, with moderate, and with severe pregnancy-induced hypertension (Mantel–Haenszel chi-square = 11.8, $p = .001$). Characterize this study in terms of whether it is observational, prospective, or retrospective. Describe each variable involved as to whether it is continuous, discrete, quantitative, qualitative, a risk factor, or a confounding variable. Explain the meaning of the reported statistic. What are your conclusions based on the given information?

33. The objective of a study by Fratiglioni et al. (A-31) was to determine the risk factors for late-onset Alzheimer's disease using a case-control approach. Ninety-eight cases and 216 controls were gathered from an ongoing population survey on aging and dementia in Stockholm. The authors reported relative risk statistics and confidence intervals for the following variables: at least one first-degree relative affected by dementia (3.2; 1.8–5.7), alcohol abuse (4.4; 1.4–13.8), manual work for men (5.3; 1.1–25.5). Characterize this study as to whether it is observational, prospective, or retrospective. Describe the variables as to whether they are continuous, discrete, quantitative, qualitative, a risk factor, or a confounding variable. Explain the meaning of the reported statistics. What are your conclusions based on the given information?

34. Beuret et al. (A-32) conducted a study to determine the influence of 38 variables on outcome after cardiopulmonary resuscitation (CPR) and to assess neuropsychological status in long-term survivors. The charts of 181 consecutive patients resuscitated in a 1100-bed university hospital over a two-year period were analyzed. Of the 181 resuscitated patients, 23 could be discharged. The authors reported odds ratios and confidence intervals on the following variables that significantly affected outcome: presence of shock or renal failure before cardiac arrest (10.6; 1.3–85.8 and 13.8; 1.7–109.2), administration of epinephrine (11.2; 3.2–39.2), and CPR of more than 15 minutes' duration (4.9; 1.7–13.7). Characterize this study as to whether it is observational, prospective, or retrospective. Describe the variables as to whether they are continuous, discrete, quantitative, qualitative, a risk factor, or a confounding variable. Explain the meaning of the reported odds ratios.

Exercises for Use With the Large Data Sets Available on Computer Disk from the Publisher

1. Refer to the data on smoking, alcohol consumption, blood pressure, and respiratory disease among 1200 adults (SMOKING, Disk 2). The variables are as follows:

Sex (A):	1 = male, 0 = female
Smoking status (B):	0 = nonsmoker, 1 = smoker
Drinking level (C):	0 = nondrinker
	1 = light to moderate drinker
	2 = heavy drinker
Symptoms of respiratory disease (D):	1 = present, 0 = absent
High blood pressure status (E):	1 = present, 0 = absent

Select a simple random sample of size 100 from this population and carry out an analysis to see if you can conclude that there is a relationship between smoking status and symptoms of respiratory disease. Let $\alpha = .05$ and determine the p value for your test. Compare your results with those of your classmates.

2. Refer to Exercise 1. Select a simple random sample of size 100 from the population and carry out a test to see if you can conclude that there is a relationship between drinking status and high blood pressure status in the population. Let $\alpha = .05$ and determine the p value. Compare your results with those of your classmates.

3. Refer to Exercise 1. Select a simple random sample of size 100 from the population and carry out a test to see if you can conclude that there is a relationship between sex and

smoking status in the population. Let $\alpha = .05$ and determine the p value. Compare your results with those of your classmates.

4. Refer to Exercise 1. Select a simple random sample of size 100 from the population and carry out a test to see if you can conclude that there is a relationship between sex and drinking level in the population. Let $\alpha = .05$ and find the p value. Compare your results with those of your classmates.

REFERENCES

References Cited

1. Karl Pearson, "On the Criterion That a Given System of Deviations from the Probable in the Case of a Correlated System of Variables Is Such That It Can Be Reasonably Supposed to Have Arisen from Random Sampling," *The London, Edinburgh and Dublin Philosophical Magazine and Journal of Science*, Fifth Series, *50* (1900), 157–175. Reprinted in *Karl Pearson's Early Statistical Papers*, Cambridge University Press, 1948.

2. H. O. Lancaster, *The Chi-Squared Distribution*, Wiley, New York, 1969.

3. Harald Cramer, *Mathematical Methods of Statistics*, Princeton University Press, Princeton, N.J., 1958.

4. Ram C. Dahiya and John Gurland, "Pearson Chi-Squared Test of Fit with Random Intervals," *Biometrika*, *59* (1972), 147–153.

5. G. S. Watson, "On Chi-Square Goodness-of-Fit Tests for Continuous Distributions," *Journal of the Royal Statistical Society*, B, *20* (1958), 44–72.

6. G. S. Watson, "The χ^2 Goodness-of-Fit Test for Normal Distributions," *Biometrika*, *44* (1957), 336–348.

7. G. S. Watson, "Some Recent Results in Chi-Square Goodness-of-Fit Tests," *Biometrics*, *15* (1959), 440–468.

8. G. R. Chase, "On the Chi-Square Test When the Parameters Are Estimated Independently of the Sample," *Journal of the American Statistical Association*, *67* (1972), 609–611.

9. William G. Cochran, "The χ^2 Test of Goodness of Fit," *Annals of Mathematical Statistics*, *23* (1952), 315–345.

10. William G. Cochran, "Some Methods for Strengthening the Common χ^2 Tests," *Biometrics*, *10* (1954), 417–451.

11. John T. Roscoe and Jackson A. Byars, "An Investigation of the Restraints with Respect to Sample Size Commonly Imposed on the Use of the Chi-Square Statistic," *Journal of the American Statistical Association*, *66* (1971), 755–759.

12. James K. Yarnold, "The Minimum Expectation in X^2 Goodness-of-Fit Tests and the Accuracy of Approximations for the Null Distribution," *Journal of the American Statistical Association*, *65* (1970), 864–886.

13. Merle W. Tate and Leon A. Hyer, "Significance Values for an Exact Multinomial Test and Accuracy of the Chi-Square Approximation," U.S. Department of Health, Education and Welfare, Office of Education, Bureau of Research, August 1969.

14. Malcolm J. Slakter, "Comparative Validity of the Chi-Square and Two Modified Chi-Square Goodness-of-Fit Tests for Small but Equal Expected Frequencies," *Biometrika*, *53* (1966), 619–623.

15. Malcolm J. Slakter, "A Comparison of the Pearson Chi-Square and Kolmogorov Goodness-of-Fit Tests with Respect to Validity," *Journal of the American Statistical Association*, *60* (1965), 854–858.

16. R. C. Lewontin and J. Felsenstein, "The Robustness of Homogeneity Tests in $2 \times N$ Tables," *Biometrics*, *21* (1965), 19–33.

17. F. Yates, "Contingency Tables Involving Small Numbers and the χ^2 Tests," *Journal of the Royal Statistical Society Supplement*, *1*, 1934 (Series B), 217–235.

18. J. E. Grizzle, "Continuity Correction in the χ^2 Test for 2×2 Tables," *The American Statistician*, *21* (October 1967), 28–32.

19. H. O. Lancaster, "The Combination of Probabilities Arising from Data in Discrete Distributions," *Biometrika*, *36* (1949), 370–382.

20. E. S. Pearson, "The Choice of Statistical Test Illustrated on the Interpretation of Data in a 2×2 Table," *Biometrika*, *34* (1947), 139–167.

21. R. L. Plackett, "The Continuity Correction in 2×2 Tables," *Biometrika*, *51* (1964), 427–338.

22. R. A. Fisher, *Statistical Methods for Research Workers*, Fifth Edition, Edinburgh, Oliver and Boyd, 1934.

23. R. A. Fisher, "The Logic of Inductive Inference," *Journal of the Royal Statistical Society Series A*, *98* (1935), 39–54.

24. J. O. Irwin, "Tests of Significance for Differences between Percentages Based on Small Numbers," *Metron*, *12* (1935), 83–94.

25. F. Yates, "Contingency Tables Involving Small Numbers and the χ^2 Test," *Journal of the Royal Statistical Society, Supplement*, *1* (1934), 217–235.

26. D. J. Finney, "The Fisher–Yates Test of Significance in 2×2 Contingency Tables," *Biometrika*, *35* (1948), 145–156.

27. R. Latscha, "Tests of Significance in a 2×2 Contingency Table: Extension of Finney's Table," *Biometrika*, *40* (1955), 74–86.

28. G. A. Barnard, "A New Test for 2×2 Tables," *Nature*, *156* (1945), 177.

29. G. A. Barnard, "A New Test for 2×2 Tables," *Nature*, *156* (1945), 783–784.

30. G. A. Barnard, "Significance Tests for 2×2 Tables," *Biometrika*, *34* (1947), 123–138.

31. R. A. Fisher, "A New Test for 2×2 Tables," *Nature*, *156* (1945), 388.

32. E. S. Pearson, "The Choice of Statistical Tests Illustrated on the Interpretation of Data Classed in a 2×2 Table," *Biometrika*, *34* (1947), 139–167.

33. A. Sweetland, "A Comparison of the Chi-Square Test for 1 df and the Fisher Exact Test," Santa Monica, Calif., Rand Corporation, 1972.

34. Wendell E. Carr, "Fisher's Exact Test Extended to More Than Two Samples of Equal Size," *Technometrics*, *22* (1980), 269 270.

35. Henry R Neave, "A New Look at an Old Test," *Bulletin of Applied Statistics*, *9* (1982), 165–178.

36. William D. Dupont, "Sensitivity of Fisher's Exact Test to Minor Perturbations in 2×2 Contingency Tables," *Statistics in Medicine*, *5* (1986), 629–635.

37. O. S. Miettinen, "Simple Interval-Estimation of Risk Ratio," *American Journal of Epidemiology*, *100* (1974), 515–516.

38. O. S. Miettinen, "Estimability and Estimation in Case-Referent Studies," *American Journal of Epidemiology*, *103* (1976), 226–235.

39. John E. Freund, *Introduction to Probability*, Dickenson Publishing Company, Encino, Calif., 1973.

40. N. Mantel and W. Haenszel, "Statistical Aspects of the Analysis of Data from Retrospective Studies of Disease," *Journal of the National Cancer Institute*, *22* (1959), 719–748.

41. N. Mantel, "Chi-Square Tests with One Degree of Freedom: Extensions of the Mantel–Haenszel Procedure," *Journal of the American Statistical Association*, *58* (1963), 690–700.

Other References, Journal Articles

1. Peter Albrecht, "On the Correct Use of the Chi-Square Goodness-of-Fit Test," *Scandinavian Acturial Journal*, (1980), 149–160.

2. Kevin L. Delucchi, "The Use and Misuse of Chi-Square: Lewis and Burke Revisited," *Psychological Bulletin*, *94* (1983), 166–176.

3. Chris W. Hornick and John E. Overall, "Evaluation of Three Sample Size Formulae for 2×2 Contingency Tables," *Journal of Educational Statistics*, *5* (1980), 351–362.

4. W. C. M. Kallenberg, J. Oosterhoff, and B. F. Schriever, "The Number of Classes in Chi-Squared Goodness-of-Fit Tests," *Journal of the American Statistical Association*, *80* (1985), 959–968.

5. Don Lewis and C. J. Burke, "The Use and Misuse of the Chi-Square Test," *Psychological Bulletin*, *46* (1949), 433–489.

6. Don Lewis and C. J. Burke, "Further Discussion of the Use and Misuse of the Chi-Square Test," *Psychological Bulletin*, *47* (1950), 347–355.

7. A. J. Viollaz, "On the Reliability of the Chi-Square Test," *Metrika*, *33* (1986), 135–142.

Applications References

A-1. Diane K. Jordan, Trudy L. Burns, James E. Divelbiss, Robert F. Woolson, and Shivanand R. Patil, "Variability in Expression of Common Fragile Sites: In Search of a New Criterion," *Human Genetics*, *85* (1990), 462–466.

A-2. Sten H. Vermund, Karen F. Kelley, Robert S. Klein, Anat R. Feingold, Klaus Schreiber, Gary Munk, and Robert D. Burk, "High Risk of Human Papillomavirus Infection and Cervical Squamous Intraepithelial Lesions Among Women with Symptomatic Human Immunodeficiency Virus Infection," *American Journal of Obstetrics and Gynecology*, *165* (1991), 392–400.

A-3. Joseph W. Chow, Michael J. Fine, David M. Shlaes, John P. Quinn, David C. Hooper, Michael P. Johnson, Reuben Ramphal, Marilyn M. Wagener, Deborah K. Miyashiro, and Victor L. Yu, "*Enterobacter* Bacteremia: Clinical Features and Emergence of Antibiotic Resistance During Therapy," *Annals of Internal Medicine*, *115* (1991), 585–590.

A-4. John M. de Figueiredo, Heidi Boerstler, and Lisa O'Connell, "Conditions Not Attributable to a Mental Disorder: An Epidemiological Study of Family Problems," *American Journal of Psychiatry*, *148* (1991), 780–783.

A-5. Hilary Klee, Jean Faugier, Cath Hayes, and Julie Morris, "The Sharing of Injecting Equipment Among Drug Users Attending Prescribing Clinics and Those Using Needle-Exchanges," *British Journal of Addiction*, *86* (1991), 217–223.

A-6. Patty J. Hale, "Employer Response to AIDS in a Low-Prevalence Area," *Family & Community Health*, *13* (No. 2, 1990), 38–45.

A-7. Lindsay S. Alger and Judith C. Lovchik, "Comparative Efficacy of Clindamycin Versus Erythromycin in Eradication of Antenatal *Chlamydia trachomatis*," *American Journal of Obstetrics and Gynecology*, *165* (1991), 375–381.

A-8. Shoji Kodama, Koji Kanazawa, Shigeru Honma, and Kenichi Tanaka, "Age as a Prognostic Factor in Patients With Squamous Cell Carcinoma of the Uterine Cervix," *Cancer*, *68* (1991), 2481–2485.

A-9. Bikram Garcha, Personal Communication, 1990.

A-10. Lowell C. Wise, "The Erosion of Nursing Resources: Employee Withdrawal Behaviors," *Research in Nursing & Health*, *16* (1993), 67–75.

A-11. Patricia B. Sutker, Daniel K. Winstead, Z. Harry Galina, and Albert N. Allain, "Cognitive Deficits and Psychopathology Among Former Prisoners of War and Combat Veterans of the Korean Conflict," *American Journal of Psychiatry*, *148* (1991), 67–72.

A-12. Kelley S. Crozier, Virginia Graziani, John F. Ditunno, Jr., and Gerald J. Herbison, "Spinal Cord Injury: Prognosis for Ambulation Based on Sensory Examination in Patients Who Are Initially Motor Complete," *Archives of Physical Medicine and Rehabilitation*, *72* (February 1991), 119–121.

A-13. I. Levin, T. Klein, J. Goldstein, O. Kuperman, J. Kanetti, and B. Klein, "Expression of Class I Histocompatibility Antigens in Transitional Cell Carcinoma of the Urinary Bladder in Relation to Survival," *Cancer*, *68* (1991), 2591–2594.

A-14. Edward Schweizer, Karl Rickels, Warren G. Case, and David J. Greenblatt, "Carbamazepine Treatment in Patients Discontinuing Long-term Benzodiazepine Therapy," *Archives of General Psychiatry*, *48* (1991), 448–452.

A-15. Anstella Robinson and Edward Abraham, "Effects of Hemorrhage and Resuscitation on Bacterial Antigen-specific Pulmonary Plasma Cell Function," *Critical Care Medicine*, *19* (1991), 1285–1293. © by Williams & Wilkins, 1991.

A-16. Philip Boyce, Ian Hickie, and Gordon Parker, "Parents, Partners or Personality? Risk Factors for Post-natal Depression," *Journal of Affective Disorders*, *21* (1991), 245–255.

A-17. Deborah Cohen, Richard Scribner, John Clark, and David Cory, "The Potential Role of Custody Facilities in Controlling Sexually Transmitted Diseases," *American Journal of Public Health, 82* (1992), 552–556.

A-18. R. Platt, D. F. Zaleznik, C. C. Hopkins, E. P. Dellinger, A. W. Karchmer, C. S. Bryan, J. F. Burke, M. A. Wikler, S. K. Marino, K. F. Holbrook, T. D. Tosteson, and M. R. Segal, "Perioperative Antibiotic Prophylaxis for Herniorrhaphy and Breast Surgery," *New England Journal of Medicine, 322* (1990), 153–160.

A-19. M. Guillermo Herrera, Penelope Nestel, Alawia El Amin, Wafaie W. Fawzi, Kamal Ahmed Mohamed, and Leisa Weld, "Vitamin A Supplementation and Child Survival," *Lancet, 340* (August 1, 1992), 267–271. © by the Lancet Ltd. 1992.

A-20. Kent A. Sepkowitz, Edward E. Telzak, Jonathan W. M. Gold, Edward M. Bernard, Steven Blum, Melanie Carrow, Mark Dickmeyer, and Donald Armstrong, "Pneumothorax in AIDS," *Annals of Internal Medicine, 114* (1991), 455–459.

A-21. Gianni Zanghieri, Carmela Di Gregorio, Carla Sacchetti, Rossella Fante, Romano Sassatelli, Giacomo Cannizzo, Alfonso Carriero, and Maurizio Ponz de Leon, "Familial Occurrence of Gastric Cancer in the 2-Year Experience of a Population-Based Registry," *Cancer, 66* (1990), 1047–1051.

A-22. James E. Childs, Brian S. Schwartz, Tom G. Ksiazek, R. Ross Graham, James W. LeDuc, and Gregory E. Glass, "Risk Factors Associated With Antibodies to Leptospires in Inner-City Residents of Baltimore: A Protective Role for Cats," *American Journal of Public Health, 82* (1992), 597–599.

A-23. Edward E. Telzak, Michele S. Zweig Greenberg, Lawrence D. Budnick, Tejinder Singh, and Steve Blum, "Diabetes Mellitus—A Newly Described Risk Factor for Infection from *Salmonella enteritidis*," *The Journal of Infectious Diseases, 164* (1991), 538–541.

A-24. John Concato, Ralph I. Horwitz, Alvan R. Feinstein, Joann G. Elmore, and Stephen F. Schiff, "Problems of Comorbidity in Mortality after Prostatectomy," *Journal of the American Medical Association, 267* (1992), 1077–1082.

A-25. Eleanor B. Sinton, D. C. Riemann, and Michael E. Ashton, "Antisperm Antibody Detection Using Concurrent Cytofluorometry and Indirect Immunofluorescence Microscopy," *American Journal of Clinical Pathology, 95* (1991), 242–246.

A-26. I. M. Goodyer and P. M. E. Altham, "Lifetime Exit Events and Recent Social and Family Adversities in Anxious and Depressed School-Age Children and Adolescents—I," *Journal of Affective Disorders, 21* (1991), 219–228.

A-27. M. Volm and J. Mattern, "Elevated Expression of Thymidylate Synthase in Doxorubicin Resistant Human Non Small Cell Lung Carcinomas," *Anticancer Research, 12* (November–December 1992), 2293–2296.

A-28. D. Z. Braverman, G. A. Morali, J. K. Patz, and W. Z. Jacobsohn, "Is Duodenal Ulcer a Seasonal Disease? A Retrospective Endoscopic Study of 3105 Patients," *American Journal of Gastroenterology, 87* (November 1992), 1591–1593.

A-29. S. Friedler, E. J. Margalioth, I. Kafka, and H. Yaffe, "Incidence of Post-Abortion Intra-Uterine Adhesions Evaluated By Hysteroscopy—A Prospective Study," *Human Reproduction, 8* (March 1993), 442–444.

A-30. S. Lehrer, J. Stone, R. Lapinski, C. J. Lockwood, B. S. Schachter, R. Berkowitz, and G. S. Berkowitz, "Association Between Pregnancy-Induced Hypertension and Asthma During Pregnancy," *American Journal of Obstetrics and Gynecology, 168* (May 1993), 1463–1466.

A-31. L. Fratiglioni, A. Ahlbom, M. Viitanen, and B. Winblad, "Risk Factors for Late-Onset Alzheimer's Disease: A Population-Based, Case-Control Study," *Annals of Neurology, 33* (March 1993), 258–266.

A-32. P. Beuret, F. Feihl, P. Vogt, A. Perret, J. A. Romand, and C. Perret, "Cardiac Arrest: Prognostic Factors and Outcome at One Year," *Resuscitation, 25* (April 1993), 171–179.

CHAPTER 13

Nonparametric and Distribution-Free Statistics

• • • • • • • • • • • • • • •

CONTENTS

13.1 Introduction

Most of the statistical inference procedures we have discussed up to this point are classified as *parametric statistics*. One exception is our uses of chi-square: as a test of goodness-of-fit and as a test of independence. These uses of chi-square come under the heading of *nonparametric statistics*.

The obvious question now is: What is the difference? In answer, let us recall the nature of the inferential procedures that we have categorized as *parametric*. In each case, our interest was focused on estimating or testing a hypothesis about one or more population parameters. Furthermore, central to these procedures was a knowledge of the functional form of the population from which were drawn the samples providing the basis for the inference.

An example of a parametric statistical test is the widely used *t* test. The most common uses of this test are for testing a hypothesis about a single population mean or the difference between two population means. One of the assumptions underlying the valid use of this test is that the sampled population or populations are at least approximately normally distributed.

As we will learn, the procedures that we discuss in this chapter either are not concerned with population parameters or do not depend on knowledge of the sampled population. Strictly speaking, only those procedures that test hypotheses that are not statements about population parameters are classified as *nonparametric*, while those that make no assumption about the sampled population are called *distribution-free* procedures. Despite this distinction, it is customary to use the terms *nonparametric* and *distribution-free* interchangeably and to discuss the various procedures of both types under the heading of *nonparametric statistics*. We will follow this convention. This point is discussed by Kendall and Sundrum (1) and Gibbons (2).

The above discussion implies the following two advantages of nonparametric statistics.

1. They allow for the testing of hypotheses that are not statements about population parameter values. Some of the chi-square tests of goodness-of-fit and the tests of independence are examples of tests possessing this advantage.
2. Nonparametric tests may be used when the form of the sampled population is unknown.

Other advantages have been listed by several writers, for example, Gibbons (2), Blum and Fattu (3), and Moses (4). In addition to the two already mentioned, the following are most frequently given.

3. Nonparametric procedures tend to be computationally easier and consequently more quickly applied than parametric procedures. This can be a desirable feature in certain cases, but when time is not at a premium, it merits a low priority as a criterion for choosing a nonparametric test.
4. Nonparametric procedures may be applied when the data being analyzed consist merely of rankings or classifications. That is, the data may not be based on a measurement scale strong enough to allow the arithmetic operations necessary for carrying out parametric procedures. The subject of measurement scales is discussed in more detail in the next section.

Although nonparametric statistics enjoy a number of advantages, their disadvantages must also be recognized. Moses (4) has noted the following.

1. The use of nonparametric procedures with data that can be handled with a parametric procedure results in a waste of data.
2. The application of some of the nonparametric tests may be laborious for large samples.

In a general introductory textbook, space limitations prevent the presentation of more than a sampling of nonparametric procedures. Additional procedures discussed at an introductory or intermediate level may be found in the book by Daniel (5). More mathematically rigorous books have been written by Gibbons (2), Hajek (6), and Walsh (7, 8). Savage (9) has prepared a bibliography of nonparametric statistics.

13.2
Measurement Scales

As was pointed out in the previous section, one of the advantages of nonparametric statistical procedures is that they can be used with data that are based on a weak measurement scale. To understand fully the meaning of this statement, it is necessary to know and understand the meaning of measurement and the various measurement scales most frequently used. At this point the reader may wish to refer to the discussion of measurement scales in Chapter 1.

Many authorities are of the opinion that different statistical tests require different measurement scales. Although this idea appears to be followed in practice, Anderson (10), Gaito (11), Lord (12), and Armstrong (13) present some interesting alternative points of view. The subject is also discussed by Borgatta and Bohrnstedt (14).

13.3
The Sign Test

The familiar t test is not strictly valid for testing (1) the null hypothesis that a population mean is equal to some particular value, or (2) the null hypothesis that the mean of a population of differences between pairs of measurements is equal to zero unless the relevant populations are at least approximately normally distributed. Case 2 will be recognized as a situation that was analyzed by the paired comparisons test in Chapter 7. When the normality assumptions cannot be made or when the data at hand are ranks rather than measurements on an interval or ratio scale, the investigator may wish for an optional procedure. Although the t

test is known to be rather insensitive to violations of the normality assumption, there are times when an alternative test is desirable.

A frequently used nonparametric test that does not depend on the assumptions of the *t* test is the *sign test*. This test focuses on the median rather than the mean as a measure of central tendency or location. The median and mean will be equal in symmetric distributions. The only assumption underlying the test is that the distribution of the variable of interest is continuous. This assumption rules out the use of nominal data.

The sign test gets its name from the fact that pluses and minuses, rather than numerical values, provide the raw data used in the calculations. We illustrate the use of the sign test, first in the case of a single sample, and then by an example involving paired samples.

Example 13.3.1   Researchers wished to know if instruction in personal care and grooming would improve the appearance of mentally retarded girls. In a school for the mentally retarded, 10 girls selected at random received special instruction in personal care and grooming. Two weeks after completion of the course of instruction the girls were interviewed by a nurse and a social worker who assigned each girl a score based on her general appearance. The investigators believed that the scores achieved the level of an ordinal scale. They felt that although a score of, say, 8 represented a better appearance than a score of 6, they were unwilling to say that the difference between scores of 6 and 8 was equal to the difference between, say, scores of 8 and 10; or that the difference between scores of 6 and 8 represented twice as much improvement as the difference between scores of 5 and 6. The scores are shown in Table 13.3.1. We wish to know if we can conclude that the median score of the population from which we assume this sample to have been drawn is different from 5.

Solution

1. *Data* See problem statement.

2. *Assumptions* We assume that the measurements are taken on a continuous variable.

TABLE 13.3.1 General Appearance Scores of 10 Mentally Retarded Girls

Girl	Score	Girl	Score
1	4	6	6
2	5	7	10
3	8	8	7
4	8	9	6
5	9	10	6

3. *Hypotheses*

H_0: The population median is 5.

H_A: The population median is not 5.

Let $\alpha = .05$.

4. *Test Statistic* The test statistic for the sign test is either the observed number of plus signs or the observed number of minus signs. The nature of the alternative hypothesis determines which of these test statistics is appropriate. In a given test, any one of the following alternative hypotheses is possible:

$$H_A: P(+) > P(-) \qquad \text{one-sided alternative}$$
$$H_A: P(+) < P(-) \qquad \text{one-sided alternative}$$
$$H_A: P(+) \neq P(-) \qquad \text{two-sided alternative}$$

If the alternative hypothesis is

$$H_A: P(+) > P(-)$$

a sufficiently small number of minus signs causes rejection of H_0. The test statistic is the number of minus signs. Similarly, if the alternative hypothesis is

$$H_A: P(+) < P(-)$$

a sufficiently small number of plus signs causes rejection of H_0. The test statistic is the number of plus signs. If the alternative hypothesis is

$$H_A: P(+) \neq P(-)$$

either a sufficiently small number of plus signs or a sufficiently small number of minus signs causes rejection of the null hypothesis. We may take as the test statistic the less frequently occurring sign.

5. *Distribution of the Test Statistic* As a first step in determining the nature of the test statistic, let us examine the data in Table 13.3.1 to determine which scores lie above and which ones lie below the hypothesized median of 5. If we assign a plus sign to those scores that lie above the hypothesized median and a minus to those that fall below, we have the results shown in Table 13.3.2.

TABLE 13.3.2 Scores Above (+) and Below (−) the Hypothesized Median Based on Data of Example 13.3.1

Girl	1	2	3	4	5	6	7	8	9	10
Score relative to hypothesized median	−	0	+	+	+	+	+	+	+	+

If the null hypothesis were true, that is, if the median were, in fact, 5, we would expect the numbers of scores falling above and below 5 to be approximately equal. This line of reasoning suggests an alternative way in which we could have stated the null hypothesis, namely that the probability of a plus is equal to the probability of a minus, and these probabilities are each equal to .5. Stated symbolically, the hypothesis would be

$$H_0: P(+) = P(-) = .5$$

In other words, we would expect about the same number of plus signs as minus signs in Table 13.3.2 when H_0 is true. A look at Table 13.3.2 reveals a preponderance of pluses; specifically, we observe eight pluses, one minus, and one zero, which was assigned to the score that fell exactly on the median. The usual procedure for handling zeros is to eliminate them from the analysis and reduce n, the sample size, accordingly. If we follow this procedure our problem reduces to one consisting of nine observations of which eight are plus and one is minus.

Since the number of pluses and minuses is not the same, we wonder if the distribution of signs is sufficiently disproportionate to cast doubt on our hypothesis. Stated another way, we wonder if this small a number of minuses could have come about by chance alone when the null hypothesis is true; or if the number is so small that something other than chance (that is, a false null hypothesis) is responsible for the results.

Based on what we learned in Chapter 4, it seems reasonable to conclude that the observations in Table 13.3.2 constitute a set of n independent random variables from the Bernoulli population with parameter, p. If we let $k =$ the test statistic, the sampling distribution of k is the binomial probability distribution with parameter $p = .5$ if the null hypothesis is true.

6. *Decision Rule*   The decision rule depends on the alternative hypothesis.

For H_A: $P(+) > P(-)$, reject H_0 if, when H_0 is true, the probability of observing k or fewer minus signs is less than or equal to α.

For H_A: $P(+) < P(-)$, reject H_0 if the probability of observing, when H_0 is true, k or fewer plus signs is equal to or less than α.

For H_A: $P(+) \neq P(-)$, reject H_0 if (given that H_0 is true) the probability of obtaining a value of k as extreme as or more extreme than was actually computed is equal to or less than $\alpha/2$.

For this example the decision rule is: Reject H_0 if the p value for the computed test statistic is less than or equal to .05.

7. *Calculation of Test Statistic*   We may determine the probability of observing x or fewer minus signs when given a sample of size n and parameter p by evaluating the following expression:

$$P(k \leq x | n, p) = \sum_{k=0}^{x} {}_n C_k p^k q^{n-k} \tag{13.3.1}$$

For our example we would compute

$$_9C_0(.5)^0(.5)^{9-0} + _9C_1(.5)^1(.5)^{9-1} = .00195 + .01758 = .0195$$

8. *Statistical Decision*   In Table B we find

$$P(k \leq 1 | 9, .5) = .0195$$

With a two-sided test either a sufficiently small number of minuses or a sufficiently small number of pluses would cause rejection of the null hypothesis. Since, in our example, there are fewer minuses, we focus our attention on minuses rather than pluses. By setting α equal to .05, we are saying that if the number of minuses is so small that the probability of observing this few or fewer is less than .025 (half of α), we will reject the null hypothesis. The probability we have computed, .0195, is less than .025. We, therefore, reject the null hypothesis.

9. *Conclusion*   We conclude that the median score is not 5. The p value for this test is $2(.0195) = .0390$.

Sign Test-Paired Data   When the data to be analyzed consist of observations in matched pairs and the assumptions underlying the t test are not met, or the measurement scale is weak, the sign test may be employed to test the null hypothesis that the median difference is 0. An alternative way of stating the null hypothesis is

$$P(X_i > Y_i) = P(X_i < Y_i) = .5$$

One of the matched scores, say Y_i, is subtracted from the other score, X_i. If Y_i is less than X_i, the sign of the difference is $+$, and if Y_i is greater than X_i, the sign of the difference is $-$. If the median difference is 0, we would expect a pair picked at random to be just as likely to yield a $+$ as a $-$ when the subtraction is performed. We may state the null hypothesis, then, as

$$H_0: P(+) = P(-) = .5$$

In a random sample of matched pairs we would expect the number of $+$'s and $-$'s to be about equal. If there are more $+$'s or more $-$'s than can be accounted for by chance alone when the null hypothesis is true, we will entertain some doubt about the truth of our null hypothesis. By means of the sign test, we can decide how many of one sign constitutes more than can be accounted for by chance alone.

Example 13.3.2

A dental research team wished to know if teaching people how to brush their teeth would be beneficial. Twelve pairs of patients seen in a dental clinic were obtained by carefully matching on such factors as age, sex, intelligence, and initial oral hygiene scores. One member of each pair received instruction on how to brush the

TABLE 13.3.3 Oral Hygiene Scores of 12 Subjects Receiving Oral Hygiene Instruction (X_i) and 12 Subjects Not Receiving Instruction (Y_i)

Pair Number	Instructed (X_i)	Not Instructed (Y_i)
	Score	
1	1.5	2.0
2	2.0	2.0
3	3.5	4.0
4	3.0	2.5
5	3.5	4.0
6	2.5	3.0
7	2.0	3.5
8	1.5	3.0
9	1.5	2.5
10	2.0	2.5
11	3.0	2.5
12	2.0	2.5

teeth and on other oral hygiene matters. Six months later all 24 subjects were examined and assigned an oral hygiene score by a dental hygienist unaware of which subjects had received the instruction. A low score indicates a high level of oral hygiene. The results are shown in Table 13.3.3.

Solution

1. *Data*   See problem statement.

2. *Assumptions*   We assume that the population of differences between pairs of scores is a continuous variable.

3. *Hypotheses*   If the instruction produces a beneficial effect, this fact would be reflected in the scores assigned to the members of each pair. If we take the differences $X_i - Y_i$ we would expect to observe more $-$'s than $+$'s if instruction had been beneficial, since a low score indicates a higher level of oral hygiene. If, in fact, instruction is beneficial, the median of the hypothetical population of all such differences would be less than 0, that is, negative. If, on the other hand, instruction has no effect, the median of this population would be zero. The null and alternate hypotheses, then, are

   H_0: the median of the differences is zero $[P(+) = P(-)]$

   H_A: the median of the differences is negative $[P(+) < P(-)]$

   Let α be .05.

4. *Test Statistic*   The test statistic is the number of plus signs.

5. *Distribution of the Test Statistic*   The sampling distribution of k is the binomial distribution with parameters n and .5 if H_0 is true.

6. *Decision Rule*   Reject H_0 if $P(k \leq 2 | 11, .5) \leq .05$.

TABLE 13.3.4 Signs of Differences ($X_i - Y_i$) in Oral Hygiene Scores of 12
Subjects Instructed (X_i) and 12 Matched Subjects Not Instructed (Y_i)

Pair	1	2	3	4	5	6	7	8	9	10	11	12
Sign of score differences	−	0	−	+	−	−	−	−	−	−	+	−

7. *Calculation of the Test Statistic* As will be seen, the procedure here is identical to the single sample procedure once the score differences have been obtained for each pair. Performing the subtractions and observing signs yields the results shown in Table 13.3.4.

   The nature of the hypothesis indicates a one-sided test so that all of $\alpha = .05$ is associated with the rejection region, which consists of all values of k (where k is equal to the number of + signs) for which the probability of obtaining that many or fewer pluses due to chance alone when H_0 is true is equal to or less than .05. We see in Table 13.3.4 that the experiment yielded one zero, two pluses, and nine minuses. When we eliminate the zero, the effective sample size is $n = 11$ with two pluses and nine minuses. In other words, since a "small" number of plus signs will cause rejection of the null hypothesis, the value of our test statistic is $k = 2$.

8. *Statistical Decision* We want to know the probability of obtaining no more than two pluses out of eleven tries when the null hypothesis is true. As we have seen, the answer is obtained by evaluating the appropriate binomial expression. In this example we find

$$P(k \le 2 | 11, .5) = \sum_{k=0}^{2} {}_{11}C_k (.5)^k (.5)^{11-k}$$

By consulting Table B, we find this probability to be .0327. Since .0327 is less than .05, we must reject H_0.

9. *Conclusion* We conclude that the median difference is negative. That is, we conclude that the instruction was beneficial. For this test, $p = .0327$.

Sign Test With "Greater Than" Tables As has been demonstrated, the sign test may be used with a single sample or with two samples in which each member of one sample is matched with a member of the other sample to form a sample of matched pairs. We have also seen that the alternative hypothesis may lead to either a one-sided or a two-sided test. In either case we concentrate on the less frequently occurring sign and calculate the probability of obtaining that few or fewer of that sign.

   We use the least frequently occurring sign as our test statistic because the binomial probabilities in Table B are "less than or equal to" probabilities. By using the least frequently occurring sign we can obtain the probability we need directly from Table B without having to do any subtracting. If the probabilities in Table B were "greater than or equal to" probabilities, which are often found in tables of the binomial distribution, we would use the more frequently occurring sign as our test statistic in order to take advantage of the convenience of obtaining the desired probability directly from the table without having to do any subtracting. In fact, we could, in our present examples, use the more frequently occurring sign as our test statistic, but since Table B contains "less than or equal to" probabilities we would have to perform a subtraction operation to obtain the desired probability. As an illustration, consider the last example. If we use as our test statistic the most frequently occurring sign, it is 9, the number of minuses. The desired probability, then, is the probability of 9 or more minuses, when $n = 11$, and $p = .5$. That is, we want

$$P(k \geq 9 | 11, .5)$$

Since, however, Table B contains "less than or equal to" probabilities, we must obtain this probability by subtraction. That is,

$$P(k \geq 9 | 11, .5) = 1 - P(k \leq 8 | 11, .5)$$

$$= 1 - .9673$$

$$= .0327$$

which is the result obtained previously.

Sample Size   We saw in Chapter 5 that when the sample size is large and when p is close to .5, the binomial distribution may be approximated by the normal distribution. The rule of thumb used was that the normal approximation is appropriate when both np and nq are greater than 5. When $p = .5$, as was hypothesized in our two examples, a sample of size 12 would satisfy the rule of thumb. Following this guideline, one could use the normal approximation when the sign test is used to test the null hypothesis that the median or median difference is 0 and n is equal to or greater than 12. Since the procedure involves approximating a continuous distribution by a discrete distribution, the continuity correction of .5 is generally used. The test statistic then is

$$z = \frac{(k \pm .5) - .5n}{.5\sqrt{n}} \tag{13.3.2}$$

which is compared with the value of z from the standard normal distribution corresponding to the chosen level of significance. In Equation 13.3.2, $k + .5$ is used when $k < n/2$ and $k - .5$ is used when $k > n/2$.

In addition to the references already cited, the sign test is discussed in considerable detail by Dixon and Mood (15).

Computer Analysis   Many statistics software packages will perform the sign test. For example, if we were to use MINITAB to perform the test for Example 13.3.1 in which the data are stored in column 1, the command would be

```
STEST 5 C1
```

This command results in a two-sided test. The subcommands

```
ALTERNATIVE = 1    and    ALTERNATIVE = -1
```

correspond, respectively, to H_A: Median greater than the hypothesized value and H_A: Median less than the hypothesized value.

EXERCISES

13.3.1   A random sample of 15 student nurses was given a test to measure their level of authoritarianism with the following results.

Student Number	Authoritarianism Score
1	75
2	90
3	85
4	110
5	115
6	95
7	132
8	74
9	82
10	104
11	88
12	124
13	110
14	76
15	98

Test at the .05 level of significance, the null hypothesis that the median score for the population sampled is 100. Determine the p value.

13.3.2   The aim of a study by Vaubourdolle et al. (A-1) was to investigate the influence of percutaneously delivered dihydrotestosterone (DHT) on the rate of disappearance of ethanol from the plasma in order to determine if the inhibitory effect of DHT on alcohol dehydrogenase activity occurs in healthy men. Subjects were ten healthy male volunteers aged 25 to 44 years. Among the data collected were the following testosterone (T) concentrations (nmol/l) before and after DHT treatment:

Subject:	1	2	3	4	5	6	7	8	9	10
Before:	21.5	23.0	21.0	21.8	22.8	14.7	21.0	23.4	20.0	29.5
After:	9.4	17.2	13.0	6.4	4.8	4.5	10.7	15.6	12.5	7.7

SOURCE: M. Vaubourdolle, J. Guechot, O. Chazouilleres, R. E. Poupon, and J. Giboudeau, "Effect of Dihydrotestosterone on the Rate of Ethanol Elimination in Healthy Men," *Alcoholism: Clinical and Experimental Research*, *15* (No. 2, 1991), 238–240, © The Research Society on Alcoholism, 1991.

May we conclude, on the basis of these data, that DHT treatment reduces T concentration in healthy men? Let $\alpha = .01$.

13.3.3 A sample of 15 patients suffering from asthma participated in an experiment to study the effect of a new treatment on pulmonary function. Among the various measurements recorded were those of forced expiratory volume (liters) in 1 second (FEV_1) before and after application of the treatment. The results were as follows.

Subject	Before	After	Subject	Before	After
1	1.69	1.69	9	2.58	2.44
2	2.77	2.22	10	1.84	4.17
3	1.00	3.07	11	1.89	2.42
4	1.66	3.35	12	1.91	2.94
5	3.00	3.00	13	1.75	3.04
6	.85	2.74	14	2.46	4.62
7	1.42	3.61	15	2.35	4.42
8	2.82	5.14			

On the basis of these data, can one conclude that the treatment is effective in increasing the FEV_1 level? Let $\alpha = .05$ and find the p value.

13.4
The Wilcoxon Signed-Rank Test for Location

Sometimes we wish to test a null hypothesis about a population mean, but for some reason neither z nor t is an appropriate test statistic. If we have a small sample ($n < 30$) from a population that is known to be grossly nonnormally distributed, and the central limit theorem is not applicable, the z statistic is ruled out. The t statistic is not appropriate because the sampled population does not sufficiently approximate a normal distribution. When confronted with such a situation we usually look for an appropriate nonparametric statistical procedure. As we have seen, the sign test may be used when our data consist of a single sample or when we have paired data. If, however, the data for analysis are measured on at least an interval scale, the sign test may be undesirable since it would not make full use of the information contained in the data. A more appropriate procedure might be the Wilcoxon (16) signed-rank test, which makes use of the magnitudes of the differences between measurements and a hypothesized location parameter rather than just the signs of the differences.

Assumptions The Wilcoxon test for location is based on the following assumptions about the data.

1. The sample is random.
2. The variable is continuous.
3. The population is symmetrically distributed about its mean μ.
4. The measurement scale is at least interval.

Hypotheses The following are the null hypotheses (along with their alternatives) that may be tested about some unknown population mean μ_0.

$$(a) \ H_0: \mu = \mu_0 \quad (b) \ H_0: \mu \geq \mu_0 \quad (c) \ H_0: \mu \leq \mu_0$$

$$H_1: \mu \neq \mu_0 \qquad H_1: \mu < \mu_0 \qquad H_1: \mu > \mu_0$$

When we use the Wilcoxon procedure we perform the following calculations.

1. Subtract the hypothesized mean μ_0 from each observation x_i, to obtain

$$d_i = x_i - \mu_0$$

If any x_i is equal to the mean, so that $d_i = 0$, eliminate that d_i from the calculations and reduce n accordingly.

2. Rank the usable d_i from the smallest to the largest without regard to the sign of d_i. That is, consider only the absolute value of the d_i, designated by $|d_i|$, when ranking them. If two or more of the $|d_i|$ are equal, assign each tied value the mean of the rank positions the tied values occupy. If, for example, the three smallest $|d_i|$ are all equal, place them in rank positions 1, 2, and 3, but assign each a rank of $(1 + 2 + 3)/3 = 2$.

3. Assign each rank the sign of the d_i that yields that rank.

4. Find T_+, the sum of the ranks with positive signs, and T_-, the sum of the ranks with negative signs.

The Test Statistic The Wilcoxon test statistic is either T_+ or T_-, depending on the nature of the alternative hypothesis. If the null hypothesis is true, that is, if the true population mean is equal to the hypothesized mean, and if the assumptions are met, the probability of observing a positive difference $d_i = x_i - \mu_0$ of a given magnitude is equal to the probability of observing a negative difference of the same magnitude. Then, in repeated sampling, when the null hypothesis is true and the assumptions are met, the expected value of T_+ is equal to the expected value of T_-. We do not expect T_+ and T_- computed from a given sample to be equal. However, when H_0 is true, we do not expect a large difference in their values. Consequently, a sufficiently small value of T_+ or a sufficiently small value of T_- will cause rejection of H_0.

When the alternative hypothesis is two-sided $(\mu \neq \mu_0)$ either a sufficiently small value of T_+ or a sufficiently small value of T_- will cause us to reject H_0: $\mu = \mu_0$. The test statistic, then, is T_+ or T_-, whichever is smaller. To simplify notation, we call the smaller of the two T.

When H_0: $\mu \geq \mu_0$ is true we expect our sample to yield a large value of T_+. Therefore when the one-sided alternative hypothesis states that the true population mean is less than the hypothesized mean $(\mu < \mu_0)$, a sufficiently small value of T_+ will cause rejection of H_0, and T_+ is the test statistic.

When H_0: $\mu \leq \mu_0$ is true we expect our sample to yield a large value of T_-. Therefore for the one-sided alternative H_A: $\mu > \mu_0$ a sufficiently small value of T_- will cause rejection of H_0 and T_- is the test statistic.

Critical Values   Critical values of the Wilcoxon test statistic are given in Appendix II Table K. Exact probability levels (P) are given to four decimal places for all possible rank totals (T) that yield a different probability level at the fourth decimal place from 0.0001 up through 0.5000. The rank totals (T) are tabulated for all sample sizes from $n = 5$ through $n = 30$. The following are the decision rules for the three possible alternative hypotheses:

a. H_A: $\mu \neq \mu_0$. Reject H_0 at the α level of significance if the calculated T is smaller than or equal to the tabulated T for n and preselected $\alpha/2$. Alternatively we may enter Table K with n and our calculated value of T to see whether the tabulated P associated with the calculated T is less than or equal to our stated level of significance. If so, we may reject H_0.

b. H_A: $\mu < \mu_0$. Reject H_0 at the α level of significance if T_+ is less than or equal to the tabulated T for n and preselected α.

c. H_A: $\mu > \mu_0$. Reject H_0 at the α level of significance if T_- is less than or equal to the tabulated T for n and preselected α.

Example 13.4.1

Cardiac output (liters/minute) was measured by thermodilution in a simple random sample of 15 postcardiac surgical patients in the left lateral position. The results were as follows:

4.91	4.10	6.74	7.27	7.42	7.50	6.56	4.64
5.98	3.14	3.23	5.80	6.17	5.39	5.77	

We wish to know if we can conclude on the basis of these data that the population mean is different from 5.05.

Solution:

1. *Data* See statement of example.

2. *Assumptions* We assume that the requirements for the application of the Wilcoxon signed-ranks test are met.

3. *Hypotheses*

H_0: $\mu = 5.05$

H_A: $\mu \neq 5.05$

Let $\alpha = 0.05$.

4. *Test Statistic* The test statistic will be T_+ or T_-, whichever is smaller. We will call the test statistic T.

5. *Distribution of the Test Statistic* Critical values of the test statistic are given in Table K of Appendix II.

6. *Decision Rule* We will reject H_0 if the computed value of T is less than or equal to 25, the critical value for $n = 15$, and $\alpha/2 = .0240$, the closest value to .0250 in Table K.

7. *Calculation of Test Statistic* The calculation of the test statistic is shown in Table 13.4.1.

8. *Statistical Decision* Since 34 is greater than 25, we are unable to reject H_0.

9. *Conclusion* We conclude that the population mean may be 5.05. From Table K we see that the p value is $p = 2(.0757) = .1514$

TABLE 13.4.1 Calculation of the Test Statistic for Example 13.4.1

Cardiac Output	$d_i = x_i - 5.05$	Rank of d_i	Signed Rank of d_i
4.91	−.14	1	−1
4.10	−.95	7	−7
6.74	+1.69	10	+10
7.27	+2.22	13	+13
7.42	+2.37	14	+14
7.50	+2.45	15	+15
6.56	+1.51	9	+9
4.64	−.41	3	−3
5.98	+.93	6	+6
3.14	−1.91	12	−12
3.23	−1.82	11	−11
5.80	+.75	5	+5
6.17	+1.12	8	+8
5.39	+.34	2	+2
5.77	+.72	4	+4
			$T_+ = 86, T_- = 34, T = 34$

Wilcoxon Matched-Pairs Signed-Ranks Test   The Wilcoxon test may be used with paired data under circumstances in which it is not appropriate to use the paired-comparisons t test described in Chapter 7. In such cases obtain each of the $n\,d_i$ values, the difference between each of the n pairs of measurements. If we let μ_D = the mean of a population of such differences, we may follow the procedure described above to test any one of the following null hypotheses: H_0: $\mu_D = 0$, H_0: $\mu_D \le 0$, and H_0: $\mu_D \ge 0$.

Computer Analysis   Many statistics software packages will perform the Wilcoxon signed-rank test. If, for example, the data of Exercise 13.4.1 are stored in column 1, we could use MINITAB to perform the test by means of the command

```
WTEST 5.05 C1
```

The subcommands

```
ALTERNATIVE -1    and    ALTERNATIVE 1
```

respectively, will perform the one-sided tests in which $<$ and $>$ appear in the alternative hypothesis.

EXERCISES

13.4.1   Sixteen laboratory animals were fed a special diet from birth through age 12 weeks. Their weight gains (in grams) were as follows:

63	68	79	65	64	63	65	64	76	74	66
66	67	73	69	76						

Can we conclude from these data that the diet results in a mean weight gain of less than 70 grams? Let $\alpha = .05$, and find the p value.

13.4.2   A psychologist selects a random sample of 25 handicapped students. Their manual dexterity scores were as follows:

33	53	22	40	24	56	36	28	38	42	35	52	52
36	47	41	32	20	42	34	53	37	35	47	42	

Do these data provide sufficient evidence to indicate that the mean score for the population is not 45? Let $\alpha = .05$. Find the p value.

13.4.3   In a study by Davis et al. (A-2) maternal language directed toward children with mental retardation and children matched either for language ability or chronological age was compared in free-play and instruction situations. Results were consistent with the hypothesis that mothers of children with retardation match their verbal behavior to their children's language ability. Among the data collected were the following measurements on number of utterances per minute during free play by mothers of children with retardation (A) and mothers of age-matched children who were not mentally retarded (B).

A: 21.90 15.80 16.50 15.00 14.25 17.10 13.50 14.60 18.75 19.80
B: 13.95 13.35   9.40 11.85 12.45   9.95   9.10   8.00 14.65 12.20

SOURCE: Hilton Davis, Ph.D. Used with permission.

May we conclude, on the basis of these data, that among mothers of mentally retarded children, the average number of utterances per minute during free play is higher than among mothers whose children are not mentally retarded? Let $\alpha = .01$.

13.5
The Median Test

A nonparametric procedure that may be used to test the null hypothesis that two independent samples have been drawn from populations with equal medians is the median test. The test, attributed mainly to Mood (17) and Westenberg (18), is also discussed by Brown and Mood (19) and Moses (4) as well as in several other references already cited.

We illustrate the procedure by means of an example.

Example 13.5.1

Do urban and rural male junior high school students differ with respect to their level of mental health?

Solution

1. *Data*   Members of a random sample of 12 male students from a rural junior high school and an independent random sample of 16 male students from an urban junior high school were given a test to measure their level of mental health. The results are shown in Table 13.5.1.

   To determine if we can conclude that there is a difference we perform a hypothesis test that makes use of the median test. Suppose we choose a .05 level of significance.

2. *Assumptions*   The assumptions underlying the test are (a) the samples are selected independently and at random from their respective populations, (b) the populations are of the same form, differing only in location, and (c) the variable of interest is continuous. The level of measurement must be, at least, ordinal. The two samples do not have to be of equal size.

3. *Hypotheses*

$$H_0: M_U = M_R$$

$$H_A: M_U \neq M_R$$

TABLE 13.5.1 Level of Mental Health Scores of Junior High Boys

		School	
Urban	**Rural**	**Urban**	**Rural**
35	29	25	50
26	50	27	37
27	43	45	34
21	22	46	31
27	42	33	
38	47	26	
23	42	46	
25	32	41	

M_U is the median score of the sampled population of urban students and M_R is the median score of the sampled population of rural students. Let $\alpha = .05$.

4. *Test Statistic*   As will be shown in the discussion that follows, the test statistic is X^2 as computed, for example, by Equation 12.4.1 for a 2×2 contingency table.

5. *Distribution of the Test Statistic*   When H_0 is true and the assumptions are met, X^2 is distributed approximately as χ^2 with 1 degree of freedom.

6. *Decision Rule*   Reject H_0 if the computed value of X^2 is ≥ 3.841 (since $\alpha = .05$).

7. *Calculation of Test Statistic*   The first step in calculating the test statistic is to compute the common median of the two samples combined. This is done by arranging the observations in ascending order and, since the total number of observations is even, obtaining the mean of the two middle numbers. For our example the median is $(33 + 34)/2 = 33.5$.

We now determine for each group the number of observations falling above and below the common median. The resulting frequencies are arranged in a 2×2 table. For the present example we obtain Table 13.5.2.

If the two samples are, in fact, from populations with the same median, we would expect about one half the scores in each sample to be above the combined median and about one half to be below. If the conditions relative to sample size and expected frequencies for a 2×2 contingency table as discussed Chapter 12 are met, the chi-square test with 1 degree of freedom may be used to test the null

TABLE 13.5.2 Level of Mental Health Scores of Junior High School Boys

	Urban	**Rural**	**Total**
Number of scores above median	6	8	14
Number of scores below median	10	4	14
Total	16	12	28

hypothesis of equal population medians. For our examples we have, by Formula 12.4.1,

$$X^2 = \frac{28[(6)(4) - (8)(10)]^2}{(16)(12)(14)(14)} = 2.33$$

8. *Statistical Decision* Since 2.33 < 3.841, the critical value of χ^2 with $\alpha = .05$ and 1 degree of freedom, we are unable to reject the null hypothesis on the basis of these data.

9. *Conclusion* We conclude that the two samples may have been drawn from populations with equal medians. Since 2.33 < 2.706, we have $p > .10$.

Handling Values Equal to the Median Sometimes one or more observed values will be exactly equal to the common median and, hence, will fall neither above nor below it. We note that if $n_1 + n_2$ is odd, at least one value will always be exactly equal to the median. This raises the question of what to do with observations of this kind. One solution is to drop them from the analysis if $n_1 + n_2$ is large and there are only a few values that fall at the combined median. Or we may dichotomize the scores into those that exceed the median and those that do not, in which case the observations that equal the median will be counted in the second category. Alternative procedures are suggested by Senders (20) and Hays and Winkler (21).

Median Test Extension The median test extends logically to the case where it is desired to test the null hypothesis that $k \geq 3$ samples are from populations with equal medians. For this test a $2 \times k$ contingency table may be constructed by using the frequencies that fall above and below the median computed from combined samples. If conditions as to sample size and expected frequencies are met, X^2 may be computed and compared with the critical χ^2 with $k - 1$ degrees of freedom.

EXERCISES

13.5.1 Fifteen patient records from each of two hospitals were reviewed and assigned a score designed to measure level of care. The scores were as follows:

Hospital A: 99, 85, 73, 98, 83, 88, 99, 80, 74, 91, 80, 94, 94, 98, 80
Hospital B: 78, 74, 69, 79, 57, 78, 79, 68, 59, 91, 89, 55, 60, 55, 79

Would you conclude, at the .05 level of significance, that the two population medians are different? Determine the p value.

13.5.2 The following serum albumin values were obtained from 17 normal and 13 hospitalized subjects.

Serum Albumin (g / 100 ml)			
Normal Subjects		Hospitalized Subjects	
2.4	3.0	1.5	3.1
3.5	3.2	2.0	1.3
3.1	3.5	3.4	1.5
4.0	3.8	1.7	1.8
4.2	3.9	2.0	2.0
3.4	4.0	3.8	1.5
4.5	3.5	3.5	
5.0	3.6		
2.9			

Would you conclude at the .05 level of significance that the medians of the two populations sampled are different? Determine the p value.

13.6
The Mann – Whitney Test

The median test discussed in the preceding section does not make full use of all the information present in the two samples when the variable of interest is measured on at least an ordinal scale. By reducing an observation's information content to merely that of whether or not it falls above or below the common median is a waste of information. If, for testing the desired hypothesis, there is available a procedure that makes use of more of the information inherent in the data, that procedure should be used if possible. Such a nonparametric procedure that can often be used instead of the median test is the Mann–Whitney test (22). Since this test is based on the ranks of the observations it utilizes more information than does the median test.

Assumptions   The assumptions underlying the Mann–Whitney test are as follows:

1. The two samples, of size n and m, respectively, available for analysis have been independently and randomly drawn from their respective populations.
2. The measurement scale is at least ordinal.
3. The variable of interest is continuous.
4. If the populations differ at all, they differ only with respect to their medians.

Hypotheses   When these assumptions are met we may test the null hypothesis that the two populations have equal medians against either of the three possible alternatives: (1) the populations do not have equal medians (two-sided test), (2) the median of population 1 is larger than the median of population 2 (one-sided test), or (3) the median of population 1 is smaller than the median of population 2 (one-sided test). If the two populations are symmetric, so that within each population the mean and median are the same, the conclusions we reach regarding the two population medians will also apply to the two population means. The following example illustrates the use of the Mann–Whitney test.

Example 13.6.1

A researcher designed an experiment to assess the effects of prolonged inhalation of cadmium oxide. Fifteen laboratory animals served as experimental subjects, while 10 similar animals served as controls. The variable of interest was hemoglobin level following the experiment. The results are shown in Table 13.6.1. We wish to know if we can conclude that prolonged inhalation of cadmium oxide reduces hemoglobin level.

Solution

1. *Data*   See Table 13.6.1.

2. *Assumptions*   We presume that the assumptions of the Mann–Whitney test are met.

3. *Hypotheses*   The null and alternative hypotheses are as follows:

$$H_0: M_X \geq M_Y$$

$$H_A: M_X < M_Y$$

where M_X is the median of a population of animals exposed to cadmium oxide

TABLE 13.6.1 Hemoglobin Determinations
(Grams) for 25 Laboratory Animals

Exposed Animals (X)	Unexposed Animals (Y)
14.4	17.4
14.2	16.2
13.8	17.1
16.5	17.5
14.1	15.0
16.6	16.0
15.9	16.9
15.6	15.0
14.1	16.3
15.3	16.8
15.7	
16.7	
13.7	
15.3	
14.0	

TABLE 13.6.2 Original Data and Ranks, Example 13.6.1

X	Rank	Y	Rank
13.7	1		
13.8	2		
14.0	3		
14.1	4.5		
14.1	4.5		
14.2	6		
14.4	7		
		15.0	8.5
		15.0	8.5
15.3	10.5		
15.3	10.5		
15.6	12		
15.7	13		
15.9	14		
		16.0	15
		16.2	16
		16.3	17
16.5	18		
16.6	19		
16.7	20		
		16.8	21
		16.9	22
		17.1	23
		17.4	24
		17.5	25
Total		145	

and M_Y is the median of a population of animals not exposed to the substance. Suppose we let $\alpha = .05$.

4. *Test Statistic* To compute the test statistic we combine the two samples and rank all observations from smallest to largest while keeping track of the sample to which each observation belongs. Tied observations are assigned a rank equal to the mean of the rank positions for which they are tied. The results of this step are shown in Table 13.6.2.

   The test statistic is

$$T = S - \frac{n(n + 1)}{2} \tag{13.6.1}$$

where n is the number of sample X observations and S is the sum of the ranks assigned to the sample observations from the population of X values. The choice of which sample's values we label X is arbitrary.

5. *Distribution of Test Statistic* Critical values from the distribution of the test statistic are given in Table L for various levels of α.

6. *Decision Rule*   If the median of the X population is, in fact, smaller than the median of the Y population, as specified in the alternative hypothesis, we would expect (for equal sample sizes) the sum of the ranks assigned to the observations from the X population to be smaller than the sum of the ranks assigned to the observations from the Y population. The test statistic is based on this rationale in such a way that a sufficiently small value of T will cause rejection of H_0: $M_X \geq M_Y$.

In general, for one-sided tests of the type illustrated here the decision rule is:

Reject H_0: $M_X \geq M_Y$ if the computed T is less than w_α, where w_α is the critical value of T obtained by entering Appendix II Table L with n, the number of X observations; m, the number of Y observations; and α, the chosen level of significance.

If we use the Mann–Whitney procedure to test

$$H_0: M_X \leq M_Y$$

against

$$H_A: M_X > M_Y$$

sufficiently large values of T will cause rejection so that the decision rule is:

Reject H_0: $M_X < M_Y$ if computed T is greater than $w_{1-\alpha}$, where $W_{1-\alpha} = nm - W_\alpha$.

For the two-sided test situation with

$$H_0: M_X = M_Y$$

$$H_A: M_X \neq M_Y$$

Computed values of T that are either sufficiently large or sufficiently small will cause rejection of H_0: the decision rule for this case, then, is:

Reject H_0: $M_X = M_Y$ if the computed value of T is either less than $w_{\alpha/2}$ or greater than $w_{1-(\alpha/2)}$, where $w_{\alpha/2}$ is the critical value of T for n, m, and $\alpha/2$ given in Appendix II Table L, and $w_{1-(\alpha/2)} = nm - w_{\alpha/2}$.

For this example the decision rule is:

Reject H_0 if the computed value of T is smaller than 45, the critical value of the test statistic for $n = 15$, $m = 10$, and $\alpha = .05$ found in Table L.

7. *Calculation of Test Statistic*   For our present example we have, as shown in Table 13.6.2, $S = 145$, so that

$$T = 145 - \frac{15(15 + 1)}{2} = 25$$

8. *Statistical Decision*   When we enter Table L with $n = 15$, $m = 10$, and $\alpha = .05$, we find the critical value of w_α to be 45. Since $25 < 45$, we reject H_0.

9. *Conclusion*   We conclude that M_X is smaller than M_Y. This leads to the conclusion that prolonged inhalation of cadmium oxide does reduce the hemoglobin level.

Since $22 < 25 < 30$, we have for this test $.005 > p > .001$.

Large Sample Approximation   When either n or m is greater than 20 we cannot use Appendix Table L to obtain critical values for the Mann–Whitney test. When this is the case we may compute

$$z = \frac{T - mn/2}{\sqrt{nm(n + m + 1)/12}} \tag{13.6.2}$$

and compare the result, for significance, with critical values of the standard normal distribution.

If a large proportion of the observations are tied, a correction factor proposed by Noether (23) may be used.

Many statistics software packages will perform the Mann–Whitney test. With the data of two samples stored in columns 1 and 2, for example, MINITAB will perform a two-sided test in response to the command

```
MANN-WHITNEY C1 C2
```

The subcommands

```
ALTERNATIVE -1    and    ALTERNATIVE 1
```

will perform, respectively, one-sided tests with $<$ and $>$ in the alternative.

EXERCISES

13.6.1   The purpose of a study by Demotes-Mainard et al. (A-3) was to compare the pharmacokinetics of both total and unbound cefpiramide (a cephalosporin) in healthy volunteers and patients with alcoholic cirrhosis. Among the data collected were the following total plasma clearance (ml/min) values following a single 1 gram intravenous injection of cefpiramide.

Volunteers: 21.7, 29.3, 25.3, 22.8, 21.3, 31.2, 29.2, 28.7, 17.2, 25.7, 32.3
Patients with alcoholic cirrhosis: 18.1, 12.3, 8.8, 10.3, 8.5, 29.3, 8.1, 6.9, 7.9, 14.6, 11.1

SOURCE: Fabienne Demotes-Mainard, Ph.D. Used with permission.

May we conclude, on the basis of these data, that patients with alcoholic cirrhosis and patients without the disease differ with regard to the variable of interest? Let $\alpha = .01$.

13.6.2   Lebranchu et al. (A-4) conducted a study in which the subjects were nine patients with common variable immunodeficiency (CVI) and 12 normal controls. Among the data collected were the following on number of CD4 + T cells per mm^3 of peripheral blood.

CVI patients: 623, 437, 370, 300, 330, 527, 290, 730, 1000
Controls: 710, 1260, 717, 590, 930, 995, 630, 977, 530, 710, 1275, 825

SOURCE: Dr. Yvon Lebranchu. Used with permission.

May we conclude, on the basis of these data, that CVI patients have a reduced level of CD4 + cells? Let $\alpha = .01$.

13.6.3   The purpose of a study by Liu et al. (A-5) was to characterize the mediator, cellular, and permeability changes occurring immediately and 19 hours following bronchoscopic segmental challenge of the peripheral airways with ragweed antigen in allergic, mildly asthmatic subjects. In addition to the subjects with asthma, the study included normal subjects who had no asthmatic symptoms. Among the data collected were the following measurements on percent of fluid recovered from antigen-challenged sites following bronchoalveolar lavage (BAL).

Normal subjects: 70, 55, 63, 68, 73, 77, 67
Asthmatic subjects: 64, 25, 70, 35, 43, 49, 62, 56, 43, 66

SOURCE: Mark C. Liu, M.D. Used with permission.

May we conclude, on the basis of these data, that under the conditions described, we can expect to recover less fluid from asthmatic subjects? Let $\alpha = .05$.

13.7
The Kolmogorov – Smirnov
Goodness-of-Fit Test

When one wishes to know how well the distribution of sample data conforms to some theoretical distribution, a test known as the Kolmogorov–Smirnov goodness-of-fit test provides an alternative to the chi-square goodness-of-fit test discussed in Chapter 12. The test gets its name from A. Kolmogorov and N. V. Smirnov, two Russian mathematicians who introduced two closely related tests in the 1930s.

Kolmogorov's work (24) is concerned with the one-sample case as discussed here. Smirnov's work (25) deals with the case involving two samples in which interest centers on testing the hypothesis that the distributions of the two parent populations are identical. The test for the first situation is frequently referred to as the Kolmogorov–Smirnov one-sample test. The test for the two-sample case, commonly referred to as the Kolmogorov–Smirnov two-sample test, will not be discussed here. Those interested in this topic may refer to Daniel (5).

The Test Statistic   In using the Kolmogorov–Smirnov goodness-of-fit test a comparison is made between some theoretical cumulative distribution function, $F_T(x)$, and a sample cumulative distribution function, $F_S(x)$. The sample is a random sample from a population with unknown cumulative distribution function $F(x)$. It will be recalled (Section 4.2) that a cumulative distribution function gives the probability that X is equal to or less than a particular value, x. That is, by means of the sample cumulative distribution function, $F_S(x)$, we may estimate $P(X \leq x)$. If there is close agreement between the theoretical and sample cumulative distributions, the hypothesis that the sample was drawn from the population with the specified cumulative distribution function, $F_T(x)$, is supported. If, however, there is a discrepancy between the theoretical and observed cumulative distribution functions too great to be attributed to chance alone, when H_0 is true, the hypothesis is rejected.

The difference between the theoretical cumulative distribution function, $F_T(x)$, and the sample cumulative distribution function, $F_S(x)$, is measured by the statistic D, which is the greatest vertical distance between $F_S(x)$ and $F_T(x)$. When a two-sided test is appropriate, that is, when the hypotheses are

$$H_0: F(x) = F_T(x) \qquad \text{for all } x \text{ from } -\infty \text{ to } +\infty$$

$$H_A: F(x) \neq F_T(x) \qquad \text{for at least one } x$$

the test statistic is

$$D = \sup_x \left| F_s(x) - F_t(x) \right| n \qquad (13.7.1)$$

which is read, "D equals the supremum, (greatest) over all x, of the absolute value of the difference $F_S(x)$ minus $F_T(x)$."

The null hypothesis is rejected at the α level of significance if the computed value of D exceeds the value shown in Table M for $1 - \alpha$ (two-sided) and the sample size n. Tests in which the alternative is one sided are possible. Numerical examples are given by Goodman (26).

Assumptions   The assumptions underlying the Kolmogorov–Smirnov test include the following:

1. The sample is a random sample.
2. The hypothesized distribution $F_T(x)$ is continuous.

Noether (23) has shown that when values of D are based on a discrete theoretical distribution, the test is conservative. When the test is used with discrete data, then, the investigator should bear in mind that the true probability of commuting a type I error is at most equal to α, the stated level of significance. The test is also conservative if one or more parameters have to be estimated from sample data.

Example 13.7.1

Fasting, blood glucose determinations made on 36 nonobese, apparently healthy, adult males are shown in Table 13.7.1. We wish to know if we may conclude that these data are not from a normally distributed population with a mean of 80 and a standard deviation of 6.

Solution

1. *Data* See Table 13.7.1.

2. *Assumptions* The sample available is a simple random sample from a continuous population distribution.

3. *Hypotheses* The appropriate hypotheses are

$$H_0: F(x) = F_T(x) \qquad \text{for all } x \text{ from } -\infty \text{ to } +\infty$$

$$H_A: F(x) \neq F_T(x) \qquad \text{for at least one } x$$

Let $\alpha = .05$.

4. *Test Statistic* See Equation 13.7.1.

5. *Distribution of Test Statistic* Critical values of the test statistic for selected values of α are given in Table M.

6. *Decision Rule* Reject H_0 if the computed value of D exceeds .221, the critical value of D for $n = 36$ and $\alpha = .05$.

7. *Calculation of Test Statistic* Our first step is to compute values of $F_S(x)$ as shown in Table 13.7.2.

   Each value of $F_S(x)$ is obtained by dividing the corresponding cumulative frequency by the sample size. For example, the first value of $F_S(x) = 2/36 = .0556$.

TABLE 13.7.1 Fasting Blood Glucose Values (mg / 100 ml) for 36 Nonobese, Apparently Healthy, Adult Males

75	92	80	80	84	72
84	77	81	77	75	81
80	92	72	77	78	76
77	86	77	92	80	78
68	78	92	68	80	81
87	76	80	87	77	86

TABLE 13.7.2 Values of $F_S(x)$ for Example 13.7.1

x	Frequency	Cumulative Frequency	$F_S(x)$
68	2	2	.0556
72	2	4	.1111
75	2	6	.1667
76	2	8	.2222
77	6	14	.3889
78	3	17	.4722
80	6	23	.6389
81	3	26	.7222
84	2	28	.7778
86	2	30	.8333
87	2	32	.8889
92	4	36	1.0000
	$\overline{36}$		

We obtain values of $F_T(x)$ by first converting each observed value of x to a value of the standard normal variable, z. From Table D we then find the area between $-\infty$ and z. From these areas we are able to compute values of $F_T(x)$. The procedure, which is similar to that used to obtain expected relative frequencies in the chi-square goodness-of-fit test, is summarized in Table 13.7.3.

The test statistic D may be computed algebraically, or it may be determined graphically by actually measuring the largest vertical distance between the curves of $F_S(x)$ and $F_T(x)$ on a graph. The graphs of the two distributions are shown in Figure 13.7.1.

Examination of the graphs of $F_S(x)$ and $F_T(x)$ reveals that $D \approx .16 = (.72 - .56)$. Now let us compute the value of D algebraically. The possible

TABLE 13.7.3 Steps in Calculation of $F_T(x)$ for Example 13.7.1

x	$z = (x - 80) / 6$	$F_T(x)$
68	-2.00	.0228
72	-1.33	.0918
75	$-.83$	.2033
76	$-.67$	.2514
77	$-.50$	.3085
78	$-.33$	.3707
80	$.00$	.5000
81	$.17$	.5675
84	$.67$	.7486
86	1.00	.8413
87	1.17	.8790
92	2.00	.9772

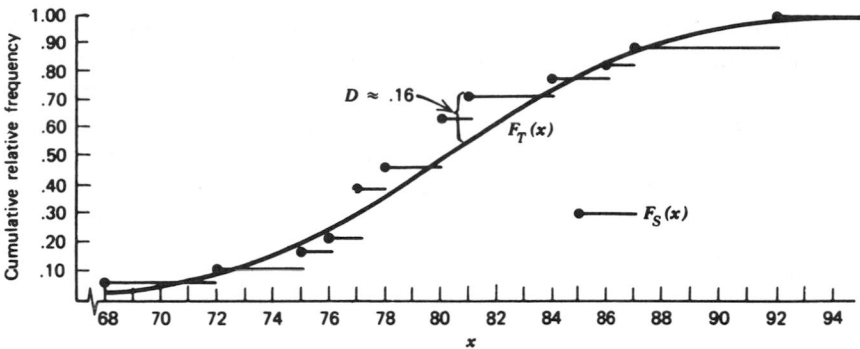

Figure 13.7.1 $F_S(x)$ and $F_T(x)$ for Example 13.7.1.

values of $|F_S(x) - F_T(x)|$ are shown in Table 13.7.4. This table shows that the exact value of D is .1547.

8. *Statistical Decision*   Reference to Table M reveals that a computed D of .1547 is not significant at any reasonable level. Therefore, we are not willing to reject H_0.

9. *Conclusion*   The sample may have come from the specified distribution. Since we have a two-sided test, and since .1547 < .174, we have $p > .20$.

A Precaution   The reader should be aware that in determining the value of D *it is not always sufficient to compute and choose from the possible values of* $|F_S(x) - F_T(x)|$. *The largest vertical distance between* $F_S(x)$ *and* $F_T(x)$ *may not occur at an observed value, x, but at some other value of X*. Such a situation is illustrated in Figure 13.7.2. We see

TABLE 13.7.4 Calculation of $|F_S(x) - F_T(x)|$ for Example 13.7.1

x	$F_S(x)$	$F_T(x)$	$|F_S(x) - F_T(x)|$
68	.0556	.0228	.0328
72	.1111	.0918	.0193
75	.1667	.2033	.0366
76	.2222	.2514	.0292
77	.3889	.3085	.0804
78	.4722	.3707	.1015
80	.6389	.5000	.1389
81	.7222	.5675	.1547
84	.7778	.7486	.0292
86	.8333	.8413	.0080
87	.8889	.8790	.0099
92	1.0000	.9772	.0228

that if only values of $|F_S(x) - F_T(x)|$ at the left end-points of the horizontal bars are considered we would incorrectly compute D as $|.2 - .4| = .2$. One can see by examining the graph, however, that the largest vertical distance between $F_S(x)$ and $F_T(x)$ occurs at the right end-point of the horizontal bar originating at the point corresponding to $x = .4$, and the correct value of D is $|.5 - .2| = .3$.

One can determine the correct value of D algebraically by computing, in addition to the differences $|F_S(x) - F_T(x)|$, the differences $|F_S(x_{i-1}) - F_T(x_i)|$ for all values of $i = 1, 2, \ldots, r + 1$, where $r =$ the number of different values of x and $F_S(x_0) = 0$. The correct value of the test statistic will then be

$$D = \underset{1 \le i \le r}{\text{maximum}} \left\{ \text{maximum} \left[|F_S(x_i) - F_T(x_i)|, |F_S(x_{i-1}) - F_T(x_i)| \right] \right\} \quad (13.7.2)$$

Advantages and Disadvantages   The advantages and disadvantages of the Kolmogorov–Smirnov goodness-of-fit test in comparison with the chi-square test have been discussed by Goodman (26), Massey (27), Birnbaum (28), and Slakter (29). The following are some important points of comparison.

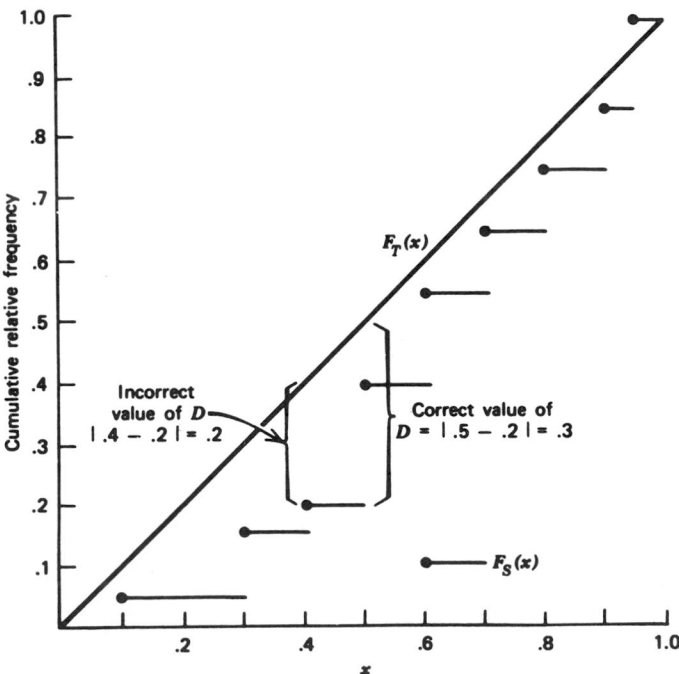

Figure 13.7.2 Graph of fictitious data showing correct calculation of D.

1. The Kolmogorov–Smirnov test does not require that the observations be grouped as is the case with the chi-square test. The consequence of this difference is that the Kolmogorov–Smirnov test makes use of all the information present in a set of data.

2. The Kolmogorov–Smirnov test can be used with any size sample. It will be recalled that certain minimum sample sizes are required for the use of the chi-square test.

3. As has been noted the Kolmogorov–Smirnov test is not applicable when parameters have to be estimated from the sample. The chi-square test may be used in these situations by reducing the degrees of freedom by 1 for each parameter estimated.

4. The problem of the assumption of a continuous theoretical distribution has already been mentioned.

EXERCISES

13.7.1 The weights at autopsy of the brains of 25 adults suffering from a certain disease were as follows.

Weight of Brain (Grams)				
859	1073	1041	1166	1117
962	1051	1064	1141	1202
973	1001	1016	1168	1255
904	1012	1002	1146	1233
920	1039	1086	1140	1348

Can one conclude from these data that the sampled population is not normally distributed with a mean of 1050 and a standard deviation of 50? Determine the p value for this test.

13.7.2 IQs of a sample of 30 adolescents arrested for drug abuse in a certain metropolitan jurisdiction were as follows.

IQ					
95	100	91	106	109	110
98	104	97	100	107	119
92	106	103	106	105	112
101	91	105	102	101	110
101	95	102	104	107	118

Do these data provide sufficient evidence that the sampled population of IQ scores is not normally distributed with a mean of 105 and a standard deviation of 10? Determine the p value.

13.7.3 For a sample of apparently normal subjects who served as controls in an experiment, the following systolic blood pressure readings were recorded at the beginning of the experiment.

162	177	151	167
130	154	179	146
147	157	141	157
153	157	134	143
141	137	151	161

Can one conclude on the basis of these data that the population of blood pressures from which the sample was drawn is not normally distributed with $\mu = 150$ and $\sigma = 12$? Determine the p value.

13.8
The Kruskal–Wallis One-Way Analysis of Variance by Ranks

In Chapter 8 we discuss how one-way analysis of variance may be used to test the null hypothesis that several population means are equal. When the assumptions underlying this technique are not met, that is, when the populations from which the samples are drawn are not normally distributed with equal variances, or when the data for analysis consist only of ranks, a nonparametric alternative to the one-way analysis of variance may be used to test the hypothesis of equal location parameters. As was pointed out in Section 13.5, the median test may be extended to accommodate the situation involving more than two samples. A deficiency of this test, however, is the fact that it uses only a small amount of the information available. The test uses only information as to whether or not the observations are above or below a single number, the median of the combined samples. The test does not directly use measurements of known quantity. Several nonparametric analogs to analysis of variance are available that use more information by taking into account the magnitude of each observation relative to the magnitude of every other observation. Perhaps the best known of these procedures is the Kruskal–Wallis one-way analysis of variance by ranks (30).

The Kruskal–Wallis Procedure The application of the test involves the following steps.

1. The $n_1, n_2, \ldots, n_k$ observations from the k samples are combined into a single series of size n and arranged in order of magnitude from smallest to largest. The observations are then replaced by ranks from 1, which is assigned to the smallest observation, to n, which is assigned to the largest observation. When two or more observations have the same value, each observation is given the mean of the ranks for which it is tied.

2. The ranks assigned to observations in each of the k groups are added separately to give k rank sums.

3. The test statistic

$$H = \frac{12}{n(n+1)} \sum_{j=1}^{k} \frac{R_j^2}{n_j} - 3(n+1) \qquad (13.8.1)$$

is computed.

In Equation 13.8.1

$$k = \text{the number of samples}$$

$$n_j = \text{the number of observations in the } j\text{th sample}$$

$$n = \text{the number of observations in all samples combined}$$

$$R_j = \text{the sum of the ranks in the } j\text{th sample}$$

4. When there are three samples and five or fewer observations in each sample, the significance of the computed H is determined by consulting Appendix II Table N. When there are more than five observations in one or more of the samples, H is compared with tabulated values of χ^2 with $k-1$ degrees of freedom. The adequacy of the chi-square approximation for small samples is discussed by Gabriel and Lachenbruch (31).

Example 13.8.1

The effects of two drugs on reaction time to a certain stimulus were studied in three samples of experimental animals. Sample III served as a control while the animals in sample I were treated with drug A and those in sample II were treated with drug B prior to the application of the stimulus. Table 13.8.1 shows the reaction times in seconds of the 13 animals.

Can we conclude that the three populations represented by the three samples differ with respect to reaction time? We can so conclude if we can reject the null hypothesis that the three populations do not differ in their reaction times.

TABLE 13.8.1 Reaction Time in Seconds of 13 Experimental Animals

	Sample	
I	II	III
17	8	2
20	7	5
40	9	4
31	8	3
35		

Solution

1. *Data*   See Table 13.8.1.

2. *Assumptions*   The samples are independent random samples from their respective populations. The measurement scale employed is at least ordinal. The distributions of the values in the sampled populations are identical except for the possibility that one or more of the populations are composed of values that tend to be larger than those of the other populations.

3. *Hypotheses*

H_0:   The population centers are all equal.

H_A: At least one of the populations tends to exhibit larger values than at least one of the other populations.

Let $\alpha = .01$.

4. *Test Statistic*   See Equation 13.8.1.

5. *Distribution of Test Statistic*   Critical values of H for various sample sizes and α levels are given in Table N.

6. *Decision Rule*   The null hypothesis will be rejected if the computed value of H is so large that the probability of obtaining a value that large or larger when H_0 is true is equal to or less than the chosen significance level, α.

7. *Calculation of Test Statistic*   When the three samples are combined into a single series and ranked, the table of ranks shown in Table 13.8.2 may be constructed.

The null hypothesis implies that the observations in the three samples constitute a single sample of size 13 from a single population. If this is true, we would expect the ranks to be well distributed among the three groups. Consequently, we would expect the total sum of ranks to be divided among the three groups in proportion to group size. Departures from these conditions are reflected in the magnitude of the test statistic H.

From the data in Table 13.8.2 and Equation 13.8.1 we obtain

$$H = \frac{12}{13(13 + 1)}\left[\frac{(55)^2}{5} + \frac{(26)^2}{4} + \frac{(10)^2}{4}\right] - 3(13 + 1)$$

$$= 10.68$$

TABLE 13.8.2 The Data of Table 13.8.1 Replaced by Ranks

	Sample	
I	**II**	**III**
9	6.5	1
10	5	4
13	8	3
11	6.5	2
12		
$R_1 = 55$	$R_2 = 26$	$R_3 = 10$

8. *Statistical Decision* Table N shows that when the n_j's are 5, 4, and 4, the probability of obtaining a value of $H \geq 10.68$ is less than .009. The null hypothesis can be rejected at the .01 level of significance.

9. *Conclusion* We conclude that there is a difference in the average reaction time among the three populations. For this test, $p < .009$.

Ties It will be noted that the two tied values in sample II were each assigned the rank of 6.5. We may adjust the value of H for this tie by dividing it by

$$1 - \frac{\sum T}{n^3 - n} \tag{13.8.2}$$

where $T = t^3 - t$. The letter t is used to designate the number of tied observations in a group of tied values. In our example there is only one group of tied values but, in general, there may be several groups of tied values resulting in several values of T. Since there were only two tied observations in our group of ties, we have $T = 2^3 - 2 = 6$ and $\sum T = 6$, so that Expression 13.8.2 is

$$1 - \frac{6}{13^3 - 13} = .9973$$

and

$$\frac{H}{1 - \dfrac{\sum T}{n^3 - n}} = \frac{10.68}{.9973} = 10.71$$

which, of course, is also significant at the .01 level.

As is the case here, the effect of the adjustment for ties is usually negligible. Note also that the effect of the adjustment is to increase H, so that if the unadjusted H is significant at the chosen level, there is no need to apply the adjustment.

More Than Three Samples/Large Samples Now let us illustrate the procedure when there are more than three samples and at least one of the n_j's is greater than 5.

Example 13.8.2 Table 13.8.3 shows the net book value of equipment capital per bed for a sample of hospitals from each of five types of hospitals. We wish to determine, by means of the Kruskal–Wallis test, if we can conclude that the average net book value of equipment capital per bed differs among the five types of hospitals. The ranks of the 41 values, along with the sum of ranks for each sample, are shown in the table.

TABLE 13.8.3 Net Book Value of Equipment Per Bed by Hospital Type

| | | Type Hospital | | |
A	B	C	D	E
\$1735(11)	\$5260(35)	\$2790(20)	\$3475(26)	\$6090(40)
1520(2)	4455(28)	2400(12)	3115(22)	6000(38)
1476(1)	4480(29)	2655(16)	3050(21)	5894(37)
1688(7)	4325(27)	2500(13)	3125(23)	5705(36)
1702(10)	5075(32)	2755(19)	3275(24)	6050(39)
2667(17)	5225(34)	2592(14)	3300(25)	6150(41)
1575(4)	4613(30)	2601(15)	2730(18)	5110(33)
1602(5)	4887(31)	1648(6)		
1530(3)		1700(9)		
1698(8)				
$R_1 = 68$	$R_2 = 246$	$R_3 = 124$	$R_4 = 159$	$R_5 = 264$

Solution: From the sums of the ranks we compute

$$H = \frac{12}{41(41 + 1)}\left[\frac{(68)^2}{10} + \frac{(246)^2}{8} + \frac{(124)^2}{9} + \frac{(159)^2}{7} + \frac{(264)^2}{7}\right]$$
$$- 3(41 + 1)$$
$$= 36.39$$

Reference to Table F with $k - 1 = 4$ degrees of freedom indicates that the probability of obtaining a value of H as large or larger than 36.39, due to chance alone, when there is no difference among the populations, is less than .005. We conclude, then, that there is a difference among the five populations with respect to the average value of the variable of interest.

Computer Analysis   The MINITAB software package computes the Kruskal–Wallis test statistic and provides additional information. The MINITAB printout for the reaction time data in Table 13.8.1 is shown as Figure 13.8.1.

```
LEVEL           NOBS          MEDIAN          AVE. RANK
1               5             11.000          11.0
2               4             6.500           6.5
3               4             2.500           2.5
OVERALL         13                            7.0
H = 10.68
H(ADJ. FOR TIES) = 10.71
```

Figure 13.8.1   MINITAB Computer Printout, Kruskal–Wallis test of reaction time data in Table 13.8.1.

We enter the reaction time data of Table 13.8.1 into column 1 and the group codes into column 2 as follows:

```
  MTB > READ REACTION TIME INTO C1, CODE FOR GROUP INTO C2
DATA > 17 1
DATA > 20 1
DATA > 40 1
DATA > 31 1
DATA > 35 1
DATA > 8 2
DATA > 7 2
DATA > 9 2
DATA > 8 2
DATA > 2 3
DATA > 5 3
DATA > 4 3
DATA > 3 3
DATA > END
```

The following command produces the analysis and the accompanying printout.

```
KRUSKAL WALLIS FOR DATA IN C1 SUBSCRIPTS IN C2
```

EXERCISES

For the following exercises, perform the test at the indicated level of significance and determine the p value.

13.8.1 In a study of complaints of fatigue among men with brain injury (BI), Walker et al. (A-6) obtained Zung depression scores from three samples of subjects: brain injured with complaint of fatigue, brain injured without complaint of fatigue, and age-matched normal controls. The results were as follows:

BI, fatigue:	46, 61, 51, 36, 51, 45, 54, 51, 69, 54, 51, 38, 64
BI, no fatigue:	39, 44, 58, 29, 40, 48, 65, 41, 46
Controls:	36, 34, 41, 29, 31, 26, 33

SOURCE: Gary C. Walker, M. D. Used with permission.

May we conclude, on the basis of these data, that the populations represented by these samples differ with respect to Zung depression scores? Let $\alpha = .01$.

13.8.2 The following are outpatient, charges ($-\$100$) made to patients for a certain surgical procedure by samples of hospitals located in three different areas of the country.

	Area	
I	**II**	**III**
$80.75	$58.63	$84.21
78.15	72.70	101.76
85.40	64.20	107.74
71.94	62.50	115.30
82.05	63.24	126.15

Can we conclude at the .05 level of significance that the three areas differ with respect to the charges?

13.8.3 Du Toit et al. (A-7) postulated that low-dose heparin (10 IU/kg/hr) administered as a continuous IV infusion may prevent or ameliorate the induction of thrombin-induced disseminated intravascular coagulation in baboons under general anesthesia. Animals in group A received thrombin only, those in group B were pretreated with heparin before thrombin administration, and those in group C received heparin two hours after disseminated intravascular coagulation was induced with thrombin. Five hours after the animals were anesthetized the following measurements for activated partial thromboplastin time (aPTT) were obtained.

Group A: 115, 181, 181, 128, 107, 84, 76, 118, 96, 110, 110
Group B: 99, 83, 92, 64, 130, 66, 89, 54, 80, 76
Group C: 92, 75, 74, 74, 94, 79, 89, 73, 61, 62, 84, 60, 62, 67, 67

SOURCE: Dr. Hendrik J. Du Toit. Used with permission.

Test for a significant difference among the three groups. Let $\alpha = .05$.

13.8.4 The effects of unilateral left hemisphere (LH) and right hemisphere (RH) lesions on the accuracy of choice and speed of response in a four-choice reaction time task were examined by Tartaglione et al. (A-8). The subjects consisted of 30 controls (group 1), 30 LH brain-damaged patients (group 2), and 30 RH brain-damaged patients (group 3). The following table shows the number of errors made by the subjects during one phase of the experiment.

Group	Number of Errors	Group	Number of Errors
1	5	2	3
1	2	2	4
1	2	2	4
1	5	2	5
1	0	2	41
1	6	2	17
1	1	2	33
1	0	2	20
1	0	2	48
1	1	2	7
1	10	2	7
1	5	2	11
1	4	2	17
1	3	2	15
1	5	2	22
1	1	2	6

Group	Number of Errors	Group	Number of Errors
1	2	3	0
1	2	3	0
1	2	3	0
1	1	3	0
1	5	3	0
1	1	3	0
1	1	3	0
1	4	3	0
1	1	3	0
1	6	3	0
1	3	3	1
1	2	3	1
1	2	3	1
1	6	3	2
2	0	3	2
2	0	3	4
2	0	3	3
2	0	3	3
2	0	3	0
2	1	3	4
2	1	3	4
2	8	3	4
2	1	3	5
2	1	3	5
2	49	3	6
2	2	3	7
2	3	3	7
2	3	3	23
		3	10
		3	8

SOURCE: Antonio Tartaglione, M. D. Used with permission.

May we conclude, on the basis of these data, that the three populations represented by these samples differ with respect to number of errors? Let $\alpha = .05$.

13.8.5 Warde et al. (A-9) studied the incidence of respiratory complications and hypoxic episodes during inhalation induction with isoflurane in healthy unpremedicated children undergoing elective surgery under general anesthesia. The children were divided at random into three groups differing with respect to the manner in which isoflurane was administered. The times required for induction of anesthesia were as follows.

Group A	Group B	Group C
8.0	11.75	6.5
7.75	7.25	7.75
8.25	9.25	7.25
5.75	8.75	4.75
9.0	11.0	7.5
11.0	12.0	5.5
13.0	12.0	6.5
8.75	8.75	6.75
6.75	6.75	7.5

Table (*continued*)

Group A	Group B	Group C
8.5	10.5	7.75
11.5	8.0	8.75
7.75	11.0	8.75
16.75	9.5	10.0
8.75	7.75	7.5
6.75	10.25	5.0
8.25	12.0	6.25
10.75	8.25	6.25
10.0	8.0	9.0
8.25	15.0	9.5
8.25	7.0	6.75
7.75	14.25	5.5
13.75	9.75	4.0
7.25	15.25	9.5
		7.25
		5.25
		6.25
		6.5
		9.75
		6.5

SOURCE: Dr. Declan J. Warde. Used with permission.

May we conclude, on the basis of these data, that the three populations represented by these samples differ with respect to induction time? Let $\alpha = .01$.

13.8.6 A study aimed at exploring the platelet imipramine binding characteristics in manic patients and to compare the results with equivalent data for healthy controls and depressed patients was conducted by Ellis et al. (A-10). Among the data collected were the following maximal imipramine binding (B_{max}) values for three diagnostic groups and a healthy control group.

Diagnosis	B_{max} (fmol / mg pr.)
Mania	439, 481, 617, 680, 1038, 883, 600, 562, 303, 492, 1075, 947, 726, 652, 988, 568
Healthy Control	509, 494, 952, 697, 329, 329, 518, 328, 516, 664, 450, 794, 774, 247, 395, 860, 751, 896, 470, 643, 505, 455, 471, 500, 504, 780, 864, 467, 766, 518, 642, 845, 639, 640, 670, 437, 806, 725, 526, 1123
Unipolar Depression	1074, 372, 473, 797, 385, 769, 797, 485, 334, 670, 510, 299, 333, 303, 768, 392, 475, 319, 301, 556, 300, 339, 488, 1114, 761, 571, 306, 80, 607, 1017, 286, 511, 147, 476, 416, 528, 419, 328, 1220, 438, 238, 867, 1657, 790, 479, 179, 530, 446, 328, 348, 773, 697, 520, 341, 604, 420, 397
Bipolar Depression	654, 548, 426, 136, 718, 1010

SOURCE: Dr. P. M. Ellis. Used with permission.

May we conclude, on the basis of these data, that the five populations represented by these samples differ with respect to B_{max} values? Let $\alpha = .05$.

13.8.7 The following table shows the pesticide residue levels (ppb) in blood samples from four populations of human subjects. Use the Kruskal–Wallis test to test at the .05 level of significance the null hypothesis that there is no difference among the populations with respect to average level of pesticide residue.

	Population		
A	**B**	**C**	**D**
10	4	15	7
37	35	5	11
12	32	10	10
31	19	12	8
11	33	6	2
9	18	6	5
44	11	9	4
12	7	11	5
15	32	9	2
42	17	14	6
23	8	15	3

13.8.8 Hepatic γ-glutamyl transpeptidase (GGTP) activity was measured in 22 patients undergoing percutaneous liver biopsy. The results were as follows:

Subject	Diagnosis	Hepatic GGTP (μ / G Protein)
1	Normal liver	27.7
2	Primary biliary cirrhosis	45.9
3	Alcoholic liver disease	85.3
4	Primary biliary cirrhosis	39.0
5	Normal liver	25.8
6	Persistent hepatitis	39.6
7	Chronic active hepatitis	41.8
8	Alcoholic liver disease	64.1
9	Persistent hepatitis	41.1
10	Persistent hepatitis	35.3
11	Alcoholic liver disease	71.5
12	Primary biliary cirrhosis	40.9
13	Normal liver	38.1
14	Primary biliary cirrhosis	40.4
15	Primary biliary cirrhosis	34.0
16	Alcoholic liver disease	74.4
17	Alcoholic liver disease	78.2
18	Persistent hepatitis	32.6
19	Chronic active hepatitis	46.3
20	Normal liver	39.6
21	Chronic active hepatitis	52.7
22	Chronic active hepatitis	57.2

Can we conclude from these sample data that the average population GGTP level differs among the five diagnostic groups? Let $\alpha = .05$ and find the p value.

13.9
The Friedman Two-Way Analysis of Variance by Ranks

Just as we may on occasion have need of a nonparametric analog to the parametric one-way analysis of variance, we may also find it necessary to analyze the data in a two-way classification by nonparametric methods analogous to the two-way analysis of variance. Such a need may arise because the assumptions necessary for parametric analysis of variance are not met, because the measurement scale employed is weak, or because results are needed in a hurry. A test frequently employed under these circumstances is the Friedman two-way analysis of variance by ranks (32, 33). This test is appropriate whenever the data are measured on, at least, an ordinal scale and can be meaningfully arranged in a two-way classification as is given for the randomized block experiment discussed in Chapter 8. The following example illustrates this procedure.

Example 13.9.1   A physical therapist conducted a study to compare three models of low-volt electrical stimulators. Nine other physical therapists were asked to rank the stimulators in order of preference. A rank of 1 indicates first preference. The results are shown in Table 13.9.1. We wish to know if we can conclude that the models are not preferred equally.

Solution:

1. *Data*   See Table 13.9.1.

2. *Assumptions*   The observations appearing in a given block are independent of the observations appearing in each of the other blocks, and within each block measurement on at least an ordinal scale is achieved.

TABLE 13.9.1 Physical Therapists' Rankings of Three Models of Low-Volt Electrical Stimulators

Therapist	Model		
	A	**B**	**C**
1	2	3	1
2	2	3	1
3	2	3	1
4	1	3	2
5	3	2	1
6	1	2	3
7	2	3	1
8	1	3	2
9	1	3	2
R_j	15	25	14

3. *Hypotheses*   In general, the hypotheses are

H_0: The treatments all have identical effects.

H_A: At least one treatment tends to yield larger
observations than at least one of the other treatments.

For our present example we state the hypotheses as follows:

H_0: The three models are equally preferred.

H_A: The three models are not equally preferred.

Let $\alpha = .05$.

4. *Test Statistic*   By means of the Friedman test we will be able to determine if it is reasonable to assume that the columns of ranks have been drawn from the same population. If the null hypothesis is true we would expect the observed distribution of ranks within any column to be the result of chance factors and, hence, we would expect the numbers 1, 2, and 3 to occur with approximately the same frequency in each column. If, on the other hand, the null hypothesis is false (that is, the models are not equally preferred), we would expect a preponderance of relatively high (or low) ranks in at least one column. This condition would be reflected in the sums of the ranks. The Friedman test will tell us whether or not the observed sums of ranks are so discrepant that it is not likely they are a result of chance when H_0 is true.

Since the data already consist of ranking within blocks (rows), our first step is to sum the ranks within each column (treatment). These sums are the R_j's shown in Table 13.9.1. A test statistic, denoted by Friedman as χ_r^2 is computed as follows:

$$\chi_r^2 = \frac{12}{nk(n+1)} \sum_{j=1}^{k} (R_j)^2 - 3n(k+1) \qquad (13.9.1)$$

where n = the number of rows (blocks) and k = the number of columns (treatments).

5. *Distribution of Test Statistic*   Critical values for various values of n and k are given in Appendix II Table O.

6. *Decision Rule*   Reject H_0 if the probability of obtaining (when H_0 is true) a value of χ_r^2 as large as or larger than actually computed is less than or equal to α.

7. *Calculation of Test Statistic*   Using the data in Table 13.9.1 and Equation 13.9.1, we compute

$$\chi_r^2 = \frac{12}{9(3)(3+1)} \left[(15)^2 + (25)^2 + (14)^2 \right] - 3(9)(3+1)$$

$$= 8.222$$

8. *Statistical Decision*   When we consult Appendix II Table Oa, we find that the probability of obtaining a value of X_r^2 as large as 8.222 due to chance alone, when the null hypothesis is true, is .016. We are able, therefore, to reject the null hypothesis.

9. *Conclusion*   We conclude that the three models of low-volt electrical stimulator are not equally preferred. For this test, $p = .016$.

Ties   When the original data consist of measurements on an interval or a ratio scale instead of ranks, the measurements are assigned ranks based on their relative magnitudes within blocks. If ties occur each value is assigned the mean of the ranks for which it is tied.

Large Samples   When the values of k and or n exceed those given in Table O, the critical value of χ_r^2 is obtained by consulting the χ^2 table (Table F) with the chosen α and $k - 1$ degrees of freedom.

Example 13.9.2

Table 13.9.2 shows the responses, in percent decrease in salivary flow, of 16 experimental animals following different dose levels of atropine. The ranks (in parentheses) and the sum of the ranks are also given in the table. We wish to see if we may conclude that the different dose levels produce different responses. That is, we wish to test the null hypothesis of no difference in response among the four dose levels.

TABLE 13.9.2 Percent Decrease in Salivary Flow of Experimental Animals Following Different Dose Levels of Atropine

Animal Number	Dose Level			
	A	**B**	**C**	**D**
1	29(10)	48(2)	75(3)	100(4)
2	72(2)	30(1)	100(3.5)	100(3.5)
3	70(1)	100(4)	86(2)	96(3)
4	54(2)	35(1)	90(3)	99(4)
5	5(1)	43(3)	32(2)	81(4)
6	17(1)	40(2)	76(3)	81(4)
7	74(1)	100(3)	100(3)	100(3)
8	6(1)	34(2)	60(3)	81(4)
9	16(1)	39(2)	73(3)	79(4)
10	52(2)	34(1)	88(3)	96(4)
11	8(1)	42(3)	31(2)	79(4)
12	29(1)	47(2)	72(3)	99(4)
13	71(1)	100(3.5)	97(2)	100(3.5)
14	7(1)	33(2)	58(3)	79(4)
15	68(1)	99(4)	84(2)	93(3)
16	70(2)	30(1)	99(3.5)	99(3.5)
R_j	20	36.5	44	59.5

Solution: From the data we compute

$$\chi_r^2 = \frac{12}{16(4)(4+1)}\left[(20)^2 + (36.5)^2 + (44)^2 + (59.5)^2\right] - 3(16)(4+1)$$

$$= 30.32$$

Reference to Table F indicates that with $k - 1 = 3$ degrees of freedom the probability of getting a value of χ_r^2 as large as 30.32 due to chance alone is, when H_0 is true, less than .005. We reject the null hypothesis and conclude that the different dose levels do produce different responses.

Many statistics software packages, including MINITAB, will perform the Friedman test. To use MINITAB we form three columns of data. For example, suppose that column 1 contains numbers that indicate the treatment to which the observations belong, column 2 contains numbers indicating the blocks to which the observations belong, and column 3 contains the observations. The command, then, is

```
FRIEDMAN C3 C1 C2
```

EXERCISES

For the following exercises perform the test at the indicated level of significance and determine the p value.

13.9.1   The following table shows the scores made by nine randomly selected student nurses on final examinations in three subject areas.

Student Number	Subject Area		
	Fundamentals	Physiology	Anatomy
1	98	95	77
2	95	71	79
3	76	80	91
4	95	81	84
5	83	77	80
6	99	70	93
7	82	80	87
8	75	72	81
9	88	81	83

Test the null hypothesis that student nurses constituting the population from which the above sample was drawn perform equally well in all three subject areas against the alternative hypothesis that they perform better in, at least, one area. Let $\alpha = .05$.

13.9.2 Fifteen randomly selected physical therapy students were given the following instructions: "Assume that you will marry a person with one of the following handicaps (the handicaps were listed and designated by the letters A to J). Rank these handicaps from 1 to 10 according to your first, second, third (and so on) choice of a handicap for your marriage partner." The results are shown in the following table.

Student Number	A	B	C	D	E	F	G	H	I	J
1	1	3	5	9	8	2	4	6	7	10
2	1	4	5	7	8	2	3	6	9	10
3	2	3	7	8	9	1	4	6	5	10
4	1	4	7	8	9	2	3	6	5	10
5	1	4	7	8	10	2	3	6	5	9
6	2	3	7	9	8	1	4	5	6	10
7	2	4	6	9	8	1	3	7	5	10
8	1	5	7	9	10	2	3	4	6	8
9	1	4	5	7	8	2	3	6	9	10
10	2	3	6	8	9	1	4	7	5	10
11	2	4	5	8	9	1	3	7	6	10
12	2	3	6	8	10	1	4	5	7	9
13	3	2	6	9	8	1	4	7	5	10
14	2	5	7	8	9	1	3	4	6	10
15	2	3	6	7	8	1	5	4	9	10

Test the null hypothesis of no preference for handicaps against the alternative that some handicaps are preferred over others. Let $\alpha = .05$.

13.9.3 Ten subjects with exercise-induced asthma participated in an experiment to compare the protective effect of a drug administered in four dose levels. Saline was used as a control. The variable of interest was change in FEV_1 after administration of the drug or saline. The results were as follows:

Subject	Saline	Dose Level of Drug (mg / ml)			
		2	10	20	40
1	−.68	−.32	−.14	−.21	−.32
2	−1.55	−.56	−.31	−.21	−.16
3	−1.41	−.28	−.11	−.08	−.83
4	−.76	−.56	−.24	−.41	−.08
5	−.48	−.25	−.17	−.04	−.18
6	−3.12	−1.99	−1.22	−.55	−.75
7	−1.16	−.88	−.87	−.54	−.84
8	−1.15	−.31	−.18	−.07	−.09
9	−.78	−.24	−.39	−.11	−.51
10	−2.12	−.35	−.28	+.11	−.41

Can one conclude on the basis of these data that different dose levels have different effects? Let $\alpha = .05$ and find the p value.

13.10
The Spearman Rank Correlation Coefficient

Several nonparametric measures of correlation are available to the researcher. Refer to Kendall (34), Kruskal (35), and Hotelling and Pabst (36) for detailed discussions of the various methods.

A frequently used procedure that is attractive because of the simplicity of the calculations involved is due to Spearman (37). The measure of correlation computed by this method is called the Spearman rank correlation coefficient and is designated by r_s. This procedure makes use of the two sets of ranks that may be assigned to the sample values of X and Y, the independent and continuous variables of a bivariate distribution.

Hypotheses   The usually tested hypotheses and their alternatives are as follows:

a. H_0: X and Y are mutually independent.
H_A: X and Y are not mutually independent.

b. H_0: X and Y are mutually independent.
H_A: There is a tendency for large values of X and large values of Y to be paired together.

c. H_0: X and Y are mutually independent.
H_A: There is a tendency for large values of X to be paired with small values of Y.

The hypotheses specified in (a) lead to a two-sided test and are used when it is desired to detect any departure from independence. The one-sided tests indicated by (b) and (c) are used, respectively, when investigators wish to know if they can conclude that the variables are directly or inversely correlated.

The Procedure   The hypothesis-testing procedure involves the following steps.

1. Rank the values of X from 1 to n (numbers of pairs of values of X and Y in the sample). Rank the values of Y from 1 to n.

2. Compute d_i for each pair of observations by subtracting the rank of Y_i from the rank of X_i.

3. Square each d_i and compute Σd_i^2, the sum of the squared values.

4. Compute

$$r_s = 1 - \frac{6 \sum d_i^2}{n(n^2 - 1)} \tag{13.10.1}$$

5. If n is between 4 and 30 compare the computed value of r_s with the critical values, r_s^*, of Table P, Appendix II. For the two-sided test, H_0 is rejected at the

α significance level if r_s is greater than r_s^* or less than $-r_s^*$ where r_s^* is at the intersection of the column headed $\alpha/2$ and the row corresponding to n. For the one-sided test with H_A specifying direct correlation, H_0 is rejected at the α significance level if r_s is greater than r_s^* for α and n. The null hypothesis is rejected at the α significance level in the other one-sided test if r_s is less than $-r_s^*$ for α and n.

6. If n is greater than 30, one may compute

$$z = r_s\sqrt{n-1} \tag{13.10.2}$$

and use Table D to obtain critical values.

7. Tied observations present a problem. Glasser and Winter (38) point out that the use of Table P is strictly valid only when the data do not contain any ties (unless some random procedure for breaking ties is employed). In practice, however, the table is frequently used after some other method for handling ties has been employed. If the number of ties is large, the following correction for ties may be employed.

$$T = \frac{t^3 - t}{12} \tag{13.10.3}$$

where t = the number of observations that are tied for some particular rank. When this correction factor is used r_s is computed from

$$r_s = \frac{\sum x^2 + \sum y^2 - \sum d_i^2}{2\sqrt{\sum x^2 \sum y^2}} \tag{13.10.4}$$

instead of from Equation 13.10.1.
    In Equation 13.10.4

$$\sum x^2 = \frac{n^3 - n}{12} - \sum T_x$$

$$\sum y^2 = \frac{n^3 - n}{12} - \sum T_y$$

T_x = the sum of the values of T for the
various tied ranks in X, and

T_y = the sum of the values of T for the
various tied ranks in Y

Most authorities agree that unless the number of ties is excessive the correction makes very little difference in the value of r_s. When the number of ties is small, we can follow the usual procedure of assigning the tied observations the mean of the ranks for which they are tied and proceed with steps 2 to 6. Edgington (39) discusses the problem of ties in some detail.

Example 13.10.1

In a study of the relationship between age and the EEG, data were collected on 20 subjects between the ages of 20 and 60 years. Table 13.10.1 shows the age and a particular EEG output value for each of the 20 subjects. The investigator wishes to know if it can be concluded that this particular EEG output is inversely correlated with age.

Solution

1. *Data* See Table 13.10.1.

2. *Assumptions* We presume that the sample available for analysis is a simple random sample and that both X and Y are measured on at least the ordinal scale.

3. *Hypotheses*

   H_0: This EEG output and age are mutually independent.

   H_A: There is a tendency for this EEG output to decrease with age.

   Suppose we let $\alpha = .05$.

4. *Test Statistic* See Equation 13.10.1.

5. *Distribution of Test Statistic* Critical values of the test statistic are given in Table P.

6. *Decision Rule* For the present test we will reject H_0 if the computed value of r_s is less than $-.3789$.

TABLE 13.10.1 Age and EEG Output Value for 20 Subjects

Subject Number	Age (X)	EEG Output Value (Y)
1	20	98
2	21	75
3	22	95
4	24	100
5	27	99
6	30	65
7	31	64
8	33	70
9	35	85
10	38	74
11	40	68
12	42	66
13	44	71
14	46	62
15	48	69
16	51	54
17	53	63
18	55	52
19	58	67
20	60	55

TABLE 13.10.2 Ranks for Data of Example 13.10.1

Subject Number	Rank(X)	Rank(Y)	d_i	d_i^2
1	1	18	-17	289
2	2	15	-13	169
3	3	17	-14	196
4	4	20	-16	256
5	5	19	-14	196
6	6	7	-1	1
7	7	6	1	1
8	8	12	-4	16
9	9	16	-7	49
10	10	14	-4	16
11	11	10	1	1
12	12	8	4	16
13	13	13	0	0
14	14	4	10	100
15	15	11	4	16
16	16	2	14	196
17	17	5	12	144
18	18	1	17	289
19	19	9	10	100
20	20	3	17	289
			$\sum d_i^2 = 2340$	

7. *Calculation of Test Statistic*   When the X and Y values are ranked we have the results shown in Table 13.10.2. The d_i, d_i^2 and $\sum d_i^2$ are shown in the same table.

Substitution of the data from Table 13.10.2 into Equation 13.10.1 gives

$$r_s = 1 - \frac{6(2340)}{20\left[(20)^2 - 1\right]} = -.76$$

8. *Statistical Decision*   Since our computed $r_s = -.76$ is less than the critical r_s^* we reject the null hypothesis,

9. *Conclusion*   We conclude that the two variables are inversely related. Since $-.76 < -0.6586$, we have for this test $p < .001$.

Let us now illustrate the procedure for a sample with $n > 30$ and some tied observations.

Example 13.10.2

In Table 13.10.3 are shown the ages and concentrations (ppm) of a certain mineral in the tissue of 35 subjects on whom autopsies were performed as part of a large research project.

The ranks, d_i, d_i^2 and $\sum d_i^2$ are shown in Table 13.10.4. Let us test, at the .05 level of significance, the null hypothesis that X and Y are mutually independent against the two-sided alternative that they are not mutually independent.

TABLE 13.10.3 Age and Mineral Concentration (PPM) in Tissue of 35 Subjects

Subject Number	Age (X)	Mineral Concentration (Y)	Subject Number	Age (X)	Mineral Concentration (Y)
1	82	169.62	19	50	4.48
2	85	48.94	20	71	46.93
3	83	41.16	21	54	30.91
4	64	63.95	22	62	34.27
5	82	21.09	23	47	41.44
6	53	5.40	24	66	109.88
7	26	6.33	25	34	2.78
8	47	4.26	26	46	4.17
9	37	3.62	27	27	6.57
10	49	4.82	28	54	61.73
11	65	108.22	29	72	47.59
12	40	10.20	30	41	10.46
13	32	2.69	31	35	3.06
14	50	6.16	32	75	49.57
15	62	23.87	33	50	5.55
16	33	2.70	34	76	50.23
17	36	3.15	35	28	6.81
18	53	60.59			

TABLE 13.10.4 Ranks for Data of Example 13.10.2

Subject Number	Rank (X)	Rank (Y)	d_i	d_i^2	Subject Number	Rank (X)	Rank (Y)	d_i	d_i^2
1	32.5	35	-2.5	6.25	19	17	9	8	64.00
2	35	27	8	64.00	20	28	25	3	9.00
3	34	23	11	121.00	21	21.5	21	.5	.25
4	25	32	-7	49.00	22	23.5	22	1.5	2.25
5	32.5	19	13.5	182.25	23	13.5	24	-10.5	110.25
6	19.5	11	8.5	72.25	24	27	34	-7	49.00
7	1	14	-13	169.00	25	6	3	3	9.00
8	13.5	8	5.5	30.25	26	12	7	5	25.00
9	9	6	3	9.00	27	2	15	-13	169.00
10	15	10	5	25.00	28	21.5	31	-9.5	90.25
11	26	33	-7	49.00	29	29	26	3	9.00
12	10	17	-7	49.00	30	11	18	-7	49.00
13	4	1	3	9.00	31	7	4	3	9.00
14	17	13	4	16.00	32	30	28	2	4.00
15	23.5	20	3.5	12.25	33	17	12	5	25.00
16	5	2	3	9.00	34	31	29	2	4.00
17	8	5	3	9.00	35	3	16	-13	169.00
18	19.5	30	-10.5	110.25				$\Sigma d_i^2 =$	1788.5

Solution: From the data in Table 13.10.4 we compute

$$r_s = 1 - \frac{6(1788.5)}{35[35^2 - 1]} = .75$$

To test the significance of r_s we compute

$$z = .75\sqrt{35 - 1} = 4.37$$

Since 4.37 is greater than $z = 3.89$, $p < 2(.0001) = .0002$, and we reject H_0 and conclude that the two variables under study are not mutually independent.

For comparative purposes let us correct for ties using Equation 13.10.3 and then compute r_s by Equation 13.10.4.

In the rankings of X we had six groups of ties that were broken by assigning the values 13.5, 17, 19.5, 21.5, 23.5, and 32.5. In five of the groups two observations tied, and in one group three observations tied. We, therefore, compute five values of

$$T_x = \frac{2^3 - 2}{12} = \frac{6}{12} = .5$$

and one value of

$$T_x = \frac{3^3 - 3}{12} = \frac{24}{12} = 2$$

From these computations, we have $\Sigma T_x = 5(.5) + 2 = 4.5$, so that

$$\Sigma x^2 = \frac{35^3 - 35}{12} - 4.5 = 3565.5$$

Since no ties occurred in the Y rankings, we have $\Sigma T_y = 0$ and

$$\Sigma y^2 = \frac{35^3 - 35}{12} - 0 = 3570.0$$

From Table 13.10.4 we have $\Sigma d_i^2 = 1788.5$. From these data we may now compute by Equation 13.10.4

$$r_s = \frac{3565.5 + 3570.0 - 1788.5}{2\sqrt{(3565.5)(3570)}} = .75$$

We see that in this case the correction for ties does not make any difference in the value of r_s.

EXERCISES

For the following exercises perform the test at the indicated level of significance and determine the p value.

13.10.1 The following table shows 15 randomly selected geographic areas ranked by population density and age-adjusted death rate. Can we conclude at the .05 level of significance that population density and age-adjusted death rate are not mutually independent?

	Rank By	
Area	Population Density (X)	Age-Adjusted Death Rate (Y)
1	8	10
2	2	14
3	12	4
4	4	15
5	9	11
6	3	1
7	10	12
8	5	7
9	6	8
10	14	5
11	7	6
12	1	2
13	13	9
14	15	3
15	11	13

13.10.2 The following table shows 10 communities ranked by DMF teeth per 100 children and fluoride concentration in ppm in the public water supply.

	Rank By	
Community	DMF Teeth Per 100 Children (X)	Fluoride Concentration (Y)
1	8	1
2	9	3
3	7	4
4	3	9
5	2	8
6	4	7
7	1	10
8	5	6
9	6	5
10	10	2

Do these data provide sufficient evidence to indicate that the number of DMF teeth per 100 children tends to decrease as fluoride concentration increases? Let $\alpha = .05$.

13.10.3 The purpose of a study by McAtee and Mack (A-11) was to investigate possible relations between performance on the atypical approach parameters of the Design Copying (DC) subtest of the Sensory Integration and Praxis Tests (SIPT) and scores on the Southern California Sensory Integration Tests (SCSIT). The subjects were children seen in a private occupational therapy clinic. The following are the scores of 24 children for the SIPT-DC parameter of Boundary and the Imitation of Postures (IP) subtest of the SCSIT.

Boundary	IP	Boundary	IP
3	−1.9	1	−1.1
3	.8	5	−.6
8	−.5	2	−.3
2	−.9	2	.9
7	.1	6	−1.3
2	.3	2	.8
3	−.7	2	−.7
2	.3	2	.3
3	−1.7	0	1.3
4	−1.6	1	.5
5	−1.6	3	.2
0	.8	2	.2

SOURCE: Shay McAtee, M. A., OTR. Used with permission.

May we conclude, on the basis of these data, that scores on the two variables are correlated? Let $\alpha = .01$.

13.10.4 Barbera et al. (A-12) conducted a study to investigate whether or not the pathologic features in the lungs of patients with chronic obstructive pulmonary disease (COPD) are related to the gas exchange response during exercise. Subjects were patients undergoing surgical resection of a lobe or lung because of a localized lung neoplasm. Among the data collected were PaO_2 measurements during exercise (E) and at rest (R) and emphysema scores (ES). The results for these variables were as follows:

Patient No.	PaO₂		ES
	R	**E**	
1	87	95	12.5
2	84	93	25.0
3	82	78	11.3
4	69	79	30.0
5	85	77	7.5
6	74	89	5.0
7	90	87	3.8
8	97	110	.0
9	67	61	70.0
10	78	69	18.8
11	101	113	5.0
12	79	82	32.5
13	84	93	.0
14	70	85	7.5
15	86	91	5.0
16	66	79	10.0
17	69	87	27.5
Mean ± SEM	81 ± 3	86 ± 3	16.0 ± 4.4

SOURCE: Joan A. Barbera, Josep Roca, Josep Ramirez, Peter D. Wagner, Pietat Ussetti, and Robert Rodriguez-Roisin, "Gas Exchange During Exercise in Mild Chronic Obstructive Pulmonary Disease: Correlation With Lung Structure," *American Review of Respiratory Disease, 144* (1991), 520–525.

Compute r_s for PaO_2 during exercise and ES and test for significance at the .01 level.

13.10.5 Refer to Exercise 13.10.4. Compute r_s for PaO_2 at rest and ES and test for significance at the .01 level.

13.10.6 As part of a study by Miller and Tricker (A-13) 76 prominent health and fitness professionals rated 17 health promotion target markets on the basis of importance in the past 10 years and the next 10 years. Their mean ratings scored on a Likert-like scale (5 = extremely important, 4 = very important, 3 = important, 2 = somewhat important, 1 = unimportant) were as follows:

	Next 10 Years	Past 10 Years
Market	**Mean Rating**	**Mean Rating**
Women	4.36	3.23
Elderly	4.25	2.61
Employees/large business	4.22	3.66
Children	4.17	2.63
Retirees	4.15	2.08
Blue-collar workers	4.03	2.15
Drug/alcohol abusers	4.03	2.95
Employees/small business	3.90	2.11
Heart/lung disease patients	3.83	3.41
General public	3.81	2.84
Obese/eating disorder	3.80	2.97
Disadvantaged minorities	3.56	2.00
Leisure/recreation seekers	3.52	2.95
At-home market	3.51	2.12
Injured (back/limbs)	3.42	2.51
Athletes	3.13	3.30
Mentally ill	2.83	1.88

SOURCE: Cheryl Miller and Ray Tricker, "Past and Future Priorities in Health Promotion in the United States: A survey of Experts," *American Journal of Health Promotion*, 5 (1991), 360–367. Used by permission.

Compute r_s for the two sets of ratings and test for significance. Let $\alpha = .05$.

13.10.7 Seventeen patients with a history of congestive heart failure participated in a study to assess the effects of exercise on various bodily functions. During a period of exercise the following data were collected on the percent change in plasma norepinephrine (Y) and the percent change in oxygen consumption (X).

Subject	X	Y
1	500	525
2	475	130
3	390	325
4	325	190
5	325	90
6	205	295
7	200	180
8	75	74
9	230	420

Table (*continued*)

Subject	X	Y
10	50	60
11	175	105
12	130	148
13	76	75
14	200	250
15	174	102
16	201	151
17	125	130

On the basis of these data can one conclude that there is an association between the two variables? Let $\alpha = .05$.

13.11
Nonparametric Regression Analysis

When the assumptions underlying simple linear regression analysis as discussed in Chapter 9 are not met, we may employ nonparametric procedures. In this section we present estimators of the slope and intercept that are easy-to-calculate alternatives to the least-squares estimators described in Chapter 9.

Theil's Slope Estimator   Theil (40) proposes a method for obtaining a point estimate of the slope coefficient β. We assume that the data conform to the classic regression model

$$y_i = \alpha + \beta x_i + e_i, \qquad i = 1, \ldots, n$$

where the x_i are known constants, α and β are unknown parameters, and y_i is an observed value of the continuous random variable Y at x_i. For each value of x_i, we assume a subpopulation of Y values, and the e_i are mutually independent. The x_i are all distinct (no ties), and we take $x_1 < x_2 < \cdots < x_n$.

The data consist of n pairs of sample observations, $(x_1, y_1), (x_2, y_2), \ldots, (x_n, y_n)$, where the ith pair represents measurements taken on the ith unit of association.

To obtain Theil's estimator of β, we first form all possible sample slopes $S_{ij} = (y_j - y_i)/(x_j - x_i)$, where $i < j$. There will be $N = {}_nC_2$ values of S_{ij}. The estimator of β, which we designate by $\hat{\beta}$, is the median of S_{ij} values. That is,

$$\hat{\beta} = \text{median} \left\{ S_{ij} \right\} \qquad\qquad (13.11.1)$$

The following example illustrates the calculation of $\hat{\beta}$.

**Example
13.11.1**   In Table 13.11.1 are the plasma testosterone (ng/ml) levels (Y) and seminal citric acid (mg/ml) levels in a sample of eight adult males. We wish to compute the estimate of the population regression slope coefficient by Theil's method.

TABLE 13.11.1 Plasma Testosterone and Seminal Citric Acid Levels in Adult Males

Testosterone:	230	175	315	290	275	150	360	425
Citric acid:	421	278	618	482	465	105	550	750

Solution: The $N = {}_8C_2 = 28$ ordered values of S_{ij} are shown in Table 13.11.2.

If we let $i = 1$ and $j = 2$, the indicators of the first and second values of Y and X in Table 13.11.1, we may compute S_{12} as follows:

$$S_{12} = (175 - 230)/(278 - 421) = -.3846$$

When all the slopes are computed in a similar manner and ordered as in Table 13.11.2, $-.3846$ winds up as the tenth value in the ordered array.

The median of the S_{ij} values is .4878. Consequently, our estimate of the population slope coefficient is $\hat{\beta} = .4878$.

An Estimator of the Intercept Coefficient   Dietz (41) recommends two intercept estimators. The first, designated $\hat{\alpha}_{1,M}$, is the median of the n terms $Y_i - \hat{\beta}x_i$ in which $\hat{\beta}$ is the Theil estimator. It is recommended when the researcher is not willing to assume that the error terms are symmetric about 0. If the researcher is willing to assume a symmetric distribution of error terms, Dietz recommends the estimator $\hat{\alpha}_{2,M}$, which is the median of the $n(n + 1)/2$ pairwise averages of the $y_i - \hat{\beta}x_i$ terms. We illustrate the calculation of each in the following example.

TABLE 13.11.2 Ordered Values of S_{IJ} for Example 13.11.1

− .6618	.5037
.1445	.5263
.1838	.5297
.2532	.5348
.2614	.5637
.3216	.5927
.325	.6801
.3472	.8333
.3714	.8824
.3846	.9836
.4118	1.0000
.4264	1.0078
.4315	1.0227
.4719	1.0294

Example 13.11.2   Refer to Example 13.11.1. Let us compute $\hat{\alpha}_{1,M}$ and $\hat{\alpha}_{2,M}$ from the data on testosterone and citric acid levels.

Solution: The ordered $y_i - .4878x_i$ terms are: 13.5396, 24.6362, 39.3916, 48.1730, 54.8804, 59.1500, 91.7100, and 98.7810. The median, 51.5267, is the estimator $\hat{\alpha}_{1,M}$. The $8(8 + 1)/2 = 36$ ordered pairwise averages of the $y_i - .4878x_i$ are

13.5396	49.2708	75.43
19.0879	51.5267	76.8307
24.6362	52.6248	78.9655
26.4656	53.6615	91.71
30.8563	54.8804	95.2455
32.0139	56.1603	98.781
34.21	57.0152	
36.3448	58.1731	
36.4046	59.15	
39.3916	61.7086	
39.7583	65.5508	
41.8931	69.0863	
43.7823	69.9415	
47.136	73.2952	
48.173	73.477	

The median of these averages, 53.1432, is the estimator $\hat{\alpha}_{2,M}$. The estimating equation, then, is $y_i = 53.1432 + .4878x_i$ if we are willing to assume that the distribution of error terms is symmetric about 0. If we are not willing to make the assumption of symmetry, the estimating equation is $y_i = 51.5267 + .4878x_i$.

For a more extensive discussion of nonparametric regression analysis, see the book on nonparametric statistics by Daniel (5).

EXERCISES

13.11.1 The following are the heart rates (HR: beats/minute) and oxygen consumption values ($VO_{2>}$: cal/kg/24 h) for nine infants with chronic congestive heart failure:

HR(X):	163	164	156	151	152	167	165	153	155
$VO_2(Y)$:	53.9	57.4	41.0	40.0	42.0	64.4	59.1	49.9	43.2

Compute $\hat{\beta}$, $\hat{\alpha}_{1,M>}$, and $\hat{\alpha}_{2,M}$.

13.11.2 The following are the body weights (grams) and total surface area (cm^2) of nine laboratory animals:

Body weight (X): 660.2 706.0 924.0 936.0 992.1 888.9 999.4 890.3 841.2
Surface area (Y): 781.7 888.7 1038.1 1040.0 1120.0 1071.5 1134.5 965.3 925.0

Compute the slope estimator and two intercept estimators.

13.12
Summary

This chapter is concerned with nonparametric statistical tests. These tests may be used either when the assumptions underlying the parametric tests are not realized or when the data to be analyzed are measured on a scale too weak for the arithmetic procedures necessary for the parametric tests.

Nine nonparametric tests are described and illustrated. Except for the Kolmogorov–Smirvon goodness-of-fit test, each test provides a nonparametric alternative to a well-known parametric test. There are a number of other nonparametric tests available, many of which are described and illustrated in the references cited at the end of this chapter.

REVIEW QUESTIONS AND EXERCISES

1. Define nonparametric statistics.

2. What is meant by the term distribution-free statistical tests?

3. What are some of the advantages of using nonparametric statistical tests?

4. What are some of the disadvantages of the nonparametric tests?

5. Describe a situation in your particular area of interest where each of the following tests could be used. Use real or realistic data and test an appropriate hypothesis using each test.
   a. The sign test
   b. The median test
   c. The Wilcoxon Test
   d. The Mann–Whitney test
   e. The Kolmogorov–Smirnov goodness-of-fit test
   f. The Kruskal–Wallis one-way analysis of variance by ranks
   g. The Friedman two-way analysis of variance by ranks
   h. The Spearman rank correlation coefficient
   i. Nonparametric regression analysis

6. The following are the ranks of the ages (X) of 20 surgical patients and the dose (Y) of an analgesic agent required to block one spinal segment.

Rank of Age in Years (X)	Rank of Dose Requirement (Y)	Rank of Age in Years (X)	Rank of Dose Requirement (Y)
1	1	11	13
2	7	12	5
3	2	13	11
4	4	14	16
5	6	15	20
6	8	16	18
7	3	17	19
8	15	18	17
9	9	19	10
10	12	20	14

Compute r_s and test (two-sided) for significance. Let $\alpha = .05$. Determine the p value for this test.

7. The following pulmonary function data were collected on children with muscular dystrophy before and after a period of respiratory therapy. Scores are expressed as percent of predicted normal values for height, weight, and body surface measurement.

Forced Vital Capacity (liters)									
Before:	74	65	84	89	84	65	78	86	83	82
After:	79	78	100	92	104	70	81	84	85	90

Use the sign test to determine whether one should conclude that the therapy is effective. Let $\alpha = .05$. What is the p value?

8. Three methods of reducing skin bacterial load by bathing were compared. Bacteria counts were made on the right foot of subjects before and after treatment. The variable of interest was percent reduction of bacteria. Twenty-seven nursing student volunteers participated in the experiment. The three methods of bathing the foot were whirlpool agitation, spraying, and soaking. The results were as follows:

Whirlpool		Spraying		Soaking	
91	80	18	16	6	10
87	92	22	15	6	12
88	81	20	26	8	5
84	93	29	19	9	9
86		25		13	

Can one conclude on the basis of these data that the three methods are not equally effective? Let $\alpha = .05$. What is the p value for this test?

9. Ten subjects with bronchial asthma participated in an experiment to evaluate the relative effectiveness of three drugs. The following table shows the change in FEV_1

(forced expired volume in 1 second) values (expressed as liters) two hours after drug administration:

Subject	Drug		
	A	B	C
1	.00	.13	.26
2	.04	.17	.23
3	.02	.20	.21
4	.02	.27	.19
5	.04	.11	.36
6	.03	.18	.25
7	.05	.21	.32
8	.02	.23	.38
9	.00	.24	.30
10	.12	.08	.30

Are these data sufficient to indicate a difference in drug effectiveness? Let $\alpha = .05$. What is the p value for this test?

10. Sera from two groups of subjects following streptococcal infection were assayed for neutralizing antibodies to streptolysin O (ASO). The results were as follows:

ASO (Measured in Todd units)	
Group A	Group B
324	558
275	108
349	291
604	863
566	303
810	640
340	358
295	503
357	646
580	689
344	250
655	540
380	630
503	190
314	

Do these data provide sufficient evidence to indicate a difference in population medians? Let $\alpha = .05$. What is the p-value for this test? Use both the median test and the Mann–Whitney test and compare the results.

11. The following are the $PaCO_2$ (mm Hg) values in 16 patients with bronchopulmonary disease:

$$39, 40, 45, 48, 49, 56, 60, 75, 42, 48, 32, 37, 32, 33, 33, 36$$

Use the Kolomogorov–Smirnov test to the test the null hypothesis that $PaCO_2$ values in the sampled population are normally distributed with $\mu = 44$ and $\sigma = 12$.

12. The following table shows the caloric intake (cal/day/kg) and oxygen consumption, VO_2 (ml/min/kg) in 10 infants:

Caloric Intake (X)	$VO_2(Y)$
50	7.0
70	8.0
90	10.5
120	11.0
40	9.0
100	10.8
150	12.0
110	10.0
75	9.5
160	11.9

Test the null hypothesis that the two variables are mutually independent against the alternative that they are directly related. Let $\alpha = .05$. What is the p value for this test?

13. The following are the estriol levels (mg/24 hour urine specimens) of 16 pregnant women and the birth weights (grams $\times$ 100) of their babies.

Estroil Levels	Birth Weight
15	31
17	31
17	32
18	31
20	32
22	31
25	32
16	33
17	34
17	29
17	28
15	28
10	26
26	33
28	35
25	39

Test the null hypothesis that the two variables are mutually independent against the alternative that they are directly related. Let the probability of committing a type I error be .05. What is the p value?

14. The following are the college grade point averages of 12 students receiving a B.S. degree in nursing and their scores on the state certification examination:

GPA:	2.5	2.2	3.0	2.8	2.8	2.5	2.3	3.1	3.7	2.9	2.7	2.4
EXAM SCORE:	84	85	91	83	87	89	86	95	93	79	90	85

Can we conclude at the .05 level of significance that the two variables are not mutually independent? What is the p value for the test?

REFERENCES

References Cited

1. M. G. Kendall and R. M. Sundrum, "Distribution–free Methods and Order Properties," *Review of the International Statistical Institute*, *21:3* (1953), 124–134.

2. Jean Dickinson Gibbons, *Nonparametric Statistical Inference*, Marcel Dekker, New York, 1985.

3. J. R. Blum and N. A. Fattu, "Nonparametric Methods," *Review of Educational Research*, *24*, (1954), 467–487.

4. I. E. Moses, "Nonparametric Statistics for Psychological Research," *Psychological Bulletin*, *49* (1952), 122–143.

5. Wayne W. Daniel, *Applied Nonparametric Statistics*, Second edition, PWS-Kent, Boston, 1989.

6. Jaroslav Hajek, *A Course in Nonparametric Statistics*, Holden–Day, San Francisco, 1969.

7. John Edward Walsh, *Handbook of Nonparametric Statistics*, Van Nostrand, Princeton, N.J. 1962.

8. John E. Walsh, *Handbook of Nonparametric Statistics*, II, Van Nostrand, Princeton, N.J., 1965.

9. I. R. Savage, *Bibliography of Nonparametric Statistics*, Harvard University Press, Cambridge, Mass., 1962.

10. N. H. Anderson, "Scales and Statistics: Parametric and Nonparametric," *Psychological Bulletin*, *58* (1961), 305–316.

11. J. Gaito, "Nonparametric Methods in Psychological Research," *Psychological Reports*, *5* (1959), 115–125.

12. F. M. Lord, "On the Statistical Treatment of Football Numbers," *American Psychologist*, *8* (1953), 750–751.

13. Gordon D. Armstrong "Parametric Statistics and Ordinal Data: A Pervasive Misconception," *Nursing Research*, *30* (1981), 60–62.

14. Edgar F. Borgatta and George W. Bohrnstedt, "Level of Measurement Once Over Again," *Sociological Methods & Research*, *9* (1980), 147–160.

15. W. J. Dixon and A. M. Mood, "The Statistical Sign Test," *Journal of the American Statistical Association*, *41* (1946), 557–566.

16. Frank Wilcoxon, "Individual Comparisons by Ranking Methods," *Biometrics*, *1* (1945), 80–83.

17. A. M. Mood, *Introduction to the Theory of Statistics*, McGraw-Hill, New York, 1950.

18. J. Westenberg, "Significance Test for Median and Interquartile Range in Samples from Continuous Populations of Any Form," *Proceedings Koninklijke Nederlandse Akademie Van Wetenschappen*, *51* (1948), 252–261.

19. G. W. Brown and A. M. Mood, "On Median Tests for Linear Hypotheses," *Proceedings of the Second Berkeley Symposium on Mathematical Statistics and Probability*, University of California Press, Berkeley, 1951, pp. 159–166.

20. V. L. Senders, *Measurement and Statistics*, Oxford University Press, New York, 1958.

21. William L. Hays and Robert L. Winkler, *Statistics: Probability, Inference, and Decision*, Holt, Rinehart and Winston, New York, 1971.

22. H. B. Mann and D. R. Whitney, "On a Test of Whether One of Two Random Variables Is Stochastically Larger Than the Other," *Annals of Mathematical Statistics*, *18* (1947), 50–60.

23. Gottfried E. Noether, *Elements of Nonparametric Statistics*, Wiley, New York, 1967.

24. A. N. Kolmogorov, "Sulla Determinazione Empirial di una Legge di Distribuizione," *Giornale dell' Institute Italiano degli Altuari*, *4* (1933), 83–91.

25. N. V. Smirnov, "Estimate of Deviation Between Empirical Distribution Functions in Two Independent Samples," (in Russian) *Bulletin Moscow University*, *2* (1939), 3–16.

26. L. A. Goodman, "Kolmogorov–Smirnov Tests for Psychological Research," *Psychological Bulletin*, *51* (1954), 160–168.

27. F. J. Massey, "The Kolmogorov–Smirnov Test for Goodness of Fit," *Journal of the American Statistical Association*, *46* (1951), 68–78.

28. Z. W. Birnbaum, "Numerical Tabulation of the Distribution of Kolmogorov's Statistic for Finite Sample Size," *Journal of the American Statistical Association*, *47* (1952), 425–441.

29. M. J. Slakter, "A Comparison of the Pearson Chi-Square and Kolmogorov Goodness-of-Fit Tests with Respect to Validity," *Journal of the American Statistical Association*, *60* (1965), 854–858.

30. W. H. Kruskal and W. A. Wallis, "Use of Ranks in One-Criterion Analysis of Variance," *Journal of the American Statistical Association 47* (1952), 583–621; errata, ibid., *48* (1953), 907–911.

31. K. R. Gabriel and P. A. Lachenbruch, "Nonparametric ANOVA in Small Samples: A Monte Carlo Study of the Adequacy of the Asymptotic Approximation," *Biometrics*, *25* (1969), 593–596.

32. M. Friedman, "The Use of Ranks to Avoid the Assumption of Normality Implicit in the Analysis of Variance," *Journal of the American Statistical Association*, *32* (1937), 675–701.

33. M. Friedman, "A Comparison of Alternative Tests of Significance for the Problem of *m* Rankings," *Annals of Mathematical Statistics*, *II* (1940), 86–92.

34. M. G. Kendall, *Rank Correlation Methods*, Second Edition, Hafner, New York, 1955.

35. W. H. Kruskal, "Ordinal Measures of Association," *Journal of the American Statistical Association*, *53* (1958), 814–861.

36. Harold Hotelling and Margaret R. Pabst, "Rank Correlation and Tests of Significance Involving No Assumption of Normality," *Annals of Mathematical Statistics*, *7* (1936), 29–43.

37. C. Spearman, "The Proof and Measurement of Association Between Two Things," *American Journal of Psychology*, *15* (1904), 72–101.

38. G. J. Glasser and R. F. Winter, "Critical Values of the Coefficient of Rank Correlation for Testing the Hypothesis of Independence," *Biometrika*, *48* (1961), 444–448.

39. Eugene S. Edgington, *Statistical Inference: The Distribution-Free Approach*, McGraw-Hill, New York, 1969.

40. H. Theil, "A Rank-Invariant Method of Linear and Polynomial Regression Analysis. III," *Koninklijke Nederlandse Akademie Van Wetenschappen*, *Proceedings*, Series A, *53* (1950), 1397–1412.

41. E. Jacquelin Dietz, "Teaching Regression in a Nonparametric Statistic Course," *The American Statistician*, *43* (1989), 35–40.

Additional References: Journal Articles

1. Wayne W. Daniel, *On Nonparametric and Robust Tests for Dispersion: A Selected Bibliography*, Vance Bibliographies, Monticello, Ill., December 1979.

2. Wayne W. Daniel, *Goodness-of-fit: A Selected Bibliography for the Statistician and the Researcher*, Vance Bibliographies, Monticello, Ill., May 1980.

3. Wayne W. Daniel and Carol E. Coogler, "Some Quick and Easy Statistical Procedures for the Physical Therapist," *Physical Therapy*, *54* (1974), 135–140.

4. Wayne W. Daniel and Beaufort B. Longest, "Some Practical Statistical Procedures," *Journal of Nursing Administration*, *5* (1975), 23–27.

5. Olive Jean Dunn, "Multiple Comparisons Using Rank Sums," *Technometrics*, *6* (1964), 241–252.

6. B. J. McDonald and W. A. Thomspon, "Rank Sum Multiple Comparisons in One- and Two-Way Classifications," *Biometrika*, *54* (1967), 487–498.

Applications References

A-1. M. Vaubourdolle, J. Guechot, O. Chazouilleres, R. E. Poupon, and J. Giboudeau, "Effect of Dihydrotestosterone on the Rate of Ethanol Elimination in Healthy Men," *Alcoholism: Clinical and Experimental Research*, *15* (No. 2, 1991), 238–240.

A-2. Hilton Davis, Amanda Stroud, and Lynette Green, "Maternal Language Environment of Children With Mental Retardation," *American Journal on Mental Retardation*, *93* (1988), 144–153.

A-3. F. Demotes-Mainard, G. Vinçon, M. Amouretti, F. Dumas, J. Necciari, G. Kieffer, and B. Begaud, "Pharmacokinetics and Protein Binding of Cefpiramide in Patients With Alcoholic Cirrhosis," *Clinical Pharmacology and Therapeutics*, *49* (1991), 263–269.

A-4. Y. Lebranchu, G. Thibault, D. Degenne, and P. Bardos, "Abnormalities in CD4+ T Lymphocyte Subsets in Patients With Common Variable Immunodeficiency," *Clinical Immunology and Immunopathology*, *61* (1991), 83–92.

A-5. Mark C. Liu, Walter C. Hubbard, David Proud, Becky A. Stealey, Stephen J. Galli, Anne Kagey-Sobotka, Eugene R. Bleeker, and Lawrence M. Lichtenstein, "Immediate and Late Inflammatory Responses to Ragweed Antigen Challenge of the Peripheral Airways in Allergic Asthamtics," *American Review of Respiratory Disease*, *144* (1991), 51–58.

A-6. Gary C. Walker, Diana D. Cardenas, Mark R. Guthrie, Alvin McLean, Jr., and Marvin M. Brooke, "Fatigue and Depression in Brain-Injured Patients Correlated With Quadriceps Strength and Endurance," *Archives of Physical Medicine and Rehabilitation*, *72* (1991), 469–472.

A-7. Hendrik J. Du Toit, André R. Coetzee, and Derek O. Chalton, "Heparin Treatment in Thrombin-Induced Disseminated Intravascular Coagulation in the Baboon," *Critical Care Medicine*, *19* (1991), 1195–1200.

A-8. Antonio Tartaglione, Maria Laura Inglese, Fabio Bandini, Luciano Spadavecchia, Kerry Hamsher, and Emilio Favale, "Hemisphere Asymmetry in Decision Making Abilities: An Experimental Study in Unilateral Brain Damage," *Brain*, *114* (1991), 1441–1456.

A-9. D. Warde, H. Nagi, and S. Raftery, "Respiratory Complications and Hypoxic Episodes During Inhalation Induction With Isoflurane in Children," *British Journal of Anaesthesia*, *66* (1991), 327–330.

A-10. Peter E. Ellis, Graham W. Mellsop, Ruth Beetson, and Russell R. Cooke, "Platelet Tritiated Imipramine Binding in Patients Suffering from Mania," *Journal of Affective Disorders*, *22* (1991), 105–110.

A-11. Shay McAtee and Wendy Mack, "Relations Between Design Copying and Other Tests of Sensory Integrative Dysfunction: A Pilot Study," *The American Journal of Occupational Therapy*, *44* (1990), 596–601.

A-12. Joan A. Barbera, Josep Roca, Josep Ramirez, Peter D. Wagner, Pietat Ussetti, and Robert Rodriguez-Roisin, "Gas Exchange During Exercise in Mild Chronic Obstructive Pulmonary Disease: Correlation With Lung Structure," *American Review of Respiratory Disease*, *144* (1991), 520–525.

A-13. Cheryl Miller and Ray Tricker, "Past and Future Priorities in Health Promotion in the United States: A Survey of Experts," *American Journal of Health Promotion*, *5* (1991), 360–367.

Vital Statistics

• •

CONTENTS

14.1 Introduction

The private physician arrives at a diagnosis and treatment plan for an individual patient by means of a case history, a physical examination, and various laboratory tests. The community may be thought of as a living complex organism for which the public health team is the physician. To carry out this role satisfactorily the public health team must also make use of appropriate tools and techniques for evaluating the health status of the community. Traditionally these tools and techniques have consisted of the community's vital statistics, which include the counts of births, deaths, illnesses, and the various rates and ratios that may be computed from them.

In succeeding sections we give some of the more useful and widely used rates and ratios. Before proceeding, however, let us distinguish between the terms *rate* and *ratio* by defining each as follows.

1. *Rate* Although there are some exceptions, the term *rate* usually is reserved to refer to those calculations that imply the probability of the occurrence of some

634   **Chapter 14 • Vital Statistics**

event. A rate is expressed in the form

$$\left(\frac{a}{a + b}\right)k \qquad (14.1.1)$$

where

a = the frequency with which an event has occurred during some specified period of time

$a + b$ = the number of persons exposed to the risk of the event during the same period of time

k = some number such as 10, 100, 1000, 10,000, or 100,000

As indicated by Expression 14.1.1 the numerator of a rate is a component part of the denominator. The purpose of the multiplier, k, called the base, is to avoid results involving the very small numbers that may arise in the calculation of rates and to facilitate comprehension of the rate. The value chosen for k will depend on the magnitudes of the numerator and denominator.

2. *Ratio*   A ratio is a fraction of the form

$$\left(\frac{c}{d}\right)k \qquad (14.1.2)$$

where k is some base as already defined and both c and d refer to the frequency of occurrence of some event or item. In the case of a ratio, as opposed to a rate, the numerator is not a component part of the denominator. We can speak, for example, of the person–doctor ratio or the person–hospital-bed ratio of a certain geographic area. The values of k most frequently used in ratios are 1 and 100.

14.2
Death Rates and Ratios

The rates and ratios discussed in this section are concerned with the occurrence of death. Death rates express the relative frequency of the occurrence of death within some specified interval of time in a specific population. The denominator of a death rate is referred to as the population at risk. The numerator represents only those deaths that occurred in the population specified by the denominator.

1. *Annual Crude Death Rate*   The annual crude death rate is defined as

$$\frac{\text{total number of deaths during year (January 1 to December 31)}}{\text{total population as of July 1}} \cdot k$$

where the value of k is usually chosen as 1000. This is the most widely used rate for measuring the overall health of a community. To compare the crude death rates of two communities is hazardous, unless it is known that the communities are comparable with respect to the many characteristics, other than health conditions, that influence the death rate. Variables that enter into the picture include age, race, sex, and socioeconomic status. When two populations must be compared on the basis of death rates, adjustments may be made to reconcile the population differences with respect to these variables. The same precautions should be exercised when comparing the annual death rates for the same community for two different years.

2. *Annual Specific Death Rates* It is usually more meaningful and enlightening to observe the death rates of small, well-defined subgroups of the total population. Rates of this type are called *specific death rates* and are defined as

$$\frac{\text{total number of deaths in a specific subgroup during a year}}{\text{total population in the specific subgroup as of July 1}} \cdot k$$

where k is usually equal to 1000. Subgroups for which specific death rates may be computed include those groups that may be distinguished on the basis of sex, race, and age. Specific rates may be computed for two or more characteristics simultaneously. For example, we may compute the death rate for white males, thus obtaining a race–sex specific rate. Cause-specific death rates may also be computed by including in the numerator only those deaths due to a particular cause of death, say cancer, heart disease, or accidents. Because of the small fraction that results, the base, k, for a cause-specific rate is usually 100,000 or 1,000,000.

3. *Adjusted or Standardized Death Rates* As we have already pointed out, the usefulness of the crude death rate is restricted by the fact that it does not reflect the composition of the population with respect to certain characteristics by which it is influenced. We have seen that by means of specific death rates various segments of the population may be investigated individually. If, however, we attempt to obtain an overall impression of the health of a population by looking at individual specific death rates, we are soon overwhelmed by their great number.

What is wanted is a single figure that measures the forces of mortality in a population while holding constant one or more of the compositional factors such as age, race, or sex. Such a figure, called an *adjusted death rate*, is available. It is most commonly obtained by what is known as the *direct method* of adjustment. The method consists essentially of applying to a *standard population* specific rates observed in the population of interest. From the resulting expected numbers we may compute an overall rate that tells us what the rate for the population of interest would be if that population had the same composition as the standard population. This method is not restricted to the computation of adjusted death rates only, but it may be used to obtain other adjusted rates, for example, an adjusted birth rate. If two or more populations are adjusted in this manner, they are then directly comparable on the basis of the adjustment factors. Opinions differ as to what population should be used as the standard. The population of the United States as of the last decennial census is frequently used. For adjustment calculations a population of 1,000,000, reflecting the composition of the standard population and called the *standard million*, is usually used. In the following example we illustrate the direct method of adjustment to obtain an age-adjusted death rate.

Example 14.2.1

The 1970 crude death rate for Georgia was 9.1 deaths per 1000 population. Let us obtain an age-adjusted death rate for Georgia by using the 1970 United States census as the standard population. In other words, we want a death rate that could have been expected in Georgia if the age composition of the Georgia population had been the same as that of the United States in 1970.

Solution: The data necessary for the calculations are shown in Table 14.2.1.

The procedure for calculating an age-adjusted death rate by the direct method consists of the following steps.

1. The population of interest is listed (column 2) according to age group (column 1).
2. The deaths in the population of interest are listed (column 3) by age group.
3. The age-specific death rates (column 4) for each age group are calculated by dividing column 3 by column 2 and multiplying by 100,000.
4. The standard population (column 5) is listed by age group.

TABLE 14.2.1 Calculation of age-adjusted death rate for Georgia, 1970, by direct method

1 Age (years)	2 Population[a]	3 Deaths[a]	4 Age-specific Death Rates (per 100,000)	5 Standard Population Based on U.S. Population 1970[b]	6 Number of Expected Deaths in Standard Population
0 to 4	424,600	2,483	584.8	84,416	494
5 to 14	955,000	449	47.0	200,508	94
15 to 24	863,000	1,369	158.6	174,406	277
25 to 34	608,100	1,360	223.6	122,569	274
35 to 44	518,400	2,296	442.9	113,614	503
45 to 54	486,400	4,632	952.3	114,265	1.088
55 to 64	384,400	7,792	2,027.1	91,480	1,854
65 to 74	235,900	9,363	3,969.1	61,195	2,429
75 and over	132,900	12,042	9,060.9	37,547	3,402
Total	4,608,700	41,786[c]		1,000,000	10,415

[a] *Georgia Vital and Morbidity Statistics* 1970, Georgia Department of Public Health, Atlanta, Georgia.
[b] *1970 Census of Population*, PC(1)-B1, Table 49.
[c] Excludes 44 deaths at unknown age.

5. The expected number of deaths in the standard population for each group (column 6) is computed by multiplying column 4 by column 5 and dividing by 100,000. The entries in column 6 are the deaths that would be expected in the standard population if the persons in this population had been exposed to the same risk of death experienced by the population being adjusted.

6. The entries in column 6 are summed to obtain the total number of expected deaths in the standard population.

7. The age-adjusted death rate is computed in the same manner as a crude death rate. That is, the age-adjusted death rate is equal to

$$\frac{\text{total number of expected deaths}}{\text{total standard population}} \cdot 1000$$

In the present example we have an age-adjusted death rate of

$$\frac{10,415}{1,000,000} \cdot 1000 = 10.4$$

We see, then, that by adjusting the 1970 population of Georgia to the age distribution of the standard population, we obtain an adjusted death rate that is 1.3 per 1000 greater than the crude death rate (10.4 − 9.1). This increase in the death rate following adjustment reflects the fact that in 1970 the population of Georgia was slightly younger than the population of the United States as a whole. For example, only 8 percent of the Georgia population was 65 years of age or older whereas 10 percent of the United States population was in that age group.

---

4. *Maternal Mortality Rate*   This rate is defined as

$$\frac{\text{deaths from all puerperal causes during a year}}{\text{total live births during the year}} \cdot k$$

where k is taken as 1000 or 100,000. The preferred denominator for this rate is the number of women who were pregnant during the year. This denominator, however, is impossible to determine.

A death from a puerperal cause is a death that can be ascribed to some phase of childbearing. Because of the decline in the maternal mortality rate in the United States, it is more convenient to use $k = 100,000$. In some countries, however, $k = 1000$ results in a more convenient rate. The decline in the maternal mortality rate in this country also has had the effect of reducing its usefulness as a discriminator among communities with varying qualities of medical care and health facilities.

Some limitations of the maternal mortality rate include the following.

a. Fetal deaths are not included in the denominator. This results in an inflated rate, since a mother can die from a puerperal cause without producing a live birth.

b. A maternal death can be counted only once, although twins or larger multiple births may have occurred. Such cases cause the denominator to be too large and, hence, there is a too small rate.

c. Under-registration of live births, which result in a too small denominator, causes the rate to be too large.

d. A maternal death may occur in a year later than the year in which the birth occurred. Although there are exceptions, in most cases the transfer of maternal deaths will balance out in a given year.

5. *Infant Mortality Rate*   This rate is defined as

$$\frac{\text{number of deaths under 1 year of age during a year}}{\text{total number of live births during the year}} \cdot k$$

where k is generally taken as 1000. Use and interpretation of this rate must be made in light of its limitations, which are similar to those that characterize the maternal mortality rate. Many of the infants who die in a given calendar year were born during the previous year; and, similarly, many children born in a given calendar year will die the during the following year. In populations with a stable birthrate this does not pose a serious problem. In periods of rapid change, however, some adjustment should be made. One way to make an adjustment is to allocate the infant deaths to the calendar year in which the infants were born before computing the rate.

6. *Neonatal Mortality Rate*   In an effort to better understand the nature of infant deaths, rates for ages less than a year are frequently computed. Of these, the one most frequently computed is the *neonatal mortality rate*, which is defined as

$$\frac{\text{number of deaths under 28 days of age during a year}}{\text{total number of live births during the year}} \cdot k$$

where $k = 1000$.

7. *Fetal Death Rate*   This rate is defined as

$$\frac{\text{total number of fetal deaths during a year}}{\text{total deliveries during the year}} \cdot k$$

where k is usually taken to be 1000. A fetal death is defined as a product of conception that shows no sign of life after complete birth. There are several problems associated with the use and interpretation of this rate. There is variation among reporting areas with respect to the duration of gestation. Some areas report all fetal deaths regardless of length of gestation while others have a minimum gestation period that must be reached before reporting is required. Another objection to the fetal death rate is that it does not take into account the extent to which a community is trying to reproduce. The ratio to be considered next has been proposed to overcome this objection.

8. *Fetal Death Ratio* This ratio is defined as

$$\frac{\text{total number of fetal deaths during a year}}{\text{total number of live births during the year}} \cdot k$$

where k is taken as 100 or 1000.

Some authorities have suggested that the number of fetal deaths as well as live births be included in the denominator in an attempt to include all pregnancies in the computation of the ratio. The objection to this suggestion rests on the incompleteness of fetal death reporting.

9. *Perinatal Mortality Rate* Since fetal deaths occurring late in pregnancy and neonatal deaths frequently have the same underlying causes, it has been suggested that the two be combined to obtain what is known as the *perinatal mortality rate*. This rate is computed as

$$\frac{\begin{array}{c}(\text{number of fetal deaths of 28 weeks or more}) \\ + (\text{infant deaths under 7 days})\end{array}}{\begin{array}{c}(\text{number of fetal deaths of 28 weeks or more}) \\ + (\text{number of live births})\end{array}} \cdot k$$

where $k = 1000$.

10. *Cause-of-Death Ratio* This ratio is defined as

$$\frac{\text{number of deaths due to a specific disease during a year}}{\text{total number of deaths due to all causes during the year}} \cdot k$$

where $k = 100$. This index is used to measure the relative importance of a given cause of death. It should be used with caution in comparing one community with another. A higher cause-of-death ratio in one community than that in another may be because the first community has a low mortality from other causes.

11. *Proportional Mortality Ratio* This index has been suggested as a single measure for comparing the overall health conditions of different communities. It is defined as

$$\frac{\text{number of deaths of persons 50 years of age and older}}{\text{total number of deaths}} \cdot k$$

where $k = 100$. The specified class is usually an age group such as 50 years and over, or a cause of death category, such as accidents. The proportional mortality ratio exhibits certain defects as noted by Linder and Grove (1).

EXERCISES

14.2.1 The following annual data were reported for a certain geographic area:

	Total	Number	
		White	Nonwhite
Estimated population as of July 1	597,500	361,700	235,800
Total live births	12,437	6,400	6,037
Immature births	1,243	440	803
Fetal deaths:	592	365	227
Total			
Under 20 weeks gestation	355	269	86
20 to 27 weeks gestation	103	42	61
28 weeks and more	123	49	74
Unknown length of gestation	11	5	6
Deaths	6,219	3,636	2,583
Total all ages			
Under 1 year	267	97	170
Under 28 days	210	79	131
Deaths from immaturity	16	12	4
Maternal deaths	2	—	2
Cause of death			
Malignant neoplasms	948	626	322
Ischaemic heart disease	1,697	1,138	559

Source: *Georgia Vital and Morbidity Statistics 1970*, Georgia Department of Public Health, Atlanta, p. 47.

From these data compute the following rates and ratios: (a) crude death rate, (b) race-specific death rates for white and nonwhite, (c) maternal mortality rate, (d) infant mortality rate, (e) neonatal mortality rate, (f) fetal death ratio, (g) cause of death ratios for malignant neoplasms and ischaemic heart disease.

14.2.2 The following table shows the deaths and estimated population by age for the state of Georgia for 1971. Use these data to compute the age-adjusted death rate for Georgia, 1971. Use the same standard population that was used in Example 14.2.1.

Age (years)	Estimated Population	Deaths
0 to 4	423,700	2,311
5 to 14	947,900	480
15 to 24	891,300	1,390
25 to 34	623,700	1,307
35 to 44	520,000	2,137
45 to 54	494,200	4,640
55 to 64	388,600	7,429
65 to 74	243,000	9,389
75 and over	136,000	12,411
Total	4,668,400	41,494[a]

[a]Excludes 42 deaths at unknown age.

Source: Statistics Sections, Office of Evaluation and Research, Georgia Department of Human Resources, Atlanta.

14.3
Measures of Fertility

The term *fertility* as used by American demographers refers to the actual bearing of children as opposed to the capacity to bear children, for which phenomenon the term *fecundity* is used. A knowledge of the "rate" of childbearing in a community is important to the health worker in planning services and facilities for mothers, infants, and children. The following are the six basic measures of fertility.

1. *Crude Birth Rate*   This rate is the most widely used of the fertility measures. It is obtained from

$$\frac{\text{total number of live births during a year}}{\text{total population as of July 1}} \cdot k$$

where $k = 1000$. For an illustration of the computation of this and the other five rates, see Table 14.3.1.

2. *General Fertility Rate*   This rate is defined as

$$\frac{\text{number of live births during a year}}{\text{total number of women of childbearing age}} \cdot k$$

where $k = 1000$ and the childbearing age is usually defined as ages 15 through 44 or ages 15 through 49. The attractive feature of this rate, when compared to the crude birth rate, is the fact that the denominator approximates the number of persons actually exposed to the risk of bearing a child.

3. *Age-Specific Fertility Rate*   Since the rate of childbearing is not uniform throughout the childbearing ages, a rate that permits the analysis of fertility rates for shorter maternal age intervals is desirable. The rate used is the age-specific fertility rate, which is defined as

$$\frac{\text{number of births to women of a certain age in a year}}{\text{total number of women of the specified age}} \cdot k$$

where $k = 1000$. Age-specific rates may be computed for single years of age, or any age interval. Rates for five-year age groups are the ones most frequently computed. Specific fertility rates may be computed also for other population subgroups such as those defined by race, socioeconomic status, and various demographic characteristics.

TABLE 14.3.1 Illustration of procedures for computing six basic measures of fertility, for Georgia, 1970

1	2	3	4	5	6	7
Age of Woman (years)	Number of Women in Population[a]	Number of Births to Women of Specified Age[b]	Age-Specfic Birthrate per 1000 Women	Standard Population Based on U.S. Population 1970[c]	Expected Births	Cumulative Fertility Rate
15 to 19	220,100	21,790	99.0	193.762	19,182	495.0
20 to 24	209,500	37,051	176.9	173,583	30,707	1,379.5
25 to 29	170,100	22,135	130.1	140,764	18,313	2,030.0
30 to 34	139,100	9,246	66.5	119,804	7,967	2,362.5
35 to 39	135,400	3,739	27.6	116,925	3,227	2,500.5
40 to 49	261,700	1,044	4.0	255,162	1,021	2,540.5
Total	1,135,900	95,005		1,000,000	80,417	

Computation of six basic rates:
  (1) Crude birth rate = total births divided by total population
        = (95,584/4,608,700)(1000) = 21.
  (2) General fertility rate = (95,584/1,135,900)(1000) = 84.1.
  (3) Age-specific fertility rates = entries in column 3 divided by entries in column 2 multiplied by 1000 for each age group. Results appear in column 4.
  (4) Total fertility rate = the sum of each age-specific rate multiplied by the age interval width = (99.0)(5) + (176.9)(5) + (130.1)(5) + (66.5)(5) + (27.6)(5) + (4.0)(10) = 2,540.5.
  (5) Cumulative fertility rate = age-specific birth rate multiplied by age interval width cumulated by age. See column 7.
  (6) Standardized general fertility rate = (80,417/1,000,000)(1000) = 80.4.

[a]Statistics Section, Office of Evaluation and Research, Georgia Department of Human Resources, Atlanta.

[b]*Georgia Vital and Morbidity Statistics 1970*, Georgia Department of Public Health, Atlanta.

[c]1970 Census of Population, PC(1)-B1.

4. *Total Fertility Rate*   If the age-specific fertility rates for all ages are added and multiplied by the interval into which the ages were grouped, the result is called the *total fertility rate*. The resulting figure is an estimate of the number of children a cohort of 1000 women would have if, during their reproductive years, they reproduced at the rates represented by the age-specific fertility rates from which the total fertility rate is computed.

5. *Cumulative Fertility Rate*   The cumulative fertility rate is computed in the same manner as the total fertility rate except that the adding process can terminate at the end of any desired age group. The numbers in column 7 of Table 14.3.1 are the cumulative fertility rates through the ages indicated in column 1. The final entry in the cumulative fertility rate column is the total fertility rate.

6. *Standardized Fertility Rate*   Just as the crude death rate may be standardized or adjusted, so may we standardize the general fertility rate. The procedure is identical to that discussed in Section 14.2 for adjusting the crude death rate. The necessary computations for computing the age-standardized fertility rate are shown in Table 14.3.1.

EXERCISES

14.3.1 The data in the following table are for the state of Georgia for 1971.

Age of Woman (years)	Number of Women in Population	Number of Births to Women of Specified Age
15 to 19	225,200	21,834
20 to 24	217,600	35,997
25 to 29	173,400	21,670
30 to 34	143,300	8,935
35 to 39	134,100	3,464
40 to 49	267,800	925[a]

[a]May include some births to women over 49 years of age.

SOURCE: Statistics Section, Office of Evaluation and Research, Georgia Department of Human Resources, Atlanta.

From the above data compute the following rates:

a. Age-specific fertility rates for each age group.
b. Total fertility rate.
c. Cumulative fertility rate through each age group.
d. General fertility rate standardized by age.

Use the standard population shown in Table 14.3.1

14.3.2 There were a total of 95,546 live births in Georgia in 1971. The estimated total population as of July 1, 1971, was 4,668,400, and the number of women between the ages of 15 and 49 was 1,161,400. Use these data to compute:

a. The crude birth rate.
b. The general fertility rate.

14.4
Measures of Morbidity

Another area that concerns the health worker who is analyzing the health of a community is *morbidity*. The word *morbidity* refers to the community's status with respect to disease. Data for the study of the morbidity of a community are not, as a rule, as readily available and complete as are the data on births and deaths because of incompleteness of reporting and differences among states with regard to laws requiring the reporting of diseases. The two rates most frequently used in the study of diseases in a community are the *incidence rate* and the *prevalence rate*.

1. *Incidence Rate* This rate is defined as

$$\frac{\text{total number of new cases of a specific disease during a year}}{\text{total population as of July 1}} \cdot k$$

where the value of k depends on the magnitude of the numerator. A base of 1000 is used when convenient, but 100 can be used for the more common diseases, and 10,000 or 100,000 can be used for those less common or rare. This rate, which measures the degree to which new cases are occurring in the community, is useful in helping determine the need for initiation of preventive measures. It is a meaningful measure for both chronic and acute diseases.

2. *Prevalence Rate*   Although it is referred to as a rate, the *prevalence rate* is really a ratio, since it is computed from

$$\frac{\text{total number of cases, new or old, existing at a point in time}}{\text{total population at that point in time}} \cdot k$$

where the value of k is selected by the same criteria as for the incidence rate. This rate is especially useful in the study of chronic diseases, but it may also be computed for acute diseases.

3. *Case-Fatality Ratio*   This ratio is useful in determining how well the treatment program for a certain disease is succeeding. It is defined as

$$\frac{\text{total number of deaths due to a disease}}{\text{total number of cases due to the disease}} \cdot k$$

where $k = 100$. The period of time covered is arbitrary, depending on the nature of the disease, and it may cover several years for an endemic disease. Note that this ratio can be interpreted as the probability of dying following contraction of the disease in question and, as such, reveals the seriousness of the disease.

4. *Immaturity Ratio*   This ratio is defined as

$$\frac{\text{number of live births under 2500 grams during a year}}{\text{total number of live births during the year}} \cdot k$$

where $k = 100$.

5. *Secondary Attack Rate*   This rate measures the occurrence of a contagious disease among susceptible persons who have been exposed to a primary case and is defined as

$$\frac{\begin{array}{c}\text{number of additional cases among contacts of a}\\\text{primary case within the maximum incubation period}\end{array}}{\text{total number of susceptible contacts}} \cdot k$$

where $k = 100$. This rate is used to measure the spread of infection and is usually applied to closed groups such as a household or classroom where it can be reasonably assumed that all members were, indeed, contacts.

14.5 Summary

This chapter is concerned with the computation and interpretation of various rates and ratios that are useful in studying the health of a community. More specifically, we discuss the more important rates and ratios relating to births, deaths, and morbidity. Individuals who wish to continue their reading in this area should consult the references.

REFERENCES

References Cited

1. Forest E. Linder and Robert D. Grove, *Vital Statistics Rates in the United States, 1900–1940*, United States Government Printing Office, Washington, D.C., 1947.

Other References

1. Donald J. Bogue, *Principles of Demography*, Wiley, New York, 1969.

2. John P. Fox, Carrie E. Hall, and Lila R. Elveback, *Epidemiology*, Macmillan, New York, 1970, Chapter 7.

3. Bernard G. Greenberg, "Biostatistics," in Hugh Rodman Leavell and E. Gurney Clark, *Preventive Medicine*, Third Edition, McGraw-Hill, New York, 1965.

4. Mortimer Spiegelman, *Introduction to Demography*, Revised Edition, Harvard University Press, Cambridge, Mass., 1968.

Some Basic MINITAB Data Handling Commands

NOTATION

Commands are left justified, subcommands are indented.

K	denotes a constant such as 8.3 or K14
C	denotes a column, such as C12 or 'Height'
E	denotes either a constant or column
M	denotes a matrix, such as M5
[]	encloses an optional argument

SYMBOLS

* Missing Value Symbol. An * can be used as data in REA, SET and INSERT, in data files and in the Data Editor. Enclose the * in single quotes in session commands and subcommands.
# Comment Symbol. The symbol # anywhere on a line tells Minitab to ignore the rest of the line.
& Continuation Symbol. To continue a command onto another line, end the first line with the symbol &. You can use + + as a synonym for &.

GENERAL INFORMATION

HELP	explains Minitab commands, can be a command or a subcommand
INFO	[C . . . C] gives the status of worksheet
STOP	ends the current session

INPUT & OUTPUT OF DATA

READ	data [from 'filename']	into C . . . C
SET	data [from 'filename']	into C
INSERT	data [from 'filename']	[between rows K and K] of C . . . C

READ, SET and INSERT have the subcommands:
FORMAT	(Fortran format)
NOBS	= K
END	of data (optional)
NAME	for C is 'name', for C is 'name' . . . for C is 'name'
PRINT	the data in E . . . E
WRITE	[to 'filename'] the data in C . . . C

PRINT and WRITE have the subcommand:
FORMAT	(Fortran format)
SAVE	[in 'filename'] a copy of the worksheet
PORTABLE	
LOTUS	save in Lotus format
RETRIEVE	the Minitab saved worksheet [in 'filename']
PORTABLE	
LOTUS	retrieve Lotus file

EDITING & MANIPULATING DATA

LET C(K) = K	# changes the number in row K of C
DELETE	rows K . . . K of C . . . C
ERASE	all data in E . . . E
INSERT	(see Section 2)
COPY	C . . . C into C . . . C

COPY	C into K...K	
USE	rows K...K	
USE	rows where C = K...K	
OMIT	rows K...K	
OMIT	rows where C = K...K	
COPY	K...K into C	
CODE	(K...K) to K... (K...K) to K for C...C, put in C...C	
STACK	(E...E)... on (E...E), put in (C...C)	
SUBSCRIPTS	into C	
UNSTACK	(C...C) into (E...E)...(E...E)	
SUBSCRIPTS	are in C	
CONVERT	using table in C C, the data in C, and put in C	
CONCATENATE	C...C put in C	

ARITHMETIC

LET = expression

    Expressions may use

      Arithmetic operators + − * / **(exponentiation)

      Comparison operators = ~= ⟨ ⟩ <= >=

      Logical operators & | ~

    and any of the following: ABSOLUTE, SQRT, LOGTEN, LOGE, EXPO, ANTILOG, ROUND, SIN, COS, TAN, ASIN, ACOS, ATAN, SIGNS, NSCORE, PARSUMS, PARPRODUCTS, COUNT, N, NMISS, SUM, MEAN, STDEV, MEDIAN, MIN, MAX, SSQ, SORT, RANK, LAG, EQ, NE, LT, GT, LE, GE, AND, OR, NOT.

      EXAMPLES: LET C2 = SQRT(C1 − MIN(C1))
                       LET C3(5) = 4.5

Simple Arithmetic Operations

ADD	E to E...	to E, put in E
SUBTRACT	E from	E, put in E
MULTIPLY	E by E...	by E, put in E
DIVIDE	E by	E, put in E
RAISE	E to the power	E, put in E

Columnwise Functions

ABSOLUTE value	of E, put in E
SQRT	of E, put in E
LOGE	of E, put in E
LOGTEN	of E, put in E
EXPONENTIATE	E, put in E
ANTILOG	of E, put in E
ROUND to integer	E, put in E
SIN	of E, put in E
COS	of E, put in E
TAN	of E, put in E
ASIN	of E, put in E
ACOS	of E, put in E
ATAN	of E, put in E
SIGNS	of E, put in E
PARSUMS	of C, put in C
PARPRODUCTS	of C, put in C

Normal Scores

NSCORES	of C, put in C

Columnwise Statistics

COUNT the number of values in	C [put in K]
N (number of nonmissing values) in	C [put in K]
NMISS (number of missing values) in	C [put in K]
SUM	of the values in C [put in K]
MEAN	of the values in C [put in K]
STDEV	of the values in C [put in K]
MEDIAN	of the values in C [put in K]
MINIMUM	of the values in C [put in K]
MAXIMUM	of the values in C [put in K]
SSQ (uncorrected sum of sq.) for	C [put in K]

Rowwise Statistics

RCOUNT	of E...E put in C
RN	of E...E put in C
RNMISS	of E...E put in C
RSUM	of E...E put in C
RMEAN	of E...E put in C
RSTDEV	of E...E put in C
RMEDIAN	of E...E put in C
RMINIMUM	of E...E put in C
RMAXIMUM	of E...E put in C
RSSQ	of E...E put in C

Indicator Variables

INDICATOR	variables for subscripts in C, put in C...C

BASIC STATISTICS

DESCRIBE	C...C
BY	C
ZINTERVAL	[K% confidence] assuming sigma = K for C...C
ZTEST	[of mu = K] assuming sigma = K for C...C
ALTERNATIVE	= K
TINTERVAL	[K% confidence] for data in C...C
TTEST	[of mu = K] on data in C...C
ALTERNATIVE	= K
TWOSAMPLE	test and c.i. [K% confidence] samples in C C
ALTERNATIVE	= K
POOLED	procedure
TWOT	test and c.i. [K% confidence] data in C, groups in C
ALTERNATIVE	= K
POOLED	procedure
CORRELATION	between C...C [put in M]
COVARIANCE	between C...C [put in M]
CENTER	the data in C...C put in C...C
LOCATION	[subtracting K...K]
SCALE	[dividing by K...K]
MINMAX	[with K as min and K as max]

REGRESSION

REGRESS	C on K predictors C . . . C [put st. resids in C [fits in C]]	
	NOCONSTANT	in equation
	WEIGHTS	are in C
	MSE	put in K
	COEFFICIENTS	put in C
	XPXINV	put in M
	RMATRIX	put in M
	III	put in C (leverage)
	RESIDUALS	put in C (observed-fit)
	TRESIDUALS	put in C (deleted studentized)
	COOKD	put in C (Cook's distance)
	DFITS	put in C
	PREDICT	for E . . . E
	VIF	(variance inflation factors)
	DW	(Durbin-Watson statistic)
	PURE	(pure error lack-of-fit test)
	XLOF	(experimental lack-of-fit test)
	TOLERANCE	K [K]
STEPWISE	regression of C on the predictors C . . . C	
	FENTER	= K (default is four)
	FREMOVE	= K (default is four)
	FORCE	C . . . C
	ENTER	C . . . C
	REMOVE	C . . . C
	BEST	K alternative predictors (default is zero)
	STEPS	= K (default depends on output width)
BREG	C on predictors C . . . C	
	INCLUDE	predictors C . . . C
	BEST	K models
	NVARS	K [K]
	NOCONSTANT	in equation
NOCONSTANT	in REGRESS, STEPWISE and BREG commands that follow	
CONSTANT	fit a constant in REGRESS, STEPWISE and BREG	
BRIEF	K	

ANALYSIS OF VARIANCE

AOVONEWAY	aov for samples in C . . . C	
ONEWAY	aov, data in C, levels in C [put resides in C [fits in C]]	
	TUKEY	[family error rate K]
	FISHER	[individual error rate K]
	DUNNETT	[family error rate K] for control group K
	MCB	[family error rate K] best is K
TWOWAY	aov, data in C, levels in C C [put resides in C [fits in C]]	

ADDITIVE	model	
MEANS	for the factors C [C]	
ANOVA	model	
	RANDOM	factorlist
	EMS	
	FITS	put in C . . . C
	RESIDUALS	put in C . . . C
	MEANS	for termlist
	TEST	for termlist/errorterm
	RESTRICT	use restricted model

NONPARAMETRICS

RUNS	test [above and below K] for C	
STEST	sign test [median = K] for C . . . C	
	ALTERNATIVE	= K
SINTERVAL	sign c.i. [K% confidence] for C . . . C	
WTEST	Wilcoxon one-sample rank test [median = K] for C . . . C	
	ALTERNATIVE	= K
WINTERVAL	Wilcoxon c.i. [K% confidence] for C . . . C	
MANN-WHITNEY	test and c.i. [K% confidence] on C C	
	ALTERNATIVE	= K
KRUSKAL-WALLIS	test for data in C, subscripts in C	
	MOOD	median test, data in C, subscripts in C [put res. in C [fits in C]]
FRIEDMAN	data in C, treatment in C, blocks in C [put res. in C [fits in C]]	
WALSH	averages for C, put in C [indices into C C]	
WDIFF	for C and C, put in C [indices into C C]	
WSLOPE	y in C, x in C, put in C [indices into C C]	

EXPLORATORY DATA ANALYSIS

STEM-AND-LEAF	display of C . . . C	
	TRIM	outliers
	INCREMENT	= K
	BY	C
BOXPLOT	for C	
GBOXPLOT	for C (high resolution version)	
BOXPLOT and GBOXPLOT have the subcommands:		
	INCREMENT	= K
	START	at K [end at K]
	BY	C
	LINES	= K
	NOTCH	[K% confidence] sign c.i.
	LEVELS	K . . . K
	FILE	'filename' to store GBOXPLOT output

Statistical Tables

• •

LIST OF TABLES

TABLE A Random Digits

	00000 12345	00001 67890	11111 12345	11112 67890	22222 12345	22223 67890	33333 12345	33334 67890	44444 12345	44445 67890
01	85967	73152	14511	85285	36009	95892	36962	67835	63314	50162
02	07483	51453	11649	86348	76431	81594	95848	36738	25014	15460
03	96283	01898	61414	83525	04231	13604	75339	11730	85423	60698
04	49174	12074	98551	37895	93547	24769	09404	76548	05393	96770
05	97366	39941	21225	93629	19574	71565	33413	56087	40875	13351
06	90474	41469	16812	81542	81652	45554	27931	93994	22375	00953
07	28599	64109	09497	76235	41383	31555	12639	00619	22909	29563
08	25254	16210	89717	65997	82667	74624	36348	44018	64732	93589
09	28785	02760	24359	99410	77319	73408	58993	61098	04393	48245
10	84725	86576	86944	93296	10081	82454	76810	52975	10324	15457
11	41059	66456	47679	66810	15941	84602	14493	65515	19251	41642
12	67434	41045	82830	47617	36932	46728	71183	36345	41404	81110
13	72766	68816	37643	19959	57550	49620	98480	25640	67257	18671
14	92079	46784	66125	94932	64451	29275	57669	66658	30818	58353
15	29187	40350	62533	73603	34075	16451	42885	03448	37390	96328
16	74220	17612	65522	80607	19184	64164	66962	82310	18163	63495
17	03786	02407	06098	92917	40434	60602	82175	04470	78754	90775
18	75085	55558	15520	27038	25471	76107	90832	10819	56797	33751
19	09161	33015	19155	11715	00551	24909	31894	37774	37953	78837
20	75707	48992	64998	87080	39333	00767	45637	12538	67439	94914
21	21333	48660	31288	00086	79889	75532	28704	62844	92337	99695
22	65626	50061	42539	14812	48895	11196	34335	60492	70650	51108
23	84380	07389	87891	76255	89604	41372	10837	66992	93183	56920
24	46479	32072	80083	63868	70930	89654	05359	47196	12452	38234
25	59847	97197	55147	76639	76971	55928	36441	95141	42333	67483
26	31416	11231	27904	57383	31852	69137	96667	14315	01007	31929
27	82066	83436	67914	21465	99605	83114	97885	74440	99622	87912
28	01850	42782	39202	18582	46214	99228	79541	78298	75404	63648
29	32315	89276	89582	87138	16165	15984	21466	63830	30475	74729
30	59388	42703	55198	80380	67067	97155	34160	85019	03527	78140
31	58089	27632	50987	91373	07736	20436	96130	73483	85332	24384
32	61705	57285	30392	23660	75841	21931	04295	00875	09114	32101
33	18914	98982	60199	99275	41967	35208	30357	76772	92656	62318
34	11965	94089	34803	48941	69709	16784	44642	89761	66864	62803
35	85251	48111	80936	81781	93248	67877	16498	31924	51315	79921
36	66121	96986	84844	93873	46352	92183	51152	85878	30490	15974
37	53972	96642	24199	58080	35450	03482	66953	49521	63719	57615
38	14509	16594	78883	43222	23093	58645	60257	89250	63266	90858
39	37700	07688	65533	72126	23611	93993	01848	03910	38552	17472
40	85466	59392	72722	15473	73295	49759	56157	60477	83284	56367
41	52969	55863	42312	67842	05673	91878	82738	36563	79540	61935
42	42744	68315	17514	02878	97291	74851	42725	57894	81434	62041
43	26140	13336	67726	61876	29971	99294	96664	52817	90039	53211
44	95589	56319	14563	24071	06916	59555	18195	32280	79357	04224
45	39113	13217	59999	49952	83021	47709	53105	19295	88318	41626
46	41392	17622	18994	98283	07249	52289	24209	91139	30715	06604
47	54684	53645	79246	70183	87731	19185	08541	33519	07223	97413
48	89442	61001	36658	57444	95388	36682	38052	46719	09428	94012
49	36751	16778	54888	15357	68003	43564	90976	58904	40512	07725
50	98159	02564	21416	74944	53049	88749	02865	25772	89853	88714

TABLE B Cumulative Binomial Probability Distribution

$$P(X \le x | n, p) = \sum_{X=0}^{x} \binom{n}{x} p^x q^{n-x}$$

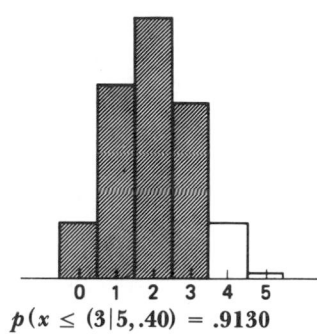

0 1 2 3 4 5

$p(x \le (3|5, .40) = .9130$

$n = 5$

x \\ p	.01	.02	.03	.04	.05	.06	.07	.08	.09	.10
0	.9510	.9039	.8587	.8154	.7738	.7339	.6957	.6591	.6240	.5905
1	.9990	.9962	.9915	.9852	.9774	.9681	.9575	.9456	.9326	.9185
2	1.0000	.9999	.9997	.9994	.9988	.9980	.9969	.9955	.9937	.9914
3	1.0000	1.0000	1.0000	1.0000	1.0000	.9999	.9999	.9998	.9997	.9995
4	1.0000	1.0000	1.0000	1.0000	1.0000	1.0000	1.0000	1.0000	1.0000	1.0000

x \\ p	.11	.12	.13	.14	.15	.16	.17	.18	.19	.20
0	.5584	.5277	.4984	.4704	.4437	.4182	.3939	.3707	.3487	.3277
1	.9035	.8875	.8708	.8533	.8352	.8165	.7973	.7776	.7576	.7373
2	.9888	.9857	.9821	.9780	.9734	.9682	.9625	.9563	.9495	.9421
3	.9993	.9991	.9987	.9983	.9978	.9971	.9964	.9955	.9945	.9933
4	1.0000	1.0000	1.0000	.9999	.9999	.9999	.9999	.9998	.9998	.9997
5	1.0000	1.0000	1.0000	1.0000	1.0000	1.0000	1.0000	1.0000	1.0000	1.0000

x \\ p	.21	.22	.23	.24	.25	.26	.27	.28	.29	.30
0	.3077	.2887	.2707	.2536	.2373	.2219	.2073	.1935	.1804	.1681
1	.7167	.6959	.6749	.6539	.6328	.6117	.5907	.5697	.5489	.5282
2	.9341	.9256	.9164	.9067	.8965	.8857	.8743	.8624	.8499	.8369
3	.9919	.9903	.9886	.9866	.9844	.9819	.9792	.9762	.9728	.9692
4	.9996	.9995	.9994	.9992	.9990	.9988	.9986	.9983	.9979	.9976
5	1.0000	1.0000	1.0000	1.0000	1.0000	1.0000	1.0000	1.0000	1.0000	1.0000

x \\ p	.31	.32	.33	.34	.35	.36	.37	.38	.39	.40
0	.1564	.1454	.1350	.1252	.1160	.1074	.0992	.0916	.0845	.0778
1	.5077	.4875	.4675	.4478	.4284	.4094	.3907	.3724	.3545	.3370
2	.8234	.8095	.7950	.7801	.7648	.7491	.7330	.7165	.6997	.6826
3	.9653	.9610	.9564	.9514	.9460	.9402	.9340	.9274	.9204	.9130
4	.9971	.9966	.9961	.9955	.9947	.9940	.9931	.9921	.9910	.9898
5	1.0000	1.0000	1.0000	1.0000	1.0000	1.0000	1.0000	1.0000	1.0000	1.0000

TABLE B (*continued*)

	$n = 5$ (*continued*)									
x \ p	.41	.42	.43	.44	.45	.46	.47	.48	.49	.50
0	.0715	.0656	.0602	.0551	.0503	.0459	.0418	.0380	.0345	.0312
1	.3199	.3033	.2871	.2714	.2562	.2415	.2272	.2135	.2002	.1875
2	.6651	.6475	.6295	.6114	.5931	.5747	.5561	.5375	.5187	.5000
3	.9051	.8967	.8879	.8786	.8688	.8585	.8478	.8365	.8247	.8125
4	.9884	.9869	.9853	.9835	.9815	.9794	.9771	.9745	.9718	.9688
5	1.0000	1.0000	1.0000	1.0000	1.0000	1.0000	1.0000	1.0000	1.0000	1.0000

	$n = 6$									
x \ p	.01	.02	.03	.04	.05	.06	.07	.08	.09	.10
0	.9415	.8858	.8330	.7828	.7351	.6899	.6470	.6064	.5679	.5314
1	.9985	.9943	.9875	.9784	.9672	.9541	.9392	.9227	.9048	.8857
2	1.0000	.9998	.9995	.9988	.9978	.9962	.9942	.9915	.9882	.9841
3	1.0000	1.0000	1.0000	1.0000	.9999	.9998	.9997	.9995	.9992	.9987
4	1.0000	1.0000	1.0000	1.0000	1.0000	1.0000	1.0000	1.0000	1.0000	.9999
5	1.0000	1.0000	1.0000	1.0000	1.0000	1.0000	1.0000	1.0000	1.0000	1.0000

x \ p	.11	.12	.13	.14	.15	.16	.17	.18	.19	.20
0	.4970	.4644	.4336	.4046	.3771	.3513	.3269	.3040	.2824	.2621
1	.8655	.8444	.8224	.7997	.7765	.7528	.7287	.7044	.6799	.6554
2	.9794	.9739	.9676	.9605	.9527	.9440	.9345	.9241	.9130	.9011
3	.9982	.9975	.9966	.9955	.9941	.9925	.9906	.9884	.9859	.9830
4	.9999	.9999	.9998	.9997	.9996	.9995	.9993	.9990	.9987	.9984
5	1.0000	1.0000	1.0000	1.0000	1.0000	1.0000	1.0000	1.0000	1.0000	.9999
6	1.0000	1.0000	1.0000	1.0000	1.0000	1.0000	1.0000	1.0000	1.0000	1.0000

x \ p	.21	.22	.23	.24	.25	.26	.27	.28	.29	.30
0	.2431	.2252	.2084	.1927	.1780	.1642	.1513	.1393	.1281	.1176
1	.6308	.6063	.5820	.5578	.5339	.5104	.4872	.4644	.4420	.4202
2	.8885	.8750	.8609	.8461	.8306	.8144	.7977	.7804	.7626	.7443
3	.9798	.9761	.9720	.9674	.9624	.9569	.9508	.9443	.9372	.9295
4	.9980	.9975	.9969	.9962	.9954	.9944	.9933	.9921	.9907	.9891
5	.9999	.9999	.9999	.9998	.9998	.9997	.9996	.9995	.9994	.9993
6	1.0000	1.0000	1.0000	1.0000	1.0000	1.0000	1.0000	1.0000	1.0000	1.0000

x \ p	.31	.32	.33	.34	.35	.36	.37	.38	.39	.40
0	.1079	.0989	.0905	.0827	.0754	.0687	.0625	.0568	.0515	.0467
1	.3988	.3780	.3578	.3381	.3191	.3006	.2828	.2657	.2492	.2333
2	.7256	.7064	.6870	.6672	.6471	.6268	.6063	.5857	.5650	.5443
3	.9213	.9125	.9031	.8931	.8826	.8714	.8596	.8473	.8343	.8208
4	.9873	.9852	.9830	.9805	.9777	.9746	.9712	.9675	.9635	.9590
5	.9991	.9989	.9987	.9985	.9982	.9978	.9974	.9970	.9965	.9959
6	1.0000	1.0000	1.0000	1.0000	1.0000	1.0000	1.0000	1.0000	1.0000	1.0000

TABLE B (*continued*)

					n = 6 (*continued*)					

p x	.41	.42	.43	.44	.45	.46	.47	.48	.49	.50
0	.0422	.0381	.0343	.0308	.0277	.0248	.0222	.0198	.0176	.0156
1	.2181	.2035	.1895	.1762	.1636	.1515	.1401	.1293	.1190	.1094
2	.5236	.5029	.4823	.4618	.4415	.4214	.4015	.3820	.3627	.3437
3	.8067	.7920	.7768	.7610	.7447	.7200	.7107	.6930	.6740	.6562
4	.9542	.9490	.9434	.9373	.9308	.9238	.9163	.9083	.8997	.8906
5	.9952	.9945	.9937	.9927	.9917	.9905	.9892	.9878	.9862	.9844
6	1.0000	1.0000	1.0000	1.0000	1.0000	1.0000	1.0000	1.0000	1.0000	1.0000

					n = 7					

p x	.01	.02	.03	.04	.05	.06	.07	.08	.09	.10
0	.9321	.8681	.8080	.7514	.6983	.6485	.6017	.5578	.5168	.4783
1	.9980	.9921	.9829	.9706	.9556	.9382	.9187	.8974	.8745	.8503
2	1.0000	.9997	.9991	.9980	.9962	.9937	.9903	.9860	.9807	.9743
3	1.0000	1.0000	1.0000	.9999	.9998	.9996	.9993	.9988	.9982	.9973
4	1.0000	1.0000	1.0000	1.0000	1.0000	1.0000	1.0000	.9999	.9999	.9998
5	1.0000	1.0000	1.0000	1.0000	1.0000	1.0000	1.0000	1.0000	1.0000	1.0000

p x	.11	.12	.13	.14	.15	.16	.17	.18	.19	.20
0	.4423	.4087	.3773	.3479	.3206	.2951	.2714	.2493	.2288	.2097
1	.8250	.7988	.7719	.7444	.7166	.6885	.6604	.6323	.6044	.5767
2	.9669	.9584	.9487	.9380	.9262	.9134	.8995	.8846	.8687	.8520
3	.9961	.9946	.9928	.9906	.9879	.9847	.9811	.9769	.9721	.9667
4	.9997	.9996	.9994	.9991	.9988	.9983	.9978	.9971	.9963	.9953
5	1.0000	1.0000	1.0000	1.0000	.9999	.9999	.9999	.9998	.9997	.9996
6	1.0000	1.0000	1.0000	1.0000	1.0000	1.0000	1.0000	1.0000	1.0000	1.0000

p x	.21	.22	.23	.24	.25	.26	.27	.28	.29	.30
0	.1920	.1757	.1605	.1465	.1335	.1215	.1105	.1003	.0910	.0824
1	.5494	.5225	.4960	.4702	.4449	.4204	.3965	.3734	.3510	.3294
2	.8343	.8159	.7967	.7769	.7564	.7354	.7139	.6919	.6696	.6471
3	.9606	.9539	.9464	.9383	.9294	.9198	.9095	.8984	.8866	.8740
4	.9942	.9928	.9912	.9893	.9871	.9847	.9819	.9787	.9752	.9712
5	.9995	.9994	.9992	.9989	.9987	.9983	.9979	.9974	.9969	.9962
6	1.0000	1.0000	1.0000	1.0000	.9999	.9999	.9999	.9999	.9998	.9998
7	1.0000	1.0000	1.0000	1.0000	1.0000	1.0000	1.0000	1.0000	1.0000	1.0000

TABLE B (*continued*)

					n = 7 (*continued*)					
x \ *p*	.31	.32	.33	.34	.35	.36	.37	.38	.39	.40
0	.0745	.0672	.0606	.0546	.0490	.0440	.0394	.0352	.0314	.0280
1	.3086	.2887	.2696	.2513	.2338	.2172	.2013	.1863	.1721	.1586
2	.6243	.6013	.5783	.5553	.5323	.5094	.4866	.4641	.4419	.4199
3	.8606	.8466	.8318	.8163	.8002	.7833	.7659	.7479	.7293	.7102
4	.9668	.9620	.9566	.9508	.9444	.9375	.9299	.9218	.9131	.9037
5	.9954	.9945	.9935	.9923	.9910	.9895	.9877	.9858	.9836	.9812
6	.9997	.9997	.9996	.9995	.9994	.9992	.9991	.9989	.9986	.9984
7	1.0000	1.0000	1.0000	1.0000	1.0000	1.0000	1.0000	1.0000	1.0000	1.0000
x \ *p*	.41	.42	.43	.44	.45	.46	.47	.48	.49	.50
0	.0249	.0221	.0195	.0173	.0152	.0134	.0117	.0103	.0090	.0078
1	.1459	.1340	.1228	.1123	.1024	.0932	.0847	.0767	.0693	.0625
2	.3983	.3771	.3564	.3362	.3164	.2973	.2787	.2607	.2433	.2266
3	.6906	.6706	.6502	.6294	.6083	.5869	.5654	.5437	.5219	.5000
4	.8937	.8831	.8718	.8598	.8471	.8337	.8197	.8049	.7895	.7734
5	.9784	.9754	.9721	.9684	.9643	.9598	.9549	.9496	.9438	.9375
6	.9981	.9977	.9973	.9968	.9963	.9956	.9949	.9941	.9932	.9922
7	1.0000	1.0000	1.0000	1.0000	1.0000	1.0000	1.0000	1.0000	1.0000	1.0000

					n = 8					
x \ *p*	.01	.02	.03	.04	.05	.06	.07	.08	.09	.10
0	.9227	.8508	.7837	.7214	.6634	.6096	.5596	.5132	.4703	.4305
1	.9973	.9897	.9777	.9619	.9428	.9208	.8965	.8702	.8423	.8131
2	.9999	.9996	.9987	.9969	.9942	.9904	.9853	.9789	.9711	.9619
3	1.0000	1.0000	.9999	.9998	.9996	.9993	.9987	.9978	.9966	.9950
4	1.0000	1.0000	1.0000	1.0000	1.0000	1.0000	.9999	.9999	.9997	.9996
5	1.0000	1.0000	1.0000	1.0000	1.0000	1.0000	1.0000	1.0000	1.0000	1.0000
x \ *p*	.11	.12	.13	.14	.15	.16	.17	.18	.19	.20
0	.3937	.3596	.3282	.2992	.2725	.2479	.2252	.2044	.1853	.1678
1	.7829	.7520	.7206	.6889	.6572	.6256	.5943	.5634	.5330	.5033
2	.9513	.9392	.9257	.9109	.8948	.8774	.8588	.8392	.8185	.7969
3	.9929	.9903	.9871	.9832	.9786	.9733	.9672	.9603	.9524	.9437
4	.9993	.9990	.9985	.9979	.9971	.9962	.9950	.9935	.9917	.9896
5	1.0000	.9999	.9999	.9998	.9998	.9997	.9995	.9993	.9991	.9988
6	1.0000	1.0000	1.0000	1.0000	1.0000	1.0000	1.0000	1.0000	.9999	.9999
7	1.0000	1.0000	1.0000	1.0000	1.0000	1.0000	1.0000	1.0000	1.0000	1.0000

TABLE B (*continued*)

					$n = 8$ (*continued*)					
$\diagdown$ p x	.21	.22	.23	.24	.25	.26	.27	.28	.29	.30
0	.1517	.1370	.1236	.1113	.1001	.0899	.0806	.0722	.0646	.0576
1	.4743	.4462	.4189	.3925	.3671	.3427	.3193	.2969	.2756	.2553
2	.7745	.7514	.7276	.7033	.6785	.6535	.6282	.6027	.5772	.5518
3	.9311	.9235	.9120	.8996	.8862	.8719	.8567	.8406	.8237	.8059
4	.9871	.9842	.9809	.9770	.9727	.9678	.9623	.9562	.9495	.9420
5	.9984	.9979	.9973	.9966	.9958	.9948	.9936	.9922	.9906	.9887
6	.9999	.9998	.9998	.9997	.9996	.9995	.9994	.9992	.9990	.9987
7	1.0000	1.0000	1.0000	1.0000	1.0000	1.0000	1.0000	1.0000	.9999	.9999
8	1.0000	1.0000	1.0000	1.0000	1.0000	1.0000	1.0000	1.0000	1.0000	1.0000

$\diagdown$ p x	.31	.32	.33	.34	.35	.36	.37	.38	.39	.40
0	.0514	.0457	.0406	.0360	.0319	.0281	.0248	.0218	.0192	.0168
1	.2360	.2178	.2006	.1844	.1691	.1548	.1414	.1289	.1172	.1064
2	.5264	.5013	.4764	.4519	.4278	.4042	.3811	.3585	.3366	.3154
3	.7874	.7681	.7481	.7276	.7064	.6847	.6626	.6401	.6172	.5941
4	.9339	.9250	.9154	.9051	.8939	.8820	.8693	.8557	.8414	.8263
5	.9866	.9841	.9813	.9782	.9747	.9707	.9664	.9615	.9561	.9502
6	.9984	.9980	.9976	.9970	.9964	.9957	.9949	.9939	.9928	.9915
7	.9999	.9999	.9999	.9998	.9998	.9997	.9996	.9996	.9995	.9993
8	1.0000	1.0000	1.0000	1.0000	1.0000	1.0000	1.0000	1.0000	1.0000	1.0000

$\diagdown$ p x	.41	.42	.43	.44	.45	.46	.47	.48	.49	.50
0	.0147	.0128	.0111	.0097	.0084	.0072	.0062	.0053	.0046	.0039
1	.0963	.0870	.0784	.0705	.0632	.0565	.0504	.0448	.0398	.0352
2	.2948	.2750	.2560	.2376	.2201	.2034	.1875	.1724	.1581	.1445
3	.5708	.5473	.5238	.5004	.4770	.4537	.4306	.4078	.3854	.3633
4	.8105	.7938	.7765	.7584	.7396	.7202	.7001	.6795	.6584	.6367
5	.9437	.9366	.9289	.9206	.9115	.9018	.8914	.8802	.8682	.8555
6	.9900	.9883	.9864	.9843	.9819	.9792	.9761	.9728	.9690	.9648
7	.9992	.9990	.9988	.9986	.9983	.9980	.9976	.9972	.9967	.9961
8	1.0000	1.0000	1.0000	1.0000	1.0000	1.0000	1.0000	1.0000	1.0000	1.0000

					$n = 9$					
$\diagdown$ p x	.01	.02	.03	.04	.05	.06	.07	.08	.09	.10
0	.9135	.8337	.7602	.6925	.6302	.5730	.5204	.4722	.4279	.3874
1	.9966	.9869	.9718	.9522	.9288	.9022	.8729	.8417	.8088	.7748
2	.9999	.9994	.9980	.9955	.9916	.9862	.9791	.9702	.9595	.9470
3	1.0000	1.0000	.9999	.9997	.9994	.9987	.9977	.9963	.9943	.9917
4	1.0000	1.0000	1.0000	1.0000	1.0000	.9999	.9998	.9997	.9995	.9991
5	1.0000	1.0000	1.0000	1.0000	1.0000	1.0000	1.0000	1.0000	1.0000	.9999
6	1.0000	1.0000	1.0000	1.0000	1.0000	1.0000	1.0000	1.0000	1.0000	1.0000

TABLE B (*continued*)

	|\ p	$n = 9$ (*continued*)								

x \\ p	.11	.12	.13	.14	.15	.16	.17	.18	.19	.20
0	.3504	.3165	.2855	.2573	.2316	.2082	.1869	.1676	.1501	.1342
1	.7401	.7049	.6696	.6343	.5995	.5652	.5315	.4988	.4670	.4362
2	.9327	.9167	.8991	.8798	.8591	.8371	.8139	.7895	.7643	.7382
3	.9883	.9842	.9791	.9731	.9661	.9580	.9488	.9385	.9270	.9144
4	.9986	.9979	.9970	.9959	.9944	.9925	.9902	.9875	.9842	.9804
5	.9999	.9998	.9997	.9996	.9994	.9991	.9987	.9983	.9977	.9969
6	1.0000	1.0000	1.0000	1.0000	1.0000	.9999	.9999	.9998	.9998	.9997
7	1.0000	1.0000	1.0000	1.0000	1.0000	1.0000	1.0000	1.0000	1.0000	1.0000

x \\ p	.21	.22	.23	.24	.25	.26	.27	.28	.29	.30
0	.1199	.1069	.0952	.0846	.0751	.0665	.0589	.0520	.0458	.0404
1	.4066	.3782	.3509	.3250	.3003	.2770	.2548	.2340	.2144	.1960
2	.7115	.6842	.6566	.6287	.6007	.5727	.5448	.5171	.4898	.4628
3	.9006	.8856	.8696	.8525	.8343	.8151	.7950	.7740	.7522	.7297
4	.9760	.9709	.9650	.9584	.9511	.9429	.9338	.9238	.9130	.9012
5	.9960	.9949	.9935	.9919	.9900	.9878	.9851	.9821	.9787	.9747
6	.9996	.9994	.9992	.9990	.9987	.9983	.9978	.9972	.9965	.9957
7	1.0000	1.0000	.9999	.9999	.9999	.9999	.9998	.9997	.9997	.9996
8	1.0000	1.0000	1.0000	1.0000	1.0000	1.0000	1.0000	1.0000	1.0000	1.0000

x \\ p	.31	.32	.33	.34	.35	.36	.37	.38	.39	.40
0	.0355	.0311	.0272	.0238	.0207	.0180	.0156	.0135	.0117	.0101
1	.1788	.1628	.1478	.1339	.1211	.1092	.0983	.0882	.0790	.0705
2	.4364	.4106	.3854	.3610	.3373	.3144	.2924	.2713	.2511	.2318
3	.7065	.6827	.6585	.6338	.6089	.5837	.5584	.5331	.5078	.4826
4	.8885	.8748	.8602	.8447	.8283	.8110	.7928	.7738	.7540	.7334
5	.9702	.9652	.9596	.9533	.9464	.9388	.9304	.9213	.9114	.9006
6	.9947	.9936	.9922	.9906	.9888	.9867	.9843	.9816	.9785	.9750
7	.9994	.9993	.9991	.9989	.9986	.9983	.9979	.9974	.9969	.9962
8	1.0000	1.0000	1.0000	.9999	.9999	.9999	.9999	.9998	.9998	.9997
9	1.0000	1.0000	1.0000	1.0000	1.0000	1.0000	1.0000	1.0000	1.0000	1.0000

x \\ p	.41	.42	.43	.44	.45	.46	.47	.48	.49	.50
0	.0087	.0074	.0064	.0054	.0046	.0039	.0033	.0028	.0023	.0020
1	.0628	.0558	.0495	.0437	.0385	.0338	.0296	.0259	.0225	.0195
2	.2134	.1961	.1796	.1641	.1495	.1358	.1231	.1111	.1001	.0898
3	.4576	.4330	.4087	.3848	.3614	.3386	.3164	.2948	.2740	.2539
4	.7122	.6903	.6678	.6449	.6214	.5976	.5735	.5491	.5246	.5000
5	.8891	.8767	.8634	.8492	.8342	.8183	.8015	.7839	.7654	.7461
6	.9710	.9666	.9617	.9563	.9502	.9436	.9363	.9283	.9196	.9102
7	.9954	.9945	.9935	.9923	.9909	.9893	.9875	.9855	.9831	.9805
8	.9997	.9996	.9995	.9994	.9992	.9991	.9989	.9986	.9984	.9980
9	1.0000	1.0000	1.0000	1.0000	1.0000	1.0000	1.0000	1.0000	1.0000	1.0000

TABLE B (*continued*)

					$n = 10$					
p x	.01	.02	.03	.04	.05	.06	.07	.08	.09	.10
0	.9044	.8171	.7374	.6648	.5987	.5386	.4840	.4344	.3894	.3487
1	.9957	.9838	.9655	.9418	.9139	.8824	.8483	.8121	.7746	.7361
2	.9999	.9991	.9972	.9938	.9885	.9812	.9717	.9599	.9460	.9298
3	1.0000	1.0000	.9999	.9996	.9990	.9980	.9964	.9942	.9912	.9872
4	1.0000	1.0000	1.0000	1.0000	.9999	.9998	.9997	.9994	.9990	.9984
5	1.0000	1.0000	1.0000	1.0000	1.0000	1.0000	1.0000	1.0000	.9999	.9999
6	1.0000	1.0000	1.0000	1.0000	1.0000	1.0000	1.0000	1.0000	1.0000	1.0000
p x	.11	.12	.13	.14	.15	.16	.17	.18	.19	.20
0	.3118	.2785	.2484	.2213	.1969	.1749	.1552	.1374	.1216	.1074
1	.6972	.6583	.6196	.5816	.5443	.5080	.4730	.4392	.4068	.3758
2	.9116	.8913	.8692	.8455	.8202	.7936	.7659	.7372	.7078	.6778
3	.9822	.9761	.9687	.9600	.9500	.9386	.9259	.9117	.8961	.8791
4	.9975	.9963	.9947	.9927	.9901	.9870	.9832	.9787	.9734	.9672
5	.9997	.9996	.9994	.9990	.9986	.9980	.9973	.9963	.9951	.9936
6	1.0000	1.0000	.9999	.9999	.9999	.9998	.9997	.9996	.9994	.9991
7	1.0000	1.0000	1.0000	1.0000	1.0000	1.0000	1.0000	1.0000	.9999	.9999
8	1.0000	1.0000	1.0000	1.0000	1.0000	1.0000	1.0000	1.0000	1.0000	1.0000
p x	.21	.22	.23	.24	.25	.26	.27	.28	.29	.30
0	.0947	.0834	.0733	.0643	.0563	.0492	.0430	.0374	.0326	.0282
1	.3464	.3185	.2921	.2673	.2440	.2222	.2019	.1830	.1655	.1493
2	.6474	.6169	.5863	.5558	.5256	.4958	.4665	.4378	.4099	.3828
3	.8609	.8413	.8206	.7988	.7759	.7521	.7274	.7021	.6761	.6496
4	.9601	.9521	.9431	.9330	.9219	.9096	.8963	.8819	.8663	.8497
5	.9918	.9896	.9870	.9839	.9803	.9761	.9713	.9658	.9596	.9527
6	.9988	.9984	.9979	.9973	.9965	.9955	.9944	.9930	.9913	.9894
7	.9999	.9998	.9998	.9997	.9996	.9994	.9993	.9990	.9988	.9984
8	1.0000	1.0000	1.0000	1.0000	1.0000	1.0000	.9999	.9999	.9999	.9999
9	1.0000	1.0000	1.0000	1.0000	1.0000	1.0000	1.0000	1.0000	1.0000	1.0000
p x	.31	.32	.33	.34	.35	.36	.37	.38	.39	.40
0	.0245	.0211	.0182	.0157	.0135	.0115	.0098	.0084	.0071	.0060
1	.1344	.1206	.1080	.0965	.0860	.0764	.0677	.0598	.0527	.0464
2	.3566	.3313	.3070	.2838	.2616	.2405	.2206	.2017	.1840	.1673
3	.6228	.5956	.5684	.5411	.5138	.4868	.4600	.4336	.4077	.3823
4	.8321	.8133	.7936	.7730	.7515	.7292	.7061	.6823	.6580	.6331
5	.9449	.9363	.9268	.9164	.9051	.8928	.8795	.8652	.8500	.8338
6	.9871	.9845	.9815	.9780	.9740	.9695	.9644	.9587	.9523	.9452
7	.9980	.9975	.9968	.9961	.9952	.9941	.9929	.9914	.9897	.9877
8	.9998	.9997	.9997	.9996	.9995	.9993	.9991	.9989	.9986	.9983
9	1.0000	1.0000	1.0000	1.0000	1.0000	1.0000	1.0000	.9999	.9999	.9999
10	1.0000	1.0000	1.0000	1.0000	1.0000	1.0000	1.0000	1.0000	1.0000	1.0000

TABLE B (*continued*)

				$n = 10$ (*continued*)						
x \ p	.41	.42	.43	.44	.45	.46	.47	.48	.49	.50
0	.0051	.0043	.0036	.0030	.0025	.0021	.0017	.0014	.0012	.0010
1	.0406	.0355	.0309	.0269	.0233	.0201	.0173	.0148	.0126	.0107
2	.1517	.1372	.1236	.1111	.0996	.0889	.0791	.0702	.0621	.0547
3	.3575	.3335	.3102	.2877	.2660	.2453	.2255	.2067	.1888	.1719
4	.6078	.5822	.5564	.5304	.5044	.4784	.4526	.4270	.4018	.3770
5	.8166	.7984	.7793	.7593	.7384	.7168	.6943	.6712	.6474	.6230
6	.9374	.9288	.9194	.9092	.8980	.8859	.8729	.8590	.8440	.8281
7	.9854	.9828	.9798	.9764	.9726	.9683	.9634	.9580	.9520	.9453
8	.9979	.9975	.9969	.9963	.9955	.9946	.9935	.9923	.9909	.9893
9	.9999	.9998	.9998	.9997	.9997	.9996	.9995	.9994	.9992	.9990
10	1.0000	1.0000	1.0000	1.0000	1.0000	1.0000	1.0000	1.0000	1.0000	1.0000

				$n = 11$						
x \ p	.01	.02	.03	.04	.05	.06	.07	.08	.09	.10
0	.8953	.8007	.7153	.6382	.5688	.5063	.4501	.3996	.3544	.3138
1	.9948	.9805	.9587	.9308	.8981	.8618	.8228	.7819	.7399	.6974
2	.9998	.9988	.9963	.9917	.9848	.9752	.9630	.9481	.9305	.9104
3	1.0000	1.0000	.9998	.9993	.9984	.9970	.9947	.9915	.9871	.9815
4	1.0000	1.0000	1.0000	1.0000	.9999	.9997	.9995	.9990	.9983	.9972
5	1.0000	1.0000	1.0000	1.0000	1.0000	1.0000	1.0000	.9999	.9998	.9997
6	1.0000	1.0000	1.0000	1.0000	1.0000	1.0000	1.0000	1.0000	1.0000	1.0000

x \ p	.11	.12	.13	.14	.15	.16	.17	.18	.19	.20
0	.2775	.2451	.2161	.1903	.1673	.1469	.1288	.1127	.0985	.0859
1	.6548	.6127	.5714	.5311	.4922	.4547	.4189	.3849	.3526	.3221
2	.8880	.8634	.8368	.8085	.7788	.7479	.7161	.6836	.6506	.6174
3	.9744	.9659	.9558	.9440	.9306	.9154	.8987	.8803	.8603	.8389
4	.9958	.9939	.9913	.9881	.9841	.9793	.9734	.9666	.9587	.9496
5	.9995	.9992	.9988	.9982	.9973	.9963	.9949	.9932	.9910	.9883
6	1.0000	.9999	.9999	.9998	.9997	.9995	.9993	.9990	.9986	.9980
7	1.0000	1.0000	1.0000	1.0000	1.0000	1.0000	.9999	.9999	.9998	.9998
8	1.0000	1.0000	1.0000	1.0000	1.0000	1.0000	1.0000	1.0000	1.0000	1.0000

x \ p	.21	.22	.23	.24	.25	.26	.27	.28	.29	.30
0	.0748	.0650	.0564	.0489	.0422	.0364	.0314	.0270	.0231	.0198
1	.2935	.2667	.2418	.2186	.1971	.1773	.1590	.1423	.1270	.1130
2	.5842	.5512	.5186	.4866	.4552	.4247	.3951	.3665	.3390	.3127
3	.8160	.7919	.7667	.7404	.7133	.6854	.6570	.6281	.5989	.5696
4	.9393	.9277	.9149	.9008	.8854	.8687	.8507	.8315	.8112	.7897
5	.9852	.9814	.9769	.9717	.9657	.9588	.9510	.9423	.9326	.9218
6	.9973	.9965	.9954	.9941	.9924	.9905	.9881	.9854	.9821	.9784
7	.9997	.9995	.9993	.9991	.9988	.9984	.9979	.9973	.9966	.9957
8	1.0000	1.0000	.9999	.9999	.9999	.9998	.9998	.9997	.9996	.9994
9	1.0000	1.0000	1.0000	1.0000	1.0000	1.0000	1.0000	1.0000	1.0000	1.0000

TABLE B (*continued*)

				$n = 11$ (*continued*)						
p / x	.31	.32	.33	.34	.35	.36	.37	.38	.39	.40
0	.0169	.0144	.0122	.0104	.0088	.0074	.0062	.0052	.0044	.0036
1	.1003	.0888	.0784	.0690	.0606	.0530	.0463	.0403	.0350	.0302
2	.2877	.2639	.2413	.2201	.2001	.1814	.1640	.1478	.1328	.1189
3	.5402	.5110	.4821	.4536	.4256	.3981	.3714	.3455	.3204	.2963
4	.7672	.7437	.7193	.6941	.6683	.6419	.6150	.5878	.5603	.5328
5	.9099	.8969	.8829	.8676	.8513	.8339	.8153	.7957	.7751	.7535
6	.9740	.9691	.9634	.9570	.9499	.9419	.9330	.9232	.9124	.9006
7	.9946	.9933	.9918	.9899	.9878	.9852	.9823	.9790	.9751	.9707
8	.9992	.9990	.9987	.9984	.9980	.9974	.9968	.9961	.9952	.9941
9	.9999	.9999	.9999	.9998	.9998	.9997	.9996	.9995	.9994	.9993
10	1.0000	1.0000	1.0000	1.0000	1.0000	1.0000	1.0000	1.0000	1.0000	10000

p / x	.41	.42	.43	.44	.45	.46	.47	.48	.49	.50
0	.0030	.0025	.0021	.0017	.0014	.0011	.0009	.0008	.0006	.0005
1	.0261	.0224	.0192	.0164	.0139	.0118	.0100	.0084	.0070	.0059
2	.1062	.0945	.0838	.0740	.0652	.0572	.0501	.0436	.0378	.0327
3	.2731	.2510	.2300	.2100	.1911	.1734	.1567	.1412	.1267	.1133
4	.5052	.4777	.4505	.4236	.3971	.3712	.3459	.3213	.2974	.2744
5	.7310	.7076	.6834	.6586	.6331	.6071	.5807	.5540	.5271	.5000
6	.8879	.8740	.8592	.8432	.8262	.8081	.7890	.7688	.7477	.7256
7	.9657	.9601	.9539	.9468	.9390	.9304	.9209	.9105	.8991	.8867
8	.9928	.9913	.9896	.9875	.9852	.9825	.9794	.9759	.9718	.9673
9	.9991	.9988	.9986	.9982	.9978	.9973	.9967	.9960	.9951	.9941
10	.9999	.9999	.9999	.9999	.9998	.9998	.9998	.9997	.9996	.9995
11	1.0000	1.0000	1.0000	1.0000	1.0000	1.0000	1.0000	1.0000	1.0000	1.0000

				$n = 12$						
p / x	.01	.02	.03	.04	.05	.06	.07	.08	.09	.10
0	.8864	.7847	.6938	.6127	.5404	.4759	.4186	.3677	.3225	.2824
1	.9938	.9769	.9514	.9191	.8816	.8405	.7967	.7513	.7052	.6590
2	.9998	.9985	.9952	.9893	.9804	.9684	.9532	.9348	.9134	.8891
3	1.0000	.9999	.9997	.9990	.9978	.9957	.9925	.9880	.9820	.9744
4	1.0000	1.0000	1.0000	.9999	.9998	.9996	.9991	.9984	.9973	.9957
5	1.0000	1.0000	1.0000	1.0000	1.0000	1.0000	.9999	.9998	.9997	.9995
6	1.0000	1.0000	1.0000	1.0000	1.0000	1.0000	1.0000	1.0000	1.0000	.9999
7	1.0000	1.0000	1.0000	1.0000	1.0000	1.0000	1.0000	1.0000	1.0000	1.0000

TABLE B (*continued*)

					$n = 12$ (*continued*)					

x \ p	.11	.12	.13	.14	.15	.16	.17	.18	.19	.20
0	.2470	.2157	.1880	.1637	.1422	.1234	.1069	.0924	.0798	.0687
1	.6133	.5686	.5252	.4834	.4435	.4055	.3696	.3359	.3043	.2749
2	.8623	.8333	.8023	.7697	.7358	.7010	.6656	.6298	.5940	.5583
3	.9649	.9536	.9403	.9250	.9078	.8886	.8676	.8448	.8205	.7946
4	.9935	.9905	.9867	.9819	.9761	.9690	.9607	.9511	.9400	.9274
5	.9991	.9986	.9978	.9967	.9954	.9935	.9912	.9884	.9849	.9806
6	.9999	.9998	.9997	.9996	.9993	.9990	.9985	.9979	.9971	.9961
7	1.0000	1.0000	1.0000	1.0000	.9999	.9999	.9998	.9997	.9996	.9994
8	1.0000	1.0000	1.0000	1.0000	1.0000	1.0000	1.0000	1.0000	1.0000	.9999
9	1.0000	1.0000	1.0000	1.0000	1.0000	1.0000	1.0000	1.0000	1.0000	1.0000

x \ p	.21	.22	.23	.24	.25	.26	.27	.28	.29	.30
0	.0591	.0507	.0434	.0371	.0317	.0270	.0229	.0194	.0164	.0138
1	.2476	.2224	.1991	.1778	.1584	.1406	.1245	.1100	.0968	.0850
2	.5232	.4886	.4550	.4222	.3907	.3603	.3313	.3037	.2775	.2528
3	.7674	.7390	.7096	.6795	.6488	.6176	.5863	.5548	.5235	.4925
4	.9134	.8979	.8808	.8623	.8424	.8210	.7984	.7746	.7496	.7237
5	.9755	.9696	.9626	.9547	.9456	.9354	.9240	.9113	.8974	.8822
6	.9948	.9932	.9911	.9887	.9857	.9822	.9781	.9733	.9678	.9614
7	.9992	.9989	.9984	.9979	.9972	.9964	.9953	.9940	.9924	.9905
8	.9999	.9999	.9998	.9997	.9996	.9995	.9993	.9990	.9987	.9983
9	1.0000	1.0000	1.0000	1.0000	1.0000	.9999	.9999	.9999	.9998	.9998
10	1.0000	1.0000	1.0000	1.0000	1.0000	1.0000	1.0000	1.0000	1.0000	1.0000

x \ p	.31	.32	.33	.34	.35	.36	.37	.38	.39	.40
0	.0116	.0098	.0082	.0068	.0057	.0047	.0039	.0032	.0027	.0022
1	.0744	.0650	.0565	.0491	.0424	.0366	.0315	.0270	.0230	.0196
2	.2296	.2078	.1876	.1687	.1513	.1352	.1205	.1069	.0946	.0834
3	.4619	.4319	.4027	.3742	.3467	.3201	.2947	.2704	.2472	.2253
4	.6968	.6692	.6410	.6124	.5833	.5541	.5249	.4957	.4668	.4382
5	.8657	.8479	.8289	.8087	.7873	.7648	.7412	.7167	.6913	.6652
6	.9542	.9460	.9368	.9266	.9154	.9030	.8894	.8747	.8589	.8418
7	.9882	.9856	.9824	.9787	.9745	.9696	.9641	.9578	.9507	.9427
8	.9978	.9972	.9964	.9955	.9944	.9930	.9915	.9896	.9873	.9847
9	.9997	.9996	.9995	.9993	.9992	.9989	.9986	.9982	.9978	.9972
10	1.0000	1.0000	1.0000	.9999	.9999	.9999	.9999	.9998	.9998	.9997
11	1.0000	1.0000	1.0000	1.0000	1.0000	1.0000	1.0000	1.0000	1.0000	1.0000

TABLE B (*continued*)

n = 12 (*continued*)

x \ p	.41	.42	.43	.44	.45	.46	.47	.48	.49	.50
0	.0018	.0014	.0012	.0010	.0008	.0006	.0005	.0004	.0003	.0002
1	.0166	.0140	.0118	.0099	.0083	.0069	.0057	.0047	.0039	.0032
2	.0733	.0642	.0560	.0487	.0421	.0363	.0312	.0267	.0227	.0193
3	.2047	.1853	.1671	.1502	.1345	.1199	.1066	.0943	.0832	.0730
4	.4101	.3825	.3557	.3296	.3044	.2802	.2570	.2348	.2138	.1938
5	.6384	.6111	.5833	.5552	.5269	.4986	.4703	.4423	.4145	.3872
6	.8235	.8041	.7836	.7620	.7393	.7157	.6911	.6657	.6396	.6128
7	.9338	.9240	.9131	.9012	.8883	.8742	.8589	.8425	.8249	.8062
8	.9817	.9782	.9742	.9696	.9644	.9585	.9519	.9445	.9362	.9270
9	.9965	.9957	.9947	.9935	.9921	.9905	.9886	.9863	.9837	.9807
10	.9996	.9995	.9993	.9991	.9989	.9986	.9983	.9979	.9974	.9968
11	1.0000	1.0000	1.0000	.9999	.9999	.9999	.9999	.9999	.9998	.9998
12	1.0000	1.0000	1.0000	1.0000	1.0000	1.0000	1.0000	1.0000	1.0000	1.0000

n = 13

x \ p	.01	.02	.03	.04	.05	.06	.07	.08	.09	.10
0	.8775	.7690	.6730	.5882	.5133	.4474	.3893	.3383	.2935	.2542
1	.9928	.9730	.9436	.9068	.8646	.8186	.7702	.7206	.6707	.6213
2	.9997	.9980	.9938	.9865	.9755	.9608	.9422	.9201	.8946	.8661
3	1.0000	.9999	.9995	.9986	.9969	.9940	.9897	.9837	.9758	.9658
4	1.0000	1.0000	1.0000	.9999	.9997	.9993	.9987	.9976	.9959	.9935
5	1.0000	1.0000	1.0000	1.0000	1.0000	.9999	.9999	.9997	.9995	.9991
6	1.0000	1.0000	1.0000	1.0000	1.0000	1.0000	1.0000	1.0000	.9999	.9999
7	1.0000	1.0000	1.0000	1.0000	1.0000	1.0000	1.0000	1.0000	1.0000	1.0000

x \ p	.11	.12	.13	.14	.15	.16	.17	.18	.19	.20
0	.2198	.1898	.1636	.1408	.1209	.1037	.0887	.0758	.0646	.0550
1	.5730	.5262	.4814	.4386	.3983	.3604	.3249	.2920	.2616	.2336
2	.8349	.8015	.7663	.7296	.6920	.6537	.6152	.5769	.5389	.5017
3	.9536	.9391	.9224	.9033	.8820	.8586	.8333	.8061	.7774	.7473
4	.9903	.9861	.9807	.9740	.9658	.9562	.9449	.9319	.9173	.9009
5	.9985	.9976	.9964	.9947	.9925	.9896	.9861	.9817	.9763	.9700
6	.9998	.9997	.9995	.9992	.9987	.9981	.9973	.9962	.9948	.9930
7	1.0000	1.0000	.9999	.9999	.9998	.9997	.9996	.9994	.9991	.9988
8	1.0000	1.0000	1.0000	1.0000	1.0000	1.0000	1.0000	.9999	.9999	.9998
9	1.0000	1.0000	1.0000	1.0000	1.0000	1.0000	1.0000	1.0000	1.0000	1.0000

TABLE B (*continued*)

					$n = 13$ (*continued*)					
x \ p	.21	.22	.23	.24	.25	.26	.27	.28	.29	.30
0	.0467	.0396	.0334	.0282	.0238	.0200	.0167	.0140	.0117	.0097
1	.2080	.1846	.1633	.1441	.1267	.1111	.0971	.0846	.0735	.0637
2	.4653	.4301	.3961	.3636	.3326	.3032	.2755	.2495	.2251	.2025
3	.7161	.6839	.6511	.6178	.5843	.5507	.5174	.4845	.4522	.4206
4	.8827	.8629	.8415	.8184	.7940	.7681	.7411	.7130	.6840	.6543
5	.9625	.9538	.9438	.9325	.9198	.9056	.8901	.8730	.8545	.8346
6	.9907	.9880	.9846	.9805	.9757	.9701	.9635	.9560	.9473	.9376
7	.9983	.9976	.9968	.9957	.9944	.9927	.9907	.9882	.9853	.9818
8	.9998	.9996	.9995	.9993	.9990	.9987	.9982	.9976	.9969	.9960
9	1.0000	1.0000	.9999	.9999	.9999	.9998	.9997	.9996	.9995	.9993
10	1.0000	1.0000	1.0000	1.0000	1.0000	1.0000	1.0000	1.0000	.9999	.9999
11	1.0000	1.0000	1.0000	1.0000	1.0000	1.0000	1.0000	1.0000	1.0000	1.0000

x \ p	.31	.32	.33	.34	.35	.36	.37	.38	.39	.40
0	.0080	.0066	.0055	.0045	.0037	.0030	.0025	.0020	.0016	.0013
1	.0550	.0473	.0406	.0347	.0296	.0251	.0213	.0179	.0151	.0126
2	.1815	.1621	.1443	.1280	.1132	.0997	.0875	.0765	.0667	.0579
3	.3899	.3602	.3317	.3043	.2783	.2536	.2302	.2083	.1877	.1686
4	.6240	.5933	.5624	.5314	.5005	.4699	.4397	.4101	.3812	.3530
5	.8133	.7907	.7669	.7419	.7159	.6889	.6612	.6327	.6038	.5744
6	.9267	.9146	.9012	.8865	.8705	.8532	.8346	.8147	.7935	.7712
7	.9777	.9729	.9674	.9610	.9538	.9456	.9365	.9262	.9149	.9023
8	.9948	.9935	.9918	.9898	.9874	.9846	.9813	.9775	.9730	.9679
9	.9991	.9988	.9985	.9980	.9975	.9968	.9960	.9949	.9937	.9922
10	.9999	.9999	.9998	.9997	.9997	.9995	.9994	.9992	.9990	.9987
11	1.0000	1.0000	1.0000	1.0000	1.0000	1.0000	.9999	.9999	.9999	.9999
12	1.0000	1.0000	1.0000	1.0000	1.0000	1.0000	1.0000	1.0000	1.0000	1.0000

x \ p	.41	.42	.43	.44	.45	.46	.47	.48	.49	.50
0	.0010	.0008	.0007	.0005	.0004	.0003	.0003	.0002	.0002	.0001
1	.0105	.0088	.0072	.0060	.0049	.0040	.0033	.0026	.0021	.0017
2	.0501	.0431	.0370	.0316	.0269	.0228	.0192	.0162	.0135	.0112
3	.1508	.1344	.1193	.1055	.0929	.0815	.0712	.0619	.0536	.0461
4	.3258	.2997	.2746	.2507	.2279	.2065	.1863	.1674	.1498	.1334
5	.5448	.5151	.4854	.4559	.4268	.3981	.3701	.3427	.3162	.2905
6	.7476	.7230	.6975	.6710	.6437	.6158	.5873	.5585	.5293	.5000
7	.8886	.8736	.8574	.8400	.8212	.8012	.7800	.7576	.7341	.7095
8	.9621	.9554	.9480	.9395	.9302	.9197	.9082	.8955	.8817	.8666
9	.9904	.9883	.9859	.9830	.9797	.9758	.9713	.9662	.9604	.9539
10	.9983	.9979	.9973	.9967	.9959	.9949	.9937	.9923	.9907	.9888
11	.9998	.9998	.9997	.9996	.9995	.9993	.9991	.9989	.9986	.9983
12	1.0000	1.0000	1.0000	1.0000	1.0000	1.0000	.9999	.9999	.9999	.9999
13	1.0000	1.0000	1.0000	1.0000	1.0000	1.0000	1.0000	1.0000	1.0000	1.0000

TABLE B (*continued*)

					$n = 14$					
x \ p	.01	.02	.03	.04	.05	.06	.07	.08	.09	.10
0	.8687	.7536	.6528	.5647	.4877	.4205	.3620	.3112	.2670	.2288
1	.9916	.9690	.9355	.8941	.8470	.7963	.7436	.6900	.6368	.5846
2	.9997	.9975	.9923	.9833	.9699	.9522	.9302	.9042	.8745	.8416
3	1.0000	.9999	.9994	.9981	.9958	.9920	.9864	.9786	.9685	.9559
4	1.0000	1.0000	1.0000	.9998	.9996	.9990	.9980	.9965	.9941	.9908
5	1.0000	1.0000	1.0000	1.0000	1.0000	.9999	.9998	.9996	.9992	.9985
6	1.0000	1.0000	1.0000	1.0000	1.0000	1.0000	1.0000	1.0000	.9999	.9998
7	1.0000	1.0000	1.0000	1.0000	1.0000	1.0000	1.0000	1.0000	1.0000	1.0000

x \ p	.11	.12	.13	.14	.15	.16	.17	.18	.19	.20
0	.1956	.1670	.1423	.1211	.1028	.0871	.0736	.0621	.0523	.0440
1	.5342	.4859	.4401	.3969	.3567	.3193	.2848	.2531	.2242	.1979
2	.8061	.7685	.7292	.6889	.6479	.6068	.5659	.5256	.4862	.4481
3	.9406	.9226	.9021	.8790	.8535	.8258	.7962	.7649	.7321	.6982
4	.9863	.9804	.9731	.9641	.9533	.9406	.9259	.9093	.8907	.8702
5	.9976	.9962	.9943	.9918	.9885	.9843	.9791	.9727	.9651	.9561
6	.9997	.9994	.9991	.9985	.9978	.9968	.9954	.9936	.9913	.9884
7	1.0000	.9999	.9999	.9998	.9997	.9995	.9992	.9988	.9983	.9976
8	1.0000	1.0000	1.0000	1.0000	1.0000	.9999	.9999	.9998	.9997	.9996
9	1.0000	1.0000	1.0000	1.0000	1.0000	1.0000	1.0000	1.0000	1.0000	1.0000

x \ p	.21	.22	.23	.24	.25	.26	.27	.28	.29	.30
0	.0369	.0309	.0258	.0214	.0178	.0148	.0122	.0101	.0083	.0068
1	.1741	.1527	.1335	.1163	.1010	.0874	.0754	.0648	.0556	.0475
2	.4113	.3761	.3426	.3109	.2811	.2533	.2273	.2033	.1812	.1608
3	.6634	.6281	.5924	.5568	.5213	.4864	.4521	.4187	.3863	.3552
4	.8477	.8235	.7977	.7703	.7415	.7116	.6807	.6490	.6168	.5842
5	.9457	.9338	.9203	.9051	.8883	.8699	.8498	.8282	.8051	.7805
6	.9848	.9804	.9752	.9690	.9617	.9533	.9437	.9327	.9204	.9067
7	.9967	.9955	.9940	.9921	.9897	.9868	.9833	.9792	.9743	.9685
8	.9994	.9992	.9989	.9984	.9978	.9971	.9962	.9950	.9935	.9917
9	.9999	.9999	.9998	.9998	.9997	.9995	.9993	.9991	.9988	.9983
10	1.0000	1.0000	1.0000	1.0000	1.0000	.9999	.9999	.9999	.9998	.9998
11	1.0000	1.0000	1.0000	1.0000	1.0000	1.0000	1.0000	1.0000	1.0000	1.0000

TABLE B (*continued*)

					$n = 14$ (*continued*)					
x \ p	.31	.32	.33	.34	.35	.36	.37	.38	.39	.40
0	.0055	.0045	.0037	.0030	.0024	.0019	.0016	.0012	.0010	.0008
1	.0404	.0343	.0290	.0244	.0205	.0172	.0143	.0119	.0098	.0081
2	.1423	.1254	.1101	.0963	.0839	.0729	.0630	.0543	.0466	.0398
3	.3253	.2968	.2699	.2444	.2205	.1982	.1774	.1582	.1405	.1243
4	.5514	.5187	.4862	.4542	.4227	.3920	.3622	.3334	.3057	.2793
5	.7546	.7276	.6994	.6703	.6405	.6101	.5792	.5481	.5169	.4859
6	.8916	.8750	.8569	.8374	.8164	.7941	.7704	.7455	.7195	.6925
7	.9619	.9542	.9455	.9357	.9247	.9124	.8988	.8838	.8675	.8499
8	.9895	.9869	.9837	.9800	.9757	.9706	.9647	.9580	.9503	.9417
9	.9978	.9971	.9963	.9952	.9940	.9924	.9905	.9883	.9856	.9825
10	.9997	.9995	.9994	.9992	.9989	.9986	.9981	.9976	.9969	.9961
11	1.0000	.9999	.9999	.9999	.9999	.9998	.9997	.9997	.9995	.9994
12	1.0000	1.0000	1.0000	1.0000	1.0000	1.0000	1.0000	1.0000	1.0000	.9999
13	1.0000	1.0000	1.0000	1.0000	1.0000	1.0000	1.0000	1.0000	1.0000	1.0000

x \ p	.41	.42	.43	.44	.45	.46	.47	.48	.49	.50
0	.0006	.0005	.0004	.0003	.0002	.0002	.0001	.0001	.0001	.0001
1	.0066	.0054	.0044	.0036	.0029	.0023	.0019	.0015	.0012	.0009
2	.0339	.0287	.0242	.0203	.0170	.0142	.0117	.0097	.0079	.0065
3	.1095	.0961	.0839	.0730	.0632	.0545	.0468	.0399	.0339	.0287
4	.2541	.2303	.2078	.1868	.1672	.1490	.1322	.1167	.1026	.0898
5	.4550	.4246	.3948	.3656	.3373	.3100	.2837	.2585	.2346	.2120
6	.6645	.6357	.6063	.5764	.5461	.5157	.4852	.4549	.4249	.3953
7	.8308	.8104	.7887	.7656	.7414	.7160	.6895	.6620	.6337	.6047
8	.9320	.9211	.9090	.8957	.8811	.8652	.8480	.8293	.8094	.7880
9	.9788	.9745	.9696	.9639	.9574	.9500	.9417	.9323	.9218	.9102
10	.9951	.9939	.9924	.9907	.9886	.9861	.9832	.9798	.9759	.9713
11	.9992	.9990	.9987	.9983	.9978	.9973	.9966	.9958	.9947	.9935
12	.9999	.9999	.9999	.9998	.9997	.9997	.9996	.9994	.9993	.9991
13	1.0000	1.0000	1.0000	1.0000	1.0000	1.0000	1.0000	1.0000	1.0000	.9999
14	1.0000	1.0000	1.0000	1.0000	1.0000	1.0000	1.0000	1.0000	1.0000	1.0000

					$n = 15$					
x \ p	.01	.02	.03	.04	.05	.06	.07	.08	.09	.10
0	.8601	.7386	.6333	.5421	.4633	.3953	.3367	.2863	.2430	.2059
1	.9904	.9647	.9270	.8809	.8290	.7738	.7168	.6597	.6035	.5490
2	.9996	.9970	.9906	.9797	.9638	.9429	.9171	.8870	.8531	.8159
3	1.0000	.9998	.9992	.9976	.9945	.9896	.9825	.9727	.9601	.9444
4	1.0000	1.0000	.9999	.9998	.9994	.9986	.9972	.9950	.9918	.9873
5	1.0000	1.0000	1.0000	1.0000	.9999	.9999	.9997	.9993	.9987	.9978
6	1.0000	1.0000	1.0000	1.0000	1.0000	1.0000	1.0000	.9999	.9998	.9997
7	1.0000	1.0000	1.0000	1.0000	1.0000	1.0000	1.0000	1.0000	1.0000	1.0000

TABLE B (*continued*)

					$n = 15$ (*continued*)					
x \ p	.11	.12	.13	.14	.15	.16	.17	.18	.19	.20
0	.1741	.1470	.1238	.1041	.0874	.0731	.0611	.0510	.0424	.0352
1	.4969	.4476	.4013	.3583	.3186	.2821	.2489	.2187	.1915	.1671
2	.7762	.7346	.6916	.6480	.6042	.5608	.5181	.4766	.4365	.3980
3	.9258	.9041	.8796	.8524	.8227	.7908	.7571	.7218	.6854	.6482
4	.9813	.9735	.9639	.9522	.9383	.9222	.9039	.8833	.8606	.8358
5	.9963	.9943	.9916	.9879	.9832	.9773	.9700	.9613	.9510	.9389
6	.9994	.9990	.9985	.9976	.9964	.9948	.9926	.9898	.9863	.9819
7	.9999	.9999	.9998	.9996	.9994	.9990	.9986	.9979	.9970	.9958
8	1.0000	1.0000	1.0000	1.0000	.9999	.9999	.9998	.9997	.9995	.9992
9	1.0000	1.0000	1.0000	1.0000	1.0000	1.0000	1.0000	1.0000	.9999	.9999
10	1.0000	1.0000	1.0000	1.0000	1.0000	1.0000	1.0000	1.0000	1.0000	1.0000

x \ p	.21	.22	.23	.24	.25	.26	.27	.28	.29	.30
0	.0291	.0241	.0198	.0163	.0134	.0109	.0089	.0072	.0059	.0047
1	.1453	.1259	.1087	.0935	.0802	.0685	.0583	.0495	.0419	.0353
2	.3615	.3269	.2945	.2642	.2361	.2101	.1863	.1645	.1447	.1268
3	.6105	.5726	.5350	.4978	.4613	.4258	.3914	.3584	.3268	.2969
4	.8090	.7805	.7505	.7190	.6865	.6531	.6190	.5846	.5500	.5155
5	.9252	.9095	.8921	.8728	.8516	.8287	.8042	.7780	.7505	.7216
6	.9766	.9702	.9626	.9537	.9434	.9316	.9183	.9035	.8870	.8689
7	.9942	.9922	.9896	.9865	.9827	.9781	.9726	.9662	.9587	.9500
8	.9989	.9984	.9977	.9969	.9958	.9944	.9927	.9906	.9879	.9848
9	.9998	.9997	.9996	.9994	.9992	.9989	.9985	.9979	.9972	.9963
10	1.0000	1.0000	.9999	.9999	.9999	.9998	.9998	.9997	.9995	.9993
11	1.0000	1.0000	1.0000	1.0000	1.0000	1.0000	1.0000	1.0000	.9999	.9999
12	1.0000	1.0000	1.0000	1.0000	1.0000	1.0000	1.0000	1.0000	1.0000	1.0000

x \ p	.31	.32	.33	.34	.35	.36	.37	.38	.39	.40
0	.0038	.0031	.0025	.0020	.0016	.0012	.0010	.0008	.0006	.0005
1	.0296	.0248	.0206	.0171	.0142	.0117	.0096	.0078	.0064	.0052
2	.1107	.0962	.0833	.0719	.0617	.0528	.0450	.0382	.0322	.0271
3	.2686	.2420	.2171	.1940	.1727	.1531	.1351	.1187	.1039	.0905
4	.4813	.4477	.4148	.3829	.3519	.3222	.2938	.2668	.2413	.2173
5	.6916	.6607	.6291	.5968	.5643	.5316	.4989	.4665	.4346	.4032
6	.8491	.8278	.8049	.7806	.7548	.7278	.6997	.6705	.6405	.6098
7	.9401	.9289	.9163	.9023	.8868	.8698	.8513	.8313	.8098	.7869
8	.9810	.9764	.9711	.9649	.9578	.9496	.9403	.9298	.9180	.9050
9	.9952	.9938	.9921	.9901	.9876	.9846	.9810	.9768	.9719	.9662
10	.9991	.9988	.9984	.9978	.9972	.9963	.9953	.9941	.9925	.9907
11	.9999	.9998	.9997	.9996	.9995	.9994	.9991	.9989	.9985	.9981
12	1.0000	1.0000	1.0000	1.0000	.9999	.9999	.9999	.9998	.9998	.9997
13	1.0000	1.0000	1.0000	1.0000	1.0000	1.0000	1.0000	1.0000	1.0000	1.0000

TABLE B (*continued*)

<table>
<tr><td colspan="11" align="center">n = 15 (continued)</td></tr>
<tr><td>p
x</td><td>.41</td><td>.42</td><td>.43</td><td>.44</td><td>.45</td><td>.46</td><td>.47</td><td>.48</td><td>.49</td><td>.50</td></tr>
<tr><td>0</td><td>.0004</td><td>.0003</td><td>.0002</td><td>.0002</td><td>.0001</td><td>.0001</td><td>.0001</td><td>.0001</td><td>.0000</td><td>.0000</td></tr>
<tr><td>1</td><td>.0042</td><td>.0034</td><td>.0027</td><td>.0021</td><td>.0017</td><td>.0013</td><td>.0010</td><td>.0008</td><td>.0006</td><td>.0005</td></tr>
<tr><td>2</td><td>.0227</td><td>.0189</td><td>.0157</td><td>.0130</td><td>.0107</td><td>.0087</td><td>.0071</td><td>.0057</td><td>.0046</td><td>.0037</td></tr>
<tr><td>3</td><td>.0785</td><td>.0678</td><td>.0583</td><td>.0498</td><td>.0424</td><td>.0359</td><td>.0303</td><td>.0254</td><td>.0212</td><td>.0176</td></tr>
<tr><td>4</td><td>.1948</td><td>.1739</td><td>.1546</td><td>.1367</td><td>.1204</td><td>.1055</td><td>.0920</td><td>.0799</td><td>.0690</td><td>.0592</td></tr>
<tr><td>5</td><td>.3726</td><td>.3430</td><td>.3144</td><td>.2869</td><td>.2608</td><td>.2359</td><td>.2125</td><td>.1905</td><td>.1699</td><td>.1509</td></tr>
<tr><td>6</td><td>.5786</td><td>.5470</td><td>.5153</td><td>.4836</td><td>.4522</td><td>.4211</td><td>.3905</td><td>.3606</td><td>.3316</td><td>.3036</td></tr>
<tr><td>7</td><td>.7626</td><td>.7370</td><td>.7102</td><td>.6824</td><td>.6535</td><td>.6238</td><td>.5935</td><td>.5626</td><td>.5314</td><td>.5000</td></tr>
<tr><td>8</td><td>.8905</td><td>.8746</td><td>.8573</td><td>.8385</td><td>.8182</td><td>.7966</td><td>.7735</td><td>.7490</td><td>.7233</td><td>.6964</td></tr>
<tr><td>9</td><td>.9596</td><td>.9521</td><td>.9435</td><td>.9339</td><td>.9231</td><td>.9110</td><td>.8976</td><td>.8829</td><td>.8667</td><td>.8491</td></tr>
<tr><td>10</td><td>.9884</td><td>.9857</td><td>.9826</td><td>.9789</td><td>.9745</td><td>.9695</td><td>.9637</td><td>.9570</td><td>.9494</td><td>.9408</td></tr>
<tr><td>11</td><td>.9975</td><td>.9968</td><td>.9960</td><td>.9949</td><td>.9937</td><td>.9921</td><td>.9903</td><td>.9881</td><td>.9855</td><td>.9824</td></tr>
<tr><td>12</td><td>.9996</td><td>.9995</td><td>.9993</td><td>.9991</td><td>.9989</td><td>.9986</td><td>.9982</td><td>.9977</td><td>.9971</td><td>.9963</td></tr>
<tr><td>13</td><td>1.0000</td><td>1.0000</td><td>.9999</td><td>.9999</td><td>.9999</td><td>.9998</td><td>.9998</td><td>.9997</td><td>.9996</td><td>.9995</td></tr>
<tr><td>14</td><td>1.0000</td><td>1.0000</td><td>1.0000</td><td>1.0000</td><td>1.0000</td><td>1.0000</td><td>1.0000</td><td>1.0000</td><td>1.0000</td><td>1.0000</td></tr>
<tr><td colspan="11" align="center">n = 16</td></tr>
<tr><td>p
x</td><td>.01</td><td>.02</td><td>.03</td><td>.04</td><td>.05</td><td>.06</td><td>.07</td><td>.08</td><td>.09</td><td>.10</td></tr>
<tr><td>0</td><td>.8515</td><td>.7238</td><td>.6143</td><td>.5204</td><td>.4401</td><td>.3716</td><td>.3131</td><td>.2634</td><td>.2211</td><td>.1853</td></tr>
<tr><td>1</td><td>.9891</td><td>.9601</td><td>.9182</td><td>.8673</td><td>.8108</td><td>.7511</td><td>.6902</td><td>.6299</td><td>.5711</td><td>.5147</td></tr>
<tr><td>2</td><td>.9995</td><td>.9963</td><td>.9887</td><td>.9758</td><td>.9571</td><td>.9327</td><td>.9031</td><td>.8688</td><td>.8306</td><td>.7892</td></tr>
<tr><td>3</td><td>1.0000</td><td>.9998</td><td>.9989</td><td>.9968</td><td>.9930</td><td>.9868</td><td>.9779</td><td>.9658</td><td>.9504</td><td>.9316</td></tr>
<tr><td>4</td><td>1.0000</td><td>1.0000</td><td>.9999</td><td>.9997</td><td>.9991</td><td>.9981</td><td>.9962</td><td>.9932</td><td>.9889</td><td>.9830</td></tr>
<tr><td>5</td><td>1.0000</td><td>1.0000</td><td>1.0000</td><td>1.0000</td><td>.9999</td><td>.9998</td><td>.9995</td><td>.9990</td><td>.9981</td><td>.9967</td></tr>
<tr><td>6</td><td>1.0000</td><td>1.0000</td><td>1.0000</td><td>1.0000</td><td>1.0000</td><td>1.0000</td><td>.9999</td><td>.9999</td><td>.9997</td><td>.9995</td></tr>
<tr><td>7</td><td>1.0000</td><td>1.0000</td><td>1.0000</td><td>1.0000</td><td>1.0000</td><td>1.0000</td><td>1.0000</td><td>1.0000</td><td>1.0000</td><td>.9999</td></tr>
<tr><td>8</td><td>1.0000</td><td>1.0000</td><td>1.0000</td><td>1.0000</td><td>1.0000</td><td>1.0000</td><td>1.0000</td><td>1.0000</td><td>1.0000</td><td>1.0000</td></tr>
<tr><td>p
x</td><td>.11</td><td>.12</td><td>.13</td><td>.14</td><td>.15</td><td>.16</td><td>.17</td><td>.18</td><td>.19</td><td>.20</td></tr>
<tr><td>0</td><td>.1550</td><td>.1293</td><td>.1077</td><td>.0895</td><td>.0743</td><td>.0614</td><td>.0507</td><td>.0418</td><td>.0343</td><td>.0281</td></tr>
<tr><td>1</td><td>.4614</td><td>.4115</td><td>.3653</td><td>.3227</td><td>.2839</td><td>.2487</td><td>.2170</td><td>.1885</td><td>.1632</td><td>.1407</td></tr>
<tr><td>2</td><td>.7455</td><td>.7001</td><td>.6539</td><td>.6074</td><td>.5614</td><td>.5162</td><td>.4723</td><td>.4302</td><td>.3899</td><td>.3518</td></tr>
<tr><td>3</td><td>.9093</td><td>.8838</td><td>.8552</td><td>.8237</td><td>.7899</td><td>.7540</td><td>.7164</td><td>.6777</td><td>.6381</td><td>.5981</td></tr>
<tr><td>4</td><td>.9752</td><td>.9652</td><td>.9529</td><td>.9382</td><td>.9209</td><td>.9012</td><td>.8789</td><td>.8542</td><td>.8273</td><td>.7982</td></tr>
<tr><td>5</td><td>.9947</td><td>.9918</td><td>.9880</td><td>.9829</td><td>.9765</td><td>.9685</td><td>.9588</td><td>.9473</td><td>.9338</td><td>.9183</td></tr>
<tr><td>6</td><td>.9991</td><td>.9985</td><td>.9976</td><td>.9962</td><td>.9944</td><td>.9920</td><td>.9888</td><td>.9847</td><td>.9796</td><td>.9733</td></tr>
<tr><td>7</td><td>.9999</td><td>.9998</td><td>.9996</td><td>.9993</td><td>.9989</td><td>.9984</td><td>.9976</td><td>.9964</td><td>.9949</td><td>.9930</td></tr>
<tr><td>8</td><td>1.0000</td><td>1.0000</td><td>.9999</td><td>.9999</td><td>.9998</td><td>.9997</td><td>.9996</td><td>.9993</td><td>.9990</td><td>.9985</td></tr>
<tr><td>9</td><td>1.0000</td><td>1.0000</td><td>1.0000</td><td>1.0000</td><td>1.0000</td><td>1.0000</td><td>.9999</td><td>.9999</td><td>.9998</td><td>.9998</td></tr>
<tr><td>10</td><td>1.0000</td><td>1.0000</td><td>1.0000</td><td>1.0000</td><td>1.0000</td><td>1.0000</td><td>1.0000</td><td>1.0000</td><td>1.0000</td><td>1.0000</td></tr>
</table>

TABLE B (*continued*)

					$n = 16$ (*continued*)					
x\p	.21	.22	.23	.24	.25	.26	.27	.28	.29	.30
0	.0230	.0188	.0153	.0124	.0100	.0081	.0065	.0052	.0042	.0033
1	.1209	.1035	.0883	.0750	.0635	.0535	.0450	.0377	.0314	.0261
2	.3161	.2827	.2517	.2232	.1971	.1733	.1518	.1323	.1149	.0994
3	.5582	.5186	.4797	.4417	.4050	.3697	.3360	.3041	.2740	.2459
4	.7673	.7348	.7009	.6659	.6302	.5940	.5575	.5212	.4853	.4499
5	.9008	.8812	.8595	.8359	.8103	.7831	.7542	.7239	.6923	.6598
6	.9658	.9568	.9464	.9342	.9204	.9049	.8875	.8683	.8474	.8247
7	.9905	.9873	.9834	.9786	.9729	.9660	.9580	.9486	.9379	.9256
8	.9979	.9970	.9959	.9944	.9925	.9902	.9873	.9837	.9794	.9743
9	.9996	.9994	.9992	.9988	.9984	.9977	.9969	.9959	.9945	.9929
10	.9999	.9999	.9999	.9998	.9997	.9996	.9994	.9992	.9989	.9984
11	1.0000	1.0000	1.0000	1.0000	1.0000	.9999	.9999	.9999	.9998	.9997
12	1.0000	1.0000	1.0000	1.0000	1.0000	1.0000	1.0000	1.0000	1.0000	1.0000

x\p	.31	.32	.33	.34	.35	.36	.37	.38	.39	.40
0	.0026	.0021	.0016	.0013	.0010	.0008	.0006	.0005	.0004	.0003
1	.0216	.0178	.0146	.0120	.0098	.0079	.0064	.0052	.0041	.0033
2	.0856	.0734	.0626	.0533	.0451	.0380	.0319	.0266	.0222	.0183
3	.2196	.1953	.1730	.1525	.1339	.1170	.1018	.0881	.0759	.0651
4	.4154	.3819	.3496	.3187	.2892	.2613	.2351	.2105	.1877	.1666
5	.6264	.5926	.5584	.5241	.4900	.4562	.4230	.3906	.3592	.3288
6	.8003	.7743	.7469	.7181	.6881	.6572	.6254	.5930	.5602	.5272
7	.9119	.8965	.8795	.8609	.8406	.8187	.7952	.7702	.7438	.7161
8	.9683	.9612	.9530	.9436	.9329	.9209	.9074	.8924	.8758	.8577
9	.9908	.9883	.9852	.9815	.9771	.9720	.9659	.9589	.9509	.9417
10	.9979	.9972	.9963	.9952	.9938	.9921	.9900	.9875	.9845	.9809
11	.9996	.9995	.9993	.9990	.9987	.9983	.9977	.9970	.9962	.9951
12	1.0000	.9999	.9999	.9999	.9998	.9997	.9996	.9995	.9993	.9991
13	1.0000	1.0000	1.0000	1.0000	1.0000	1.0000	1.0000	.9999	.9999	.9999
14	1.0000	1.0000	1.0000	1.0000	1.0000	1.0000	1.0000	1.0000	1.0000	1.0000

TABLE B (*continued*)

					$n = 16$ (*continued*)					
p x	.41	.42	.43	.44	.45	.46	.47	.48	.49	.50
0	.0002	.0002	.0001	.0001	.0001	.0001	.0000	.0000	.0000	.0000
1	.0026	.0021	.0016	.0013	.0010	.0008	.0006	.0005	.0003	.0003
2	.0151	.0124	.0101	.0082	.0066	.0053	.0042	.0034	.0027	.0021
3	.0556	.0473	.0400	.0336	.0281	.0234	.0194	.0160	.0131	.0106
4	.1471	.1293	.1131	.0985	.0853	.0735	.0630	.0537	.0456	.0384
5	.2997	.2720	.2457	.2208	.1976	.1759	.1559	.1374	.1205	.1051
6	.4942	.4613	.4289	.3971	.3660	.3359	.3068	.2790	.2524	.2272
7	.6872	.6572	.6264	.5949	.5629	.5306	.4981	.4657	.4335	.4018
8	.8381	.8168	.7940	.7698	.7441	.7171	.6889	.6596	.6293	.5982
9	.9313	.9195	.9064	.8919	.8759	.8584	.8393	.8186	.7964	.7728
10	.9766	.9716	.9658	.9591	.9514	.9426	.9326	.9214	.9089	.8949
11	.9938	.9922	.9902	.9879	.9851	.9817	.9778	.9732	.9678	.9616
12	.9988	.9984	.9979	.9973	.9965	.9956	.9945	.9931	.9914	.9894
13	.9998	.9998	.9997	.9996	.9994	.9993	.9990	.9987	.9984	.9979
14	1.0000	1.0000	1.0000	1.0000	.9999	.9999	.9999	.9999	.9998	.9997
15	1.0000	1.0000	1.0000	1.0000	1.0000	1.0000	1.0000	1.0000	1.0000	1.0000

					$n = 17$					
p x	.01	.02	.03	.04	.05	.06	.07	.08	.09	.10
0	.8429	.7093	.5958	.4996	.4181	.3493	.2912	.2423	.2012	.1668
1	.9877	.9554	.9091	.8535	.7922	.7283	.6638	.6005	.5396	.4818
2	.9994	.9956	.9866	.9714	.9497	.9218	.8882	.8497	.8073	.7618
3	1.0000	.9997	.9986	.9960	.9912	.9836	.9727	.9581	.9397	.9174
4	1.0000	1.0000	.9999	.9996	.9988	.9974	.9949	.9911	.9855	.9779
5	1.0000	1.0000	1.0000	1.0000	.9999	.9997	.9993	.9985	.9973	.9953
6	1.0000	1.0000	1.0000	1.0000	1.0000	1.0000	.9999	.9998	.9996	.9992
7	1.0000	1.0000	1.0000	1.0000	1.0000	1.0000	1.0000	1.0000	1.0000	.9999
8	1.0000	1.0000	1.0000	1.0000	1.0000	1.0000	1.0000	1.0000	1.0000	1.0000

p x	.11	.12	.13	.14	.15	.16	.17	.18	.19	.20
0	.1379	.1138	.0937	.0770	.0631	.0516	.0421	.0343	.0278	.0225
1	.4277	.3777	.3318	.2901	.2525	.2187	.1887	.1621	.1387	.1182
2	.7142	.6655	.6164	.5676	.5198	.4734	.4289	.3867	.3468	.3096
3	.8913	.8617	.8290	.7935	.7556	.7159	.6749	.6331	.5909	.5489
4	.9679	.9554	.9402	.9222	.9013	.8776	.8513	.8225	.7913	.7582
5	.9925	.9886	.9834	.9766	.9681	.9577	.9452	.9305	.9136	.8943
6	.9986	.9977	.9963	.9944	.9917	.9882	.9837	.9780	.9709	.9623
7	.9998	.9996	.9993	.9989	.9983	.9973	.9961	.9943	.9920	.9891
8	1.0000	.9999	.9999	.9998	.9997	.9995	.9992	.9988	.9982	.9974
9	1.0000	1.0000	1.0000	1.0000	1.0000	.9999	.9999	.9998	.9997	.9995
10	1.0000	1.0000	1.0000	1.0000	1.0000	1.0000	1.0000	1.0000	1.0000	.9999
11	1.0000	1.0000	1.0000	1.0000	1.0000	1.0000	1.0000	1.0000	1.0000	1.0000

TABLE B (*continued*)

n = 17 (*continued*)

p x	.21	.22	.23	.24	.25	.26	.27	.28	.29	.30
0	.0182	.0146	.0118	.0094	.0075	.0060	.0047	.0038	.0030	.0023
1	.1004	.0849	.0715	.0600	.0501	.0417	.0346	.0286	.0235	.0193
2	.2751	.2433	.2141	.1877	.1637	.1422	.1229	.1058	.0907	.0774
3	.5073	.4667	.4272	.3893	.3530	.3186	.2863	.2560	.2279	.2019
4	.7234	.6072	.6500	.6121	.5739	.5357	.4977	.4601	.4210	.3887
5	.8727	.8490	.8230	.7951	.7653	.7339	.7011	.6671	.6323	.5968
6	.9521	.9402	.9264	.9106	.8929	.8732	.8515	.8279	.8024	.7752
7	.9853	.9806	.9749	.9680	.9598	.9501	.9389	.9261	.9116	.8954
8	.9963	.9949	.9930	.9906	.9876	.9839	.9794	.9739	.9674	.9597
9	.9993	.9989	.9984	.9978	.9969	.9958	.9943	.9925	.9902	.9873
10	.9999	.9998	.9997	.9996	.9994	.9991	.9987	.9982	.9976	.9968
11	1.0000	1.0000	1.0000	.9999	.9999	.9998	.9998	.9997	.9995	.9993
12	1.0000	1.0000	1.0000	1.0000	1.0000	1.0000	1.0000	1.0000	.9999	.9999
13	1.0000	1.0000	1.0000	1.0000	1.0000	1.0000	1.0000	1.0000	1.0000	1.0000

p x	.31	.32	.33	.34	.35	.36	.37	.38	.39	.40
0	.0018	.0014	.0011	.0009	.0007	.0005	.0004	.0003	.0002	.0002
1	.0157	.0128	.0104	.0083	.0067	.0054	.0043	.0034	.0027	.0021
2	.0657	.0556	.0468	.0392	.0327	.0272	.0225	.0185	.0151	.0123
3	.1781	.1563	.1366	.1188	.1028	.0885	.0759	.0648	.0550	.0464
4	.3547	.3222	.2913	.2622	.2348	.2094	.1858	.1640	.1441	.1260
5	.5610	.5251	.4895	.4542	.4197	.3861	.3535	.3222	.2923	.2639
6	.7464	.7162	.6847	.6521	.6188	.5848	.5505	.5161	.4818	.4478
7	.8773	.8574	.8358	.8123	.7872	.7605	.7324	.7029	.6722	.6405
8	.9508	.9405	.9288	.9155	.9006	.8841	.8659	.8459	.8243	.8011
9	.9838	.9796	.9746	.9686	.9617	.9536	.9443	.9336	.9216	.9081
10	.9957	.9943	.9926	.9905	.9880	.9849	.9811	.9766	.9714	.9652
11	.9991	.9987	.9983	.9977	.9970	.9960	.9949	.9934	.9916	.9894
12	.9998	.9998	.9997	.9996	.9994	.9992	.9989	.9985	.9981	.9975
13	1.0000	1.0000	1.0000	.9999	.9999	.9999	.9998	.9998	.9997	.9995
14	1.0000	1.0000	1.0000	1.0000	1.0000	1.0000	1.0000	1.0000	1.0000	.9999
15	1.0000	1.0000	1.0000	1.0000	1.0000	1.0000	1.0000	1.0000	1.0000	1.0000

TABLE B (*continued*)

					$n = 17$ (*continued*)					
p x	.41	.42	.43	.44	.45	.46	.47	.48	.49	.50
0	.0001	.0001	.0001	.0001	.0000	.0000	.0000	.0000	.0000	.0000
1	.0016	.0013	.0010	.0008	.0006	.0004	.0003	.0002	.0002	.0001
2	.0100	.0080	.0065	.0052	.0041	.0032	.0025	.0020	.0015	.0012
3	.0390	.0326	.0271	.0224	.0184	.0151	.0123	.0099	.0080	.0064
4	.1096	.0949	.0817	.0699	.0596	.0505	.0425	.0356	.0296	.0245
5	.2372	.2121	.1887	.1670	.1471	.1288	.1122	.0972	.0838	.0717
6	.4144	.3818	.3501	.3195	.2902	.2623	.2359	.2110	.1878	.1662
7	.6080	.5750	.5415	.5079	.4743	.4410	.4082	.3761	.3448	.3145
8	.7762	.7498	.7220	.6928	.6626	.6313	.5992	.5665	.5333	.5000
9	.8930	.8764	.8581	.8382	.8166	.7934	.7686	.7423	.7145	.6855
10	.9580	.9497	.9403	.9295	.9174	.9038	.8888	.8721	.8538	.8338
11	.9867	.9835	.9797	.9752	.9699	.9637	.9566	.9483	.9389	.9283
12	.9967	.9958	.9946	.9931	.9914	.9892	.9866	.9835	.9798	.9755
13	.9994	.9992	.9989	.9986	.9981	.9976	.9969	.9960	.9950	.9936
14	.9999	.9999	.9998	.9998	.9997	.9996	.9995	.9993	.9991	.9988
15	1.0000	1.0000	1.0000	1.0000	1.0000	1.0000	.9999	.9999	.9999	.9999
16	1.0000	1.0000	1.0000	1.0000	1.0000	1.0000	1.0000	1.0000	1.0000	1.0000

					$n = 18$					
p x	.01	.02	.03	.04	.05	.06	.07	.08	.09	.10
0	.8345	.6951	.5780	.4796	.3972	.3283	.2708	.2229	.1831	.1501
1	.9862	.9505	.8997	.8393	.7735	.7055	.6378	.5719	.5091	.4503
2	.9993	.9948	.9843	.9667	.9419	.9102	.8725	.8298	.7832	.7338
3	1.0000	.9996	.9982	.9950	.9891	.9799	.9667	.9494	.9277	.9018
4	1.0000	1.0000	.9998	.9994	.9985	.9966	.9933	.9884	.9814	.9718
5	1.0000	1.0000	1.0000	.9999	.9998	.9995	.9990	.9979	.9962	.9936
6	1.0000	1.0000	1.0000	1.0000	1.0000	1.0000	.9999	.9997	.9994	.9988
7	1.0000	1.0000	1.0000	1.0000	1.0000	1.0000	1.0000	1.0000	.9999	.9998
8	1.0000	1.0000	1.0000	1.0000	1.0000	1.0000	1.0000	1.0000	1.0000	1.0000
p x	.11	.12	.13	.14	.15	.16	.17	.18	.19	.20
0	.1227	.1002	.0815	.0662	.0536	.0434	.0349	.0281	.0225	.0180
1	.3958	.3460	.3008	.2602	.2241	.1920	.1638	.1391	.1176	.0991
2	.6827	.6310	.5794	.5287	.4797	.4327	.3881	.3462	.3073	.2713
3	.8718	.8382	.8014	.7618	.7202	.6771	.6331	.5888	.5446	.5010
4	.9595	.9442	.9257	.9041	.8794	.8518	.8213	.7884	.7533	.7164
5	.9898	.9846	.9778	.9690	.9581	.9449	.9292	.9111	.8903	.8671
6	.9979	.9966	.9946	.9919	.9882	.9833	.9771	.9694	.9600	.9487
7	.9997	.9994	.9989	.9983	.9973	.9959	.9940	.9914	.9880	.9837
8	1.0000	.9999	.9998	.9997	.9995	.9992	.9987	.9980	.9971	.9957
9	1.0000	1.0000	1.0000	1.0000	.9999	.9999	.9998	.9996	.9994	.9991
10	1.0000	1.0000	1.0000	1.0000	1.0000	1.0000	1.0000	.9999	.9999	.9998
11	1.0000	1.0000	1.0000	1.0000	1.0000	1.0000	1.0000	1.0000	1.0000	1.0000

TABLE B (*continued*)

				$n = 18$ (*continued*)						
x \ p	.21	.22	.23	.24	.25	.26	.27	.28	.29	.30
0	.0144	.0114	.0091	.0072	.0056	.0044	.0035	.0027	.0021	.0016
1	.0831	.0694	.0577	.0478	.0395	.0324	.0265	.0216	.0176	.0142
2	.2384	.2084	.1813	.1570	.1353	.1161	.0991	.0842	.0712	.0600
3	.4586	.4175	.3782	.3409	.3057	.2728	.2422	.2140	.1881	.1646
4	.6780	.6387	.5988	.5586	.5187	.4792	.4406	.4032	.3671	.3327
5	.8414	.8134	.7832	.7512	.7174	.6824	.6462	.6093	.5719	.5344
6	.9355	.9201	.9026	.8829	.8610	.8370	.8109	.7829	.7531	.7217
7	.9783	.9717	.9637	.9542	.9431	.9301	.9153	.8986	.8800	.8593
8	.9940	.9917	.9888	.9852	.9807	.9751	.9684	.9605	.9512	.9404
9	.9986	.9980	.9972	.9961	.9946	.9927	.9903	.9873	.9836	.9790
10	.9997	.9996	.9994	.9991	.9988	.9982	.9975	.9966	.9954	.9939
11	1.0000	.9999	.9999	.9998	.9998	.9997	.9995	.9993	.9990	.9986
12	1.0000	1.0000	1.0000	1.0000	1.0000	.9999	.9999	.9999	.9998	.9997
13	1.0000	1.0000	1.0000	1.0000	1.0000	1.0000	1.0000	1.0000	1.0000	1.0000

x \ p	.31	.32	.33	.34	.35	.36	.37	.38	.39	.40
0	.0013	.0010	.0007	.0006	.0004	.0003	.0002	.0002	.0001	.0001
1	.0114	.0092	.0073	.0058	.0046	.0036	.0028	.0022	.0017	.0013
2	.0502	.0419	.0348	.0287	.0236	.0193	.0157	.0127	.0103	.0082
3	.1432	.1241	.1069	.0917	.0783	.0665	.0561	.0472	.0394	.0328
4	.2999	.2691	.2402	.2134	.1886	.1659	.1451	.1263	.1093	.0942
5	.4971	.4602	.4241	.3889	.3550	.3224	.2914	.2621	.2345	.2088
6	.6889	.6550	.6202	.5849	.5491	.5133	.4776	.4424	.4079	.3743
7	.8367	.8122	.7859	.7579	.7283	.6973	.6651	.6319	.5979	.5634
8	.9280	.9139	.8981	.8804	.8609	.8396	.8165	.7916	.7650	.7368
9	.9736	.9671	.9595	.9506	.9403	.9286	.9153	.9003	.8837	.8653
10	.9920	.9896	.9867	.9831	.9788	.9736	.9675	.9603	.9520	.9424
11	.9980	.9973	.9964	.9953	.9938	.9920	.9898	.9870	.9837	.9797
12	.9996	.9995	.9992	.9989	.9986	.9981	.9974	.9966	.9956	.9942
13	.9999	.9999	.9999	.9998	.9997	.9996	.9995	.9993	.9990	.9987
14	1.0000	1.0000	1.0000	1.0000	1.0000	.9999	.9999	.9999	.9998	.9998
15	1.0000	1.0000	1.0000	1.0000	1.0000	1.0000	1.0000	1.0000	1.0000	1.0000

TABLE B (*continued*)

						$n = 18$ (*continued*)					

p x	.41	.42	.43	.44	.45	.46	.47	.48	.49	.50
0	.0001	.0001	.0000	.0000	.0000	.0000	.0000	.0000	.0000	.0000
1	.0010	.0008	.0006	.0004	.0003	.0002	.0002	.0001	.0001	.0001
2	.0066	.0052	.0041	.0032	.0025	.0019	.0015	.0011	.0009	.0007
3	.0271	.0223	.0182	.0148	.0120	.0096	.0077	.0061	.0048	.0038
4	.0807	.0687	.0582	.0490	.0411	.0342	.0283	.0233	.0190	.0154
5	.1849	.1628	.1427	.1243	.1077	.0928	.0795	.0676	.0572	.0481
6	.3418	.3105	.2807	.2524	.2258	.2009	.1778	.1564	.1368	.1189
7	.5287	.4938	.4592	.4250	.3915	.3588	.3272	.2968	.2678	.2403
8	.7072	.6764	.6444	.6115	.5778	.5438	.5094	.4751	.4409	.4073
9	.8451	.8232	.7996	.7742	.7473	.7188	.6890	.6579	.6258	.5927
10	.9314	.9189	.9049	.8893	.8720	.8530	.8323	.8098	.7856	.7597
11	.9750	.9693	.9628	.9551	.9463	.9362	.9247	.9117	.8972	.8811
12	.9926	.9906	.9882	.9853	.9817	.9775	.9725	.9666	.9598	.9519
13	.9983	.9978	.9971	.9962	.9951	.9937	.9921	.9900	.9875	.9846
14	.9997	.9996	.9994	.9993	.9990	.9987	.9983	.9977	.9971	.9962
15	1.0000	.9999	.9999	.9999	.9999	.9998	.9997	.9996	.9995	.9993
16	1.0000	1.0000	1.0000	1.0000	1.0000	1.0000	1.0000	1.0000	.9999	.9999
17	1.0000	1.0000	1.0000	1.0000	1.0000	1.0000	1.0000	1.0000	1.0000	1.0000

						$n = 19$					

p x	.01	.02	.03	.04	.05	.06	.07	.08	.09	.10
0	.8262	.6812	.5606	.4604	.3774	.3086	.2519	.2051	.1666	.1351
1	.9847	.9454	.8900	.8249	.7547	.6829	.6121	.5440	.4798	.4203
2	.9991	.9939	.9817	.9616	.9335	.8979	.8561	.8092	.7585	.7054
3	1.0000	.9995	.9978	.9939	.9868	.9757	.9602	.9398	.9147	.8850
4	1.0000	1.0000	.9998	.9993	.9980	.9956	.9915	.9853	.9765	.9648
5	1.0000	1.0000	1.0000	.9999	.9998	.9994	.9986	.9971	.9949	.9914
6	1.0000	1.0000	1.0000	1.0000	1.0000	.9999	.9998	.9996	.9991	.9983
7	1.0000	1.0000	1.0000	1.0000	1.0000	1.0000	1.0000	.9999	.9999	.9997
8	1.0000	1.0000	1.0000	1.0000	1.0000	1.0000	1.0000	1.0000	1.0000	1.0000

p x	.11	.12	.13	.14	.15	.16	.17	.18	.19	.20
0	.1092	.0881	.0709	.0569	.0456	.0364	.0290	.0230	.0182	.0144
1	.3658	.3165	.2723	.2331	.1985	.1682	.1419	.1191	.0996	.0829
2	.6512	.5968	.5432	.4911	.4413	.3941	.3500	.3090	.2713	.2369
3	.8510	.8133	.7725	.7292	.6841	.6380	.5915	.5451	.4995	.4551
4	.9498	.9315	.9096	.8842	.8556	.8238	.7893	.7524	.7136	.6733
5	.9865	.9798	.9710	.9599	.9463	.9300	.9109	.8890	.8643	.8369
6	.9970	.9952	.9924	.9887	.9837	.9772	.9690	.9589	.9468	.9324
7	.9995	.9991	.9984	.9974	.9959	.9939	.9911	.9874	.9827	.9767
8	.9999	.9998	.9997	.9995	.9992	.9986	.9979	.9968	.9953	.9933
9	1.0000	1.0000	1.0000	.9999	.9999	.9998	.9996	.9993	.9990	.9984
10	1.0000	1.0000	1.0000	1.0000	1.0000	1.0000	.9999	.9999	.9998	.9997
11	1.0000	1.0000	1.0000	1.0000	1.0000	1.0000	1.0000	1.0000	1.0000	1.0000

TABLE B (*continued*)

					n = 19 (*continued*)					

x \ p	.21	.22	.23	.24	.25	.26	.27	.28	.29	.30
0	.0113	.0089	.0070	.0054	.0042	.0033	.0025	.0019	.0015	.0011
1	.0687	.0566	.0465	.0381	.0310	.0251	.0203	.0163	.0131	.0104
2	.2058	.1778	.1529	.1308	.1113	.0943	.0795	.0667	.0557	.0462
3	.4123	.3715	.3329	.2968	.2631	.2320	.2035	.1776	.1542	.1332
4	.6319	.5900	.5480	.5064	.4654	.4256	.3871	.3502	.3152	.2822
5	.8071	.7749	.7408	.7050	.6677	.6295	.5907	.5516	.5125	.4739
6	.9157	.8966	.8751	.8513	.8251	.7968	.7664	.7343	.7005	.6655
7	.9693	.9604	.9497	.9371	.9225	.9059	.8871	.8662	.8432	.8180
8	.9907	.9873	.9831	.9778	.9713	.9634	.9541	.9432	.9306	.9161
9	.9977	.9966	.9953	.9934	.9911	.9881	.9844	.9798	.9742	.9674
10	.9995	.9993	.9989	.9984	.9977	.9968	.9956	.9940	.9920	.9895
11	.9999	.9999	.9998	.9997	.9995	.9993	.9990	.9985	.9980	.9972
12	1.0000	1.0000	1.0000	.9999	.9999	.9999	.9998	.9997	.9996	.9994
13	1.0000	1.0000	1.0000	1.0000	1.0000	1.0000	1.0000	1.0000	.9999	.9999
14	1.0000	1.0000	1.0000	1.0000	1.0000	1.0000	1.0000	1.0000	1.0000	1.0000

x \ p	.31	.32	.33	.34	.35	.36	.37	.38	.39	.40
0	.0009	.0007	.0005	.0004	.0003	.0002	.0002	.0001	.0001	.0001
1	.0083	.0065	.0051	.0040	.0031	.0024	.0019	.0014	.0011	.0008
2	.0382	.0314	.0257	.0209	.0170	.0137	.0110	.0087	.0069	.0055
3	.1144	.0978	.0831	.0703	.0591	.0495	.0412	.0341	.0281	.0230
4	.2514	.2227	.1963	.1720	.1500	.1301	.1122	.0962	.0821	.0696
5	.4359	.3990	.3634	.3293	.2968	.2661	.2373	.2105	.1857	.1629
6	.6294	.5927	.5555	.5182	.4812	.4446	.4087	.3739	.3403	.3081
7	.7909	.7619	.7312	.6990	.6656	.6310	.5957	.5599	.5238	.4878
8	.8997	.8814	.8611	.8388	.8145	.7884	.7605	.7309	.6998	.6675
9	.9595	.9501	.9392	.9267	.9125	.8965	.8787	.8590	.8374	.8139
10	.9863	.9824	.9777	.9720	.9653	.9574	.9482	.9375	.9253	.9115
11	.9962	.9949	.9932	.9911	.9886	.9854	.9815	.9769	.9713	.9648
12	.9991	.9988	.9983	.9977	.9969	.9959	.9946	.9930	.9909	.9884
13	.9998	.9998	.9997	.9995	.9993	.9991	.9987	.9983	.9977	.9969
14	1.0000	1.0000	.9999	.9999	.9999	.9998	.9998	.9997	.9995	.9994
15	1.0000	1.0000	1.0000	1.0000	1.0000	1.0000	1.0000	1.0000	.9999	.9999
16	1.0000	1.0000	1.0000	1.0000	1.0000	1.0000	1.0000	1.0000	1.0000	1.0000

TABLE B (*continued*)

				$n = 19$ (*continued*)						
x \ p	.41	.42	.43	.44	.45	.46	.47	.48	.49	.50
0	.0000	.0000	.0000	.0000	.0000	.0000	.0000	.0000	.0000	.0000
1	.0006	.0005	.0004	.0003	.0002	.0001	.0001	.0001	.0001	.0000
2	.0043	.0033	.0026	.0020	.0015	.0012	.0009	.0007	.0005	.0004
3	.0187	.0151	.0122	.0097	.0077	.0061	.0048	.0037	.0029	.0022
4	.0587	.0492	.0410	.0340	.0280	.0229	.0186	.0150	.0121	.0096
5	.1421	.1233	.1063	.0912	.0777	.0658	.0554	.0463	.0385	.0318
6	.2774	.2485	.2213	.1961	.1727	.1512	.1316	.1138	.0978	.0835
7	.4520	.4168	.3824	.3491	.3169	.2862	.2570	.2294	.2036	.1796
8	.6340	.5997	.5647	.5294	.4940	.4587	.4238	.3895	.3561	.3238
9	.7886	.7615	.7328	.7026	.6710	.6383	.6046	.5701	.5352	.5000
10	.8960	.8787	.8596	.8387	.8159	.7913	.7649	.7369	.7073	.6762
11	.9571	.9482	.9379	.9262	.9129	.8979	.8813	.8628	.8425	.8204
12	.9854	.9817	.9773	.9720	.9658	.9585	.9500	.9403	.9291	.9165
13	.9960	.9948	.9933	.9914	.9891	.9863	.9829	.9788	.9739	.9682
14	.9991	.9988	.9984	.9979	.9972	.9964	.9954	.9940	.9924	.9904
15	.9999	.9998	.9997	.9996	.9995	.9993	.9990	.9987	.9983	.9978
16	1.0000	1.0000	1.0000	.9999	.9999	.9999	.9999	.9998	.9997	.9996
17	1.0000	1.0000	1.0000	1.0000	1.0000	1.0000	1.0000	1.0000	1.0000	1.0000

				$n = 20$						
x \ p	.01	.02	.03	.04	.05	.06	.07	.08	.09	.10
0	.8179	.6676	.5438	.4420	.3585	.2901	.2342	.1887	.1516	.1216
1	.9831	.9401	.8802	.8103	.7358	.6605	.5869	.5169	.4516	.3917
2	.9990	.9929	.9790	.9561	.9245	.8850	.8390	.7879	.7334	.6769
3	1.0000	.9994	.9973	.9926	.9841	.9710	.9529	.9294	.9007	.8670
4	1.0000	1.0000	.9997	.9990	.9974	.9944	.9893	.9817	.9710	.9568
5	1.0000	1.0000	1.0000	.9999	.9997	.9991	.9981	.9962	.9932	.9887
6	1.0000	1.0000	1.0000	1.0000	1.0000	.9999	.9997	.9994	.9987	.9976
7	1.0000	1.0000	1.0000	1.0000	1.0000	1.0000	1.0000	.9999	.9998	.9996
8	1.0000	1.0000	1.0000	1.0000	1.0000	1.0000	1.0000	1.0000	1.0000	.9999
9	1.0000	1.0000	1.0000	1.0000	1.0000	1.0000	1.0000	1.0000	1.0000	1.0000

TABLE B (*continued*)

					$n = 20$ (*continued*)					
x \ p	.11	.12	.13	.14	.15	.16	.17	.18	.19	.20
0	.0972	.0776	.0617	.0490	.0388	.0306	.0241	.0189	.0148	.0115
1	.3376	.2891	.2461	.2084	.1756	.1471	.1227	.1018	.0841	.0692
2	.6198	.5631	.5080	.4550	.4049	.3580	.3146	.2748	.2386	.2061
3	.8290	.7873	.7427	.6959	.6477	.5990	.5504	.5026	.4561	.4114
4	.9390	.9173	.8917	.8625	.8298	.7941	.7557	.7151	.6729	.6296
5	.9825	.9740	.9630	.9493	.9327	.9130	.8902	.8644	.8357	.8042
6	.9959	.9933	.9897	.9847	.9781	.9696	.9591	.9463	.9311	.9133
7	.9992	.9986	.9976	.9962	.9941	.9912	.9873	.9823	.9759	.9679
8	.9999	.9998	.9995	.9992	.9987	.9979	.9967	.9951	.9929	.9900
9	1.0000	1.0000	.9999	.9999	.9998	.9996	.9993	.9989	.9983	.9974
10	1.0000	1.0000	1.0000	1.0000	1.0000	.9999	.9999	.9998	.9996	.9994
11	1.0000	1.0000	1.0000	1.0000	1.0000	1.0000	1.0000	1.0000	.9999	.9999
12	1.0000	1.0000	1.0000	1.0000	1.0000	1.0000	1.0000	1.0000	1.0000	1.0000

x \ p	.21	.22	.23	.24	.25	.26	.27	.28	.29	.30
0	.0090	.0069	.0054	.0041	.0032	.0024	.0018	.0014	.0011	.0008
1	.0566	.0461	.0374	.0302	.0243	.0195	.0155	.0123	.0097	.0076
2	.1770	.1512	.1284	.1085	.0913	.0763	.0635	.0526	.0433	.0355
3	.3690	.3289	.2915	.2569	.2252	.1962	.1700	.1466	.1256	.1071
4	.5858	.5420	.4986	.4561	.4148	.3752	.3375	.3019	.2685	.2375
5	.7703	.7343	.6965	.6573	.6172	.5765	.5357	.4952	.4553	.4164
6	.8929	.8699	.8442	.8162	.7858	.7533	.7190	.6831	.6460	.6080
7	.9581	.9464	.9325	.9165	.8982	.8775	.8545	.8293	.8018	.7723
8	.9862	.9814	.9754	.9680	.9591	.9485	.9360	.9216	.9052	.8867
9	.9962	.9946	.9925	.9897	.9861	.9817	.9762	.9695	.9615	.9520
10	.9991	.9987	.9981	.9972	.9961	.9945	.9926	.9900	.9868	.9829
11	.9998	.9997	.9996	.9994	.9991	.9986	.9981	.9973	.9962	.9949
12	1.0000	1.0000	.9999	.9999	.9998	.9997	.9996	.9994	.9991	.9987
13	1.0000	1.0000	1.0000	1.0000	1.0000	1.0000	.9999	.9999	.9998	.9997
14	1.0000	1.0000	1.0000	1.0000	1.0000	1.0000	1.0000	1.0000	1.0000	1.0000

TABLE B (*continued*)

					$n = 20$ (*continued*)					
p \ *x*	.31	.32	.33	.34	.35	.36	.37	.38	.39	.40
0	.0006	.0004	.0003	.0002	.0002	.0001	.0001	.0001	.0001	.0000
1	.0060	.0047	.0036	.0028	.0021	.0016	.0012	.0009	.0007	.0005
2	.0289	.0235	.0189	.0152	.0121	.0096	.0076	.0060	.0047	.0036
3	.0908	.0765	.0642	.0535	.0444	.0366	.0300	.0245	.0198	.0160
4	.2089	.1827	.1589	.1374	.1182	.1011	.0859	.0726	.0610	.0510
5	.3787	.3426	.3082	.2758	.2454	.2171	.1910	.1671	.1453	.1256
6	.5695	.5307	.4921	.4540	.4166	.3803	.3453	.3118	.2800	.2500
7	.7409	.7078	.6732	.6376	.6010	.5639	.5265	.4892	.4522	.4159
8	.8660	.8432	.8182	.7913	.7624	.7317	.6995	.6659	.6312	.5956
9	.9409	.9281	.9134	.8968	.8782	.8576	.8350	.8103	.7837	.7553
10	.9780	.9721	.9650	.9566	.9468	.9355	.9225	.9077	.8910	.8725
11	.9931	.9909	.9881	.9846	.9804	.9753	.9692	.9619	.9534	.9435
12	.9982	.9975	.9966	.9955	.9940	.9921	.9898	.9868	.9833	.9790
13	.9996	.9994	.9992	.9989	.9985	.9979	.9972	.9963	.9951	.9935
14	.9999	.9999	.9999	.9998	.9997	.9996	.9994	.9991	.9988	.9984
15	1.0000	1.0000	1.0000	1.0000	1.0000	.9999	.9999	.9998	.9998	.9997
16	1.0000	1.0000	1.0000	1.0000	1.0000	1.0000	1.0000	1.0000	1.0000	1.0000

p \ *x*	.41	.42	.43	.44	.45	.46	.47	.48	.49	.50
0	.0000	.0000	.0000	.0000	.0000	.0000	.0000	.0000	.0000	.0000
1	.0004	.0003	.0002	.0002	.0001	.0001	.0001	.0000	.0000	.0000
2	.0028	.0021	.0016	.0012	.0009	.0007	.0005	.0004	.0003	.0002
3	.0128	.0102	.0080	.0063	.0049	.0038	.0029	.0023	.0017	.0013
4	.0423	.0349	.0286	.0233	.0189	.0152	.0121	.0096	.0076	.0059
5	.1079	.0922	.0783	.0660	.0553	.0461	.0381	.0313	.0255	.0207
6	.2220	.1959	.1719	.1499	.1299	.1119	.0958	.0814	.0688	.0577
7	.3804	.3461	.3132	.2817	.2520	.2241	.1980	.1739	.1518	.1316
8	.5594	.5229	.4864	.4501	.4143	.3793	.3454	.3127	.2814	.2517
9	.7252	.6936	.6606	.6264	.5914	.5557	.5196	.4834	.4474	.4119
10	.8520	.8295	.8051	.7788	.7507	.7209	.6896	.6568	.6229	.5881
11	.9321	.9190	.9042	.8877	.8692	.8489	.8266	.8024	.7762	.7483
12	.9738	.9676	.9603	.9518	.9420	.9306	.9177	.9031	.8867	.8684
13	.9916	.9893	.9864	.9828	.9786	.9735	.9674	.9603	.9520	.9423
14	.9978	.9971	.9962	.9950	.9936	.9917	.9895	.9867	.9834	.9793
15	.9996	.9994	.9992	.9989	.9985	.9980	.9973	.9965	.9954	.9941
16	.9999	.9999	.9999	.9998	.9997	.9996	.9995	.9993	.9990	.9987
17	1.0000	1.0000	1.0000	1.0000	1.0000	.9999	.9999	.9999	.9999	.9998
18	1.0000	1.0000	1.0000	1.0000	1.0000	1.0000	1.0000	1.0000	1.0000	1.0000

TABLE B (*continued*)

	$n = 25$									
x \ p	.01	.02	.03	.04	.05	.06	.07	.08	.09	.10
0	.7778	.6035	.4670	.3604	.2774	.2129	.1630	.1244	.0946	.0718
1	.9742	.9114	.8280	.7358	.6424	.5527	.4696	.3947	.3286	.2712
2	.9980	.9868	.9620	.9235	.8729	.8129	.7466	.6768	.6063	.5371
3	.9999	.9986	.9938	.9835	.9659	.9402	.9064	.8649	.8169	.7636
4	1.0000	.9999	.9992	.9972	.9928	.9850	.9726	.9549	.9314	.9020
5	1.0000	1.0000	.9999	.9996	.9988	.9969	.9935	.9877	.9790	.9666
6	1.0000	1.0000	1.0000	1.0000	.9998	.9995	.9987	.9972	.9946	.9905
7	1.0000	1.0000	1.0000	1.0000	1.0000	.9999	.9998	.9995	.9989	.9977
8	1.0000	1.0000	1.0000	1.0000	1.0000	1.0000	1.0000	.9999	.9998	.9995
9	1.0000	1.0000	1.0000	1.0000	1.0000	1.0000	1.0000	1.0000	1.0000	.9999
10	1.0000	1.0000	1.0000	1.0000	1.0000	1.0000	1.0000	1.0000	1.0000	1.0000

x \ p	.11	.12	.13	.14	.15	.16	.17	.18	.19	.20
0	.0543	.0409	.0308	.0230	.0172	.0128	.0095	.0070	.0052	.0038
1	.2221	.1805	.1457	.1168	.0931	.0737	.0580	.0454	.0354	.0274
2	.4709	.4088	.3517	.3000	.2537	.2130	.1774	.1467	.1204	.0982
3	.7066	.6475	.5877	.5286	.4711	.4163	.3648	.3171	.2734	.2340
4	.8669	.8266	.7817	.7332	.6821	.6293	.5759	.5228	.4708	.4207
5	.9501	.9291	.9035	.8732	.8385	.7998	.7575	.7125	.6653	.6167
6	.9844	.9757	.9641	.9491	.9305	.9080	.8815	.8512	.8173	.7800
7	.9959	.9930	.9887	.9827	.9745	.9639	.9505	.9339	.9141	.8909
8	.9991	.9983	.9970	.9950	.9920	.9879	.9822	.9748	.9652	.9532
9	.9998	.9996	.9993	.9987	.9979	.9965	.9945	.9917	.9878	.9827
10	1.0000	.9999	.9999	.9997	.9995	.9991	.9985	.9976	.9963	.9944
11	1.0000	1.0000	1.0000	1.0000	.9999	.9998	.9997	.9994	.9990	.9985
12	1.0000	1.0000	1.0000	1.0000	1.0000	1.0000	.9999	.9999	.9998	.9996
13	1.0000	1.0000	1.0000	1.0000	1.0000	1.0000	1.0000	1.0000	1.0000	.9999
14	1.0000	1.0000	1.0000	1.0000	1.0000	1.0000	1.0000	1.0000	1.0000	1.0000

TABLE B (*continued*)

						$n = 25$ (*continued*)				
x \ p	.21	.22	.23	.24	.25	.26	.27	.28	.29	.30
0	.0028	.0020	.0015	.0010	.0008	.0005	.0004	.0003	.0002	.0001
1	.0211	.0162	.0123	.0093	.0070	.0053	.0039	.0029	.0021	.0016
2	.0796	.0640	.0512	.0407	.0321	.0252	.0196	.0152	.0117	.0090
3	.1987	.1676	.1403	.1166	.0962	.0789	.0642	.0519	.0417	.0332
4	.3730	.3282	.2866	.2484	.2137	.1826	.1548	.1304	.1090	.0905
5	.5675	.5184	.4701	.4233	.3783	.3356	.2956	.2585	.2245	.1935
6	.7399	.6973	.6529	.6073	.5611	.5149	.4692	.4247	.3817	.3407
7	8642	.8342	.8011	.7651	.7265	.6858	.6435	.6001	.5560	.5118
8	.9386	.9212	.9007	.8772	.8506	.8210	.7885	.7535	.7162	.6769
9	.9760	.9675	.9569	.9440	.9287	.9107	.8899	.8662	.8398	.8106
10	.9918	.9883	.9837	.9778	.9703	.9611	.9498	.9364	.9205	.9022
11	.9976	.9964	.9947	.9924	.9893	.9852	.9801	.9736	.9655	.9558
12	.9994	.9990	.9985	.9977	.9966	.9951	.9931	.9904	.9870	.9825
13	.9999	.9998	.9996	.9994	.9991	.9986	.9979	.9970	.9957	.9940
14	1.0000	1.0000	.9999	.9999	.9998	.9997	.9995	.9992	.9988	.9982
15	1.0000	1.0000	1.0000	1.0000	1.0000	.9999	.9999	.9998	.9997	.9995
16	1.0000	1.0000	1.0000	1.0000	1.0000	1.0000	1.0000	1.0000	.9999	.9999
17	1.0000	1.0000	1.0000	1.0000	1.0000	1.0000	1.0000	1.0000	1.0000	1.0000
x \ p	.31	.32	.33	.34	.35	.36	.37	.38	.39	.40
0	.0001	.0001	.0000	.0000	.0000	.0000	.0000	.0000	.0000	.0000
1	.0011	.0008	.0006	.0004	.0003	.0002	.0002	.0001	.0001	.0001
2	.0068	.0051	.0039	.0029	.0021	.0016	.0011	.0008	.0006	.0004
3	.0263	.0207	.0162	.0126	.0097	.0074	.0056	.0043	.0032	.0024
4	.0746	.0610	.0496	.0400	.0320	.0255	.0201	.0158	.0123	.0095
5	.1656	.1407	.1187	.0994	.0826	.0682	.0559	.0454	.0367	.0294
6	.3019	.2657	.2321	.2013	.1734	.1483	.1258	.1060	.0886	.0736
7	.4681	.4253	.3837	.3439	.3061	.2705	.2374	.2068	.1789	.1536
8	.6361	.5943	.5518	.5092	.4668	.4252	.3848	.3458	.3086	.2735
9	.7787	.7445	.7081	.6700	.6303	.5896	.5483	.5067	.4653	.4246
10	.8812	.8576	.8314	.8025	.7712	.7375	.7019	.6645	.6257	.5858
11	.9440	.9302	.9141	.8956	.8746	.8510	.8249	.7964	.7654	.7323
12	.9770	.9701	.9617	.9515	.9396	.9255	.9093	.8907	.8697	.8462
13	.9917	.9888	.9851	.9804	.9745	.9674	.9588	.9485	.9363	.9222
14	.9974	.9964	.9950	.9931	.9907	.9876	.9837	.9788	.9729	.9656
15	.9993	.9990	.9985	.9979	.9971	.9959	.9944	.9925	.9900	.9868
16	.9998	.9998	.9996	.9995	.9992	.9989	.9984	.9977	.9968	.9957
17	1.0000	1.0000	.9999	.9999	.9998	.9997	.9996	.9994	.9992	.9988
18	1.0000	1.0000	1.0000	1.0000	1.0000	.9999	.9999	.9999	.9998	.9997
19	1.0000	1.0000	1.0000	1.0000	1.0000	1.0000	1.0000	1.0000	1.0000	.9999
20	1.0000	1.0000	1.0000	1.0000	1.0000	1.0000	1.0000	1.0000	1.0000	1.0000

TABLE B (*continued*)

					$n = 25$ (*continued*)					
p x	.41	.42	.43	.44	.45	.46	.47	.48	.49	.50
0	.0000	.0000	.0000	.0000	.0000	.0000	.0000	.0000	.0000	.0000
1	.0000	.0000	.0000	.0000	.0000	.0000	.0000	.0000	.0000	.0000
2	.0003	.0002	.0002	.0001	.0001	.0000	.0000	.0000	.0000	.0000
3	.0017	.0013	.0009	.0007	.0005	.0003	.0002	.0002	.0001	.0001
4	.0073	.0055	.0042	.0031	.0023	.0017	.0012	.0009	.0006	.0005
5	.0233	.0184	.0144	.0112	.0086	.0066	.0050	.0037	.0028	.0020
6	.0606	.0495	.0401	.0323	.0258	.0204	.0160	.0124	.0096	.0073
7	.1308	.1106	.0929	.0773	.0639	.0523	.0425	.0342	.0273	.0216
8	.2407	.2103	.1823	.1569	.1340	.1135	.0954	.0795	.0657	.0539
9	.3849	.3465	.3098	.2750	.2424	.2120	.1840	.1585	.1354	.1148
10	.5452	.5044	.4637	.4235	.3843	.3462	.3098	.2751	.2426	.2122
11	.6971	.6603	.6220	.5826	.5426	.5022	.4618	.4220	.3829	.3450
12	.8203	.7920	.7613	.7285	.6937	.6571	.6192	.5801	.5402	.5000
13	.9059	.8873	.8664	.8431	.8173	.7891	.7587	.7260	.6914	.6550
14	.9569	.9465	.9344	.9203	.9040	.8855	.8647	.8415	.8159	.7878
15	.9829	.9780	.9720	.9647	.9560	.9457	.9337	.9197	.9036	.8852
16	.9942	.9922	.9897	.9866	.9826	.9778	.9719	.9648	.9562	.9461
17	.9983	.9977	.9968	.9956	.9942	.9923	.9898	.9868	.9830	.9784
18	.9996	.9994	.9992	.9988	.9984	.9977	.9969	.9959	.9945	.9927
19	.9999	.9999	.9998	.9997	.9996	.9995	.9992	.9989	.9985	.9980
20	1.0000	1.0000	1.0000	1.0000	.9999	.9999	.9998	.9998	.9997	.9995
21	1.0000	1.0000	1.0000	1.0000	1.0000	1.0000	1.0000	1.0000	.9999	.9999
22	1.0000	1.0000	1.0000	1.0000	1.0000	1.0000	1.0000	1.0000	1.0000	1.0000

TABLE C Cumulative Poisson Distribution $P(X \le X|\lambda)$. 1000 Times the Probability of X or Fewer Occurrences of Event that has Average Number of Occurrences Equal to λ

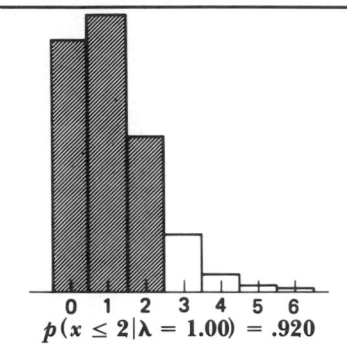

$p(x \le 2|\lambda = 1.00) = .920$

x \ λ	.02	.04	.06	.08	.10	.15	.20	.25
0	980	961	942	923	905	861	819	779
1	1000	999	998	997	995	990	982	974
2		1000	1000	1000	1000	999	999	998
3						1000	1000	1000

x \ λ	.30	.35	.40	.45	.50	.55	.60	.65
0	741	705	670	638	607	577	549	522
1	963	951	938	925	910	894	878	861
2	996	994	992	989	986	982	977	972
3	1000	1000	999	999	998	998	997	998
4			1000	1000	1000	1000	1000	999
5								1000

x \ λ	.70	.75	.80	.85	.90	.95	1.0	1.1
0	497	472	449	427	407	387	368	333
1	844	827	809	791	772	754	736	699
2	966	959	953	945	937	929	920	900
3	994	993	991	989	987	984	981	974
4	999	999	999	998	998	997	996	995
5	1000	1000	1000	1000	1000	1000	999	999
6							1000	1000

TABLE C (*continued*)

λ / x	1.2	1.3	1.4	1.5	1.6	1.7	1.8	1.9
0	301	273	247	223	202	183	165	150
1	663	627	592	558	525	493	463	434
2	879	857	833	809	783	757	731	704
3	966	957	946	934	921	907	891	875
4	992	989	986	981	976	970	964	956
5	998	998	997	996	994	992	990	987
6	1000	1000	999	999	999	998	997	997
7			1000	1000	1000	1000	999	999
8							1000	1000

λ / x	2.0	2.2	2.4	2.6	2.8	3.0	3.2	3.4
0	135	111	091	074	061	050	041	033
1	406	355	308	267	231	199	171	147
2	677	623	570	518	469	423	380	340
3	857	819	779	736	692	647	603	558
4	947	928	904	877	848	815	781	744
5	983	975	964	951	935	916	895	871
6	995	993	988	983	976	966	955	942
7	999	998	997	995	992	988	983	977
8	1000	1000	999	999	998	997	994	992
9			1000	1000	999	999	998	997
10					1000	1000	1000	999
11								1000

λ / x	3.6	3.8	.40	4.2	4.4	4.6	4.8	5.0
0	027	022	018	015	012	010	008	007
1	126	107	092	078	066	056	048	040
2	303	269	238	210	185	163	143	125
3	515	473	433	395	359	326	294	265
4	706	668	629	590	551	513	476	440
5	844	816	785	753	720	686	651	616
6	927	909	889	867	844	818	791	762
7	969	960	949	936	921	905	887	867
8	988	984	979	972	964	955	944	932
9	996	994	992	989	985	980	975	968
10	999	998	997	996	994	992	990	986
11	1000	999	999	999	998	997	996	995
12		1000	1000	1000	999	999	999	998
13					1000	1000	1000	999
14								1000

TABLE C (*continued*)

λ x	5.2	5.4	5.6	5.8	6.0	6.2	6.4	6.6
0	006	005	004	003	002	002	002	001
1	034	029	024	021	017	015	012	010
2	109	095	082	072	062	054	046	040
3	238	213	191	170	151	134	119	105
4	406	373	342	313	285	259	235	213
5	581	546	512	478	446	414	384	355
6	732	702	670	638	606	574	542	511
7	845	822	797	771	744	716	687	658
8	918	903	886	867	847	826	803	780
9	960	951	941	929	916	902	886	869
10	982	977	972	965	957	949	939	927
11	993	990	988	984	980	975	969	963
12	997	996	995	993	991	989	986	982
13	999	999	998	997	996	995	994	992
14	1000	999	999	999	999	998	997	997
15		1000	1000	1000	999	999	999	999
16					1000	1000	1000	999
17								1000

λ x	6.8	7.0	7.2	7.4	7.6	7.8	8.0	8.5
0	001	001	001	001	001	000	000	000
1	009	007	006	005	004	004	003	002
2	034	030	025	022	019	016	014	009
3	093	082	072	063	055	048	042	030
4	192	173	156	140	125	112	100	074
5	327	301	276	253	231	210	191	150
6	480	450	420	392	365	338	313	256
7	628	599	569	539	510	481	453	386
8	755	729	703	676	648	620	593	523
9	850	830	810	788	765	741	717	653
10	915	901	887	871	854	835	816	763
11	955	947	937	926	915	902	888	849
12	978	973	967	961	954	945	936	909
13	990	987	984	980	976	971	966	949
14	996	994	993	991	989	986	983	973
15	998	998	997	996	995	993	992	986
16	999	999	999	998	998	997	996	993
17	1000	1000	999	999	999	999	998	997
18			1000	1000	1000	1000	999	999
19							1000	999
20								1000

TABLE C (*continued*)

x \ λ	9.0	9.5	10.0	10.5	11.0	11.5	12.0	12.5
1	001	001	000	000	000	000	000	000
2	006	004	003	002	001	001	001	000
3	021	015	010	007	005	003	002	002
4	055	040	029	021	015	011	008	005
5	116	089	067	050	038	028	020	015
6	207	165	130	102	079	060	046	035
7	324	269	220	179	143	114	090	070
8	456	392	333	279	232	191	155	125
9	587	522	458	397	341	289	242	201
10	706	645	583	521	460	402	347	297
11	803	752	697	639	579	520	462	406
12	876	836	792	742	689	633	576	519
13	926	898	864	825	781	733	682	628
14	959	940	917	888	854	815	772	725
15	978	967	951	932	907	878	844	806
16	989	982	973	960	944	924	899	869
17	995	991	986	978	968	954	937	916
18	998	996	993	988	982	974	963	948
19	999	998	997	994	991	986	979	969
20	1000	999	998	997	995	992	988	983
21		1000	999	999	998	996	994	991
22			1000	999	999	998	997	995
23				1000	1000	999	999	998
24						1000	999	999
25							1000	999
26								1000

TABLE C (*continued*)

λ / x	13.0	13.5	14.0	14.5	15	16	17	18
3	001	001	000	000	000	000	000	000
4	004	003	002	001	001	000	000	000
5	011	008	006	004	003	001	001	000
6	026	019	014	010	008	004	002	001
7	054	041	032	024	018	010	005	003
8	100	079	062	048	037	022	013	007
9	166	135	109	088	070	043	026	015
10	252	211	176	145	118	077	049	030
11	353	304	260	220	185	127	085	055
12	463	409	358	311	268	193	135	092
13	573	518	464	413	363	275	201	143
14	675	623	570	518	466	368	281	208
15	764	718	669	619	568	467	371	287
16	835	798	756	711	664	566	468	375
17	890	861	827	790	749	659	564	469
18	930	908	883	853	819	742	655	562
19	957	942	923	901	875	812	736	651
20	975	965	952	936	917	868	805	731
21	986	980	971	960	947	911	861	799
22	992	989	983	976	967	942	905	855
23	996	994	991	986	981	963	937	899
24	998	997	995	992	989	978	959	932
25	999	998	997	996	994	987	975	955
26	1000	999	999	998	997	993	985	972
27		1000	999	999	998	996	991	983
28			1000	999	999	998	995	990
29				1000	1000	999	997	994
30						999	999	997
31						1000	999	998
32							1000	999
33								1000

TABLE C (*continued*)

x \ λ	19	20	21	22	23	24	25
6	001	000	000	000	000	000	000
7	002	001	000	000	000	000	000
8	004	002	001	001	000	000	000
9	009	005	003	002	001	000	000
10	018	011	006	004	002	001	001
11	035	021	013	008	004	003	001
12	061	039	025	015	009	005	003
13	098	066	043	028	017	011	006
14	150	105	072	048	031	020	012
15	215	157	111	077	052	034	022
16	292	221	163	117	082	056	038
17	378	297	227	169	123	087	060
18	469	381	302	232	175	128	092
19	561	470	384	306	238	180	134
20	647	559	471	387	310	243	185
21	725	644	558	472	389	314	247
22	793	721	640	556	472	392	318
23	849	787	716	637	555	473	394
24	893	843	782	712	635	554	473
25	927	888	838	777	708	632	553
26	951	922	883	832	772	704	629
27	969	948	917	877	827	768	700
28	980	966	944	913	873	823	763
29	988	978	963	940	908	868	818
30	993	987	976	959	936	904	863
31	996	992	985	973	956	932	900
32	998	995	991	983	971	953	929
33	999	997	994	989	981	969	950
34	999	999	997	994	988	979	966
35	1000	999	998	996	993	987	978
36		1000	999	998	996	992	985
37			999	999	997	995	991
38			1000	999	999	997	994
39				1000	999	998	997
40					1000	999	998
41						999	999
42						1000	999
43							1000

TABLE D Normal Curve Areas $P(z \leq z_0)$ Entries in the Body of the Table are Areas between $-\infty$ and z

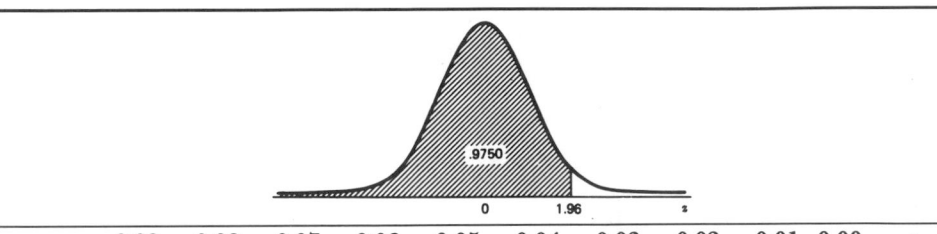

z	−0.09	−0.08	−0.07	−0.06	−0.05	−0.04	−0.03	−0.02	−0.01	0.00	z
−3.80	.0001	.0001	.0001	.0001	.0001	.0001	.0001	.0001	.0001	.0001	−3.80
−3.70	.0001	.0001	.0001	.0001	.0001	.0001	.0001	.0001	.0001	.0001	−3.70
−3.60	.0001	.0001	.0001	.0001	.0001	.0001	.0001	.0001	.0002	.0002	−3.60
−3.50	.0002	.0002	.0002	.0002	.0002	.0002	.0002	.0002	.0002	.0002	−3.50
−3.40	.0002	.0003	.0003	.0003	.0003	.0003	.0003	.0003	.0003	.0003	−3.40
−3.30	.0003	.0004	.0004	.0004	.0004	.0004	.0004	.0005	.0005	.0005	−3.30
−3.20	.0005	.0005	.0005	.0006	.0006	.0006	.0006	.0006	.0007	.0007	−3.20
−3.10	.0007	.0007	.0008	.0008	.0008	.0008	.0009	.0009	.0009	.0010	−3.10
−3.00	.0010	.0010	.0011	.0011	.0011	.0012	.0012	.0013	.0013	.0013	−3.00
−2.90	.0014	.0014	.0015	.0015	.0016	.0016	.0017	.0018	.0018	.0019	−2.90
−2.80	.0019	.0020	.0021	.0021	.0022	.0023	.0023	.0024	.0025	.0026	−2.80
−2.70	.0026	.0027	.0028	.0029	.0030	.0031	.0032	.0033	.0034	.0035	−2.70
−2.60	.0036	.0037	.0038	.0039	.0040	.0041	.0043	.0044	.0045	.0047	−2.60
−2.50	.0048	.0049	.0051	.0052	.0054	.0055	.0057	.0059	.0060	.0062	−2.50
−2.40	.0064	.0066	.0068	.0069	.0071	.0073	.0075	.0078	.0080	.0082	−2.40
−2.30	.0084	.0087	.0089	.0091	.0094	.0096	.0099	.0102	.0104	.0107	−2.30
−2.20	.0110	.0113	.0116	.0119	.0122	.0125	.0129	.0132	.0136	.0139	−2.20
−2.10	.0143	.0146	.0150	.0154	.0158	.0162	.0166	.0170	.0174	.0179	−2.10
−2.00	.0183	.0188	.0192	.0197	.0202	.0207	.0212	.0217	.0222	.0228	−2.00
−1.90	.0233	.0239	.0244	.0250	.0256	.0262	.0268	.0274	.0281	.0287	−1.90
−1.80	.0294	.0301	.0307	.0314	.0322	.0329	.0336	.0344	.0351	.0359	−1.80
−1.70	.0367	.0375	.0384	.0392	.0401	.0409	.0418	.0427	.0436	.0446	−1.70
−1.60	.0455	.0465	.0475	.0485	.0495	.0505	.0516	.0526	.0537	.0548	−1.60
−1.50	.0559	.0571	.0582	.0594	.0606	.0618	.0630	.0643	.0655	.0668	−1.50
−1.40	.0681	.0694	.0708	.0721	.0735	.0749	.0764	.0778	.0793	.0808	−1.40
−1.30	.0823	.0838	.0853	.0869	.0885	.0901	.0918	.0934	.0951	.0968	−1.30
−1.20	.0985	.1003	.1020	.1038	.1056	.1075	.1093	.1112	.1131	.1151	−1.20
−1.10	.1170	.1190	.1210	.1230	.1251	.1271	.1292	.1314	.1335	.1357	−1.10
−1.00	.1379	.1401	.1423	.1446	.1469	.1492	.1515	.1539	.1562	.1587	−1.00
−0.90	.1611	.1635	.1660	.1685	.1711	.1736	.1762	.1788	.1814	.1841	−0.90
−0.80	.1867	.1894	.1922	.1949	.1977	.2005	.2033	.2061	.2090	.2119	−0.80
−0.70	.2148	.2177	.2206	.2236	.2266	.2296	.2327	.2358	.2389	.2420	−0.70
−0.60	.2451	.2483	.2514	.2546	.2578	.2611	.2643	.2676	.2709	.2743	−0.60
−0.50	.2776	.2810	.2843	.2877	.2912	.2946	.2981	.3015	.3050	.3085	−0.50
−0.40	.3121	.3156	.3192	.3228	.3264	.3300	.3336	.3372	.3409	.3446	−0.40
−.030	.3483	.3520	.3557	.3594	.3632	.3669	.3707	.3745	.3783	.3821	−0.30
−0.20	.3859	.3897	.3936	.3974	.4013	.4052	.4090	.4129	.4168	.4207	−0.20
−0.10	.4247	.4286	.4325	.4364	.4404	.4443	.4483	.4522	.4562	.4602	−0.10
0.00	.4641	.4681	.4721	.4761	.4801	.4840	.4880	.4920	.4960	.5000	0.00

TABLE D (*continued*)

z	0.00	0.01	0.02	0.03	0.04	0.05	0.06	0.07	0.08	0.09	z
0.00	.5000	.5040	.5080	.5120	.5160	.5199	.5239	.5279	.5319	.5359	0.00
0.10	.5398	.5438	.5478	.5517	.5557	.5596	.5636	.5675	.5714	.5753	0.10
0.20	.5793	.5832	.5871	.5910	.5948	.5987	.6026	.6064	.6103	.6141	0.20
0.30	.6179	.6217	.6255	.6293	.6331	.6368	.6406	.6443	.6480	.6517	0.30
0.40	.6554	.6591	.6628	.6664	.6700	.6736	.6772	.6808	.6844	.6879	0.40
0.50	.6915	.6950	.6985	.7019	.7054	.7088	.7123	.7157	.7190	.7224	0.50
0.60	.7257	.7291	.7324	.7357	.7389	.7422	.7454	.7486	.7517	.7549	0.60
0.70	.7580	.7611	.7642	.7673	.7704	.7734	.7764	.7794	.7823	.7852	0.70
0.80	.7881	.7910	.7939	.7967	.7995	.8023	.8051	.8078	.8106	.8133	0.80
0.90	.8159	.8186	.8212	.8238	.8264	.8289	.8315	.8340	.8365	.8389	0.90
1.00	.8413	.8438	.8461	.8485	.8508	.8531	.8554	.8577	.8599	.8621	1.00
1.10	.8643	.8665	.8686	.8708	.8729	.8749	.8770	.8790	.8810	.8830	1.10
1.20	.8849	.8869	.8888	.8907	.8925	.8944	.8962	.8980	.8997	.9015	1.20
1.30	.9032	.9049	.9066	.9082	.9099	.9115	.9131	.9147	.9162	.9177	1.30
1.40	.9192	.9207	.9222	.9236	.9251	.9265	.9279	.9292	.9306	.9319	1.40
1.50	.9332	.9345	.9357	.9370	.9382	.9394	.9406	.9418	.9429	.9441	1.50
1.60	.9452	.9463	.9474	.9484	.9495	.9505	.9515	.9525	.9535	.9545	1.60
1.70	.9554	.9564	.9573	.9582	.9591	.9599	.9608	.9616	.9625	.9633	1.70
1.80	.9641	.9649	.9656	.9664	.9671	.9678	.9686	.9693	.9699	.9706	1.80
1.90	.9713	.9719	.9726	.9732	.9738	.9744	.9750	.9756	.9761	.9767	1.90
2.00	.9772	.9778	.9783	.9788	.9793	.9798	.9803	.9808	.9812	.9817	2.00
2.10	.9821	.9826	.9830	.9834	.9838	.9842	.9846	.9850	.9854	.9857	2.10
2.20	.9861	.9864	.9868	.9871	.9875	.9878	.9881	.9884	.9887	.9890	2.20
2.30	.9893	.9896	.9898	.9901	.9904	.9906	.9909	.9911	.9913	.9916	2.30
2.40	.9918	.9920	.9922	.9925	.9927	.9929	.9931	.9932	.9934	.9936	2.40
2.50	.9938	.9940	.9941	.9943	.9945	.9946	.9948	.9949	.9951	.9952	2.50
2.60	.9953	.9955	.9956	.9957	.9959	.9960	.9961	.9962	.9963	.9964	2.60
2.70	.9965	.9966	.9967	.9968	.9969	.9970	.9971	.9972	.9973	.9974	2.70
2.80	.9974	.9975	.9976	.9977	.9977	.9978	.9979	.9979	.9980	.9981	2.80
2.90	.9981	.9982	.9982	.9983	.9984	.9984	.9985	.9985	.9986	.9986	2.90
3.00	.9987	.9987	.9987	.9988	.9988	.9989	.9989	.9989	.9990	.9990	3.00
3.10	.9990	.9991	.9991	.9991	.9992	.9992	.9992	.9992	.9993	.9993	3.10
3.20	.9993	.9993	.9994	.9994	.9994	.9994	.9994	.9995	.9995	.9995	3.20
3.30	.9995	.9995	.9995	.9996	.9996	.9996	.9996	.9996	.9996	.9997	3.30
3.40	.9997	.9997	.9997	.9997	.9997	.9997	.9997	.9997	.9997	.9998	3.40
3.50	.9998	.9998	.9998	.9998	.9998	.9998	.9998	.9998	.9998	.9998	3.50
3.60	.9998	.9998	.9999	.9999	.9999	.9999	.9999	.9999	.9999	.9999	3.60
3.70	.9999	.9999	.9999	.9999	.9999	.9999	.9999	.9999	.9999	.9999	3.70
3.80	.9999	.9999	.9999	.9999	.9999	.9999	.9999	.9999	.9999	.9999	3.80

TABLE E Percentiles of the t Distribution

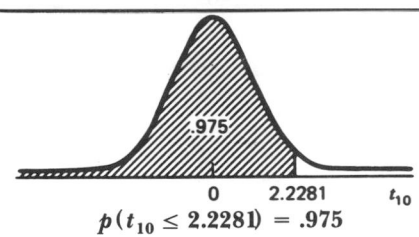

$p(t_{10} \le 2.2281) = .975$

d.f.	$t_{.90}$	$t_{.95}$	$t_{.975}$	$t_{.99}$	$t_{.995}$
1	3.078	6.3138	12.706	31.821	63.657
2	1.886	2.9200	4.3027	6.965	9.9248
3	1.638	2.3534	3.1825	4.541	5.8409
4	1.533	2.1318	2.7764	3.747	4.6041
5	1.476	2.0150	2.5706	3.365	4.0321
6	1.440	1.9432	2.4469	3.143	3.7074
7	1.415	1.8946	2.3646	2.998	3.4995
8	1.397	1.8595	2.3060	2.896	3.3554
9	1.383	1.8331	2.2622	2.821	3.2498
10	1.372	1.8125	2.2281	2.764	3.1693
11	1.363	1.7959	2.2010	2.718	3.1058
12	1.356	1.7823	2.1788	2.681	3.0545
13	1.350	1.7709	2.1604	2.650	3.0123
14	1.345	1.7613	2.1448	2.624	2.9768
15	1.341	1.7530	2.1315	2.602	2.9467
16	1.337	1.7459	2.1199	2.583	2.9208
17	1.333	1.7396	2.1098	2.567	2.8982
18	1.330	1.7341	2.1009	2.552	2.8784
19	1.328	1.7291	2.0930	2.539	2.8609
20	1.325	1.7247	2.0860	2.528	2.8453
21	1.323	1.7207	2.0796	2.518	2.8314
22	1.321	1.7171	2.0739	2.508	2.8188
23	1.319	1.7139	2.0687	2.500	2.8073
24	1.318	1.7109	2.0639	2.492	2.7969
25	1.316	1.7081	2.0595	2.485	2.7874
26	1.315	1.7056	2.0555	2.479	2.7787
27	1.314	1.7033	2.0518	2.473	2.7707
28	1.313	1.7011	2.0484	2.467	2.7633
29	1.311	1.6991	2.0452	2.462	2.7564
30	1.310	1.6973	2.0423	2.457	2.7500
35	1.3062	1.6896	2.0301	2.438	2.7239
40	1.3031	1.6839	2.0211	2.423	2.7045
45	1.3007	1.6794	2.0141	2.412	2.6896
50	1.2987	1.6759	2.0086	2.403	2.6778
60	1.2959	1.6707	2.0003	2.390	2.6603
70	1.2938	1.6669	1.9945	2.381	2.6480
80	1.2922	1.6641	1.9901	2.374	2.6388
90	1.2910	1.6620	1.9867	2.368	2.6316
100	1.2901	1.6602	1.9840	2.364	2.6260
120	1.2887	1.6577	1.9799	2.358	2.6175
140	1.2876	1.6558	1.9771	2.353	2.6114
160	1.2869	1.6545	1.9749	2.350	2.6070
180	1.2863	1.6534	1.9733	2.347	2.6035
200	1.2858	1.6525	1.9719	2.345	2.6006
∞	1.282	1.645	1.96	2.326	2.576

TABLE F Percentiles of the Chi-square Distribution

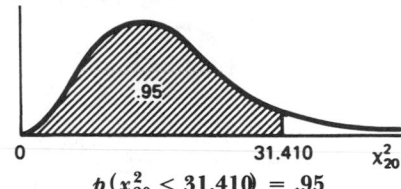

$$p(x_{20}^2 \leq 31.410) = .95$$

d.f.	$\chi_{.005}^2$	$\chi_{.025}^2$	$\chi_{.05}^2$	$\chi_{.90}^2$	$\chi_{.95}^2$	$\chi_{.975}^2$	$\chi_{.99}^2$	$\chi_{.995}^2$
1	.0000393	.000982	.00393	2.706	3.841	5.024	6.635	7.879
2	.0100	.0506	.103	4.605	5.991	7.378	9.210	10.597
3	.0717	.216	.352	6.251	7.815	9.348	11.345	12.838
4	.207	.484	.711	7.779	9.488	11.143	13.277	14.860
5	.412	.831	1.145	9.236	11.070	12.832	15.086	16.750
6	.676	1.237	1.635	10.645	12.592	14.449	16.812	18.548
7	.989	1.690	2.167	12.017	14.067	16.013	18.475	20.278
8	1.344	2.180	2.733	13.362	15.507	17.535	20.090	21.955
9	1.735	2.700	3.325	14.684	16.919	19.023	21.666	23.589
10	2.156	3.247	3.940	15.987	18.307	20.483	23.209	25.188
11	2.603	3.816	4.575	17.275	19.675	21.920	24.725	26.757
12	3.074	4.404	5.226	18.549	21.026	23.336	26.217	28.300
13	3.565	5.009	5.892	19.812	22.362	24.736	27.688	29.819
14	4.075	5.629	6.571	21.064	23.685	26.119	29.141	31.319
15	4.601	6.262	7.261	22.307	24.996	27.488	30.578	32.801
16	5.142	6.908	7.962	23.542	26.296	28.845	32.000	34.267
17	5.697	7.564	8.672	24.769	27.587	30.191	33.409	35.718
18	6.265	8.231	9.390	25.989	28.869	31.526	34.805	37.156
19	6.844	8.907	10.117	27.204	30.144	32.852	36.191	38.582
20	7.434	9.591	10.851	28.412	31.410	34.170	37.566	39.997
21	8.034	10.283	11.591	29.615	32.671	35.479	38.932	41.401
22	8.643	10.982	12.338	30.813	33.924	36.781	40.289	42.796
23	9.260	11.688	13.091	32.007	35.172	38.076	41.638	44.181
24	9.886	12.401	13.848	33.196	36.415	39.364	42.980	45.558
25	10.520	13.120	14.611	34.382	37.652	40.646	44.314	46.928
26	11.160	13.844	15.379	35.563	38.885	41.923	45.642	48.290
27	11.808	14.573	16.151	36.741	40.113	43.194	46.963	49.645
28	12.461	15.308	16.928	37.916	41.337	44.461	48.278	50.993
29	13.121	16.047	17.708	39.087	42.557	45.722	49.588	52.336
30	13.787	16.791	18.493	40.256	43.773	46.979	50.892	53.672
35	17.192	20.569	22.465	46.059	49.802	53.203	57.342	60.275
40	20.707	24.433	26.509	51.805	55.758	59.342	63.691	66.766
45	24.311	28.366	30.612	57.505	61.656	65.410	69.957	73.166
50	27.991	32.357	34.764	63.167	67.505	71.420	76.154	79.490
60	35.535	40.482	43.188	74.397	79.082	83.298	88.379	91.952
70	43.275	48.758	51.739	85.527	90.531	95.023	100.425	104.215
80	51.172	57.153	60.391	96.578	101.879	106.629	112.329	116.321
90	59.196	65.647	69.126	107.565	113.145	118.136	124.116	128.299
100	67.328	74.222	77.929	118.498	124.342	129.561	135.807	140.169

TABLE G Percentiles of the F Distribution

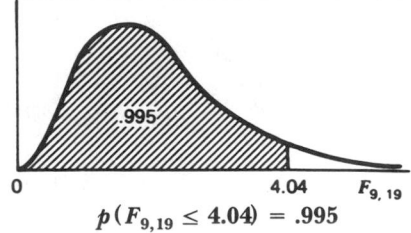

$$p(F_{9,19} \le 4.04) = .995$$

$F_{.995}$

Denominator Degrees of Freedom	Numerator Degrees of Freedom								
	1	2	3	4	5	6	7	8	9
1	16211	20000	21615	22500	23056	23437	23715	23925	24091
2	198.5	199.0	199.2	199.2	199.3	199.3	199.4	199.4	199.4
3	55.55	49.80	47.47	46.19	45.39	44.84	44.43	44.13	43.88
4	31.33	26.28	24.26	23.15	22.46	21.97	21.62	21.35	21.14
5	22.78	18.31	16.53	15.56	14.94	14.51	14.20	13.96	13.77
6	18.63	14.54	12.92	12.03	11.46	11.07	10.79	10.57	10.39
7	16.24	12.40	10.88	10.05	9.52	9.16	8.89	8.68	8.51
8	14.69	11.04	9.60	8.81	8.30	7.95	7.69	7.50	7.34
9	13.61	10.11	8.72	7.96	7.47	7.13	6.88	6.69	6.54
10	12.83	9.43	8.08	7.34	6.87	6.54	6.30	6.12	5.97
11	12.23	8.91	7.60	6.88	6.42	6.10	5.86	5.68	5.54
12	11.75	8.51	7.23	6.52	6.07	5.76	5.52	5.35	5.20
13	11.37	8.19	6.93	6.23	5.79	5.48	5.25	5.08	4.94
14	11.06	7.92	6.68	6.00	5.56	5.26	5.03	4.86	4.72
15	10.80	7.70	6.48	5.80	5.37	5.07	4.85	4.67	4.54
16	10.58	7.51	6.30	5.64	5.21	4.91	4.69	4.52	4.38
17	10.38	7.35	6.16	5.50	5.07	4.78	4.56	4.39	4.25
18	10.22	7.21	6.03	5.37	4.96	4.66	4.44	4.28	4.14
19	10.07	7.09	5.92	5.27	4.85	4.56	4.34	4.18	4.04
20	9.94	6.99	5.82	5.17	4.76	4.47	4.26	4.09	3.96
21	9.83	6.89	5.73	5.09	4.68	4.39	4.18	4.01	3.88
22	9.73	6.81	5.65	5.02	4.61	4.32	4.11	3.94	3.81
23	9.63	6.73	5.58	4.95	4.54	4.26	4.05	3.88	3.75
24	9.55	6.66	5.52	4.89	4.49	4.20	3.99	3.83	3.69
25	9.48	6.60	5.46	4.84	4.43	4.15	3.94	3.78	3.64
26	9.41	6.54	5.41	4.79	4.38	4.10	3.89	3.73	3.60
27	9.34	6.49	5.36	4.74	4.34	4.06	3.85	3.69	3.56
28	9.28	6.44	5.32	4.70	4.30	4.02	3.81	3.65	3.52
29	9.23	6.40	5.28	4.66	4.26	3.98	3.77	3.61	3.48
30	9.18	6.35	5.24	4.62	4.23	3.95	3.74	3.58	3.45
40	8.83	6.07	4.98	4.37	3.99	3.71	3.51	3.35	3.22
60	8.49	5.79	4.73	4.14	3.76	3.49	3.29	3.13	3.01
120	8.18	5.54	4.50	3.92	3.55	3.28	3.09	2.93	2.81
∞	7.88	5.30	4.28	3.72	3.35	3.09	2.90	2.74	2.62

TABLE G (*continued*)

Denominator Degrees of Freedom	Numerator Degrees of Freedom									
	10	12	15	20	24	30	40	60	120	∞
1	24224	24426	24630	24836	24940	25044	25148	25253	25359	25465
2	199.4	199.4	199.4	199.4	199.5	199.5	199.5	199.5	199.5	199.5
3	43.69	43.39	43.08	42.78	42.62	42.47	42.31	42.15	41.99	41.83
4	20.97	20.70	20.44	20.17	20.03	19.89	19.75	19.61	19.47	19.32
5	13.62	13.38	13.15	12.90	12.78	12.66	12.53	12.40	12.27	12.14
6	10.25	10.03	9.81	9.59	9.47	9.36	9.24	9.12	9.00	8.88
7	8.38	8.18	7.97	7.75	7.65	7.53	7.42	7.31	7.19	7.08
8	7.21	7.01	6.81	6.61	6.50	6.40	6.29	6.18	6.06	5.95
9	6.42	6.23	6.03	5.83	5.73	5.62	5.52	5.41	5.30	5.19
10	5.85	5.66	5.47	5.27	5.17	5.07	4.97	4.86	4.75	4.64
11	5.42	5.24	5.05	4.86	4.76	4.65	4.55	4.44	4.34	4.23
12	5.09	4.91	4.72	4.53	4.43	4.33	4.23	4.12	4.01	3.90
13	4.82	4.64	4.46	4.27	4.17	4.07	3.97	3.87	3.76	3.65
14	4.60	4.43	4.25	4.06	3.96	3.86	3.76	3.66	3.55	3.44
15	4.42	4.25	4.07	3.88	3.79	3.69	3.58	3.48	3.37	3.26
16	4.27	4.10	3.92	3.73	3.64	3.54	3.44	3.33	3.22	3.11
17	4.14	3.97	3.79	3.61	3.51	3.41	3.31	3.21	3.10	2.98
18	4.03	3.86	3.68	3.50	3.40	3.30	3.20	3.10	2.99	2.87
19	3.93	3.76	3.59	3.40	3.31	3.21	3.11	3.00	2.89	2.78
20	3.85	3.68	3.50	3.32	3.22	3.12	3.02	2.92	2.81	2.69
21	3.77	3.60	3.43	3.24	3.15	3.05	2.95	2.84	2.73	2.61
22	3.70	3.54	3.36	3.18	3.08	2.98	2.88	2.77	2.66	2.55
23	3.64	3.47	3.30	3.12	3.02	2.92	2.82	2.71	2.60	2.48
24	3.59	3.42	3.25	3.06	2.97	2.87	2.77	2.66	2.55	2.43
25	3.54	3.37	3.20	3.01	2.92	2.82	2.72	2.61	2.50	2.38
26	3.49	3.33	3.15	2.97	2.87	2.77	2.67	2.56	2.45	2.33
27	3.45	3.28	3.11	2.93	2.83	2.73	2.63	2.52	2.41	2.29
28	3.41	3.25	3.07	2.89	2.79	2.69	2.59	2.48	2.37	2.25
29	3.38	3.21	3.04	2.86	2.76	2.66	2.56	2.45	2.33	2.21
30	3.34	3.18	3.01	2.82	2.73	2.63	2.52	2.42	2.30	2.18
40	3.12	2.95	2.78	2.60	2.50	2.40	2.30	2.18	2.06	1.93
60	2.90	2.74	2.57	2.39	2.29	2.19	2.08	1.96	1.83	1.69
120	2.71	2.54	2.37	2.19	2.09	1.98	1.87	1.75	1.61	1.43
∞	2.52	2.36	2.19	2.00	1.90	1.79	1.67	1.53	1.36	1.00

TABLE G (*continued*)

$$F_{.99}$$

Denominator Degrees of Freedom	Numerator Degrees of Freedom								
	1	2	3	4	5	6	7	8	9
1	4052	4999.5	5403	5625	5764	5859	5928	5981	6022
2	98.50	99.00	99.17	99.25	99.30	99.33	99.36	99.37	99.39
3	34.12	30.82	29.46	28.71	28.24	27.91	27.67	27.49	27.35
4	21.20	18.00	16.69	15.98	15.52	15.21	14.98	14.80	14.66
5	16.26	13.27	12.06	11.39	10.97	10.67	10.46	10.29	10.16
6	13.75	10.92	9.78	9.15	8.75	8.47	8.26	8.10	7.98
7	12.25	9.55	8.45	7.85	7.46	7.19	6.99	6.84	6.72
8	11.26	8.65	7.59	7.01	6.63	6.37	6.18	6.03	5.91
9	10.56	8.02	6.99	6.42	6.06	5.80	5.61	5.47	5.35
10	10.04	7.56	6.55	5.99	5.64	5.39	5.20	5.06	4.94
11	9.65	7.21	6.22	5.67	5.32	5.07	4.89	4.74	4.63
12	9.33	6.93	5.95	5.41	5.06	4.82	4.64	4.50	4.39
13	9.07	6.70	5.74	5.21	4.86	4.62	4.44	4.30	4.19
14	8.86	6.51	5.56	5.04	4.69	4.46	4.28	4.14	4.03
15	8.68	6.36	5.42	4.89	4.56	4.32	4.14	4.00	3.89
16	8.53	6.23	5.29	4.77	4.44	4.20	4.03	3.89	3.78
17	8.40	6.11	5.18	4.67	4.34	4.10	3.93	3.79	3.68
18	8.29	6.01	5.09	4.58	4.25	4.01	3.84	3.71	3.60
19	8.18	5.93	5.01	4.50	4.17	3.94	3.77	3.63	3.52
20	8.10	5.85	4.94	4.43	4.10	3.87	3.70	3.56	3.46
21	8.02	5.78	4.87	4.37	4.04	3.81	3.64	3.51	3.40
22	7.95	5.72	4.82	4.31	3.99	3.76	3.59	3.45	3.35
23	7.88	5.66	4.76	4.26	3.94	3.71	3.54	3.41	3.30
24	7.82	5.61	4.72	4.22	3.90	3.67	3.50	3.36	3.26
25	7.77	5.57	4.68	4.18	3.85	3.63	3.46	3.32	3.22
26	7.72	5.53	4.64	4.14	3.82	3.59	3.42	3.29	3.18
27	7.68	5.49	4.60	4.11	3.78	3.56	3.39	3.26	3.15
28	7.64	5.45	4.57	4.07	3.75	3.53	3.36	3.23	3.12
29	7.60	5.42	4.54	4.04	3.73	3.50	3.33	3.20	3.09
30	7.56	5.39	4.51	4.02	3.70	3.47	3.30	3.17	3.07
40	7.31	5.18	4.31	3.83	3.51	3.29	3.12	2.99	2.89
60	7.08	4.98	4.13	3.65	3.34	3.12	2.95	2.82	2.72
120	6.85	4.79	3.95	3.48	3.17	2.96	2.79	2.66	2.56
∞	6.63	4.61	3.78	3.32	3.02	2.80	2.64	2.51	2.41

TABLE G (*continued*)

Denominator Degrees of Freedom	Numerator Degrees of Freedom									
	10	12	15	20	24	30	40	60	120	∞
1	6056	6106	6157	6209	6235	6261	6287	6313	6339	6366
2	99.40	99.42	99.43	99.45	99.46	99.47	99.47	99.48	99.49	99.50
3	27.23	27.05	26.87	26.69	26.60	26.50	26.41	26.32	26.22	26.13
4	14.55	14.37	14.20	14.02	13.93	13.84	13.75	13.65	13.56	13.46
5	10.05	9.89	9.72	9.55	9.47	9.38	9.29	9.20	9.11	9.02
6	7.87	7.72	7.56	7.40	7.31	7.23	7.14	7.06	6.97	6.88
7	6.62	6.47	6.31	6.16	6.07	5.99	5.91	5.82	5.74	5.65
8	5.81	5.67	5.52	5.36	5.28	5.20	5.12	5.03	4.95	4.86
9	5.26	5.11	4.96	4.81	4.73	4.65	4.57	4.48	4.40	4.31
10	4.85	4.71	4.56	4.41	4.33	4.25	4.17	4.08	4.00	3.91
11	4.54	4.40	4.25	4.10	4.02	3.94	3.86	3.78	3.69	3.60
12	4.30	4.16	4.01	3.86	3.78	3.70	3.62	3.54	3.45	3.36
13	4.10	3.96	3.82	3.66	3.59	3.51	3.43	3.34	3.25	3.17
14	3.94	3.80	3.66	3.51	3.43	3.35	3.27	3.18	3.09	3.00
15	3.80	3.67	3.52	3.37	3.29	3.21	3.13	3.05	2.96	2.87
16	3.69	3.55	3.41	3.26	3.18	3.10	3.02	2.93	2.84	2.75
17	3.59	3.46	3.31	3.16	3.08	3.00	2.92	2.83	2.75	2.65
18	3.51	3.37	3.23	3.08	3.00	2.92	2.84	2.75	2.66	2.57
19	3.43	3.30	3.15	3.00	2.92	2.84	2.76	2.67	2.58	2.49
20	3.37	3.23	3.09	2.94	2.86	2.78	2.69	2.61	2.52	2.42
21	3.31	3.17	3.03	2.88	2.80	2.72	2.64	2.55	2.46	2.36
22	3.26	3.12	2.98	2.83	2.75	2.67	2.58	2.50	2.40	2.31
23	3.21	3.07	2.93	2.78	2.70	2.62	2.54	2.45	2.35	2.26
24	3.17	3.03	2.89	2.74	2.66	2.58	2.49	2.40	2.31	2.21
25	3.13	2.99	2.85	2.70	2.62	2.54	2.45	2.36	2.27	2.17
26	3.09	2.96	2.81	2.66	2.58	2.50	2.42	2.33	2.23	2.13
27	3.06	2.93	2.78	2.63	2.55	2.47	2.38	2.29	2.20	2.10
28	3.03	2.90	2.75	2.60	2.52	2.44	2.35	2.26	2.17	2.06
29	3.00	2.87	2.73	2.57	2.49	2.41	2.33	2.23	2.14	2.03
30	2.98	2.84	2.70	2.55	2.47	2.39	2.30	2.21	2.11	2.01
40	2.80	2.66	2.52	2.37	2.29	2.20	2.11	2.02	1.92	1.80
60	2.63	2.50	2.35	2.20	2.12	2.03	1.94	1.84	1.73	1.60
120	2.47	2.34	2.19	2.03	1.95	1.86	1.76	1.66	1.53	1.38
∞	2.32	2.18	2.04	1.88	1.79	1.70	1.59	1.47	1.32	1.00

TABLE G (*continued*)

Denominator Degrees of Freedom	$F_{.975}$ Numerator Degrees of Freedom								
	1	2	3	4	5	6	7	8	9
1	647.8	799.5	864.2	899.6	921.8	937.1	948.2	956.7	963.3
2	38.51	39.00	39.17	39.25	39.30	39.33	39.36	39.37	39.39
3	17.44	16.04	15.44	15.10	14.88	14.73	14.62	14.54	14.47
4	12.22	10.65	9.98	9.60	9.36	9.20	9.07	8.98	8.90
5	10.01	8.43	7.76	7.39	7.15	6.98	6.85	6.76	6.68
6	8.81	7.26	6.60	6.23	5.99	5.82	5.70	5.60	5.52
7	8.07	6.54	5.89	5.52	5.29	5.12	4.99	4.90	4.82
8	7.57	6.06	5.42	5.05	4.82	4.65	4.53	4.43	4.36
9	7.21	5.71	5.08	4.72	4.48	4.32	4.20	4.10	4.03
10	6.94	5.46	4.83	4.47	4.24	4.07	3.95	3.85	3.78
11	6.72	5.26	4.63	4.28	4.04	3.88	3.76	3.66	3.59
12	6.55	5.10	4.47	4.12	3.89	3.73	3.61	3.51	3.44
13	6.41	4.97	4.35	4.00	3.77	3.60	3.48	3.39	3.31
14	6.30	4.86	4.24	3.89	3.66	3.50	3.38	3.29	3.21
15	6.20	4.77	4.15	3.80	3.58	3.41	3.29	3.20	3.12
16	6.12	4.69	4.08	3.73	3.50	3.34	3.22	3.12	3.05
17	6.04	4.62	4.01	3.66	3.44	3.28	3.16	3.06	2.98
18	5.98	4.56	3.95	3.61	3.38	3.22	3.10	3.01	2.93
19	5.92	4.51	3.90	3.56	3.33	3.17	3.05	2.96	2.88
20	5.87	4.46	3.86	3.51	3.29	3.13	3.01	2.91	2.84
21	5.83	4.42	3.82	3.48	3.25	3.09	2.97	2.87	2.80
22	5.79	4.38	3.78	3.44	3.22	3.05	2.93	2.84	2.76
23	5.75	4.35	3.75	3.41	3.18	3.02	2.90	2.81	2.73
24	5.72	4.32	3.72	3.38	3.15	2.99	2.87	2.78	2.70
25	5.69	4.29	3.69	3.35	3.13	2.97	2.85	2.75	2.68
26	5.66	4.27	3.67	3.33	3.10	2.94	2.82	2.73	2.65
27	5.63	4.24	3.65	3.31	3.08	2.92	2.80	2.71	2.63
28	5.61	4.22	3.63	3.29	3.06	2.90	2.78	2.69	2.61
29	5.59	4.20	3.61	3.27	3.04	2.88	2.76	2.67	2.59
30	5.57	4.18	3.59	3.25	3.03	2.87	2.75	2.65	2.57
40	5.42	4.05	3.46	3.13	2.90	2.74	2.62	2.53	2.45
60	5.29	3.93	3.34	3.01	2.79	2.63	2.51	2.41	2.33
120	5.15	3.80	3.23	2.89	2.67	2.52	2.39	2.30	2.22
∞	5.02	3.69	3.12	2.79	2.57	2.41	2.29	2.19	2.11

TABLE G (*continued*)

Denominator Degrees of Freedom	10	12	15	20	24	30	40	60	120	∞
				Numerator Degrees of Freedom						
1	968.6	976.7	984.9	993.1	997.2	1001	1006	1010	1014	1018
2	39.40	39.41	39.43	39.45	39.46	39.46	39.47	39.48	39.49	39.50
3	14.42	14.34	14.25	14.17	14.12	14.08	14.04	13.99	13.95	13.90
4	8.84	8.75	8.66	8.56	8.51	8.46	8.41	8.36	8.31	8.26
5	6.62	6.52	6.43	6.33	6.28	6.23	6.18	6.12	6.07	6.02
6	5.46	5.37	5.27	5.17	5.12	5.07	5.01	4.96	4.90	4.85
7	4.76	4.67	4.57	4.47	4.42	4.36	4.31	4.25	4.20	4.14
8	4.30	4.20	4.10	4.00	3.95	3.89	3.84	3.78	3.73	3.67
9	3.96	3.87	3.77	3.67	3.61	3.56	3.51	3.45	3.39	3.33
10	3.72	3.62	3.52	3.42	3.37	3.31	3.26	3.20	3.14	3.08
11	3.53	3.43	3.33	3.23	3.17	3.12	3.06	3.00	2.94	2.88
12	3.37	3.28	3.18	3.07	3.02	2.96	2.91	2.85	2.79	2.72
13	3.25	3.15	3.05	2.95	2.89	2.84	2.78	2.72	2.66	2.60
14	3.15	3.05	2.95	2.84	2.79	2.73	2.67	2.61	2.55	2.49
15	3.06	2.96	2.86	2.76	2.70	2.64	2.59	2.52	2.46	2.40
16	2.99	2.89	2.79	2.68	2.63	2.57	2.51	2.45	2.38	2.32
17	2.92	2.82	2.72	2.62	2.56	2.50	2.44	2.38	2.32	2.25
18	2.87	2.77	2.67	2.56	2.50	2.44	2.38	2.32	2.26	2.19
19	2.82	2.72	2.62	2.51	2.45	2.39	2.33	2.27	2.20	2.13
20	2.77	2.68	2.57	2.46	2.41	2.35	2.29	2.22	2.16	2.09
21	2.73	2.64	2.53	2.42	2.37	2.31	2.25	2.18	2.11	2.04
22	2.70	2.60	2.50	2.39	2.33	2.27	2.21	2.14	2.08	2.00
23	2.67	2.57	2.47	2.36	2.30	2.24	2.18	2.11	2.04	1.97
24	2.64	2.54	2.44	2.33	2.27	2.21	2.15	2.08	2.01	1.94
25	2.61	2.51	2.41	2.30	2.24	2.18	2.12	2.05	1.98	1.91
26	2.59	2.49	2.39	2.28	2.22	2.16	2.09	2.03	1.95	1.88
27	2.57	2.47	2.36	2.25	2.19	2.13	2.07	2.00	1.93	1.85
28	2.55	2.45	2.34	2.23	2.17	2.11	2.05	1.98	1.91	1.83
29	2.53	2.43	2.32	2.21	2.15	2.09	2.03	1.96	1.89	1.81
30	2.51	2.41	2.31	2.20	2.14	2.07	2.01	1.94	1.87	1.79
40	2.39	2.29	2.18	2.07	2.01	1.94	1.88	1.80	1.72	1.64
60	2.27	2.17	2.06	1.94	1.88	1.82	1.74	1.67	1.58	1.48
120	2.16	2.05	1.94	1.82	1.76	1.69	1.61	1.53	1.43	1.31
∞	2.05	1.94	1.83	1.71	1.64	1.57	1.48	1.39	1.27	1.00

TABLE G (*continued*)

$F_{.95}$

Denominator Degrees of Freedom	Numerator Degrees of Freedom								
	1	**2**	**3**	**4**	**5**	**6**	**7**	**8**	**9**
1	161.4	199.5	215.7	224.6	230.2	234.0	236.8	238.9	240.5
2	18.51	19.00	19.16	19.25	19.30	19.33	19.35	19.37	19.38
3	10.13	9.55	9.28	9.12	9.01	8.94	8.89	8.85	8.81
4	7.71	6.94	6.59	6.39	6.26	6.16	6.09	6.04	6.00
5	6.61	5.79	5.41	5.19	5.05	4.95	4.88	4.82	4.77
6	5.99	5.14	4.76	4.53	4.39	4.28	4.21	4.15	4.10
7	5.59	4.74	4.35	4.12	3.97	3.87	3.79	3.73	3.68
8	5.32	4.46	4.07	3.84	3.69	3.58	3.50	3.44	3.39
9	5.12	4.26	3.86	3.63	3.48	3.37	3.29	3.23	3.18
10	4.96	4.10	3.71	3.48	3.33	3.22	3.14	3.07	3.02
11	4.84	3.98	3.59	3.36	3.20	3.09	3.01	2.95	2.90
12	4.75	3.89	3.49	3.26	3.11	3.00	2.91	2.85	2.80
13	4.67	3.81	3.41	3.18	3.03	2.92	2.83	2.77	2.71
14	4.60	3.74	3.34	3.11	2.96	2.85	2.76	2.70	2.65
15	4.54	3.68	3.29	3.06	2.90	2.79	2.71	2.64	2.59
16	4.49	3.63	3.24	3.01	2.85	2.74	2.66	2.59	2.54
17	4.45	3.59	3.20	2.96	2.81	2.70	2.61	2.55	2.49
18	4.41	3.55	3.16	2.93	2.77	2.66	2.58	2.51	2.46
19	4.38	3.52	3.13	2.90	2.74	2.63	2.54	2.48	2.42
20	4.35	3.49	3.10	2.87	2.71	2.60	2.51	2.45	2.39
21	4.32	3.47	3.07	2.84	2.68	2.57	2.49	2.42	2.37
22	4.30	3.44	3.05	2.82	2.66	2.55	2.46	2.40	2.34
23	4.28	3.42	3.03	2.80	2.64	2.53	2.44	2.37	2.32
24	4.26	3.40	3.01	2.78	2.62	2.51	2.42	2.36	2.30
25	4.24	3.39	2.99	2.76	2.60	2.49	2.40	2.34	2.28
26	4.23	3.37	2.98	2.74	2.59	2.47	2.39	2.32	2.27
27	4.21	3.35	2.96	2.73	2.57	2.46	2.37	2.31	2.25
28	4.20	3.34	2.95	2.71	2.56	2.45	2.36	2.29	2.24
29	4.18	3.33	2.93	2.70	2.55	2.43	2.35	2.28	2.22
30	4.17	3.32	2.92	2.69	2.53	2.42	2.33	2.27	2.21
40	4.08	3.23	2.84	2.61	2.45	2.34	2.25	2.18	2.12
60	4.00	3.15	2.76	2.53	2.37	2.25	2.17	2.10	2.04
120	3.92	3.07	2.68	2.45	2.29	2.17	2.09	2.02	1.96
∞	3.84	3.00	2.60	2.37	2.21	2.10	2.01	1.94	1.88

TABLE G (*continued*)

Denominator Degrees of Freedom	Numerator Degrees of Freedom									
	10	12	15	20	24	30	40	60	120	∞
1	241.9	243.9	245.9	248.0	249.1	250.1	251.1	252.2	253.3	254.3
2	19.40	19.41	19.43	19.45	19.45	19.46	19.47	19.48	19.49	19.50
3	8.79	8.74	8.70	8.66	8.64	8.62	8.59	8.57	8.55	8.53
4	5.96	5.91	5.86	5.80	5.77	5.75	5.72	5.69	5.66	5.63
5	4.74	4.68	4.62	4.56	4.53	4.50	4.46	4.43	4.40	4.36
6	4.06	4.00	3.94	3.87	3.84	3.81	3.77	3.74	3.70	3.67
7	3.64	3.57	3.51	3.44	3.41	3.38	3.34	3.30	3.27	3.23
8	3.35	3.28	3.22	3.15	3.12	3.08	3.04	3.01	2.97	2.93
9	3.14	3.07	3.01	2.94	2.90	2.86	2.83	2.79	2.75	2.71
10	2.98	2.91	2.85	2.77	2.74	2.70	2.66	2.62	2.58	2.54
11	2.85	2.79	2.72	2.65	2.61	2.57	2.53	2.49	2.45	2.40
12	2.75	2.69	2.62	2.54	2.51	2.47	2.43	2.38	2.34	2.30
13	2.67	2.60	2.53	2.46	2.42	2.38	2.34	2.30	2.25	2.21
14	2.60	2.53	2.46	2.39	2.35	2.31	2.27	2.22	2.18	2.13
15	2.54	2.48	2.40	2.33	2.29	2.25	2.20	2.16	2.11	2.07
16	2.49	2.42	2.35	2.28	2.24	2.19	2.15	2.11	2.06	2.01
17	2.45	2.38	2.31	2.23	2.19	2.15	2.10	2.06	2.01	1.96
18	2.41	2.34	2.27	2.19	2.15	2.11	2.06	2.02	1.97	1.92
19	2.38	2.31	2.23	2.16	2.11	2.07	2.03	1.98	1.93	1.88
20	2.35	2.28	2.20	2.12	2.08	2.04	1.99	1.95	1.90	1.84
21	2.32	2.25	2.18	2.10	2.05	2.01	1.96	1.92	1.87	1.81
22	2.30	2.23	2.15	2.07	2.03	1.98	1.94	1.89	1.84	1.78
23	2.27	2.20	2.13	2.05	2.01	1.96	1.91	1.86	1.81	1.76
24	2.25	2.18	2.11	2.03	1.98	1.94	1.89	1.84	1.79	1.73
25	2.24	2.16	2.09	2.01	1.96	1.92	1.87	1.82	1.77	1.71
26	2.22	2.15	2.07	1.99	1.95	1.90	1.85	1.80	1.75	1.69
27	2.20	2.13	2.06	1.97	1.93	1.88	1.84	1.79	1.73	1.67
28	2.19	2.12	2.04	1.96	1.91	1.87	1.82	1.77	1.71	1.65
29	2.18	2.10	2.03	1.94	1.90	1.85	1.81	1.75	1.70	1.64
30	2.16	2.09	2.01	1.93	1.89	1.84	1.79	1.74	1.68	1.62
40	2.08	2.00	1.92	1.84	1.79	1.74	1.69	1.64	1.58	1.51
60	1.99	1.92	1.84	1.75	1.70	1.65	1.59	1.53	1.47	1.39
120	1.91	1.83	1.75	1.66	1.61	1.55	1.50	1.43	1.35	1.25
∞	1.83	1.75	1.67	1.57	1.52	1.46	1.39	1.32	1.22	1.00

TABLE G (*continued*)

Denominator Degrees of Freedom	$F_{.90}$ Numerator Degrees of Freedom								
	1	2	3	4	5	6	7	8	9
1	39.86	49.50	53.59	55.83	57.24	58.20	58.91	59.44	59.86
2	8.53	9.00	9.16	9.24	9.29	9.33	9.35	9.37	9.38
3	5.54	5.46	5.39	5.34	5.31	5.28	5.27	5.25	5.24
4	4.54	4.32	4.19	4.11	4.05	4.01	3.98	3.95	3.94
5	4.06	3.78	3.62	3.52	3.45	3.40	3.37	3.34	3.32
6	3.78	3.46	3.29	3.18	3.11	3.05	3.01	2.98	2.96
7	3.59	3.26	3.07	2.96	2.88	2.83	2.78	2.75	2.72
8	3.46	3.11	2.92	2.81	2.73	2.67	2.62	2.59	2.56
9	3.36	3.01	2.81	2.69	2.61	2.55	2.51	2.47	2.44
10	3.29	2.92	2.73	2.61	2.52	2.46	2.41	2.38	2.35
11	3.23	2.86	2.66	2.54	2.45	2.39	2.34	2.30	2.27
12	3.18	2.81	2.61	2.48	2.39	2.33	2.28	2.24	2.21
13	3.14	2.76	2.56	2.43	2.35	2.28	2.23	2.20	2.16
14	3.10	2.73	2.52	2.39	2.31	2.24	2.19	2.15	2.12
15	3.07	2.70	2.49	2.36	2.27	2.21	2.16	2.12	2.09
16	3.05	2.67	2.46	2.33	2.24	2.18	2.13	2.09	2.06
17	3.03	2.64	2.44	2.31	2.22	2.15	2.10	2.06	2.03
18	3.01	2.62	2.42	2.29	2.20	2.13	2.08	2.04	2.00
19	2.99	2.61	2.40	2.27	2.18	2.11	2.06	2.02	1.98
20	2.97	2.59	2.38	2.25	2.16	2.09	2.04	2.00	1.96
21	2.96	2.57	2.36	2.23	2.14	2.08	2.02	1.98	1.95
22	2.95	2.56	2.35	2.22	2.13	2.06	2.01	1.97	1.93
23	2.94	2.55	2.34	2.21	2.11	2.05	1.99	1.95	1.92
24	2.93	2.54	2.33	2.19	2.10	2.04	1.98	1.94	1.91
25	2.92	2.53	2.32	2.18	2.09	2.02	1.97	1.93	1.89
26	2.91	2.52	2.31	2.17	2.08	2.01	1.96	1.92	1.88
27	2.90	2.51	2.30	2.17	2.07	2.00	1.95	1.91	1.87
28	2.89	2.50	2.29	2.16	2.06	2.00	1.94	1.90	1.87
29	2.89	2.50	2.28	2.15	2.06	1.99	1.93	1.89	1.86
30	2.88	2.49	2.28	2.14	2.05	1.98	1.93	1.88	1.85
40	2.84	2.44	2.23	2.09	2.00	1.93	1.87	1.83	1.79
60	2.79	2.39	2.18	2.04	1.95	1.87	1.82	1.77	1.74
120	2.75	2.35	2.13	1.99	1.90	1.82	1.77	1.72	1.68
∞	2.71	2.30	2.08	1.94	1.85	1.77	1.72	1.67	1.63

TABLE G (*continued*)

Denominator Degrees of Freedom	Numerator Degrees of Freedom									
	10	12	15	20	24	30	40	60	120	∞
1	60.19	60.71	61.22	61.74	62.00	62.26	62.53	62.79	63.06	63.33
2	9.39	9.41	9.42	9.44	9.45	9.46	9.47	9.47	9.48	9.49
3	5.23	5.22	5.20	5.18	5.18	5.17	5.16	5.15	5.14	5.13
4	3.92	3.90	3.87	3.84	3.83	3.82	3.80	3.79	3.78	3.76
5	3.30	3.27	3.24	3.21	3.19	3.17	3.16	3.14	3.12	3.10
6	2.94	2.90	2.87	2.84	2.82	2.80	2.78	2.76	2.74	2.72
7	2.70	2.67	2.63	2.59	2.58	2.56	2.54	2.51	2.49	2.47
8	2.54	2.50	2.46	2.42	2.40	2.38	2.36	2.34	2.32	2.29
9	2.42	2.38	2.34	2.30	2.28	2.25	2.23	2.21	2.18	2.16
10	2.32	2.28	2.24	2.20	2.18	2.16	2.13	2.11	2.08	2.06
11	2.25	2.21	2.17	2.12	2.10	2.08	2.05	2.03	2.00	1.97
12	2.19	2.15	2.10	2.06	2.04	2.01	1.99	1.96	1.93	1.90
13	2.14	2.10	2.05	2.01	1.98	1.96	1.93	1.90	1.88	1.85
14	2.10	2.05	2.01	1.96	1.94	1.91	1.89	1.86	1.83	1.80
15	2.06	2.02	1.97	1.92	1.90	1.87	1.85	1.82	1.79	1.76
16	2.03	1.99	1.94	1.89	1.87	1.84	1.81	1.78	1.75	1.72
17	2.00	1.96	1.91	1.86	1.84	1.81	1.78	1.75	1.72	1.69
18	1.98	1.93	1.89	1.84	1.81	1.78	1.75	1.72	1.69	1.66
19	1.96	1.91	1.86	1.81	1.79	1.76	1.73	1.70	1.67	1.63
20	1.94	1.89	1.84	1.79	1.77	1.74	1.71	1.68	1.64	1.61
21	1.92	1.87	1.83	1.78	1.75	1.72	1.69	1.66	1.62	1.59
22	1.90	1.86	1.81	1.76	1.73	1.70	1.67	1.64	1.60	1.57
23	1.89	1.84	1.80	1.74	1.72	1.69	1.66	1.62	1.59	1.55
24	1.88	1.83	1.78	1.73	1.70	1.67	1.64	1.61	1.57	1.53
25	1.87	1.82	1.77	1.72	1.69	1.66	1.63	1.59	1.56	1.52
26	1.86	1.81	1.76	1.71	1.68	1.65	1.61	1.58	1.54	1.50
27	1.85	1.80	1.75	1.70	1.67	1.64	1.60	1.57	1.53	1.49
28	1.84	1.79	1.74	1.69	1.66	1.63	1.59	1.56	1.52	1.48
29	1.83	1.78	1.73	1.68	1.65	1.62	1.58	1.55	1.51	1.47
30	1.82	1.77	1.72	1.67	1.64	1.61	1.57	1.54	1.50	1.46
40	1.76	1.71	1.66	1.61	1.57	1.54	1.51	1.47	1.42	1.38
60	1.71	1.66	1.60	1.54	1.51	1.48	1.44	1.40	1.35	1.29
120	1.65	1.60	1.55	1.48	1.45	1.41	1.37	1.32	1.26	1.19
∞	1.60	1.55	1.49	1.42	1.38	1.34	1.30	1.24	1.17	1.00

TABLE H Percentage Points of the Studentized Range for 2 through 20 Treatments Upper 5% Points

Error df	2	3	4	5	6	7	8	9	10
1	17.97	26.98	32.82	37.08	40.41	43.12	45.40	47.36	49.07
2	6.08	8.33	9.80	10.88	11.74	12.44	13.03	13.54	13.99
3	4.50	5.91	6.82	7.50	8.04	8.48	8.85	9.18	9.46
4	3.93	5.04	5.76	6.29	6.71	7.05	7.35	7.60	7.83
5	3.64	4.60	5.22	5.67	6.03	6.33	6.58	6.80	6.99
6	3.46	4.34	4.90	5.30	5.63	5.90	6.12	6.32	6.49
7	3.34	4.16	4.68	5.06	5.36	5.61	5.82	6.00	6.16
8	3.26	4.04	4.53	4.89	5.17	5.40	5.60	5.77	5.92
9	3.20	3.95	4.41	4.76	5.02	5.24	5.43	5.59	5.74
10	3.15	3.88	4.33	4.65	4.91	5.12	5.30	5.46	5.60
11	3.11	3.82	4.26	4.57	4.82	5.03	5.20	5.35	5.49
12	3.08	3.77	4.20	4.51	4.75	4.95	5.12	5.27	5.39
13	3.06	3.73	4.15	4.45	4.69	4.88	5.05	5.19	5.32
14	3.03	3.70	4.11	4.41	4.64	4.83	4.99	5.13	5.25
15	3.01	3.67	4.08	4.37	4.59	4.78	4.94	5.08	5.20
16	3.00	3.65	4.05	4.33	4.56	4.74	4.90	5.03	5.15
17	2.98	3.63	4.02	4.30	4.52	4.70	4.86	4.99	5.11
18	2.97	3.61	4.00	4.28	4.49	4.67	4.82	4.96	5.07
19	2.96	3.59	3.98	4.25	4.47	4.65	4.79	4.92	5.04
20	2.95	3.58	3.96	4.23	4.45	4.62	4.77	4.90	5.01
24	2.92	3.53	3.90	4.17	4.37	4.54	4.68	4.81	4.92
30	2.89	3.49	3.85	4.10	4.30	4.46	4.60	4.72	4.82
40	2.86	3.44	3.79	4.04	4.23	4.39	4.52	4.63	4.73
60	2.83	3.40	3.74	3.98	4.16	4.31	4.44	4.55	4.65
120	2.80	3.36	3.68	3.92	4.10	4.24	4.36	4.47	4.56
∞	2.77	3.31	3.63	3.86	4.03	4.17	4.29	4.39	4.47

Error df	11	12	13	14	15	16	17	18	19	20
1	50.59	51.96	53.20	54.33	55.36	56.32	57.22	58.04	58.83	59.56
2	14.39	14.75	15.08	15.38	15.65	15.91	16.14	16.37	16.57	16.77
3	9.72	9.95	10.15	10.35	10.52	10.69	10.84	10.98	11.11	11.24
4	8.03	8.21	8.37	8.52	8.66	8.79	8.91	9.03	9.13	9.23
5	7.17	7.32	7.47	7.60	7.72	7.83	7.93	8.03	8.12	8.21
6	6.65	6.79	6.92	7.03	7.14	7.24	7.34	7.43	7.51	7.59
7	6.30	6.43	6.55	6.66	6.76	6.85	6.94	7.02	7.10	7.17
8	6.05	6.18	6.29	6.39	6.48	6.57	6.65	6.73	6.80	6.87
9	5.87	5.98	6.09	6.19	6.28	6.36	6.44	6.51	6.58	6.64
10	5.72	5.83	5.93	6.03	6.11	6.19	6.27	6.34	6.40	6.47
11	5.61	5.71	5.81	5.90	5.98	6.06	6.13	6.20	6.27	6.33
12	5.51	5.61	5.71	5.80	5.88	5.95	6.02	6.09	6.15	6.21
13	5.43	5.53	5.63	5.71	5.79	5.86	5.93	5.99	6.05	6.11
14	5.36	5.46	5.55	5.64	5.71	5.79	5.85	5.91	5.97	6.03
15	5.31	5.40	5.49	5.57	5.65	5.72	5.78	5.85	5.90	5.96

TABLE H (*continued*)

Error df	11	12	13	14	15	16	17	18	19	20
16	5.26	5.35	5.44	5.52	5.59	5.66	5.73	5.79	5.84	5.90
17	5.21	5.31	5.39	5.47	5.54	5.61	5.67	5.73	5.79	5.84
18	5.17	5.27	5.35	5.43	5.50	5.57	5.63	5.69	5.74	5.79
19	5.14	5.23	5.31	5.39	5.46	5.53	5.59	5.65	5.70	5.75
20	5.11	5.20	5.28	5.36	5.43	5.49	5.55	5.61	5.66	5.71
24	5.01	5.10	5.18	5.25	5.32	5.38	5.44	5.49	5.55	5.59
30	4.92	5.00	5.08	5.15	5.21	5.27	5.33	5.38	5.43	5.47
40	4.82	4.90	4.98	5.04	5.11	5.16	5.22	5.27	5.31	5.36
60	4.73	4.81	4.88	4.94	5.00	5.06	5.11	5.15	5.20	5.24
120	4.64	4.71	4.78	4.84	4.90	4.95	5.00	5.04	5.09	5.13
∞	4.55	4.62	4.68	4.74	4.80	4.85	4.89	4.93	4.97	5.01

Upper 1% Points

Error df	2	3	4	5	6	7	8	9	10
1	90.03	135.0	164.3	185.6	202.2	215.8	227.2	237.0	245.6
2	14.04	19.02	22.29	24.72	26.63	28.20	29.53	30.68	31.69
3	8.26	10.62	12.17	13.33	14.24	15.00	15.64	16.20	16.69
4	6.51	8.12	9.17	9.96	10.58	11.10	11.55	11.93	12.27
5	5.70	6.98	7.80	8.42	8.91	9.32	9.67	9.97	10.24
6	5.24	6.33	7.03	7.56	7.97	8.32	8.61	8.87	9.10
7	4.95	5.92	6.54	7.01	7.37	7.68	7.94	8.17	8.37
8	4.75	5.64	6.20	6.62	6.96	7.24	7.47	7.68	7.86
9	4.60	5.43	5.96	6.35	6.66	6.91	7.13	7.33	7.49
10	4.48	5.27	5.77	6.14	6.43	6.67	6.87	7.05	7.21
11	4.39	5.15	5.62	5.97	6.25	6.48	6.67	6.84	6.99
12	4.32	5.05	5.50	5.84	6.10	6.32	6.51	6.67	6.81
13	4.26	4.96	5.40	5.73	5.98	6.19	6.37	6.53	6.67
14	4.21	4.89	5.32	5.63	5.88	6.08	6.26	6.41	6.54
15	4.17	4.84	5.25	5.56	5.80	5.99	6.16	6.31	6.44
16	4.13	4.79	5.19	5.49	5.72	5.92	6.08	6.22	6.35
17	4.10	4.74	5.14	5.43	5.66	5.85	6.01	6.15	6.27
18	4.07	4.70	5.09	5.38	5.60	5.79	5.94	6.08	6.20
19	4.05	4.67	5.05	5.33	5.55	5.73	5.89	6.02	6.14
20	4.02	4.64	5.02	5.29	5.51	5.69	5.84	5.97	6.09
24	3.96	4.55	4.91	5.17	5.37	5.54	5.69	5.81	5.92
30	3.89	4.45	4.80	5.05	5.24	5.40	5.54	5.65	5.76
40	3.82	4.37	4.70	4.93	5.11	5.26	5.39	5.50	5.60
60	3.76	4.28	4.59	4.82	4.99	5.13	5.25	5.36	5.45
120	3.70	4.20	4.50	4.71	4.87	5.01	5.12	5.21	5.30
∞	3.64	4.12	4.40	4.60	4.76	4.88	4.99	5.08	5.16

TABLE H (*continued*)

Error df	11	12	13	14	15	16	17	18	19	20
1	253.2	260.0	266.2	271.8	277.0	281.8	286.3	290.4	294.3	298.0
2	32.59	33.40	34.13	34.81	35.43	36.00	36.53	37.03	37.50	37.95
3	17.13	17.53	17.89	18.22	18.52	18.81	19.07	19.32	19.55	19.77
4	12.57	12.84	13.09	13.32	13.53	13.73	13.91	14.08	14.24	14.40
5	10.48	10.70	10.89	11.08	11.24	11.40	11.55	11.68	11.81	11.93
6	9.30	9.48	9.65	9.81	9.95	10.08	10.21	10.32	10.43	10.54
7	8.55	8.71	8.86	9.00	9.12	9.24	9.35	9.46	9.55	9.65
8	8.03	8.18	8.31	8.44	8.55	8.66	8.76	8.85	8.94	9.03
9	7.65	7.78	7.91	8.03	8.13	8.23	8.33	8.41	8.49	8.57
10	7.36	7.49	7.60	7.71	7.81	7.91	7.99	8.08	8.15	8.23
11	7.13	7.25	7.36	7.46	7.56	7.65	7.73	7.81	7.88	7.95
12	6.94	7.06	7.17	7.26	7.36	7.44	7.52	7.59	7.66	7.73
13	6.79	6.90	7.01	7.10	7.19	7.27	7.35	7.42	7.48	7.55
14	6.66	6.77	6.87	6.96	7.05	7.13	7.20	7.27	7.33	7.39
15	6.55	6.66	6.76	6.84	6.93	7.00	7.07	7.14	7.20	7.26
16	6.46	6.56	6.66	6.74	6.82	6.90	6.97	7.03	7.09	7.15
17	6.38	6.48	6.57	6.66	6.73	6.81	6.87	6.94	7.00	7.05
18	6.31	6.41	6.50	6.58	6.65	6.73	6.79	6.85	6.91	6.97
19	6.25	6.34	6.43	6.51	6.58	6.65	6.72	6.78	6.84	6.89
20	6.19	6.28	6.37	6.45	6.52	6.59	6.65	6.71	6.77	6.82
24	6.02	6.11	6.19	6.26	6.33	6.39	6.45	6.51	6.56	6.61
30	5.85	5.93	6.01	6.08	6.14	6.20	6.26	6.31	6.36	6.41
40	5.69	5.76	5.83	5.90	5.96	6.02	6.07	6.12	6.16	6.21
60	5.53	5.60	5.67	5.73	5.78	5.84	5.89	5.93	5.97	6.01
120	5.37	5.44	5.50	5.56	5.61	5.66	5.71	5.75	5.79	5.83
∞	5.23	5.29	5.35	5.40	5.45	5.49	5.54	5.57	5.61	5.65

TABLE I Transformation of r to z (the body of the table contains values of $z = .5[\ln(1 + r) / (1 - r)] = \tanh^{-1} r$ for corresponding values of r, the correlation coefficient)

r	.00	.01	.02	.03	.04	.05	.06	.07	.08	.09
.0	.00000	.01000	.02000	.03001	.04002	.05004	.06007	.07012	.08017	.09024
.1	.10034	.11045	.12058	.13074	.14093	.15114	.16139	.17167	.18198	.19234
.2	.20273	.21317	.22366	.23419	.24477	.25541	.26611	.27686	.28768	.29857
.3	.30952	.32055	.33165	.34283	.35409	.36544	.37689	.38842	.40006	.41180
.4	.42365	.43561	.44769	.45990	.47223	.48470	.49731	.51007	.52298	.53606
.5	.54931	.56273	.57634	.59014	.60415	.61838	.63283	.64752	.66246	.67767
.6	.69315	.70892	.72500	.74142	.75817	.77530	.79281	.81074	.82911	.84795
.7	.86730	.88718	.90764	.92873	.95048	.97295	.99621	1.02033	1.04537	1.07143
.8	1.09861	1.12703	1.15682	1.18813	1.22117	1.25615	1.29334	1.33308	1.37577	1.42192
.9	1.47222	1.52752	1.58902	1.65839	1.73805	1.83178	1.94591	2.09229	2.29756	2.64665

TABLE J Significance Tests in a 2×2 Contingency Table[a]

	a	0.05	0.025	0.01	0.005
			Probability		
$A = 3\ B = 3$	3	$\mathbf{0}_{.050}$	—	—	—
$A = 4\ B = 4$	4	$\mathbf{0}_{.014}$	$\mathbf{0}_{.014}$	—	—
3	4	$\mathbf{0}_{.029}$	—	—	—
$A = 5\ B = 5$	5	$\mathbf{1}_{.024}$	$\mathbf{1}_{.024}$	$\mathbf{0}_{.004}$	$\mathbf{0}_{.004}$
	4	$\mathbf{0}_{.024}$	$\mathbf{0}_{.024}$	—	—
4	5	$\mathbf{1}_{.048}$	$\mathbf{0}_{.008}$	$\mathbf{0}_{.008}$	—
	4	$\mathbf{0}_{.040}$	—	—	—
3	5	$\mathbf{0}_{.018}$	$\mathbf{0}_{.018}$	—	—
2	5	$\mathbf{0}_{.048}$	—	—	—
$A = 6\ B = 6$	6	$\mathbf{2}_{.030}$	$\mathbf{1}_{.008}$	$\mathbf{1}_{.008}$	$\mathbf{0}_{.001}$
	5	$\mathbf{1}_{.040}$	$\mathbf{0}_{.008}$	$\mathbf{0}_{.008}$	—
	4	$\mathbf{0}_{.030}$	—	—	—
5	6	$\mathbf{1}_{.015}{}^{+}$	$\mathbf{1}_{.015}{}^{+}$	$\mathbf{0}_{.002}$	$\mathbf{0}_{.002}$
	5	$\mathbf{0}_{.013}$	$\mathbf{0}_{.013}$	—	—
	4	$\mathbf{0}_{.045}{}^{+}$	—	—	—
4	6	$\mathbf{1}_{.033}$	$\mathbf{0}_{.005}{}^{-}$	$\mathbf{0}_{.005}{}^{-}$	$\mathbf{0}_{.005}{}^{-}$
	5	$\mathbf{0}_{.024}$	$\mathbf{0}_{.024}$	—	—
3	6	$\mathbf{0}_{.012}$	$\mathbf{0}_{.012}$	—	—
	5	$\mathbf{0}_{.048}$	—	—	—
2	6	$\mathbf{0}_{.036}$	—	—	—
$A = 7\ B = 7$	7	$\mathbf{3}_{.035}{}^{-}$	$\mathbf{2}_{.010}{}^{+}$	$\mathbf{1}_{.002}$	$\mathbf{1}_{.002}$
	6	$\mathbf{1}_{.015}{}^{-}$	$\mathbf{1}_{.015}{}^{-}$	$\mathbf{0}_{.002}$	$\mathbf{0}_{.002}$
	5	$\mathbf{0}_{.010}{}^{+}$	$\mathbf{0}_{.010}{}^{+}$	—	—
	4	$\mathbf{0}_{.035}{}^{-}$	—	—	—
6	7	$\mathbf{2}_{.021}$	$\mathbf{2}_{.021}$	$\mathbf{1}_{.005}{}^{-}$	$\mathbf{1}_{.005}{}^{-}$
	6	$\mathbf{1}_{.025}{}^{+}$	$\mathbf{0}_{.004}$	$\mathbf{0}_{.004}$	$\mathbf{0}_{.004}$
	5	$\mathbf{0}_{.016}$	$\mathbf{0}_{.016}$	—	—
	4	$\mathbf{0}_{.049}$	—	—	—
5	7	$\mathbf{2}_{.045}{}^{+}$	$\mathbf{1}_{.010}{}^{+}$	$\mathbf{0}_{.001}$	$\mathbf{0}_{.001}$
	6	$\mathbf{1}_{.045}{}^{+}$	$\mathbf{0}_{.008}$	$\mathbf{0}_{.008}$	—
	5	$\mathbf{0}_{.027}$	—	—	—
4	7	$\mathbf{1}_{.024}$	$\mathbf{1}_{.024}$	$\mathbf{0}_{.003}$	$\mathbf{0}_{.003}$
	6	$\mathbf{0}_{.015}{}^{+}$	$\mathbf{0}_{.015}{}^{+}$	—	—
	5	$\mathbf{0}_{.045}{}^{+}$	—	—	—
3	7	$\mathbf{0}_{.008}$	$\mathbf{0}_{.008}$	$\mathbf{0}_{.008}$	—
	6	$\mathbf{0}_{.033}$	—	—	—
2	7	$\mathbf{0}_{.028}$	—	—	—
$A = 8\ B = 8$	8	$\mathbf{4}_{.038}$	$\mathbf{3}_{.013}$	$\mathbf{2}_{.003}$	$\mathbf{2}_{.003}$
	7	$\mathbf{2}_{.020}$	$\mathbf{2}_{.020}$	$\mathbf{1}_{.005}{}^{+}$	$\mathbf{0}_{.001}$
	6	$\mathbf{1}_{.020}$	$\mathbf{1}_{.020}$	$\mathbf{0}_{.003}$	$\mathbf{0}_{.003}$
	5	$\mathbf{0}_{.013}$	$\mathbf{0}_{.013}$	—	—
	4	$\mathbf{0}_{.038}$	—	—	—
$A = 8\ B = 7$	8	$\mathbf{3}_{.026}$	$\mathbf{2}_{.007}$	$\mathbf{2}_{.007}$	$\mathbf{1}_{.001}$
	7	$\mathbf{2}_{.035}{}^{-}$	$\mathbf{1}_{.009}$	$\mathbf{1}_{.009}$	$\mathbf{0}_{.001}$
	6	$\mathbf{1}_{.032}$	$\mathbf{0}_{.006}$	$\mathbf{0}_{.006}$	—
	5	$\mathbf{0}_{.019}$	$\mathbf{0}_{.019}$	—	—
6	8	$\mathbf{2}_{.015}{}^{-}$	$\mathbf{2}_{.015}{}^{-}$	$\mathbf{1}_{.003}$	$\mathbf{1}_{.003}$

[a]Bold type, for given a, A, and B, shows the value of b ($< a$), which is just significant at the probability level quoted (single-tail test). Small type, for given A, B, and $r = a + b$, shows the exact probability (if there is independence) that b is equal to or less than the integer shown in bold type.

TABLE J (*continued*)

	a	Probability 0.05	0.025	0.01	0.005
	7	$1_{.016}$	$1_{.016}$	$0_{.002}$	$0_{.002}$
	6	$0_{.009}$	$0_{.009}$	$0_{.009}$	—
	5	$0_{.028}$	—	—	—
5	8	$2_{.035^-}$	$1_{.007}$	$1_{.007}$	$0_{.001}$
	7	$1_{.032}$	$0_{.005^-}$	$0_{.005^-}$	$0_{.005^-}$
	6	$0_{.016}$	$0_{.016}$	—	—
	5	$0_{.044}$	—	—	—
4	8	$1_{.018}$	$1_{.018}$	$0_{.002}$	$0_{.002}$
	7	$0_{.010^+}$	$0_{.010^+}$	—	—
	6	$0_{.030}$	—	—	—
3	8	$0_{.006}$	$0_{.006}$	$0_{.006}$	—
	7	$0_{.024}$	$0_{.024}$	—	—
2	8	$0_{.022}$	$0_{.022}$	—	—
$A = 9\ B = 9$	9	$5_{.041}$	$4_{.015^-}$	$3_{.005^-}$	$3_{.005^-}$
	8	$3_{.025^-}$	$3_{.025^-}$	$2_{.008}$	$1_{.002}$
	7	$2_{.028}$	$1_{.008}$	$1_{.008}$	$0_{.001}$
	6	$1_{.025^-}$	$1_{.025^-}$	$0_{.005^-}$	$0_{.005^-}$
	5	$0_{.015^-}$	$0_{.015^-}$	—	—
	4	$0_{.041}$	—	—	—
8	9	$4_{.029}$	$3_{.009}$	$3_{.009}$	$2_{.002}$
	8	$3_{.043}$	$2_{.013}$	$1_{.003}$	$1_{.003}$
	7	$2_{.044}$	$1_{.012}$	$0_{.002}$	$0_{.002}$
	6	$1_{.036}$	$0_{.007}$	$0_{.007}$	—
	5	$0_{.020}$	$0_{.020}$	—	—
7	9	$3_{.019}$	$3_{.019}$	$2_{.005^-}$	$2_{.005^-}$
	8	$2_{.024}$	$2_{.024}$	$1_{.006}$	$0_{.001}$
	7	$1_{.020}$	$1_{.020}$	$0_{.003}$	$0_{.003}$
	6	$0_{.010^+}$	$0_{.010^+}$	—	—
	5	$0_{.029}$	—	—	—
6	9	$3_{.044}$	$2_{.011}$	$1_{.002}$	$1_{.002}$
	8	$2_{.047}$	$1_{.011}$	$0_{.001}$	$0_{.001}$
	7	$1_{.035^-}$	$0_{.006}$	$0_{.006}$	—
	6	$0_{.017}$	$0_{.017}$	—	—
	5	$0_{.042}$	—	—	—
5	9	$2_{.027}$	$1_{.005^-}$	$1_{.005^-}$	$1_{.005^-}$
	8	$1_{.023}$	$1_{.023}$	$0_{.003}$	$0_{.003}$
	7	$0_{.010^+}$	$0_{.010^+}$	—	—
	6	$0_{.028}$	—	—	—
4	9	$1_{.014}$	$1_{.014}$	$0_{.001}$	$0_{.001}$
	8	$0_{.007}$	$0_{.007}$	$0_{.007}$	—
	7	$0_{.021}$	$0_{.021}$	—	—
	6	$0_{.049}$	—	—	—
3	9	$1_{.045^+}$	$0_{.005^-}$	$0_{.005^-}$	$0_{.005^-}$
	8	$0_{.018}$	$0_{.018}$	—	—
	7	$0_{.045^+}$	—	—	—
2	9	$0_{.018}$	$0_{.018}$	—	—
$A = 10\ B = 10$	10	$6_{.043}$	$5_{.016}$	$4_{.005^+}$	$3_{.002}$
	9	$4_{.029}$	$3_{.010^-}$	$3_{.010^-}$	$2_{.003}$
	8	$3_{.035^-}$	$2_{.012}$	$1_{.003}$	$1_{.003}$
	7	$2_{.035^-}$	$1_{.010^-}$	$1_{.010^-}$	$0_{.002}$

TABLE J (*continued*)

	a	Probability 0.05	0.025	0.01	0.005
	6	$1_{.029}$	$0_{.005}{}^+$	$0_{.005}{}^+$	—
	5	$0_{.016}$	$0_{.016}$	—	—
	4	$0_{.043}$	—	—	—
$A = 10\ B = 9$	10	$5_{.033}$	$4_{.011}$	$3_{.003}$	$3_{.003}$
	9	$4_{.050}{}^-$	$3_{.017}$	$2_{.005}{}^-$	$2_{.005}{}^-$
	8	$2_{.019}$	$2_{.019}$	$1_{.004}$	$1_{.004}$
	7	$1_{.015}{}^-$	$1_{.015}{}^-$	$0_{.002}$	$0_{.002}$
	6	$1_{.040}$	$0_{.008}$	$0_{.008}$	—
	5	$0_{.022}$	$0_{.022}$	—	—
8	10	$4_{.023}$	$4_{.023}$	$3_{.007}$	$2_{.002}$
	9	$3_{.032}$	$2_{.009}$	$2_{.009}$	$1_{.002}$
	8	$2_{.031}$	$1_{.008}$	$1_{.008}$	$0_{.001}$
	7	$1_{.023}$	$1_{.023}$	$0_{.004}$	$0_{.004}$
	6	$0_{.011}$	$0_{.011}$	—	—
	5	$0_{.029}$	—	—	—
7	10	$3_{.015}{}^-$	$3_{.015}{}^-$	$2_{.003}$	$2_{.003}$
	9	$2_{.018}$	$2_{.018}$	$1_{.004}$	$1_{.004}$
	8	$1_{.013}$	$1_{.013}$	$0_{.002}$	$0_{.002}$
	7	$1_{.036}$	$0_{.006}$	$0_{.006}$	—
	6	$0_{.017}$	$0_{.017}$	—	—
	5	$0_{.041}$	—	—	—
6	10	$3_{.036}$	$2_{.008}$	$2_{.008}$	$1_{.001}$
	9	$2_{.036}$	$1_{.008}$	$1_{.008}$	$0_{.001}$
	8	$1_{.024}$	$1_{.024}$	$0_{.003}$	$0_{.003}$
	7	$0_{.010}{}^+$	$0_{.010}{}^+$	—	—
	6	$0_{.026}$	—	—	—
5	10	$2_{.022}$	$2_{.022}$	$1_{.004}$	$1_{.004}$
	9	$1_{.017}$	$1_{.017}$	$0_{.002}$	$0_{.002}$
	8	$1_{.047}$	$0_{.007}$	$0_{.007}$	—
	7	$0_{.019}$	$0_{.019}$	—	—
	6	$0_{.042}$	—	—	—
4	10	$1_{.011}$	$1_{.011}$	$0_{.001}$	$0_{.001}$
	9	$1_{.041}$	$0_{.005}{}^-$	$0_{.005}{}^-$	$0_{.005}{}^-$
	8	$0_{.015}{}^-$	$0_{.015}{}^-$	—	—
	7	$0_{.035}{}^-$	—	—	—
3	10	$1_{.038}$	$0_{.003}$	$0_{.003}$	$0_{.003}$
	9	$0_{.014}$	$0_{.014}$	—	—
	8	$0_{.035}{}^-$	—	—	—
2	10	$0_{.015}{}^+$	$0_{.015}{}^+$	—	—
	9	$0_{.045}{}^+$	—	—	—
$A = 11\ B = 11$	11	$7_{.045}{}^+$	$6_{.018}$	$5_{.006}$	$4_{.002}$
	10	$5_{.032}$	$4_{.012}$	$3_{.004}$	$3_{.004}$
	9	$4_{.040}$	$3_{.015}{}^-$	$2_{.004}$	$2_{.004}$
	8	$3_{.043}$	$2_{.015}{}^-$	$1_{.004}$	$1_{.004}$
	7	$2_{.040}$	$1_{.012}$	$0_{.002}$	$0_{.002}$
	6	$1_{.032}$	$0_{.006}$	$0_{.006}$	—
	5	$0_{.018}$	$0_{.018}$	—	—
	4	$0_{.045}{}^+$	—	—	—
10	11	$6_{.035}{}^+$	$5_{.012}$	$4_{.004}$	$4_{.004}$
	10	$4_{.021}$	$4_{.021}$	$3_{.007}$	$2_{.002}$

TABLE J (*continued*)

	a	Probability 0.05	0.025	0.01	0.005
	9	$3_{.024}$	$3_{.024}$	$2_{.007}$	$1_{.002}$
	8	$2_{.023}$	$2_{.023}$	$1_{.006}$	$0_{.001}$
	7	$1_{.017}$	$1_{.017}$	$0_{.003}$	$0_{.003}$
	6	$1_{.043}$	$0_{.009}$	$0_{.009}$	—
	5	$0_{.023}$	$0_{.023}$	—	—
9	11	$5_{.026}$	$4_{.008}$	$4_{.008}$	$3_{.002}$
	10	$4_{.038}$	$3_{.012}$	$2_{.003}$	$2_{.003}$
	9	$3_{.040}$	$2_{.012}$	$1_{.003}$	$1_{.003}$
	8	$2_{.035}-$	$1_{.009}$	$1_{.009}$	$0_{.001}$
	7	$1_{.025}-$	$1_{.025}-$	$0_{.004}$	$0_{.004}$
	6	$0_{.012}$	$0_{.012}$	—	—
	5	$0_{.030}$	—	—	—
$A = 11\ B = 8$	11	$4_{.018}$	$4_{.018}$	$3_{.005}-$	$3_{.005}-$
	10	$3_{.024}$	$3_{.024}$	$2_{.006}$	$1_{.001}$
	9	$2_{.022}$	$2_{.022}$	$1_{.005}-$	$1_{.005}-$
	8	$1_{.015}-$	$1_{.015}-$	$0_{.002}$	$0_{.002}$
	7	$1_{.037}$	$0_{.007}$	$0_{.007}$	—
	6	$0_{.017}$	$0_{.017}$	—	—
	5	$0_{.040}$	—	—	—
7	11	$4_{.043}$	$3_{.011}$	$2_{.002}$	$2_{.002}$
	10	$3_{.047}$	$2_{.013}$	$1_{.002}$	$1_{.002}$
	9	$2_{.039}$	$1_{.009}$	$1_{.009}$	$0_{.001}$
	8	$1_{.025}-$	$1_{.025}-$	$0_{.004}$	$0_{.004}$
	7	$0_{.010}+$	$0_{.010}+$	—	—
	6	$0_{.025}-$	$0_{.025}-$	—	—
6	11	$3_{.029}$	$2_{.006}$	$2_{.006}$	$1_{.001}$
	10	$2_{.028}$	$1_{.005}+$	$1_{.005}+$	$0_{.001}$
	9	$1_{.018}$	$1_{.018}$	$0_{.002}$	$0_{.002}$
	8	$1_{.043}$	$0_{.007}$	$0_{.007}$	—
	7	$0_{.017}$	$0_{.017}$	—	—
	6	$0_{.037}$	—	—	—
5	11	$2_{.018}$	$2_{.018}$	$1_{.003}$	$1_{.003}$
	10	$1_{.013}$	$1_{.013}$	$0_{.001}$	$0_{.001}$
	9	$1_{.036}$	$0_{.005}-$	$0_{.005}-$	$0_{.005}-$
	8	$0_{.013}$	$0_{.013}$	—	—
	7	$0_{.029}$	—	—	—
4	11	$1_{.009}$	$1_{.009}$	$1_{.009}$	$0_{.001}$
	10	$1_{.033}$	$0_{.004}$	$0_{.004}$	$0_{.004}$
	9	$0_{.011}$	$0_{.011}$	—	—
	8	$0_{.026}$	—	—	—
3	11	$1_{.033}$	$0_{.003}$	$0_{.003}$	$0_{.003}$
	10	$0_{.011}$	$0_{.011}$	—	—
	9	$0_{.027}$	—	—	—
2	11	$0_{.013}$	$0_{.013}$	—	—
	10	$0_{.038}$	—	—	—
$A = 12\ B = 12$	12	$8_{.047}$	$7_{.019}$	$6_{.007}$	$5_{.002}$
	11	$6_{.034}$	$5_{.014}$	$4_{.005}-$	$4_{.005}-$
	10	$5_{.045}-$	$4_{.018}$	$3_{.006}$	$2_{.002}$
	9	$4_{.050}-$	$3_{.020}$	$2_{.006}$	$1_{.001}$
	8	$3_{.050}-$	$2_{.018}$	$1_{.005}-$	$1_{.005}-$

TABLE J (*continued*)

	a	Probability 0.05	0.025	0.01	0.005
	7	$2_{.045^-}$	$1_{.014}$	$0_{.002}$	$0_{.002}$
	6	$1_{.034}$	$0_{.007}$	$0_{.007}$	—
	5	$0_{.019}$	$0_{.019}$	—	—
	4	$0_{.047}$	—	—	—
11	12	$7_{.037}$	$6_{.014}$	$5_{.005^-}$	$5_{.005^-}$
	11	$5_{.024}$	$5_{.024}$	$4_{.008}$	$3_{.002}$
	10	$4_{.029}$	$3_{.010^+}$	$2_{.003}$	$2_{.003}$
	9	$3_{.030}$	$2_{.009}$	$2_{.009}$	$1_{.002}$
	8	$2_{.026}$	$1_{.007}$	$1_{.007}$	$0_{.001}$
	7	$1_{.019}$	$1_{.019}$	$0_{.003}$	$0_{.003}$
	6	$1_{.045^-}$	$0_{.009}$	$0_{.009}$	—
	5	$0_{.024}$	$0_{.024}$	—	—
10	12	$6_{.029}$	$5_{.010^-}$	$5_{.010^-}$	$4_{.003}$
	11	$5_{.043}$	$4_{.015^+}$	$3_{.005^-}$	$3_{.005^-}$
	10	$4_{.048}$	$3_{.017}$	$2_{.005^-}$	$2_{.005^-}$
	9	$3_{.046}$	$2_{.015^-}$	$1_{.004}$	$1_{.004}$
	8	$2_{.038}$	$1_{.010^+}$	$0_{.002}$	$0_{.002}$
	7	$1_{.026}$	$0_{.005^-}$	$0_{.005^-}$	$0_{.005^-}$
	6	$0_{.012}$	$0_{.012}$	—	—
	5	$0_{.030}$	—	—	—
$A = 12 \ B = 9$	12	$5_{.021}$	$5_{.021}$	$4_{.006}$	$3_{.002}$
	11	$4_{.029}$	$3_{.009}$	$3_{.009}$	$2_{.002}$
	10	$3_{.029}$	$2_{.008}$	$2_{.008}$	$1_{.002}$
	9	$2_{.024}$	$2_{.024}$	$1_{.006}$	$0_{.001}$
	8	$1_{.016}$	$1_{.016}$	$0_{.002}$	$0_{.002}$
	7	$1_{.037}$	$0_{.007}$	$0_{.007}$	—
	6	$0_{.017}$	$0_{.017}$	—	—
	5	$0_{.039}$	—	—	—
8	12	$5_{.049}$	$4_{.014}$	$3_{.004}$	$3_{.004}$
	11	$3_{.018}$	$3_{.018}$	$2_{.004}$	$2_{.004}$
	10	$2_{.015^+}$	$2_{.015^+}$	$1_{.003}$	$1_{.003}$
	9	$2_{.040}$	$1_{.010^-}$	$1_{.010^-}$	$0_{.001}$
	8	$1_{.025^-}$	$1_{.025^-}$	$0_{.004}$	$0_{.004}$
	7	$0_{.010^+}$	$0_{.010^+}$	—	—
	6	$0_{.024}$	$0_{.024}$	—	—
7	12	$4_{.036}$	$3_{.009}$	$3_{.009}$	$2_{.002}$
	11	$3_{.038}$	$2_{.010^-}$	$2_{.010^-}$	$1_{.002}$
	10	$2_{.029}$	$1_{.006}$	$1_{.006}$	$0_{.001}$
	9	$1_{.017}$	$1_{.017}$	$0_{.002}$	$0_{.002}$
	8	$1_{.040}$	$0_{.007}$	$0_{.007}$	—
	7	$0_{.016}$	$0_{.016}$	—	—
	6	$0_{.034}$	—	—	—
6	12	$3_{.025^-}$	$3_{.025^-}$	$2_{.005^-}$	$2_{.005^-}$
	11	$2_{.022}$	$2_{.022}$	$1_{.004}$	$1_{.004}$
	10	$1_{.013}$	$1_{.013}$	$0_{.002}$	$0_{.002}$
	9	$1_{.032}$	$0_{.005^-}$	$0_{.005^-}$	$0_{.005^-}$
	8	$0_{.011}$	$0_{.011}$	—	—
	7	$0_{.025^-}$	$0_{.025^-}$	—	—
	6	$0_{.050^-}$	—	—	—
5	12	$2_{.015^-}$	$2_{.015^-}$	$1_{.002}$	$1_{.002}$

TABLE J (*continued*)

	a	Probability 0.05	0.025	0.01	0.005
	11	$1_{.010}{}^-$	$1_{.010}{}^-$	$1_{.010}{}^-$	$0_{.001}$
	10	$1_{.028}$	$0_{.003}$	$0_{.003}$	$0_{.003}$
	9	$0_{.009}$	$0_{.009}$	$0_{.009}$	—
	8	$0_{.020}$	$0_{.020}$	—	—
	7	$0_{.041}$	—	—	—
4	12	$2_{.050}$	$1_{.007}$	$1_{.007}$	$0_{.001}$
	11	$1_{.027}$	$0_{.003}$	$0_{.003}$	$0_{.003}$
	10	$0_{.008}$	$0_{.008}$	$0_{.008}$	—
	9	$0_{.019}$	$0_{.019}$	—	—
	8	$0_{.038}$	—	—	—
3	12	$1_{.029}$	$0_{.002}$	$0_{.002}$	$0_{.002}$
	11	$0_{.009}$	$0_{.009}$	$0_{.009}$	—
	10	$0_{.022}$	$0_{.022}$	—	—
	9	$0_{.044}$	—	—	—
2	12	$0_{.011}$	$0_{.011}$	—	—
	11	$0_{.033}$	—	—	—
$A = 13\ B = 13$	13	$9_{.048}$	$8_{.020}$	$7_{.007}$	$6_{.003}$
	12	$7_{.037}$	$6_{.015}{}^+$	$5_{.006}$	$4_{.002}$
	11	$6_{.048}$	$5_{.021}$	$4_{.008}$	$3_{.002}$
	10	$4_{.024}$	$4_{.024}$	$3_{.008}$	$2_{.002}$
	9	$3_{.024}$	$3_{.024}$	$2_{.008}$	$1_{.002}$
	8	$2_{.021}$	$2_{.021}$	$1_{.006}$	$0_{.001}$
	7	$2_{.048}$	$1_{.015}{}^+$	$0_{.003}$	$0_{.003}$
	6	$1_{.037}$	$0_{.007}$	$0_{.007}$	—
	5	$0_{.020}$	$0_{.020}$	—	—
	4	$0_{.048}$	—	—	—
12	13	$8_{.039}$	$7_{.015}{}^-$	$6_{.005}{}^+$	$5_{.002}$
	12	$6_{.027}$	$5_{.010}{}^-$	$5_{.010}{}^-$	$4_{.003}$
	11	$5_{.033}$	$4_{.013}$	$3_{.004}$	$3_{.004}$
	10	$4_{.036}$	$3_{.013}$	$2_{.004}$	$2_{.004}$
$A = 13\ B = 12$	9	$3_{.034}$	$2_{.011}$	$1_{.003}$	$1_{.003}$
	8	$2_{.029}$	$1_{.008}$	$1_{.008}$	$0_{.001}$
	7	$1_{.020}$	$1_{.020}$	$0_{.004}$	$0_{.004}$
	6	$1_{.046}$	$0_{.010}{}^-$	$0_{.010}{}^-$	—
	5	$0_{.024}$	$0_{.024}$	—	—
11	13	$7_{.031}$	$6_{.011}$	$5_{.003}$	$5_{.003}$
	12	$6_{.048}$	$5_{.018}$	$4_{.006}$	$3_{.002}$
	11	$4_{.021}$	$4_{.021}$	$3_{.007}$	$2_{.002}$
	10	$3_{.021}$	$3_{.021}$	$2_{.006}$	$1_{.001}$
	9	$3_{.050}{}^-$	$2_{.017}$	$1_{.004}$	$1_{.004}$
	8	$2_{.040}$	$1_{.011}$	$0_{.002}$	$0_{.002}$
	7	$1_{.027}$	$0_{.005}{}^-$	$0_{.005}{}^-$	$0_{.005}{}^-$
	6	$0_{.013}$	$0_{.013}$	—	—
	5	$0_{.030}$	—	—	—
10	13	$6_{.024}$	$6_{.024}$	$5_{.007}$	$4_{.002}$
	12	$5_{.035}{}^-$	$4_{.012}$	$3_{.003}$	$3_{.003}$
	11	$4_{.037}$	$3_{.012}$	$2_{.003}$	$2_{.003}$
	10	$3_{.033}$	$2_{.010}{}^+$	$1_{.002}$	$1_{.002}$
	9	$2_{.026}$	$1_{.006}$	$1_{.006}$	$0_{.001}$
	8	$1_{.017}$	$1_{.017}$	$0_{.003}$	$0_{.003}$

TABLE J (*continued*)

	a	Probability			
		0.05	0.025	0.01	0.005
	7	$1_{.038}$	$0_{.007}$	$0_{.007}$	—
	6	$0_{.017}$	$0_{.017}$	—	—
	5	$0_{.038}$	—	—	—
9	13	$5_{.017}$	$5_{.017}$	$4_{.005}^-$	$4_{.005}^-$
	12	$4_{.023}$	$4_{.023}$	$3_{.007}$	$2_{.001}$
	11	$3_{.022}$	$3_{.022}$	$2_{.006}$	$1_{.001}$
	10	$2_{.017}$	$2_{.017}$	$1_{.004}$	$1_{.004}$
	9	$2_{.040}$	$1_{.010}^+$	$0_{.001}$	$0_{.001}$
	8	$1_{.025}^-$	$1_{.025}^-$	$0_{.004}$	$0_{.004}$
	7	$0_{.010}^+$	$0_{.010}^+$	—	—
	6	$0_{.023}$	$0_{.023}$	—	—
	5	$0_{.049}$	—	—	—
8	13	$5_{.042}$	$4_{.012}$	$3_{.003}$	$3_{.003}$
	12	$4_{.047}$	$3_{.014}$	$2_{.003}$	$2_{.003}$
	11	$3_{.041}$	$2_{.011}$	$1_{.002}$	$1_{.002}$
	10	$2_{.029}$	$1_{.007}$	$1_{.007}$	$0_{.001}$
	9	$1_{.017}$	$1_{.017}$	$0_{.002}$	$0_{.002}$
	8	$1_{.037}$	$0_{.006}$	$0_{.006}$	—
	7	$0_{.015}^-$	$0_{.015}^-$	—	—
	6	$0_{.032}$	—	—	—
7	13	$4_{.031}$	$3_{.007}$	$3_{.007}$	$2_{.001}$
	12	$3_{.031}$	$2_{.007}$	$2_{.007}$	$1_{.001}$
	11	$2_{.022}$	$2_{.022}$	$1_{.004}$	$1_{.004}$
	10	$1_{.012}$	$1_{.012}$	$0_{.002}$	$0_{.002}$
	9	$1_{.029}$	$0_{.004}$	$0_{.004}$	$0_{.004}$
	8	$0_{.010}^+$	$0_{.010}^+$	—	—
	7	$0_{.022}$	$0_{.022}$	—	—
	6	$0_{.044}$	—	—	—
6	13	$3_{.021}$	$3_{.021}$	$2_{.004}$	$2_{.004}$
	12	$2_{.017}$	$2_{.017}$	$1_{.003}$	$1_{.003}$
	11	$2_{.046}$	$1_{.010}^-$	$1_{.010}^-$	$0_{.001}$
	10	$1_{.024}$	$1_{.024}$	$0_{.003}$	$0_{.003}$
	9	$1_{.050}^-$	$0_{.008}$	$0_{.008}$	—
	8	$0_{.017}$	$0_{.017}$	—	—
	7	$0_{.034}$	—	—	—
5	13	$2_{.012}$	$2_{.012}$	$1_{.002}$	$1_{.002}$
	12	$2_{.044}$	$1_{.008}$	$1_{.008}$	$0_{.001}$
	11	$1_{.022}$	$1_{.022}$	$0_{.002}$	$0_{.002}$
	10	$1_{.047}$	$0_{.007}$	$0_{.007}$	—
	9	$0_{.015}^-$	$0_{.015}^-$	—	—
	8	$0_{.029}$	—	—	—
$A = 13\ B = 4$	13	$2_{.044}$	$1_{.006}$	$1_{.006}$	$0_{.000}$
	12	$1_{.022}$	$1_{.022}$	$0_{.002}$	$0_{.002}$
	11	$0_{.006}$	$0_{.006}$	$0_{.006}$	—
	10	$0_{.015}^-$	$0_{.015}^-$	—	—
	9	$0_{.029}$	—	—	—
3	13	$1_{.025}$	$1_{.025}$	$0_{.002}$	$0_{.002}$
	12	$0_{.007}$	$0_{.007}$	$0_{.007}$	—
	11	$0_{.018}$	$0_{.018}$	—	—
	10	$0_{.036}$	—	—	—

TABLE J (*continued*)

	a	0.05	0.025	0.01	0.005
2	13	$0_{.010^-}$	$0_{.010^-}$	$0_{.010^-}$	—
	12	$0_{.029}$	—	—	—
$A = 14\ B = 14$	14	$10_{.049}$	$9_{.020}$	$8_{.008}$	$7_{.003}$
	13	$8_{.038}$	$7_{.016}$	$6_{.006}$	$5_{.002}$
	12	$6_{.023}$	$6_{.023}$	$5_{.009}$	$4_{.003}$
	11	$5_{.027}$	$4_{.011}$	$3_{.004}$	$3_{.004}$
	10	$4_{.028}$	$3_{.011}$	$2_{.003}$	$2_{.003}$
	9	$3_{.027}$	$2_{.009}$	$2_{.009}$	$1_{.002}$
	8	$2_{.023}$	$2_{.023}$	$1_{.006}$	$0_{.001}$
	7	$1_{.016}$	$1_{.016}$	$0_{.003}$	$0_{.003}$
	6	$1_{.038}$	$0_{.008}$	$0_{.008}$	—
	5	$0_{.020}$	$0_{.020}$	—	—
	4	$0_{.049}$	—	—	—
13	14	$9_{.041}$	$8_{.016}$	$7_{.006}$	$6_{.002}$
	13	$7_{.029}$	$6_{.011}$	$5_{.004}$	$5_{.004}$
	12	$6_{.037}$	$5_{.015^+}$	$4_{.005^+}$	$3_{.002}$
	11	$5_{.041}$	$4_{.017}$	$3_{.006}$	$2_{.001}$
	10	$4_{.041}$	$3_{.016}$	$2_{.005^-}$	$2_{.005^-}$
	9	$3_{.038}$	$2_{.013}$	$1_{.003}$	$1_{.003}$
	8	$2_{.031}$	$1_{.009}$	$1_{.009}$	$0_{.001}$
	7	$1_{.021}$	$1_{.021}$	$0_{.004}$	$0_{.004}$
	6	$1_{.048}$	$0_{.010^+}$	—	—
	5	$0_{.025^-}$	$0_{.025^-}$	—	—
12	14	$8_{.033}$	$7_{.012}$	$6_{.004}$	$6_{.004}$
	13	$6_{.021}$	$6_{.021}$	$5_{.007}$	$4_{.002}$
	12	$5_{.025^+}$	$4_{.009}$	$4_{.009}$	$3_{.003}$
	11	$4_{.026}$	$3_{.009}$	$3_{.009}$	$2_{.002}$
	10	$3_{.024}$	$3_{.024}$	$2_{.007}$	$1_{.002}$
	9	$2_{.019}$	$2_{.019}$	$1_{.005^-}$	$1_{.005^-}$
	8	$2_{.042}$	$1_{.012}$	$0_{.002}$	$0_{.002}$
	7	$1_{.028}$	$0_{.005^+}$	$0_{.005^+}$	—
	6	$0_{.013}$	$0_{.013}$	—	—
	5	$0_{.030}$	—	—	—
11	14	$7_{.026}$	$6_{.009}$	$6_{.009}$	$5_{.003}$
	13	$6_{.039}$	$5_{.014}$	$4_{.004}$	$4_{.004}$
	12	$5_{.043}$	$4_{.016}$	$3_{.005^-}$	$3_{.005^-}$
	11	$4_{.042}$	$3_{.015^-}$	$2_{.004}$	$2_{.004}$
	10	$3_{.036}$	$2_{.011}$	$1_{.003}$	$1_{.003}$
	9	$2_{.027}$	$1_{.007}$	$1_{.007}$	$0_{.001}$
	8	$1_{.017}$	$1_{.017}$	$0_{.003}$	$0_{.003}$
	7	$1_{.038}$	$0_{.007}$	$0_{.007}$	—
	6	$0_{.017}$	$0_{.017}$	—	—
	5	$0_{.038}$	—	—	—
10	14	$6_{.020}$	$6_{.020}$	$5_{.006}$	$4_{.002}$
	13	$5_{.028}$	$4_{.009}$	$4_{.009}$	$3_{.002}$
	12	$4_{.028}$	$3_{.009}$	$3_{.009}$	$2_{.002}$
	11	$3_{.024}$	$3_{.024}$	$2_{.007}$	$1_{.001}$
	10	$2_{.018}$	$2_{.018}$	$1_{.004}$	$1_{.004}$
	9	$2_{.040}$	$1_{.011}$	$0_{.002}$	$0_{.002}$
	8	$1_{.024}$	$1_{.024}$	$0_{.004}$	$0_{.004}$

TABLE J (*continued*)

	a	0.05	0.025	0.01	0.005
			Probability		
$A = 14\ B = 10$	7	$0_{.010^-}$	$0_{.010^-}$	$0_{.010^-}$	—
	6	$0_{.022}$	$0_{.022}$	—	—
	5	$0_{.047}$	—	—	—
9	14	$6_{.047}$	$5_{.014}$	$4_{.004}$	$4_{.004}$
	13	$4_{.018}$	$4_{.018}$	$3_{.005^-}$	$3_{.005^-}$
	12	$3_{.017}$	$3_{.017}$	$2_{.004}$	$2_{.004}$
	11	$3_{.042}$	$2_{.012}$	$1_{.002}$	$1_{.002}$
	10	$2_{.029}$	$1_{.007}$	$1_{.007}$	$0_{.001}$
	9	$1_{.017}$	$1_{.017}$	$0_{.002}$	$0_{.002}$
	8	$1_{.036}$	$0_{.006}$	$0_{.006}$	—
	7	$0_{.014}$	$0_{.014}$	—	—
	6	$0_{.030}$	—	—	—
8	14	$5_{.036}$	$4_{.010^-}$	$4_{.010^-}$	$3_{.002}$
	13	$4_{.039}$	$3_{.011}$	$2_{.002}$	$2_{.002}$
	12	$3_{.032}$	$2_{.008}$	$2_{.008}$	$1_{.001}$
	11	$2_{.022}$	$2_{.022}$	$1_{.005^-}$	$1_{.005^-}$
	10	$2_{.048}$	$1_{.012}$	$0_{.002}$	$0_{.002}$
	9	$1_{.026}$	$0_{.004}$	$0_{.004}$	$0_{.004}$
	8	$0_{.009}$	$0_{.009}$	$0_{.009}$	—
	7	$0_{.020}$	$0_{.020}$	—	—
	6	$0_{.040}$	—	—	—
7	14	$4_{.026}$	$3_{.006}$	$3_{.006}$	$2_{.001}$
	13	$3_{.025}$	$2_{.006}$	$2_{.006}$	$1_{.001}$
	12	$2_{.017}$	$2_{.017}$	$1_{.003}$	$1_{.003}$
	11	$2_{.041}$	$1_{.009}$	$1_{.009}$	$0_{.001}$
	10	$1_{.021}$	$1_{.021}$	$0_{.003}$	$0_{.003}$
	9	$1_{.043}$	$0_{.007}$	$0_{.007}$	—
	8	$0_{.015^-}$	$0_{.015^-}$	—	—
	7	$0_{.030}$	—	—	—
6	14	$3_{.018}$	$3_{.018}$	$2_{.003}$	$2_{.003}$
	13	$2_{.014}$	$2_{.014}$	$1_{.002}$	$1_{.002}$
	12	$2_{.037}$	$1_{.007}$	$1_{.007}$	$0_{.001}$
	11	$1_{.018}$	$1_{.018}$	$0_{.002}$	$0_{.002}$
	10	$1_{.038}$	$0_{.005^+}$	$0_{.005^+}$	—
	9	$0_{.012}$	$0_{.012}$	—	—
	8	$0_{.024}$	$0_{.024}$	—	—
	7	$0_{.044}$	—	—	—
5	14	$2_{.010^+}$	$2_{.010^+}$	$1_{.001}$	$1_{.001}$
	13	$2_{.037}$	$1_{.006}$	$1_{.006}$	$0_{.001}$
	12	$1_{.017}$	$1_{.017}$	$0_{.002}$	$0_{.002}$
	11	$1_{.038}$	$0_{.005^-}$	$0_{.005^-}$	$0_{.005^-}$
	10	$0_{.011}$	$0_{.011}$	—	—
	9	$0_{.022}$	$0_{.022}$	—	—
	8	$0_{.040}$	—	—	—
4	14	$2_{.039}$	$1_{.005^-}$	$1_{.005^-}$	$1_{.005^-}$
	13	$1_{.019}$	$1_{.019}$	$0_{.002}$	$0_{.002}$
	12	$1_{.044}$	$0_{.005^-}$	$0_{.005^-}$	$0_{.005^-}$
	11	$0_{.011}$	$0_{.011}$	—	—
	10	$0_{.023}$	$0_{.023}$	—	—
	9	$0_{.041}$	—	—	—

TABLE J (*continued*)

	a	0.05	0.025	0.01	0.005
			Probability		
3	14	$1_{.022}$	$1_{.022}$	$0_{.001}$	$0_{.001}$
	13	$0_{.006}$	$0_{.006}$	$0_{.006}$	—
	12	$0_{.015}-$	$0_{.015}-$	—	—
	11	$0_{.029}$	—	—	—
2	14	$0_{.008}$	$0_{.008}$	$0_{.008}$	—
	13	$0_{.025}$	$0_{.025}$	—	—
	12	$0_{.050}$	—	—	—
$A = 15\ B = 15$	15	$11_{.050}-$	$10_{.021}$	$9_{.008}$	$8_{.003}$
	14	$9_{.040}$	$8_{.018}$	$7_{.007}$	$6_{.003}$
	13	$7_{.025}+$	$6_{.010}+$	$5_{.004}$	$5_{.004}$
	12	$6_{.030}$	$5_{.013}$	$4_{.005}-$	$4_{.005}-$
$A = 15\ B = 15$	11	$5_{.033}$	$4_{.013}$	$3_{.005}-$	$3_{.005}-$
	10	$4_{.033}$	$3_{.013}$	$2_{.004}$	$2_{.004}$
	9	$3_{.030}$	$2_{.010}+$	$1_{.003}$	$1_{.003}$
	8	$2_{.025}+$	$1_{.007}$	$1_{.007}$	$0_{.001}$
	7	$1_{.018}$	$1_{.018}$	$0_{.003}$	$0_{.003}$
	6	$1_{.040}$	$0_{.008}$	$0_{.008}$	—
	5	$0_{.021}$	$0_{.021}$	—	—
	4	$0_{.050}-$	—	—	—
14	15	$10_{.042}$	$9_{.017}$	$8_{.006}$	$7_{.002}$
	14	$8_{.031}$	$7_{.013}$	$6_{.005}-$	$6_{.005}-$
	13	$7_{.041}$	$6_{.017}$	$5_{.007}$	$4_{.002}$
	12	$6_{.046}$	$5_{.020}$	$4_{.007}$	$3_{.002}$
	11	$5_{.048}$	$4_{.020}$	$3_{.007}$	$2_{.002}$
	10	$4_{.046}$	$3_{.018}$	$2_{.006}$	$1_{.001}$
	9	$3_{.041}$	$2_{.014}$	$1_{.004}$	$1_{.004}$
	8	$2_{.033}$	$1_{.009}$	$1_{.009}$	$0_{.001}$
	7	$1_{.022}$	$1_{.022}$	$0_{.004}$	$0_{.004}$
	6	$1_{.049}$	$0_{.011}$	—	—
	5	$0_{.025}+$	—	—	—
13	15	$9_{.035}-$	$8_{.013}$	$7_{.005}-$	$7_{.005}-$
	14	$7_{.023}$	$7_{.023}$	$6_{.009}$	$5_{.003}$
	13	$6_{.029}$	$5_{.011}$	$4_{.004}$	$4_{.004}$
	12	$5_{.031}$	$4_{.012}$	$3_{.004}$	$3_{.004}$
	11	$4_{.030}$	$3_{.011}$	$2_{.003}$	$2_{.003}$
	10	$3_{.026}$	$2_{.008}$	$2_{.008}$	$1_{.002}$
	9	$2_{.020}$	$2_{.020}$	$1_{.005}+$	$0_{.001}$
	8	$2_{.043}$	$1_{.013}$	$0_{.002}$	$0_{.002}$
	7	$1_{.029}$	$0_{.005}+$	$0_{.005}+$	—
	6	$0_{.013}$	$0_{.013}$	—	—
	5	$0_{.031}$	—	—	—
12	15	$8_{.028}$	$7_{.010}-$	$7_{.010}-$	$6_{.003}$
	14	$7_{.043}$	$6_{.016}$	$5_{.006}$	$4_{.002}$
	13	$6_{.049}$	$5_{.019}$	$4_{.007}$	$3_{.002}$
	12	$5_{.049}$	$4_{.019}$	$3_{.006}$	$2_{.002}$
	11	$4_{.045}+$	$3_{.017}$	$2_{.005}-$	$2_{.005}-$
	10	$3_{.038}$	$2_{.012}$	$1_{.003}$	$1_{.003}$
	9	$2_{.028}$	$1_{.007}$	$1_{.007}$	$0_{.001}$
	8	$1_{.018}$	$1_{.018}$	$0_{.003}$	$0_{.003}$
	7	$1_{.038}$	$0_{.007}$	$0_{.007}$	—

TABLE J (*continued*)

	a	Probability 0.05	0.025	0.01	0.005
	6	$0_{.017}$	$0_{.017}$	—	—
	5	$0_{.037}$	—	—	—
11	15	$7_{.022}$	$7_{.022}$	$6_{.007}$	$5_{.002}$
	14	$6_{.032}$	$5_{.011}$	$4_{.003}$	$4_{.003}$
	13	$5_{.034}$	$4_{.012}$	$3_{.003}$	$3_{.003}$
	12	$4_{.032}$	$3_{.010^+}$	$2_{.003}$	$2_{.003}$
	11	$3_{.026}$	$2_{.008}$	$2_{.000}$	$1_{.002}$
	10	$2_{.019}$	$2_{.019}$	$1_{.004}$	$1_{.004}$
	9	$2_{.040}$	$1_{.011}$	$0_{.002}$	$0_{.002}$
	8	$1_{.024}$	$1_{.024}$	$0_{.004}$	$0_{.004}$
	7	$1_{.049}$	$0_{.010^-}$	$0_{.010^-}$	—
	6	$0_{.022}$	$0_{.022}$	—	—
	5	$0_{.046}$	—	—	—
10	15	$6_{.017}$	$6_{.017}$	$5_{.005^-}$	$5_{.005^-}$
	14	$5_{.023}$	$5_{.023}$	$4_{.007}$	$3_{.002}$
	13	$4_{.022}$	$4_{.022}$	$3_{.007}$	$2_{.001}$
	12	$3_{.018}$	$3_{.018}$	$2_{.005^-}$	$2_{.005^-}$
	11	$3_{.042}$	$2_{.013}$	$1_{.003}$	$1_{.003}$
	10	$2_{.029}$	$1_{.007}$	$1_{.007}$	$0_{.001}$
	9	$1_{.016}$	$1_{.016}$	$0_{.002}$	$0_{.002}$
	8	$1_{.034}$	$0_{.006}$	$0_{.006}$	—
$A = 15\ B = 10$	7	$0_{.013}$	$0_{.013}$	—	—
	6	$0_{.028}$	—	—	—
9	15	$6_{.042}$	$5_{.012}$	$4_{.003}$	$4_{.003}$
	14	$5_{.047}$	$4_{.015^-}$	$3_{.004}$	$3_{.004}$
	13	$4_{.042}$	$3_{.013}$	$2_{.003}$	$2_{.003}$
	12	$3_{.032}$	$2_{.009}$	$2_{.009}$	$1_{.002}$
	11	$2_{.021}$	$2_{.021}$	$1_{.005^-}$	$1_{.005^-}$
	10	$2_{.045^-}$	$1_{.011}$	$0_{.002}$	$0_{.002}$
	9	$1_{.024}$	$1_{.024}$	$0_{.004}$	$0_{.004}$
	8	$1_{.048}$	$0_{.009}$	$0_{.009}$	—
	7	$0_{.019}$	$0_{.019}$	—	—
	6	$0_{.037}$	—	—	—
8	15	$5_{.032}$	$4_{.008}$	$4_{.008}$	$3_{.002}$
	14	$4_{.033}$	$3_{.009}$	$3_{.009}$	$2_{.002}$
	13	$3_{.026}$	$2_{.006}$	$2_{.006}$	$1_{.001}$
	12	$2_{.017}$	$2_{.017}$	$1_{.003}$	$1_{.003}$
	11	$2_{.037}$	$1_{.008}$	$1_{.008}$	$0_{.001}$
	10	$1_{.019}$	$1_{.019}$	$0_{.003}$	$0_{.003}$
	9	$1_{.038}$	$0_{.006}$	$0_{.006}$	—
	8	$0_{.013}$	$0_{.013}$	—	—
	7	$0_{.026}$	—	—	—
	6	$0_{.050^-}$	—	—	—
7	15	$4_{.023}$	$4_{.023}$	$3_{.005^-}$	$3_{.005^-}$
	14	$3_{.021}$	$3_{.021}$	$2_{.004}$	$2_{.004}$
	13	$2_{.014}$	$2_{.014}$	$1_{.002}$	$1_{.002}$
	12	$2_{.032}$	$1_{.007}$	$1_{.007}$	$0_{.001}$
	11	$1_{.015^+}$	$1_{.015^+}$	$0_{.002}$	$0_{.002}$
	10	$1_{.032}$	$0_{.005^-}$	$0_{.005^-}$	$0_{.005^-}$
	9	$0_{.010^+}$	$0_{.010^+}$	—	—

TABLE J (*continued*)

	a	Probability 0.05	0.025	0.01	0.005
	8	$0_{.020}$	$0_{.020}$	—	—
	7	$0_{.038}$	—	—	—
6	15	$3_{.015^+}$	$3_{.015^+}$	$2_{.003}$	$2_{.003}$
	14	$2_{.011}$	$2_{.011}$	$1_{.002}$	$1_{.002}$
	13	$2_{.031}$	$1_{.006}$	$1_{.006}$	$0_{.001}$
	12	$1_{.014}$	$1_{.014}$	$0_{.002}$	$0_{.002}$
	11	$1_{.029}$	$0_{.004}$	$0_{.004}$	$0_{.004}$
	10	$0_{.009}$	$0_{.009}$	$0_{.009}$	—
	9	$0_{.017}$	$0_{.017}$	—	—
	8	$0_{.032}$	—	—	—
5	15	$2_{.009}$	$2_{.009}$	$2_{.009}$	$1_{.001}$
	14	$2_{.032}$	$1_{.005^-}$	$1_{.005^-}$	$1_{.005^-}$
	13	$1_{.014}$	$1_{.014}$	$0_{.001}$	$0_{.001}$
	12	$1_{.031}$	$0_{.004}$	$0_{.004}$	$0_{.004}$
	11	$0_{.008}$	$0_{.008}$	$0_{.008}$	—
	10	$0_{.016}$	$0_{.016}$	—	—
	9	$0_{.030}$	—	—	—
4	15	$2_{.035^+}$	$1_{.004}$	$1_{.004}$	$1_{.004}$
	14	$1_{.016}$	$1_{.016}$	$0_{.001}$	$0_{.001}$
	13	$1_{.037}$	$0_{.004}$	$0_{.004}$	$0_{.004}$
	12	$0_{.009}$	$0_{.009}$	$0_{.009}$	—
	11	$0_{.018}$	$0_{.018}$	—	—
	10	$0_{.033}$	—	—	—
3	15	$1_{.020}$	$1_{.020}$	$0_{.001}$	$0_{.001}$
	14	$0_{.005^-}$	$0_{.005^-}$	$0_{.005^-}$	$0_{.005^-}$
	13	$0_{.012}$	$0_{.012}$	—	—
	12	$0_{.025^-}$	$0_{.025^-}$	—	—
	11	$0_{.043}$	—	—	—
2	15	$0_{.007}$	$0_{.007}$	$0_{.007}$	—
	14	$0_{.022}$	$0_{.022}$	—	—
	13	$0_{.044}$	—	—	—
A = 16 B = 16	16	$11_{.022}$	$11_{.022}$	$10_{.009}$	$9_{.003}$
	15	$10_{.041}$	$9_{.019}$	$8_{.008}$	$7_{.003}$
	14	$8_{.027}$	$7_{.012}$	$6_{.005^-}$	$6_{.005^-}$
	13	$7_{.033}$	$6_{.015^-}$	$5_{.006}$	$4_{.002}$
	12	$6_{.037}$	$5_{.016}$	$4_{.006}$	$3_{.002}$
	11	$5_{.038}$	$4_{.016}$	$3_{.006}$	$2_{.002}$
	10	$4_{.037}$	$3_{.015^-}$	$2_{.005^-}$	$2_{.005^-}$
	9	$3_{.033}$	$2_{.012}$	$1_{.003}$	$1_{.003}$
	8	$2_{.027}$	$1_{.008}$	$1_{.008}$	$0_{.001}$
	7	$1_{.019}$	$1_{.019}$	$0_{.003}$	$0_{.003}$
	6	$1_{.041}$	$0_{.009}$	$0_{.009}$	—
	5	$0_{.022}$	$0_{.022}$	—	—
15	16	$11_{.043}$	$10_{.018}$	$9_{.007}$	$8_{.002}$
	15	$9_{.033}$	$8_{.014}$	$7_{.005^+}$	$6_{.002}$
	14	$8_{.044}$	$7_{.019}$	$6_{.008}$	$5_{.003}$
	13	$6_{.023}$	$6_{.023}$	$5_{.009}$	$4_{.003}$
	12	$5_{.024}$	$5_{.024}$	$4_{.009}$	$3_{.003}$
	11	$4_{.023}$	$4_{.023}$	$3_{.008}$	$2_{.002}$
	10	$4_{.049}$	$3_{.020}$	$2_{.006}$	$1_{.001}$

TABLE J (*continued*)

	a	0.05	0.025	0.01	0.005
			Probability		
	9	$3_{.043}$	$2_{.016}$	$1_{.004}$	$1_{.004}$
	8	$2_{.035^-}$	$1_{.010^+}$	$0_{.002}$	$0_{.002}$
	7	$1_{.023}$	$1_{.023}$	$0_{.004}$	$0_{.004}$
	6	$0_{.011}$	$0_{.011}$	—	—
	5	$0_{.026}$	—		
14	16	$10_{.037}$	$9_{.014}$	$8_{.005^+}$	$7_{.002}$
	15	$8_{.025^+}$	$7_{.010^-}$	$7_{.010^-}$	$6_{.003}$
	14	$7_{.032}$	$6_{.013}$	$5_{.005^-}$	$5_{.005^-}$
	13	$6_{.035^+}$	$5_{.014}$	$4_{.005^+}$	$3_{.001}$
	12	$5_{.035^+}$	$4_{.014}$	$3_{.005^-}$	$3_{.005^-}$
	11	$4_{.033}$	$3_{.012}$	$2_{.004}$	$2_{.004}$
	10	$3_{.028}$	$2_{.009}$	$2_{.009}$	$1_{.002}$
	9	$2_{.021}$	$2_{.021}$	$1_{.006}$	$0_{.001}$
	8	$2_{.045^-}$	$1_{.013}$	$0_{.002}$	$0_{.002}$
	7	$1_{.030}$	$0_{.006}$	$0_{.006}$	—
	6	$0_{.013}$	$0_{.013}$	—	—
	5	$0_{.031}$	—	—	—
13	16	$9_{.030}$	$8_{.011}$	$7_{.004}$	$7_{.004}$
	15	$8_{.047}$	$7_{.019}$	$6_{.007}$	$5_{.002}$
	14	$6_{.023}$	$6_{.023}$	$5_{.008}$	$4_{.003}$
	13	$5_{.023}$	$5_{.023}$	$4_{.008}$	$3_{.003}$
	12	$4_{.022}$	$4_{.022}$	$3_{.007}$	$2_{.002}$
	11	$4_{.048}$	$3_{.018}$	$2_{.005^+}$	$1_{.001}$
	10	$3_{.039}$	$2_{.013}$	$1_{.003}$	$1_{.003}$
	9	$2_{.029}$	$1_{.008}$	$1_{.008}$	$0_{.001}$
	8	$1_{.018}$	$1_{.018}$	$0_{.003}$	$0_{.003}$
	7	$1_{.038}$	$0_{.007}$	$0_{.007}$	—
	6	$0_{.017}$	$0_{.017}$	—	—
	5	$0_{.037}$	—	—	—
12	16	$8_{.024}$	$8_{.024}$	$7_{.008}$	$6_{.002}$
	15	$7_{.036}$	$6_{.013}$	$5_{.004}$	$5_{.004}$
	14	$6_{.040}$	$5_{.015^-}$	$4_{.005^-}$	$4_{.005^-}$
	13	$5_{.039}$	$4_{.014}$	$3_{.004}$	$3_{.004}$
	12	$4_{.034}$	$3_{.012}$	$2_{.003}$	$2_{.003}$
	11	$3_{.027}$	$2_{.008}$	$2_{.008}$	$1_{.002}$
	10	$2_{.019}$	$2_{.019}$	$1_{.005^-}$	$1_{.005^-}$
	9	$2_{.040}$	$1_{.011}$	$0_{.002}$	$0_{.002}$
	8	$1_{.024}$	$1_{.024}$	$0_{.004}$	$0_{.004}$
	7	$1_{.048}$	$0_{.010^-}$	$0_{.010^-}$	—
	6	$0_{.021}$	$0_{.021}$	—	—
	5	$0_{.044}$	—	—	—
$A = 16\ B = 11$	16	$7_{.019}$	$7_{.019}$	$6_{.006}$	$5_{.002}$
	15	$6_{.027}$	$5_{.009}$	$5_{.009}$	$4_{.002}$
	14	$5_{.027}$	$4_{.009}$	$4_{.009}$	$3_{.002}$
	13	$4_{.024}$	$4_{.024}$	$3_{.008}$	$2_{.002}$
	12	$3_{.019}$	$3_{.019}$	$2_{.005^+}$	$1_{.001}$
	11	$3_{.041}$	$2_{.013}$	$1_{.003}$	$1_{.003}$
	10	$2_{.028}$	$1_{.007}$	$1_{.007}$	$0_{.001}$
	9	$1_{.016}$	$1_{.016}$	$0_{.002}$	$0_{.002}$
	8	$1_{.033}$	$0_{.006}$	$0_{.006}$	—

TABLE J (*continued*)

| | a | Probability | | | |
		0.05	0.025	0.01	0.005
	7	$\mathbf{0}_{.013}$	$\mathbf{0}_{.013}$	—	—
	6	$\mathbf{0}_{.027}$	—	—	—
10	16	$\mathbf{7}_{.046}$	$\mathbf{6}_{.014}$	$\mathbf{5}_{.004}$	$\mathbf{5}_{.004}$
	15	$\mathbf{5}_{.018}$	$\mathbf{5}_{.018}$	$\mathbf{4}_{.005^+}$	$\mathbf{3}_{.001}$
	14	$\mathbf{4}_{.018}$	$\mathbf{4}_{.018}$	$\mathbf{3}_{.005^-}$	$\mathbf{3}_{.005^-}$
	13	$\mathbf{4}_{.042}$	$\mathbf{3}_{.014}$	$\mathbf{2}_{.003}$	$\mathbf{2}_{.003}$
	12	$\mathbf{3}_{.032}$	$\mathbf{2}_{.009}$	$\mathbf{2}_{.009}$	$\mathbf{1}_{.002}$
	11	$\mathbf{2}_{.021}$	$\mathbf{2}_{.021}$	$\mathbf{1}_{.005^-}$	$\mathbf{1}_{.005^-}$
	10	$\mathbf{2}_{.042}$	$\mathbf{1}_{.011}$	$\mathbf{0}_{.002}$	$\mathbf{0}_{.002}$
	9	$\mathbf{1}_{.023}$	$\mathbf{1}_{.023}$	$\mathbf{0}_{.004}$	$\mathbf{0}_{.004}$
	8	$\mathbf{1}_{.045^-}$	$\mathbf{0}_{.008}$	$\mathbf{0}_{.008}$	—
	7	$\mathbf{0}_{.017}$	$\mathbf{0}_{.017}$	—	—
	6	$\mathbf{0}_{.035^-}$	—	—	—
9	16	$\mathbf{6}_{.037}$	$\mathbf{5}_{.010^-}$	$\mathbf{5}_{.010^-}$	$\mathbf{4}_{.002}$
	15	$\mathbf{5}_{.040}$	$\mathbf{4}_{.012}$	$\mathbf{3}_{.003}$	$\mathbf{3}_{.003}$
	14	$\mathbf{4}_{.034}$	$\mathbf{3}_{.010^-}$	$\mathbf{3}_{.010^-}$	$\mathbf{2}_{.002}$
	13	$\mathbf{3}_{.025^+}$	$\mathbf{2}_{.007}$	$\mathbf{2}_{.007}$	$\mathbf{1}_{.001}$
	12	$\mathbf{2}_{.016}$	$\mathbf{2}_{.016}$	$\mathbf{1}_{.003}$	$\mathbf{1}_{.003}$
	11	$\mathbf{2}_{.033}$	$\mathbf{1}_{.008}$	$\mathbf{1}_{.008}$	$\mathbf{0}_{.001}$
	10	$\mathbf{1}_{.017}$	$\mathbf{1}_{.017}$	$\mathbf{0}_{.002}$	$\mathbf{0}_{.002}$
	9	$\mathbf{1}_{.034}$	$\mathbf{0}_{.006}$	$\mathbf{0}_{.006}$	—
	8	$\mathbf{0}_{.012}$	$\mathbf{0}_{.012}$	—	—
	7	$\mathbf{0}_{.024}$	$\mathbf{0}_{.024}$	—	—
	6	$\mathbf{0}_{.045^+}$	—	—	—
8	16	$\mathbf{5}_{.028}$	$\mathbf{4}_{.007}$	$\mathbf{4}_{.007}$	$\mathbf{3}_{.001}$
	15	$\mathbf{4}_{.028}$	$\mathbf{3}_{.007}$	$\mathbf{3}_{.007}$	$\mathbf{2}_{.001}$
	14	$\mathbf{3}_{.021}$	$\mathbf{3}_{.021}$	$\mathbf{2}_{.005^-}$	$\mathbf{2}_{.005^-}$
	13	$\mathbf{3}_{.047}$	$\mathbf{2}_{.013}$	$\mathbf{1}_{.002}$	$\mathbf{1}_{.002}$
	12	$\mathbf{2}_{.028}$	$\mathbf{1}_{.006}$	$\mathbf{1}_{.006}$	$\mathbf{0}_{.001}$
	11	$\mathbf{1}_{.014}$	$\mathbf{1}_{.014}$	$\mathbf{0}_{.002}$	$\mathbf{0}_{.002}$
	10	$\mathbf{1}_{.027}$	$\mathbf{0}_{.004}$	$\mathbf{0}_{.004}$	$\mathbf{0}_{.004}$
	9	$\mathbf{0}_{.009}$	$\mathbf{0}_{.009}$	$\mathbf{0}_{.009}$	—
	8	$\mathbf{0}_{.017}$	$\mathbf{0}_{.017}$	—	—
	7	$\mathbf{0}_{.033}$	—	—	—
7	16	$\mathbf{4}_{.020}$	$\mathbf{4}_{.020}$	$\mathbf{3}_{.004}$	$\mathbf{3}_{.004}$
	15	$\mathbf{3}_{.017}$	$\mathbf{3}_{.017}$	$\mathbf{2}_{.003}$	$\mathbf{2}_{.003}$
	14	$\mathbf{3}_{.045^+}$	$\mathbf{2}_{.011}$	$\mathbf{1}_{.002}$	$\mathbf{1}_{.002}$
	13	$\mathbf{2}_{.026}$	$\mathbf{1}_{.005^-}$	$\mathbf{1}_{.005^-}$	$\mathbf{1}_{.005^-}$
	12	$\mathbf{1}_{.012}$	$\mathbf{1}_{.012}$	$\mathbf{0}_{.001}$	$\mathbf{0}_{.001}$
	11	$\mathbf{1}_{.024}$	$\mathbf{1}_{.024}$	$\mathbf{0}_{.003}$	$\mathbf{0}_{.003}$
	10	$\mathbf{1}_{.045^-}$	$\mathbf{0}_{.007}$	$\mathbf{0}_{.007}$	—
	9	$\mathbf{0}_{.014}$	$\mathbf{0}_{.014}$	—	—
	8	$\mathbf{0}_{.026}$	—	—	—
	7	$\mathbf{0}_{.047}$	—	—	—
6	16	$\mathbf{3}_{.013}$	$\mathbf{3}_{.013}$	$\mathbf{2}_{.002}$	$\mathbf{2}_{.002}$
	15	$\mathbf{3}_{.046}$	$\mathbf{2}_{.009}$	$\mathbf{2}_{.009}$	$\mathbf{1}_{.001}$
	14	$\mathbf{2}_{.025^+}$	$\mathbf{1}_{.004}$	$\mathbf{1}_{.004}$	$\mathbf{1}_{.004}$
	13	$\mathbf{1}_{.011}$	$\mathbf{1}_{.011}$	$\mathbf{0}_{.001}$	$\mathbf{0}_{.001}$
	12	$\mathbf{1}_{.023}$	$\mathbf{1}_{.023}$	$\mathbf{0}_{.003}$	$\mathbf{0}_{.003}$
	11	$\mathbf{1}_{.043}$	$\mathbf{0}_{.006}$	$\mathbf{0}_{.006}$	—

TABLE J (*continued*)

	a	Probability			
		0.05	0.025	0.01	0.005
$A = 16\ B = 6$	10	$0_{.012}$	$0_{.012}$	—	—
	9	$0_{.023}$	$0_{.023}$	—	—
	8	$0_{.040}$	—	—	—
5	16	$3_{.048}$	$2_{.008}$	$2_{.008}$	$1_{.001}$
	15	$2_{.028}$	$1_{.004}$	$1_{.004}$	$1_{.004}$
	14	$1_{.011}$	$1_{.011}$	$0_{.001}$	$0_{.001}$
	13	$1_{.025}{}^{+}$	$0_{.003}$	$0_{.003}$	$0_{.003}$
	12	$1_{.047}$	$0_{.006}$	$0_{.006}$	—
	11	$0_{.012}$	$0_{.012}$	—	—
	10	$0_{.023}$	$0_{.023}$	—	—
	9	$0_{.039}$	—	—	—
4	16	$2_{.032}$	$1_{.004}$	$1_{.004}$	$1_{.004}$
	15	$1_{.013}$	$1_{.013}$	$0_{.001}$	$1_{.001}$
	14	$1_{.032}$	$0_{.003}$	$0_{.003}$	$0_{.003}$
	13	$0_{.007}$	$0_{.007}$	$0_{.007}$	—
	12	$0_{.014}$	$0_{.014}$	—	—
	11	$0_{.026}$	—	—	—
	10	$0_{.043}$	—	—	—
3	16	$1_{.018}$	$1_{.018}$	$0_{.001}$	$0_{.001}$
	15	$0_{.004}$	$0_{.004}$	$0_{.004}$	$0_{.004}$
	14	$0_{.010}{}^{+}$	$0_{.010}{}^{+}$	—	—
	13	$0_{.021}$	$0_{.021}$	—	—
	12	$0_{.036}$	—	—	—
2	16	$0_{.007}$	$0_{.007}$	$0_{.007}$	—
	15	$0_{.020}$	$0_{.020}$	—	—
	14	$0_{.039}$	—	—	—
$A = 17\ B = 17$	17	$12_{.022}$	$12_{.022}$	$11_{.009}$	$10_{.004}$
	16	$11_{.043}$	$10_{.020}$	$9_{.008}$	$8_{.003}$
	15	$9_{.029}$	$8_{.013}$	$7_{.005}{}^{+}$	$6_{.002}$
	14	$8_{.035}{}^{+}$	$7_{.016}$	$6_{.007}$	$5_{.002}$
	13	$7_{.040}$	$6_{.018}$	$5_{.007}$	$4_{.003}$
	12	$6_{.042}$	$5_{.019}$	$4_{.007}$	$3_{.002}$
	11	$5_{.042}$	$4_{.018}$	$3_{.007}$	$2_{.002}$
	10	$4_{.040}$	$3_{.016}$	$2_{.005}{}^{+}$	$1_{.001}$
	9	$3_{.035}{}^{+}$	$2_{.013}$	$1_{.003}$	$1_{.003}$
	8	$2_{.029}$	$1_{.008}$	$1_{.008}$	$0_{.001}$
	7	$1_{.020}$	$1_{.020}$	$0_{.004}$	$0_{.004}$
	6	$1_{.043}$	$0_{.009}$	$0_{.009}$	—
	5	$0_{.022}$	$0_{.022}$	—	—
16	17	$12_{.044}$	$11_{.018}$	$10_{.007}$	$9_{.003}$
	16	$10_{.035}{}^{-}$	$9_{.015}{}^{-}$	$8_{.006}$	$7_{.002}$
	15	$9_{.046}$	$8_{.021}$	$7_{.009}$	$6_{.003}$
	14	$7_{.025}{}^{+}$	$6_{.011}$	$5_{.004}$	$5_{.004}$
	13	$6_{.027}$	$5_{.011}$	$4_{.004}$	$4_{.004}$
	12	$5_{.027}$	$4_{.011}$	$3_{.004}$	$3_{.004}$
	11	$4_{.025}{}^{+}$	$3_{.009}$	$3_{.009}$	$2_{.003}$
	10	$3_{.022}$	$3_{.022}$	$2_{.007}$	$1_{.002}$
	9	$3_{.046}$	$2_{.017}$	$1_{.004}$	$1_{.004}$
	8	$2_{.036}$	$1_{.011}$	$0_{.002}$	$0_{.002}$
	7	$1_{.024}$	$1_{.024}$	$0_{.005}{}^{-}$	$0_{.005}{}^{-}$

TABLE J (*continued*)

	a	0.05	0.025	0.01	0.005
	6	$0_{.011}$	$0_{.011}$	—	—
	5	$0_{.026}$	—	—	—
15	17	$11_{.038}$	$10_{.015^-}$	$9_{.006}$	$8_{.002}$
	16	$9_{.027}$	$8_{.011}$	$7_{.004}$	$7_{.004}$
	15	$8_{.035^+}$	$7_{.015^-}$	$6_{.006}$	$5_{.002}$
	14	$7_{.040}$	$6_{.017}$	$5_{.006}$	$4_{.002}$
	13	$6_{.041}$	$5_{.017}$	$4_{.006}$	$3_{.002}$
	12	$5_{.039}$	$4_{.016}$	$3_{.005^+}$	$2_{.001}$
	11	$4_{.035^+}$	$3_{.013}$	$2_{.004}$	$2_{.004}$
	10	$3_{.029}$	$2_{.010^-}$	$2_{.010^-}$	$1_{.002}$
	9	$2_{.022}$	$2_{.022}$	$1_{.006}$	$0_{.001}$
$A = 17\ B = 15$	8	$2_{.046}$	$1_{.014}$	$0_{.002}$	$0_{.002}$
	7	$1_{.030}$	$0_{.006}$	$0_{.006}$	—
	6	$0_{.014}$	$0_{.014}$	—	—
	5	$0_{.031}$	—	—	—
14	17	$10_{.032}$	$9_{.012}$	$8_{.004}$	$8_{.004}$
	16	$8_{.021}$	$8_{.021}$	$7_{.008}$	$6_{.003}$
	15	$7_{.026}$	$6_{.010^-}$	$6_{.010^-}$	$5_{.003}$
	14	$6_{.028}$	$5_{.011}$	$4_{.004}$	$4_{.004}$
	13	$5_{.027}$	$4_{.010^-}$	$4_{.010^-}$	$3_{.003}$
	12	$4_{.024}$	$4_{.024}$	$3_{.008}$	$2_{.002}$
	11	$4_{.049}$	$3_{.019}$	$2_{.006}$	$1_{.001}$
	10	$3_{.040}$	$2_{.014}$	$1_{.003}$	$1_{.003}$
	9	$2_{.029}$	$1_{.008}$	$1_{.008}$	$0_{.001}$
	8	$1_{.018}$	$1_{.018}$	$0_{.003}$	$0_{.003}$
	7	$1_{.038}$	$0_{.007}$	$0_{.007}$	—
	6	$0_{.017}$	$0_{.017}$	—	—
	5	$0_{.036}$	—	—	—
13	17	$9_{.026}$	$8_{.009}$	$8_{.009}$	$7_{.003}$
	16	$8_{.040}$	$7_{.015^+}$	$6_{.005^+}$	$5_{.002}$
	15	$7_{.045^+}$	$6_{.018}$	$5_{.006}$	$4_{.002}$
	14	$6_{.045^+}$	$5_{.018}$	$4_{.006}$	$3_{.002}$
	13	$5_{.042}$	$4_{.016}$	$3_{.005^+}$	$2_{.001}$
	12	$4_{.035^+}$	$3_{.013}$	$2_{.004}$	$2_{.004}$
	11	$3_{.028}$	$2_{.009}$	$2_{.009}$	$1_{.002}$
	10	$2_{.019}$	$2_{.019}$	$1_{.005^-}$	$1_{.005^-}$
	9	$2_{.040}$	$1_{.011}$	$0_{.002}$	$0_{.002}$
	8	$1_{.024}$	$1_{.024}$	$0_{.004}$	$0_{.004}$
	7	$1_{.047}$	$0_{.010^-}$	$0_{.010^-}$	—
	6	$0_{.021}$	$0_{.021}$	—	—
	5	$0_{.043}$	—	—	—
12	17	$8_{.021}$	$8_{.021}$	$7_{.007}$	$6_{.002}$
	16	$7_{.030}$	$6_{.011}$	$5_{.003}$	$5_{.003}$
	15	$6_{.033}$	$5_{.012}$	$4_{.004}$	$4_{.004}$
	14	$5_{.030}$	$4_{.011}$	$3_{.003}$	$3_{.003}$
	13	$4_{.026}$	$3_{.008}$	$3_{.008}$	$2_{.002}$
	12	$3_{.020}$	$3_{.020}$	$2_{.006}$	$1_{.001}$
	11	$3_{.041}$	$2_{.013}$	$1_{.003}$	$1_{.003}$
	10	$2_{.028}$	$1_{.007}$	$1_{.007}$	$0_{.001}$
	9	$1_{.016}$	$1_{.016}$	$0_{.002}$	$0_{.002}$

TABLE J (*continued*)

	a	Probability 0.05	0.025	0.01	0.005
	8	$1_{.032}$	$0_{.006}$	$0_{.006}$	—
	7	$0_{.012}$	$0_{.012}$	—	—
	6	$0_{.026}$	—	—	—
11	17	$7_{.016}$	$7_{.016}$	$6_{.005^-}$	$6_{.005^-}$
	16	$6_{.022}$	$6_{.022}$	$5_{.007}$	$4_{.002}$
	15	$5_{.022}$	$5_{.022}$	$4_{.007}$	$3_{.002}$
	14	$4_{.019}$	$4_{.019}$	$3_{.006}$	$2_{.001}$
	13	$4_{.042}$	$3_{.014}$	$2_{.004}$	$2_{.004}$
	12	$3_{.031}$	$2_{.009}$	$2_{.009}$	$1_{.002}$
	11	$2_{.020}$	$2_{.020}$	$1_{.005^-}$	$1_{.005^-}$
	10	$2_{.040}$	$1_{.011}$	$0_{.001}$	$0_{.001}$
	9	$1_{.022}$	$1_{.022}$	$0_{.004}$	$0_{.004}$
	8	$1_{.042}$	$0_{.008}$	$0_{.008}$	—
	7	$0_{.016}$	$0_{.016}$	—	—
	6	$0_{.033}$	—	—	—
10	17	$7_{.041}$	$6_{.012}$	$5_{.003}$	$5_{.003}$
	16	$6_{.047}$	$5_{.015^+}$	$4_{.004}$	$4_{.004}$
	15	$5_{.043}$	$4_{.014}$	$3_{.004}$	$3_{.004}$
	14	$4_{.034}$	$3_{.010^+}$	$2_{.002}$	$2_{.002}$
	13	$3_{.024}$	$3_{.024}$	$2_{.007}$	$1_{.001}$
	12	$3_{.049}$	$2_{.015^+}$	$1_{.003}$	$1_{.003}$
$A = 17\ B = 10$	11	$2_{.031}$	$1_{.007}$	$1_{.007}$	$0_{.001}$
	10	$1_{.016}$	$1_{.016}$	$0_{.002}$	$0_{.002}$
	9	$1_{.031}$	$0_{.005^+}$	$0_{.005^+}$	—
	8	$0_{.011}$	$0_{.011}$	—	—
	7	$0_{.022}$	$0_{.022}$	—	—
	6	$0_{.042}$	—	—	—
9	17	$6_{.032}$	$5_{.008}$	$5_{.008}$	$4_{.002}$
	16	$5_{.034}$	$4_{.010^-}$	$4_{.010^-}$	$3_{.002}$
	15	$4_{.028}$	$3_{.008}$	$3_{.008}$	$2_{.002}$
	14	$3_{.020}$	$3_{.020}$	$2_{.005^-}$	$2_{.005^-}$
	13	$3_{.042}$	$2_{.012}$	$1_{.002}$	$1_{.002}$
	12	$2_{.025^+}$	$1_{.006}$	$1_{.006}$	$0_{.001}$
	11	$2_{.048}$	$1_{.012}$	$0_{.002}$	$0_{.002}$
	10	$1_{.024}$	$1_{.024}$	$0_{.004}$	$0_{.004}$
	9	$1_{.045^-}$	$0_{.008}$	$0_{.008}$	—
	8	$0_{.016}$	$0_{.016}$	—	—
	7	$0_{.030}$	—	—	—
8	17	$5_{.024}$	$5_{.024}$	$4_{.006}$	$3_{.001}$
	16	$4_{.023}$	$4_{.023}$	$3_{.006}$	$2_{.001}$
	15	$3_{.017}$	$3_{.017}$	$2_{.004}$	$2_{.004}$
	14	$3_{.039}$	$2_{.010^-}$	$2_{.010^-}$	$1_{.002}$
	13	$2_{.022}$	$2_{.022}$	$1_{.004}$	$1_{.004}$
	12	$2_{.043}$	$1_{.010^-}$	$1_{.010^-}$	$0_{.001}$
	11	$1_{.020}$	$1_{.020}$	$0_{.003}$	$0_{.003}$
	10	$1_{.038}$	$0_{.006}$	$0_{.006}$	—
	9	$0_{.012}$	$0_{.012}$	—	—
	8	$0_{.022}$	$0_{.022}$	—	—
	7	$0_{.040}$	—	—	—
7	17	$4_{.017}$	$4_{.017}$	$3_{.003}$	$3_{.003}$

TABLE J (*continued*)

		Probability			
	a	0.05	0.025	0.01	0.005
	16	$3_{.014}$	$3_{.014}$	$2_{.003}$	$2_{.003}$
	15	$3_{.038}$	$2_{.009}$	$2_{.009}$	$1_{.001}$
	14	$2_{.021}$	$2_{.021}$	$1_{.004}$	$1_{.004}$
	13	$2_{.042}$	$1_{.009}$	$1_{.009}$	$0_{.001}$
	12	$1_{.018}$	$1_{.018}$	$0_{.002}$	$0_{.002}$
	11	$1_{.034}$	$0_{.005^-}$	$0_{.005^-}$	$0_{.005^-}$
	10	$0_{.010^-}$	$0_{.010^-}$	$0_{.010^-}$	—
	9	$0_{.019}$	$0_{.019}$	—	—
	8	$0_{.033}$	—	—	—
6	17	$3_{.011}$	$3_{.011}$	$2_{.002}$	$2_{.002}$
	16	$3_{.040}$	$2_{.008}$	$2_{.008}$	$1_{.001}$
	15	$2_{.021}$	$2_{.021}$	$1_{.003}$	$1_{.003}$
	14	$2_{.045^+}$	$1_{.009}$	$1_{.009}$	$0_{.001}$
	13	$1_{.018}$	$1_{.018}$	$0_{.002}$	$0_{.002}$
	12	$1_{.035^-}$	$0_{.005^-}$	$0_{.005^-}$	$0_{.005^-}$
	11	$0_{.009}$	$0_{.009}$	$0_{.009}$	—
	10	$0_{.017}$	$0_{.017}$	—	—
	9	$0_{.030}$	—	—	—
	8	$0_{.050^-}$	—	—	—
5	17	$3_{.043}$	$2_{.006}$	$2_{.006}$	$1_{.001}$
	16	$2_{.024}$	$2_{.024}$	$1_{.003}$	$1_{.003}$
	15	$1_{.009}$	$1_{.009}$	$1_{.009}$	$0_{.001}$
	14	$1_{.021}$	$1_{.021}$	$0_{.002}$	$0_{.002}$
	13	$1_{.039}$	$0_{.005^-}$	$0_{.005^-}$	$0_{.005^-}$
	12	$0_{.010^-}$	$0_{.010^-}$	$0_{.010^-}$	—
	11	$0_{.018}$	$0_{.018}$	—	—
	10	$0_{.030}$	—	—	—
	9	$0_{.049}$	—	—	—
4	17	$2_{.029}$	$1_{.003}$	$1_{.003}$	$1_{.003}$
	16	$1_{.011}$	$1_{.011}$	$0_{.001}$	$0_{.001}$
	15	$1_{.028}$	$0_{.003}$	$0_{.003}$	$0_{.003}$
	14	$0_{.006}$	$0_{.006}$	$0_{.006}$	—
$A = 17\ B = 4$	13	$0_{.012}$	$0_{.012}$	—	—
	12	$0_{.021}$	$0_{.021}$	—	—
	11	$0_{.035^+}$	—	—	—
3	17	$1_{.016}$	$1_{.016}$	$0_{.001}$	$0_{.001}$
	16	$1_{.046}$	$0_{.004}$	$0_{.004}$	$0_{.004}$
	15	$0_{.009}$	$0_{.009}$	$0_{.009}$	—
	14	$0_{.018}$	$0_{.018}$	—	—
	13	$0_{.031}$	—	—	—
	12	$0_{.049}$	—	—	—
2	17	$0_{.006}$	$0_{.006}$	$0_{.006}$	—
	16	$0_{.018}$	$0_{.018}$	—	—
	15	$0_{.035^+}$	—	—	—
$A = 18\ B = 18$	18	$13_{.023}$	$13_{.023}$	$12_{.010^-}$	$11_{.004}$
	17	$12_{.044}$	$11_{.020}$	$10_{.009}$	$9_{.004}$
	16	$10_{.030}$	$9_{.014}$	$8_{.006}$	$7_{.002}$
	15	$9_{.038}$	$8_{.018}$	$7_{.008}$	$6_{.003}$
	14	$8_{.043}$	$7_{.020}$	$6_{.009}$	$5_{.003}$
	13	$7_{.046}$	$6_{.022}$	$5_{.009}$	$4_{.003}$

TABLE J (*continued*)

	a	Probability 0.05	0.025	0.01	0.005
	12	$6_{.047}$	$5_{.022}$	$4_{.009}$	$3_{.003}$
	11	$5_{.046}$	$4_{.020}$	$3_{.008}$	$2_{.002}$
	10	$4_{.043}$	$3_{.018}$	$2_{.006}$	$1_{.001}$
	9	$3_{.038}$	$2_{.014}$	$1_{.004}$	$1_{.004}$
	8	$2_{.030}$	$1_{.009}$	$1_{.009}$	$0_{.001}$
	7	$1_{.020}$	$1_{.020}$	$0_{.004}$	$0_{.004}$
	6	$1_{.044}$	$0_{.010}$	$0_{.010}-$	—
	5	$0_{.023}$	$0_{.023}$	—	—
17	18	$13_{.045}+$	$12_{.019}$	$11_{.008}$	$10_{.003}$
	17	$11_{.036}$	$10_{.016}$	$9_{.007}$	$8_{.002}$
	16	$10_{.049}$	$9_{.023}$	$8_{.010}-$	$7_{.004}$
	15	$8_{.028}$	$7_{.012}$	$6_{.005}-$	$6_{.005}-$
	14	$7_{.030}$	$6_{.013}$	$5_{.005}+$	$4_{.002}$
	13	$6_{.031}$	$5_{.013}$	$4_{.005}-$	$4_{.005}-$
	12	$5_{.030}$	$4_{.012}$	$3_{.004}$	$3_{.004}$
	11	$4_{.028}$	$3_{.010}+$	$2_{.003}$	$2_{.003}$
	10	$3_{.023}$	$3_{.023}$	$2_{.008}$	$1_{.002}$
	9	$3_{.047}$	$2_{.018}$	$1_{.005}-$	$1_{.005}-$
	8	$2_{.037}$	$1_{.011}$	$0_{.002}$	$0_{.002}$
	7	$1_{.025}-$	$1_{.025}-$	$0_{.005}-$	$0_{.005}-$
	6	$0_{.011}$	$0_{.011}$	—	—
	5	$0_{.026}$	—	—	—
16	18	$12_{.039}$	$11_{.016}$	$10_{.006}$	$9_{.002}$
	17	$10_{.029}$	$9_{.012}$	$8_{.005}-$	$8_{.005}-$
	16	$9_{.038}$	$8_{.017}$	$7_{.007}$	$6_{.002}$
	15	$8_{.043}$	$7_{.019}$	$6_{.008}$	$5_{.003}$
	14	$7_{.046}$	$6_{.020}$	$5_{.008}$	$4_{.003}$
	13	$6_{.045}+$	$5_{.020}$	$4_{.007}$	$3_{.002}$
	12	$5_{.042}$	$4_{.018}$	$3_{.006}$	$2_{.002}$
	11	$4_{.037}$	$3_{.015}-$	$2_{.004}$	$2_{.004}$
	10	$3_{.031}$	$2_{.011}$	$1_{.003}$	$1_{.003}$
	9	$2_{.023}$	$2_{.023}$	$1_{.006}$	$0_{.001}$
	8	$2_{.046}$	$1_{.014}$	$0_{.002}$	$0_{.002}$
	7	$1_{.030}$	$0_{.006}$	$0_{.006}$	—
	6	$0_{.014}$	$0_{.014}$	—	—
	5	$0_{.031}$	—	—	—
15	18	$11_{.033}$	$10_{.013}$	$9_{.005}-$	$9_{.005}-$
	17	$9_{.023}$	$9_{.023}$	$8_{.009}$	$7_{.003}$
	16	$8_{.029}$	$7_{.012}$	$6_{.004}$	$6_{.004}$
	15	$7_{.031}$	$6_{.013}$	$5_{.005}-$	$5_{.005}-$
	14	$6_{.031}$	$5_{.013}$	$4_{.004}$	$4_{.004}$
	13	$5_{.029}$	$4_{.011}$	$3_{.004}$	$3_{.004}$
$A = 18\ B = 15$	12	$4_{.025}+$	$3_{.009}$	$3_{.009}$	$2_{.003}$
	11	$3_{.020}$	$3_{.020}$	$2_{.006}$	$1_{.001}$
	10	$3_{.041}$	$2_{.014}$	$1_{.004}$	$1_{.004}$
	9	$2_{.030}$	$1_{.008}$	$1_{.008}$	$0_{.001}$
	8	$1_{.018}$	$1_{.018}$	$0_{.003}$	$0_{.003}$
	7	$1_{.038}$	$0_{.007}$	$0_{.007}$	—
	6	$0_{.017}$	$0_{.017}$	—	—
	5	$0_{.036}$	—	—	—

TABLE J (*continued*)

	a	Probability			
		0.05	**0.025**	**0.01**	**0.005**
14	18	$10_{.028}$	$9_{.010^-}$	$9_{.010^-}$	$8_{.003}$
	17	$9_{.043}$	$8_{.017}$	$7_{.006}$	$6_{.002}$
	16	$8_{.050^-}$	$7_{.021}$	$6_{.008}$	$5_{.003}$
	15	$6_{.022}$	$6_{.022}$	$5_{.008}$	$4_{.003}$
	14	$6_{.049}$	$5_{.020}$	$4_{.007}$	$3_{.002}$
	13	$5_{.044}$	$4_{.017}$	$3_{.006}$	$2_{.001}$
	12	$4_{.037}$	$3_{.013}$	$2_{.004}$	$2_{.004}$
	11	$3_{.028}$	$2_{.009}$	$2_{.009}$	$1_{.002}$
	10	$2_{.020}$	$2_{.020}$	$1_{.005^-}$	$1_{.005^-}$
	9	$2_{.039}$	$1_{.011}$	$0_{.002}$	$0_{.002}$
	8	$1_{.024}$	$1_{.024}$	$0_{.004}$	$0_{.004}$
	7	$1_{.047}$	$0_{.009}$	$0_{.009}$	—
	6	$0_{.020}$	$0_{.020}$	—	—
	5	$0_{.043}$	—	—	—
13	18	$9_{.023}$	$9_{.023}$	$8_{.008}$	$7_{.002}$
	17	$8_{.034}$	$7_{.012}$	$6_{.004}$	$6_{.004}$
	16	$7_{.037}$	$6_{.014}$	$5_{.005^-}$	$5_{.005^-}$
	15	$6_{.036}$	$5_{.014}$	$4_{.004}$	$4_{.004}$
	14	$5_{.032}$	$4_{.012}$	$3_{.004}$	$3_{.004}$
	13	$4_{.027}$	$3_{.009}$	$3_{.009}$	$2_{.002}$
	12	$3_{.020}$	$3_{.020}$	$2_{.006}$	$1_{.001}$
	11	$3_{.040}$	$2_{.013}$	$1_{.003}$	$1_{.003}$
	10	$2_{.027}$	$1_{.007}$	$1_{.007}$	$0_{.001}$
	9	$1_{.015^+}$	$1_{.015^+}$	$0_{.002}$	$0_{.002}$
	8	$1_{.031}$	$0_{.006}$	$0_{.006}$	—
	7	$0_{.012}$	$0_{.012}$	—	—
	6	$0_{.025^+}$	—	—	—
12	18	$8_{.018}$	$8_{.018}$	$7_{.006}$	$6_{.002}$
	17	$7_{.026}$	$6_{.009}$	$6_{.009}$	$5_{.003}$
	16	$6_{.027}$	$5_{.009}$	$5_{.009}$	$4_{.003}$
	15	$5_{.024}$	$5_{.024}$	$4_{.008}$	$3_{.002}$
	14	$4_{.020}$	$4_{.020}$	$3_{.006}$	$2_{.001}$
	13	$4_{.042}$	$3_{.014}$	$2_{.004}$	$2_{.004}$
	12	$3_{.030}$	$2_{.009}$	$2_{.009}$	$1_{.002}$
	11	$2_{.019}$	$2_{.019}$	$1_{.005^-}$	$1_{.005^-}$
	10	$2_{.038}$	$1_{.010^+}$	$0_{.001}$	$0_{.001}$
	9	$1_{.021}$	$1_{.021}$	$0_{.003}$	$0_{.003}$
	8	$1_{.040}$	$0_{.007}$	$0_{.007}$	—
	7	$0_{.016}$	$0_{.016}$	—	—
	6	$0_{.031}$	—	—	—
11	18	$8_{.045^+}$	$7_{.014}$	$6_{.004}$	$6_{.004}$
	17	$6_{.018}$	$6_{.018}$	$5_{.006}$	$4_{.001}$
	16	$5_{.018}$	$5_{.018}$	$4_{.005^+}$	$3_{.001}$
	15	$5_{.043}$	$4_{.015^-}$	$3_{.004}$	$3_{.004}$
	14	$4_{.033}$	$3_{.011}$	$2_{.003}$	$2_{.003}$
	13	$3_{.023}$	$3_{.023}$	$2_{.007}$	$1_{.001}$
	12	$3_{.046}$	$2_{.014}$	$1_{.003}$	$1_{.003}$
	11	$2_{.029}$	$1_{.007}$	$1_{.007}$	$0_{.001}$
	10	$1_{.015^-}$	$1_{.015^-}$	$0_{.002}$	$0_{.002}$
	9	$1_{.029}$	$0_{.005^-}$	$0_{.005^-}$	$0_{.005^-}$

TABLE J (*continued*)

		Probability			
	a	0.05	0.025	0.01	0.005
	8	$\mathbf{0}_{.010^+}$	$\mathbf{0}_{.010^+}$	—	—
	7	$\mathbf{0}_{.020}$	$\mathbf{0}_{.020}$	—	—
	6	$\mathbf{0}_{.039}$	—	—	—
$A = 18\ B = 10$	18	$\mathbf{7}_{.037}$	$\mathbf{6}_{.010^+}$	$\mathbf{5}_{.003}$	$\mathbf{5}_{.003}$
	17	$\mathbf{6}_{.041}$	$\mathbf{5}_{.013}$	$\mathbf{4}_{.003}$	$\mathbf{4}_{.003}$
	16	$\mathbf{5}_{.036}$	$\mathbf{4}_{.011}$	$\mathbf{3}_{.003}$	$\mathbf{3}_{.003}$
	15	$\mathbf{4}_{.020}$	$\mathbf{3}_{.000}$	$\mathbf{3}_{.000}$	$\mathbf{2}_{.002}$
	14	$\mathbf{3}_{.019}$	$\mathbf{3}_{.019}$	$\mathbf{2}_{.005^-}$	$\mathbf{2}_{.005^-}$
	13	$\mathbf{3}_{.039}$	$\mathbf{2}_{.011}$	$\mathbf{1}_{.002}$	$\mathbf{1}_{.002}$
	12	$\mathbf{2}_{.023}$	$\mathbf{2}_{.023}$	$\mathbf{1}_{.005^+}$	$\mathbf{0}_{.001}$
	11	$\mathbf{2}_{.043}$	$\mathbf{1}_{.011}$	$\mathbf{0}_{.001}$	$\mathbf{0}_{.001}$
	10	$\mathbf{1}_{.022}$	$\mathbf{1}_{.022}$	$\mathbf{0}_{.003}$	$\mathbf{0}_{.003}$
	9	$\mathbf{1}_{.040}$	$\mathbf{0}_{.007}$	$\mathbf{0}_{.007}$	—
	8	$\mathbf{0}_{.014}$	$\mathbf{0}_{.014}$	—	—
	7	$\mathbf{0}_{.027}$	—	—	—
	6	$\mathbf{0}_{.049}$	—	—	—
9	18	$\mathbf{6}_{.029}$	$\mathbf{5}_{.007}$	$\mathbf{5}_{.007}$	$\mathbf{4}_{.002}$
	17	$\mathbf{5}_{.030}$	$\mathbf{4}_{.008}$	$\mathbf{4}_{.008}$	$\mathbf{3}_{.002}$
	16	$\mathbf{4}_{.023}$	$\mathbf{4}_{.023}$	$\mathbf{3}_{.006}$	$\mathbf{2}_{.001}$
	15	$\mathbf{3}_{.016}$	$\mathbf{3}_{.016}$	$\mathbf{2}_{.004}$	$\mathbf{2}_{.004}$
	14	$\mathbf{3}_{.034}$	$\mathbf{2}_{.009}$	$\mathbf{2}_{.009}$	$\mathbf{1}_{.002}$
	13	$\mathbf{2}_{.019}$	$\mathbf{2}_{.019}$	$\mathbf{1}_{.004}$	$\mathbf{1}_{.004}$
	12	$\mathbf{2}_{.037}$	$\mathbf{1}_{.009}$	$\mathbf{1}_{.009}$	$\mathbf{0}_{.001}$
	11	$\mathbf{1}_{.018}$	$\mathbf{1}_{.018}$	$\mathbf{0}_{.002}$	$\mathbf{0}_{.002}$
	10	$\mathbf{1}_{.033}$	$\mathbf{0}_{.005^+}$	$\mathbf{0}_{.005^+}$	—
	9	$\mathbf{0}_{.010^+}$	$\mathbf{0}_{.010^+}$	—	—
	8	$\mathbf{0}_{.020}$	$\mathbf{0}_{.020}$	—	—
	7	$\mathbf{0}_{.036}$	—	—	—
8	18	$\mathbf{5}_{.022}$	$\mathbf{5}_{.022}$	$\mathbf{4}_{.005^-}$	$\mathbf{4}_{.005^-}$
	17	$\mathbf{4}_{.020}$	$\mathbf{4}_{.020}$	$\mathbf{3}_{.004}$	$\mathbf{3}_{.004}$
	16	$\mathbf{3}_{.014}$	$\mathbf{3}_{.014}$	$\mathbf{2}_{.003}$	$\mathbf{2}_{.003}$
	15	$\mathbf{3}_{.032}$	$\mathbf{2}_{.008}$	$\mathbf{2}_{.008}$	$\mathbf{1}_{.001}$
	14	$\mathbf{2}_{.017}$	$\mathbf{2}_{.017}$	$\mathbf{1}_{.003}$	$\mathbf{1}_{.003}$
	13	$\mathbf{2}_{.034}$	$\mathbf{1}_{.007}$	$\mathbf{1}_{.007}$	$\mathbf{0}_{.001}$
	12	$\mathbf{1}_{.015^+}$	$\mathbf{1}_{.015^+}$	$\mathbf{0}_{.002}$	$\mathbf{0}_{.002}$
	11	$\mathbf{1}_{.028}$	$\mathbf{0}_{.004}$	$\mathbf{0}_{.004}$	$\mathbf{0}_{.004}$
	10	$\mathbf{1}_{.049}$	$\mathbf{0}_{.008}$	$\mathbf{0}_{.008}$	—
	9	$\mathbf{0}_{.016}$	$\mathbf{0}_{.016}$	—	—
	8	$\mathbf{0}_{.028}$	—	—	—
	7	$\mathbf{0}_{.048}$	—	—	—
7	18	$\mathbf{4}_{.015^+}$	$\mathbf{4}_{.015^+}$	$\mathbf{3}_{.003}$	$\mathbf{3}_{.003}$
	17	$\mathbf{3}_{.012}$	$\mathbf{3}_{.012}$	$\mathbf{2}_{.002}$	$\mathbf{2}_{.002}$
	16	$\mathbf{3}_{.032}$	$\mathbf{2}_{.007}$	$\mathbf{2}_{.007}$	$\mathbf{1}_{.001}$
	15	$\mathbf{2}_{.017}$	$\mathbf{2}_{.017}$	$\mathbf{1}_{.003}$	$\mathbf{1}_{.003}$
	14	$\mathbf{2}_{.034}$	$\mathbf{1}_{.007}$	$\mathbf{1}_{.007}$	$\mathbf{0}_{.001}$
	13	$\mathbf{1}_{.014}$	$\mathbf{1}_{.014}$	$\mathbf{0}_{.002}$	$\mathbf{0}_{.002}$
	12	$\mathbf{1}_{.027}$	$\mathbf{0}_{.004}$	$\mathbf{0}_{.004}$	$\mathbf{0}_{.004}$
	11	$\mathbf{1}_{.046}$	$\mathbf{0}_{.007}$	$\mathbf{0}_{.007}$	—
	10	$\mathbf{0}_{.013}$	$\mathbf{0}_{.013}$	—	—
	9	$\mathbf{0}_{.024}$	$\mathbf{0}_{.024}$	—	—

TABLE J (*continued*)

	a	0.05	0.025	0.01	0.005
			Probability		
	8	$\mathbf{0}_{.040}$	—	—	—
6	18	$\mathbf{3}_{.010^-}$	$\mathbf{3}_{.010^-}$	$\mathbf{3}_{.010^-}$	$\mathbf{2}_{.001}$
	17	$\mathbf{3}_{.035^+}$	$\mathbf{2}_{.006}$	$\mathbf{2}_{.006}$	$\mathbf{1}_{.001}$
	16	$\mathbf{2}_{.018}$	$\mathbf{2}_{.018}$	$\mathbf{1}_{.003}$	$\mathbf{1}_{.003}$
	15	$\mathbf{2}_{.038}$	$\mathbf{1}_{.007}$	$\mathbf{1}_{.007}$	$\mathbf{0}_{.001}$
	14	$\mathbf{1}_{.015^-}$	$\mathbf{1}_{.015^-}$	$\mathbf{0}_{.002}$	$\mathbf{0}_{.002}$
	13	$\mathbf{1}_{.028}$	$\mathbf{0}_{.003}$	$\mathbf{0}_{.003}$	$\mathbf{0}_{.003}$
	12	$\mathbf{1}_{.048}$	$\mathbf{0}_{.007}$	$\mathbf{0}_{.007}$	—
	11	$\mathbf{0}_{.013}$	$\mathbf{0}_{.013}$	—	—
	10	$\mathbf{0}_{.022}$	$\mathbf{0}_{.022}$	—	—
	9	$\mathbf{0}_{.037}$	—	—	—
5	18	$\mathbf{3}_{.040}$	$\mathbf{2}_{.006}$	$\mathbf{2}_{.006}$	$\mathbf{1}_{.001}$
	17	$\mathbf{2}_{.021}$	$\mathbf{2}_{.021}$	$\mathbf{1}_{.003}$	$\mathbf{1}_{.003}$
	16	$\mathbf{2}_{.048}$	$\mathbf{1}_{.008}$	$\mathbf{1}_{.008}$	$\mathbf{0}_{.001}$
$A = 18\ B = 5$	15	$\mathbf{1}_{.017}$	$\mathbf{1}_{.017}$	$\mathbf{0}_{.002}$	$\mathbf{0}_{.002}$
	14	$\mathbf{1}_{.033}$	$\mathbf{0}_{.004}$	$\mathbf{0}_{.004}$	$\mathbf{0}_{.004}$
	13	$\mathbf{0}_{.007}$	$\mathbf{0}_{.007}$	$\mathbf{0}_{.007}$	—
	12	$\mathbf{0}_{.014}$	$\mathbf{0}_{.014}$	—	—
	11	$\mathbf{0}_{.024}$	$\mathbf{0}_{.024}$	—	—
	10	$\mathbf{0}_{.038}$	—	—	—
4	18	$\mathbf{2}_{.026}$	$\mathbf{1}_{.003}$	$\mathbf{1}_{.003}$	$\mathbf{1}_{.003}$
	17	$\mathbf{1}_{.010^-}$	$\mathbf{1}_{.010^-}$	$\mathbf{1}_{.010^-}$	$\mathbf{0}_{.001}$
	16	$\mathbf{1}_{.024}$	$\mathbf{1}_{.024}$	$\mathbf{0}_{.002}$	$\mathbf{0}_{.002}$
	15	$\mathbf{1}_{.046}$	$\mathbf{0}_{.005^-}$	$\mathbf{0}_{.005^-}$	$\mathbf{0}_{.005^-}$
	14	$\mathbf{0}_{.010^-}$	$\mathbf{0}_{.010^-}$	$\mathbf{0}_{.010^-}$	—
	13	$\mathbf{0}_{.017}$	$\mathbf{0}_{.017}$	—	—
	12	$\mathbf{0}_{.029}$	—	—	—
	11	$\mathbf{0}_{.045^+}$	—	—	—
3	18	$\mathbf{1}_{.014}$	$\mathbf{1}_{.014}$	$\mathbf{0}_{.001}$	$\mathbf{0}_{.001}$
	17	$\mathbf{1}_{.041}$	$\mathbf{0}_{.003}$	$\mathbf{0}_{.003}$	$\mathbf{0}_{.003}$
	16	$\mathbf{0}_{.008}$	$\mathbf{0}_{.008}$	$\mathbf{0}_{.008}$	—
	15	$\mathbf{0}_{.015^+}$	$\mathbf{0}_{.015^+}$	—	—
	14	$\mathbf{0}_{.026}$	—	—	—
	13	$\mathbf{0}_{.042}$	—	—	—
2	18	$\mathbf{0}_{.005^+}$	$\mathbf{0}_{.005^+}$	$\mathbf{0}_{.005^+}$	—
	17	$\mathbf{0}_{.016}$	$\mathbf{0}_{.016}$	—	—
	16	$\mathbf{0}_{.032}$	—	—	—
$A = 19\ B = 19$	19	$\mathbf{14}_{.023}$	$\mathbf{14}_{.023}$	$\mathbf{13}_{.010^-}$	$\mathbf{12}_{.004}$
	18	$\mathbf{13}_{.045^-}$	$\mathbf{12}_{.021}$	$\mathbf{11}_{.009}$	$\mathbf{10}_{.004}$
	17	$\mathbf{11}_{.031}$	$\mathbf{10}_{.015^-}$	$\mathbf{9}_{.006}$	$\mathbf{8}_{.003}$
	16	$\mathbf{10}_{.039}$	$\mathbf{9}_{.019}$	$\mathbf{8}_{.009}$	$\mathbf{7}_{.003}$
	15	$\mathbf{9}_{.046}$	$\mathbf{8}_{.022}$	$\mathbf{6}_{.004}$	$\mathbf{6}_{.004}$
	14	$\mathbf{8}_{.050^-}$	$\mathbf{7}_{.024}$	$\mathbf{5}_{.004}$	$\mathbf{5}_{.004}$
	13	$\mathbf{6}_{.025^+}$	$\mathbf{5}_{.011}$	$\mathbf{4}_{.004}$	$\mathbf{4}_{.004}$
	12	$\mathbf{5}_{.024}$	$\mathbf{5}_{.024}$	$\mathbf{3}_{.003}$	$\mathbf{3}_{.003}$
	11	$\mathbf{5}_{.050^-}$	$\mathbf{4}_{.022}$	$\mathbf{3}_{.009}$	$\mathbf{2}_{.003}$
	10	$\mathbf{4}_{.046}$	$\mathbf{3}_{.019}$	$\mathbf{2}_{.006}$	$\mathbf{1}_{.002}$
	9	$\mathbf{3}_{.039}$	$\mathbf{2}_{.015^-}$	$\mathbf{1}_{.004}$	$\mathbf{1}_{.004}$
	8	$\mathbf{2}_{.031}$	$\mathbf{1}_{.009}$	$\mathbf{1}_{.009}$	$\mathbf{0}_{.002}$
	7	$\mathbf{1}_{.021}$	$\mathbf{1}_{.021}$	$\mathbf{0}_{.004}$	$\mathbf{0}_{.004}$

TABLE J (*continued*)

		Probability			
	a	**0.05**	**0.025**	**0.01**	**0.005**
	6	$1_{.045}-$	$0_{.010}-$	$0_{.010}-$	—
	5	$0_{.023}$	$0_{.023}$	—	—
18	19	$14_{.046}$	$13_{.020}$	$12_{.008}$	$11_{.003}$
	18	$12_{.037}$	$11_{.017}$	$10_{.007}$	$9_{.003}$
	17	$10_{.024}$	$10_{.024}$	$8_{.004}$	$8_{.004}$
	16	$9_{.030}$	$8_{.014}$	$7_{.006}$	$6_{.002}$
	15	$8_{.033}$	$7_{.015}+$	$6_{.000}$	$5_{.002}$
	14	$7_{.035}+$	$6_{.016}$	$5_{.006}$	$4_{.002}$
	13	$6_{.035}-$	$5_{.015}+$	$4_{.006}$	$3_{.002}$
	12	$5_{.033}$	$4_{.014}$	$3_{.005}-$	$3_{.005}-$
	11	$4_{.030}$	$3_{.011}$	$2_{.004}$	$2_{.004}$
	10	$3_{.025}-$	$3_{.025}-$	$2_{.008}$	$1_{.002}$
	9	$3_{.049}$	$2_{.019}$	$1_{.005}+$	$0_{.001}$
	8	$2_{.038}$	$1_{.012}$	$0_{.002}$	$0_{.002}$
	7	$1_{.025}+$	$0_{.005}-$	$0_{.005}-$	$0_{.005}-$
	6	$0_{.012}$	$0_{.012}$	—	—
	5	$0_{.027}$	—	—	—
17	19	$13_{.040}$	$12_{.016}$	$11_{.006}$	$10_{.002}$
	18	$11_{.030}$	$10_{.013}$	$9_{.005}+$	$8_{.002}$
	17	$10_{.040}$	$9_{.018}$	$8_{.008}$	$7_{.003}$
	16	$9_{.047}$	$8_{.022}$	$7_{.009}$	$6_{.003}$
	15	$8_{.050}-$	$7_{.023}$	$6_{.010}-$	$5_{.004}$
	14	$6_{.023}$	$6_{.023}$	$5_{.010}-$	$4_{.003}$
	13	$6_{.049}$	$5_{.022}$	$4_{.008}$	$3_{.003}$
$A = 19\ B = 17$	12	$5_{.045}-$	$4_{.019}$	$3_{.007}$	$2_{.002}$
	11	$4_{.039}$	$3_{.015}+$	$2_{.005}-$	$2_{.005}-$
	10	$3_{.032}$	$2_{.011}$	$1_{.003}$	$1_{.003}$
	9	$2_{.024}$	$2_{.024}$	$1_{.007}$	$0_{.001}$
	8	$2_{.047}$	$1_{.015}-$	$0_{.002}$	$0_{.002}$
	7	$1_{.031}$	$0_{.006}$	$0_{.006}$	—
	6	$0_{.014}$	$0_{.014}$	—	—
	5	$0_{.031}$	—	—	—
16	19	$12_{.035}-$	$11_{.013}$	$10_{.005}-$	$10_{.005}-$
	18	$10_{.024}$	$10_{.024}$	$9_{.010}-$	$8_{.004}$
	17	$9_{.031}$	$8_{.013}$	$7_{.005}+$	$6_{.002}$
	16	$8_{.035}-$	$7_{.015}+$	$6_{.006}$	$5_{.002}$
	15	$7_{.036}$	$6_{.015}+$	$5_{.006}$	$4_{.002}$
	14	$6_{.034}$	$5_{.014}$	$4_{.005}+$	$3_{.002}$
	13	$5_{.031}$	$4_{.013}$	$3_{.004}$	$3_{.004}$
	12	$4_{.027}$	$3_{.010}-$	$3_{.010}-$	$2_{.003}$
	11	$3_{.021}$	$3_{.021}$	$2_{.007}$	$1_{.002}$
	10	$3_{.042}$	$2_{.015}-$	$1_{.004}$	$1_{.004}$
	9	$2_{.030}$	$1_{.009}$	$1_{.009}$	$0_{.001}$
	8	$1_{.018}$	$1_{.018}$	$0_{.003}$	$0_{.003}$
	7	$1_{.037}$	$0_{.007}$	$0_{.007}$	—
	6	$0_{.017}$	$0_{.017}$	—	—
	5	$0_{.036}$	—	—	—
15	19	$11_{.029}$	$10_{.011}$	$9_{.004}$	$9_{.004}$
	18	$10_{.046}$	$9_{.019}$	$8_{.007}$	$7_{.002}$
	17	$8_{.023}$	$8_{.023}$	$7_{.009}$	$6_{.003}$

TABLE J (*continued*)

	a	Probability			
		0.05	0.025	0.01	0.005
	16	$7_{.025}{}^{-}$	$7_{.025}{}^{-}$	$6_{.010}{}^{-}$	$5_{.003}$
	15	$6_{.024}$	$6_{.024}$	$5_{.009}$	$4_{.003}$
	14	$5_{.022}$	$5_{.022}$	$4_{.008}$	$3_{.002}$
	13	$5_{.045}{}^{+}$	$4_{.018}$	$3_{.006}$	$2_{.002}$
	12	$4_{.037}$	$3_{.014}$	$2_{.004}$	$2_{.004}$
	11	$3_{.029}$	$2_{.009}$	$2_{.009}$	$1_{.002}$
	10	$2_{.020}$	$2_{.020}$	$1_{.005}{}^{+}$	$0_{.001}$
	9	$2_{.039}$	$1_{.011}$	$0_{.002}$	$0_{.002}$
	8	$1_{.023}$	$1_{.023}$	$0_{.004}$	$0_{.004}$
	7	$1_{.046}$	$0_{.009}$	$0_{.009}$	—
	6	$0_{.020}$	$0_{.020}$	—	—
	5	$0_{.042}$	—	—	—
14	19	$10_{.024}$	$10_{.024}$	$9_{.008}$	$8_{.003}$
	18	$9_{.037}$	$8_{.014}$	$7_{.005}{}^{-}$	$7_{.005}{}^{-}$
	17	$8_{.042}$	$7_{.017}$	$6_{.006}$	$5_{.002}$
	16	$7_{.042}$	$6_{.017}$	$5_{.006}$	$4_{.002}$
	15	$6_{.039}$	$5_{.015}{}^{+}$	$4_{.005}{}^{+}$	$3_{.001}$
	14	$5_{.034}$	$4_{.013}$	$3_{.004}$	$3_{.004}$
	13	$4_{.027}$	$3_{.009}$	$3_{.009}$	$2_{.003}$
	12	$3_{.020}$	$3_{.020}$	$2_{.006}$	$1_{.001}$
	11	$3_{.040}$	$2_{.013}$	$1_{.003}$	$1_{.003}$
	10	$2_{.027}$	$1_{.007}$	$1_{.007}$	$0_{.001}$
	9	$1_{.015}{}^{-}$	$1_{.015}{}^{-}$	$0_{.002}$	$0_{.002}$
	8	$1_{.030}$	$0_{.005}{}^{+}$	$0_{.005}{}^{+}$	—
	7	$0_{.012}$	$0_{.012}$	—	—
	6	$0_{.024}$	$0_{.024}$	—	—
	5	$0_{.049}$	—	—	—
13	19	$9_{.020}$	$9_{.020}$	$8_{.006}$	$7_{.002}$
	18	$8_{.029}$	$7_{.010}{}^{+}$	$6_{.003}$	$6_{.003}$
	17	$7_{.031}$	$6_{.011}$	$5_{.004}$	$5_{.004}$
	16	$6_{.029}$	$5_{.011}$	$4_{.003}$	$4_{.003}$
	15	$5_{.025}{}^{+}$	$4_{.009}$	$4_{.009}$	$3_{.003}$
	14	$4_{.020}$	$4_{.020}$	$3_{.006}$	$2_{.002}$
	13	$4_{.041}$	$3_{.015}{}^{-}$	$2_{.004}$	$2_{.004}$
$A = 19\ B = 13$	12	$3_{.029}$	$2_{.009}$	$2_{.009}$	$1_{.002}$
	11	$2_{.019}$	$2_{.019}$	$1_{.005}{}^{-}$	$1_{.005}{}^{-}$
	10	$2_{.036}$	$1_{.010}{}^{-}$	$1_{.010}{}^{-}$	$0_{.001}$
	9	$1_{.020}$	$1_{.020}$	$0_{.003}$	$0_{.003}$
	8	$1_{.038}$	$0_{.007}$	$0_{.007}$	—
	7	$0_{.015}{}^{-}$	$0_{.015}{}^{-}$	—	—
	6	$0_{.030}$	—	—	—
12	19	$9_{.049}$	$8_{.016}$	$7_{.005}{}^{-}$	$7_{.005}{}^{-}$
	18	$7_{.022}$	$7_{.022}$	$6_{.007}$	$5_{.002}$
	17	$6_{.022}$	$6_{.022}$	$5_{.007}$	$4_{.002}$
	16	$5_{.019}$	$5_{.019}$	$4_{.006}$	$3_{.002}$
	15	$5_{.042}$	$4_{.015}{}^{+}$	$3_{.004}$	$3_{.004}$
	14	$4_{.032}$	$3_{.011}$	$2_{.003}$	$2_{.003}$
	13	$3_{.023}$	$3_{.023}$	$2_{.006}$	$1_{.001}$
	12	$3_{.043}$	$2_{.014}$	$1_{.003}$	$1_{.003}$
	11	$2_{.027}$	$1_{.007}$	$1_{.007}$	$0_{.001}$
	10	$2_{.050}{}^{-}$	$1_{.014}$	$0_{.002}$	$0_{.002}$

TABLE J (*continued*)

	a	0.05	0.025	0.01	0.005
			Probability		
	9	$1_{.027}$	$0_{.005}-$	$0_{.005}-$	$0_{.005}-$
	8	$1_{.050}-$	$0_{.010}-$	$0_{.010}-$	—
	7	$0_{.019}$	$0_{.019}$	—	—
	6	$0_{.037}$	—	—	—
11	19	$8_{.041}$	$7_{.012}$	$6_{.003}$	$6_{.003}$
	18	$7_{.047}$	$6_{.016}$	$5_{.004}$	$5_{.004}$
	17	$6_{.043}$	$5_{.015}-$	$4_{.004}$	$4_{.004}$
	16	$5_{.035}+$	$4_{.012}$	$3_{.003}$	$3_{.003}$
	15	$4_{.027}$	$3_{.008}$	$3_{.008}$	$2_{.002}$
	14	$3_{.018}$	$3_{.018}$	$2_{.005}-$	$2_{.005}-$
	13	$3_{.035}+$	$2_{.010}+$	$1_{.002}$	$1_{.002}$
	12	$2_{.021}$	$2_{.021}$	$1_{.005}-$	$1_{.005}-$
	11	$2_{.040}$	$1_{.010}+$	$0_{.001}$	$0_{.001}$
	10	$1_{.020}$	$1_{.020}$	$0_{.003}$	$0_{.003}$
	9	$1_{.037}$	$0_{.006}$	$0_{.006}$	—
	8	$0_{.013}$	$0_{.013}$	—	—
	7	$0_{.025}-$	$0_{.025}-$	—	—
	6	$0_{.046}$	—	—	—
10	19	$7_{.033}$	$6_{.009}$	$6_{.009}$	$5_{.002}$
	18	$6_{.036}$	$5_{.011}$	$4_{.003}$	$4_{.003}$
	17	$5_{.030}$	$4_{.009}$	$4_{.009}$	$3_{.002}$
	16	$4_{.022}$	$4_{.022}$	$3_{.006}$	$2_{.001}$
	15	$4_{.047}$	$3_{.015}-$	$2_{.004}$	$2_{.004}$
	14	$3_{.030}$	$2_{.008}$	$2_{.008}$	$1_{.002}$
	13	$2_{.017}$	$2_{.017}$	$1_{.004}$	$1_{.004}$
	12	$2_{.033}$	$1_{.008}$	$1_{.008}$	$0_{.001}$
	11	$1_{.016}$	$1_{.016}$	$0_{.002}$	$0_{.002}$
	10	$1_{.029}$	$0_{.005}-$	$0_{.005}-$	$0_{.005}-$
	9	$0_{.009}$	$0_{.009}$	$0_{.009}$	—
	8	$0_{.018}$	$0_{.018}$	—	—
	7	$0_{.032}$	—	—	—
9	19	$6_{.026}$	$5_{.006}$	$5_{.006}$	$4_{.001}$
	18	$5_{.026}$	$4_{.007}$	$4_{.007}$	$3_{.001}$
	17	$4_{.020}$	$4_{.020}$	$3_{.005}-$	$3_{.005}-$
	16	$4_{.044}$	$3_{.013}$	$2_{.003}$	$2_{.003}$
	15	$3_{.028}$	$2_{.007}$	$2_{.007}$	$1_{.001}$
	14	$2_{.015}-$	$2_{.015}-$	$1_{.003}$	$1_{.003}$
	13	$2_{.029}$	$1_{.006}$	$1_{.006}$	$0_{.001}$
	12	$1_{.013}$	$1_{.013}$	$0_{.002}$	$0_{.002}$
	11	$1_{.024}$	$1_{.024}$	$0_{.004}$	$0_{.004}$
	10	$1_{.042}$	$0_{.007}$	$0_{.007}$	—
	9	$0_{.013}$	$0_{.013}$	—	—
	8	$0_{.024}$	$0_{.024}$	—	—
	7	$0_{.043}$	—	—	—
$A = 19\ B = 8$	19	$5_{.019}$	$5_{.019}$	$4_{.004}$	$4_{.004}$
	18	$4_{.017}$	$4_{.017}$	$3_{.004}$	$3_{.004}$
	17	$4_{.044}$	$3_{.011}$	$2_{.002}$	$2_{.002}$
	16	$3_{.027}$	$2_{.006}$	$2_{.006}$	$1_{.001}$
	15	$2_{.013}$	$2_{.013}$	$1_{.002}$	$1_{.002}$
	14	$2_{.027}$	$1_{.006}$	$1_{.006}$	$0_{.001}$
	13	$2_{.049}$	$1_{.011}$	$0_{.001}$	$0_{.001}$

TABLE J (*continued*)

	a	0.05	0.025	0.01	0.005
			Probability		
	12	$\mathbf{1}_{.021}$	$\mathbf{1}_{.021}$	$\mathbf{0}_{.003}$	$\mathbf{0}_{.003}$
	11	$\mathbf{1}_{.038}$	$\mathbf{0}_{.006}$	$\mathbf{0}_{.006}$	—
	10	$\mathbf{0}_{.011}$	$\mathbf{0}_{.011}$	—	—
	9	$\mathbf{0}_{.020}$	$\mathbf{0}_{.020}$	—	—
	8	$\mathbf{0}_{.034}$	—	—	—
7	19	$\mathbf{4}_{.013}$	$\mathbf{4}_{.013}$	$\mathbf{3}_{.002}$	$\mathbf{3}_{.002}$
	18	$\mathbf{4}_{.047}$	$\mathbf{3}_{.010^+}$	$\mathbf{2}_{.002}$	$\mathbf{2}_{.002}$
	17	$\mathbf{3}_{.028}$	$\mathbf{2}_{.006}$	$\mathbf{2}_{.006}$	$\mathbf{1}_{.001}$
	16	$\mathbf{2}_{.014}$	$\mathbf{2}_{.014}$	$\mathbf{1}_{.002}$	$\mathbf{1}_{.002}$
	15	$\mathbf{2}_{.028}$	$\mathbf{1}_{.005^+}$	$\mathbf{1}_{.005^+}$	$\mathbf{0}_{.001}$
	14	$\mathbf{1}_{.011}$	$\mathbf{1}_{.011}$	$\mathbf{0}_{.001}$	$\mathbf{0}_{.001}$
	13	$\mathbf{1}_{.021}$	$\mathbf{1}_{.021}$	$\mathbf{0}_{.003}$	$\mathbf{0}_{.003}$
	12	$\mathbf{1}_{.037}$	$\mathbf{0}_{.005^+}$	$\mathbf{0}_{.005^+}$	—
	11	$\mathbf{0}_{.010^-}$	$\mathbf{0}_{.010^-}$	$\mathbf{0}_{.010^-}$	—
	10	$\mathbf{0}_{.017}$	$\mathbf{0}_{.017}$	—	—
	9	$\mathbf{0}_{.030}$	—	—	—
	8	$\mathbf{0}_{.048}$	—	—	—
6	19	$\mathbf{4}_{.050^-}$	$\mathbf{3}_{.009}$	$\mathbf{3}_{.009}$	$\mathbf{2}_{.001}$
	18	$\mathbf{3}_{.031}$	$\mathbf{2}_{.005^+}$	$\mathbf{2}_{.005^+}$	$\mathbf{1}_{.001}$
	17	$\mathbf{2}_{.015^+}$	$\mathbf{2}_{.015^+}$	$\mathbf{1}_{.002}$	$\mathbf{1}_{.002}$
	16	$\mathbf{2}_{.032}$	$\mathbf{1}_{.006}$	$\mathbf{1}_{.006}$	$\mathbf{0}_{.000}$
	15	$\mathbf{1}_{.012}$	$\mathbf{1}_{.012}$	$\mathbf{0}_{.001}$	$\mathbf{0}_{.001}$
	14	$\mathbf{1}_{.023}$	$\mathbf{1}_{.023}$	$\mathbf{0}_{.003}$	$\mathbf{0}_{.003}$
	13	$\mathbf{1}_{.039}$	$\mathbf{0}_{.005^+}$	$\mathbf{0}_{.005^+}$	—
	12	$\mathbf{0}_{.010^-}$	$\mathbf{0}_{.010^-}$	$\mathbf{0}_{.010^-}$	—
	11	$\mathbf{0}_{.017}$	$\mathbf{0}_{.017}$	—	—
	10	$\mathbf{0}_{.028}$	—	—	—
	9	$\mathbf{0}_{.045^+}$	—	—	—
5	19	$\mathbf{3}_{.036}$	$\mathbf{2}_{.005^-}$	$\mathbf{2}_{.005^-}$	$\mathbf{2}_{.005^-}$
	18	$\mathbf{2}_{.018}$	$\mathbf{2}_{.018}$	$\mathbf{1}_{.002}$	$\mathbf{1}_{.002}$
	17	$\mathbf{2}_{.042}$	$\mathbf{1}_{.006}$	$\mathbf{1}_{.006}$	$\mathbf{0}_{.000}$
	16	$\mathbf{1}_{.014}$	$\mathbf{1}_{.014}$	$\mathbf{0}_{.001}$	$\mathbf{0}_{.001}$
	15	$\mathbf{1}_{.028}$	$\mathbf{0}_{.003}$	$\mathbf{0}_{.003}$	$\mathbf{0}_{.003}$
	14	$\mathbf{1}_{.047}$	$\mathbf{0}_{.006}$	$\mathbf{0}_{.006}$	—
	13	$\mathbf{0}_{.011}$	$\mathbf{0}_{.011}$	—	—
	12	$\mathbf{0}_{.019}$	$\mathbf{0}_{.019}$	—	—
	11	$\mathbf{0}_{.030}$	—	—	—
	10	$\mathbf{0}_{.047}$	—	—	—
4	19	$\mathbf{2}_{.024}$	$\mathbf{2}_{.024}$	$\mathbf{1}_{.002}$	$\mathbf{1}_{.002}$
	18	$\mathbf{1}_{.009}$	$\mathbf{1}_{.009}$	$\mathbf{1}_{.009}$	$\mathbf{0}_{.001}$
	17	$\mathbf{1}_{.021}$	$\mathbf{1}_{.021}$	$\mathbf{0}_{.002}$	$\mathbf{0}_{.002}$
	16	$\mathbf{1}_{.040}$	$\mathbf{0}_{.004}$	$\mathbf{0}_{.004}$	$\mathbf{0}_{.004}$
	15	$\mathbf{0}_{.008}$	$\mathbf{0}_{.008}$	$\mathbf{0}_{.008}$	—
	14	$\mathbf{0}_{.014}$	$\mathbf{0}_{.014}$	—	—
	13	$\mathbf{0}_{.024}$	$\mathbf{0}_{.024}$	—	—
	12	$\mathbf{0}_{.037}$	—	—	—
3	19	$\mathbf{1}_{.013}$	$\mathbf{1}_{.013}$	$\mathbf{0}_{.001}$	$\mathbf{0}_{.001}$
	18	$\mathbf{1}_{.038}$	$\mathbf{0}_{.003}$	$\mathbf{0}_{.003}$	$\mathbf{0}_{.003}$
	17	$\mathbf{0}_{.006}$	$\mathbf{0}_{.006}$	$\mathbf{0}_{.006}$	—
	16	$\mathbf{0}_{.013}$	$\mathbf{0}_{.013}$	—	—
	15	$\mathbf{0}_{.023}$	$\mathbf{0}_{.023}$	—	—

TABLE J (*continued*)

	a	0.05	0.025	0.01	0.005
2	14	$0_{.036}$	—	—	—
	19	$0_{.005^-}$	$0_{.005^-}$	$0_{.005^-}$	$0_{.005^-}$
$A = 19\ B = 2$	18	$0_{.014}$	$0_{.014}$	—	—
	17	$0_{.029}$	—	—	—
$A = 20\ B = 20$	16	$0_{.048}$	—	—	—
	20	$15_{.024}$	$15_{.024}$	$13_{.004}$	$13_{.004}$
	19	$14_{.046}$	$13_{.022}$	$12_{.010^-}$	$11_{.004}$
	18	$12_{.032}$	$11_{.015^+}$	$10_{.007}$	$9_{.003}$
	17	$11_{.041}$	$10_{.020}$	$9_{.009}$	$8_{.004}$
	16	$10_{.048}$	$9_{.024}$	$7_{.005^-}$	$7_{.005^-}$
	15	$8_{.027}$	$7_{.012}$	$6_{.005^+}$	$5_{.002}$
	14	$7_{.028}$	$6_{.013}$	$5_{.005^+}$	$4_{.002}$
	13	$6_{.028}$	$5_{.012}$	$4_{.005^-}$	$4_{.005^-}$
	12	$5_{.027}$	$4_{.011}$	$3_{.004}$	$3_{.004}$
	11	$4_{.024}$	$4_{.024}$	$3_{.009}$	$2_{.003}$
	10	$4_{.048}$	$3_{.020}$	$2_{.007}$	$1_{.002}$
	9	$3_{.041}$	$2_{.015^+}$	$1_{.004}$	$1_{.004}$
	8	$2_{.032}$	$1_{.010^-}$	$1_{.010^-}$	$0_{.002}$
	7	$1_{.022}$	$1_{.022}$	$0_{.004}$	$0_{.004}$
	6	$1_{.046}$	$0_{.010^+}$	—	—
	5	$0_{.024}$	$0_{.024}$	—	—
19	20	$15_{.047}$	$14_{.020}$	$13_{.008}$	$12_{.003}$
	19	$13_{.039}$	$12_{.018}$	$11_{.008}$	$10_{.003}$
	18	$11_{.026}$	$10_{.012}$	$9_{.005^-}$	$9_{.005^-}$
	17	$10_{.032}$	$9_{.015^-}$	$8_{.006}$	$7_{.002}$
	16	$9_{.036}$	$8_{.017}$	$7_{.007}$	$6_{.003}$
	15	$8_{.038}$	$7_{.018}$	$6_{.008}$	$5_{.003}$
	14	$7_{.039}$	$6_{.018}$	$5_{.007}$	$4_{.003}$
	13	$6_{.038}$	$5_{.017}$	$4_{.007}$	$3_{.002}$
	12	$5_{.035^+}$	$4_{.015^+}$	$3_{.005^+}$	$2_{.002}$
	11	$4_{.031}$	$3_{.012}$	$2_{.004}$	$2_{.004}$
	10	$3_{.026}$	$2_{.009}$	$2_{.009}$	$1_{.002}$
	9	$2_{.019}$	$2_{.019}$	$1_{.005^+}$	$0_{.001}$
	8	$2_{.039}$	$1_{.012}$	$0_{.002}$	$0_{.002}$
	7	$1_{.026}$	$0_{.005^+}$	$0_{.005^+}$	—
	6	$0_{.012}$	$0_{.012}$	—	—
	5	$0_{.027}$	—	—	—
18	20	$14_{.041}$	$13_{.017}$	$12_{.007}$	$11_{.003}$
	19	$12_{.032}$	$11_{.014}$	$10_{.006}$	$9_{.002}$
	18	$11_{.043}$	$10_{.020}$	$9_{.008}$	$8_{.003}$
	17	$10_{.050^-}$	$9_{.024}$	$7_{.004}$	$7_{.004}$
	16	$8_{.026}$	$7_{.011}$	$6_{.005^-}$	$6_{.005^-}$
	15	$7_{.027}$	$6_{.012}$	$5_{.004}$	$5_{.004}$
	14	$6_{.026}$	$5_{.011}$	$4_{.004}$	$4_{.004}$
	13	$5_{.024}$	$5_{.024}$	$4_{.009}$	$3_{.003}$
	12	$5_{.047}$	$4_{.020}$	$3_{.007}$	$2_{.002}$
	11	$4_{.041}$	$3_{.016}$	$2_{.005^+}$	$1_{.001}$
	10	$3_{.033}$	$2_{.012}$	$1_{.003}$	$1_{.003}$
	9	$2_{.024}$	$2_{.024}$	$1_{.007}$	$0_{.001}$
	8	$2_{.048}$	$1_{.015^-}$	$0_{.003}$	$0_{.003}$
	7	$1_{.031}$	$0_{.006}$	$0_{.006}$	—

TABLE J (*continued*)

	a	Probability 0.05	0.025	0.01	0.005
	6	$0_{.014}$	$0_{.014}$	—	—
	5	$0_{.031}$	—	—	—
17	20	$13_{.036}$	$12_{.014}$	$11_{.005}{}^{+}$	$10_{.002}$
	19	$11_{.026}$	$10_{.011}$	$9_{.004}$	$9_{.004}$
	18	$10_{.034}$	$9_{.015}{}^{-}$	$8_{.006}$	$7_{.002}$
	17	$9_{.038}$	$8_{.017}$	$7_{.007}$	$6_{.003}$
	16	$8_{.040}$	$7_{.018}$	$6_{.007}$	$5_{.003}$
	15	$7_{.039}$	$6_{.017}$	$5_{.007}$	$4_{.002}$
	14	$6_{.037}$	$5_{.016}$	$4_{.006}$	$3_{.002}$
	13	$5_{.033}$	$4_{.013}$	$3_{.005}{}^{-}$	$3_{.005}{}^{-}$
	12	$4_{.028}$	$3_{.010}{}^{+}$	$2_{.003}$	$2_{.003}$
	11	$3_{.022}$	$3_{.022}$	$2_{.007}$	$1_{.002}$
$A = 20\ B = 17$	10	$3_{.042}$	$2_{.015}{}^{+}$	$1_{.004}$	$1_{.004}$
	9	$2_{.031}$	$1_{.009}$	$1_{.009}$	$0_{.001}$
	8	$1_{.019}$	$1_{.019}$	$0_{.003}$	$0_{.003}$
	7	$1_{.037}$	$0_{.008}$	$0_{.008}$	—
	6	$0_{.017}$	$0_{.017}$	—	—
	5	$0_{.036}$	—	—	—
16	20	$12_{.031}$	$11_{.012}$	$10_{.004}$	$10_{.004}$
	19	$11_{.049}$	$10_{.021}$	$9_{.008}$	$8_{.003}$
	18	$9_{.026}$	$8_{.011}$	$7_{.004}$	$7_{.004}$
	17	$8_{.028}$	$7_{.012}$	$6_{.004}$	$6_{.004}$
	16	$7_{.028}$	$6_{.012}$	$5_{.004}$	$5_{.004}$
	15	$6_{.026}$	$5_{.011}$	$4_{.004}$	$4_{.004}$
	14	$5_{.023}$	$5_{.023}$	$4_{.009}$	$3_{.003}$
	13	$5_{.046}$	$4_{.019}$	$3_{.007}$	$2_{.002}$
	12	$4_{.038}$	$3_{.014}$	$2_{.004}$	$2_{.004}$
	11	$3_{.029}$	$2_{.010}{}^{-}$	$2_{.010}{}^{-}$	$1_{.002}$
	10	$2_{.020}$	$2_{.020}$	$1_{.005}{}^{+}$	$0_{.001}$
	9	$2_{.039}$	$1_{.011}$	$0_{.002}$	$0_{.002}$
	8	$1_{.023}$	$1_{.023}$	$0_{.004}$	$0_{.004}$
	7	$1_{.045}{}^{+}$	$0_{.009}$	$0_{.009}$	—
	6	$0_{.020}$	$0_{.020}$	—	—
	5	$0_{.041}$	—	—	—
15	20	$11_{.026}$	$10_{.009}$	$10_{.009}$	$9_{.003}$
	19	$10_{.040}$	$9_{.016}$	$8_{.006}$	$7_{.002}$
	18	$9_{.046}$	$8_{.019}$	$7_{.007}$	$6_{.002}$
	17	$8_{.047}$	$7_{.020}$	$6_{.008}$	$5_{.002}$
	16	$7_{.045}{}^{-}$	$6_{.019}$	$5_{.007}$	$4_{.002}$
	15	$6_{.040}$	$5_{.017}$	$4_{.006}$	$3_{.002}$
	14	$5_{.034}$	$4_{.013}$	$3_{.004}$	$3_{.004}$
	13	$4_{.028}$	$3_{.010}{}^{-}$	$3_{.010}{}^{-}$	$2_{.003}$
	12	$3_{.020}$	$3_{.020}$	$2_{.006}$	$1_{.001}$
	11	$3_{.039}$	$2_{.013}$	$1_{.003}$	$1_{.003}$
	10	$2_{.026}$	$1_{.007}$	$1_{.007}$	$0_{.001}$
	9	$2_{.049}$	$1_{.015}{}^{-}$	$0_{.002}$	$0_{.002}$
	8	$1_{.029}$	$0_{.005}{}^{+}$	$0_{.005}{}^{+}$	—
	7	$0_{.012}$	$0_{.012}$	—	—
	6	$0_{.024}$	$0_{.024}$	—	—
	5	$0_{.048}$	—	—	—
14	20	$10_{.022}$	$10_{.022}$	$9_{.007}$	$8_{.002}$

TABLE J (*continued*)

	a	Probability 0.05	0.025	0.01	0.005
	19	$9_{.032}$	$8_{.012}$	$7_{.004}$	$7_{.004}$
	18	$8_{.035^+}$	$7_{.014}$	$6_{.005^-}$	$6_{.005^-}$
	17	$7_{.035^-}$	$6_{.013}$	$5_{.005^-}$	$5_{.005^-}$
	16	$6_{.031}$	$5_{.012}$	$4_{.004}$	$4_{.004}$
	15	$5_{.026}$	$4_{.009}$	$4_{.009}$	$3_{.003}$
	14	$4_{.020}$	$4_{.020}$	$3_{.007}$	$2_{.002}$
	13	$4_{.040}$	$3_{.015^-}$	$2_{.004}$	$2_{.004}$
	12	$3_{.029}$	$2_{.009}$	$2_{.009}$	$1_{.002}$
	11	$2_{.018}$	$2_{.018}$	$1_{.005^-}$	$1_{.005^-}$
	10	$2_{.035^+}$	$1_{.010^-}$	$1_{.010^-}$	$0_{.001}$
	9	$1_{.019}$	$1_{.019}$	$0_{.003}$	$0_{.003}$
	8	$1_{.037}$	$0_{.007}$	$0_{.007}$	—
	7	$0_{.014}$	$0_{.014}$	—	—
	6	$0_{.029}$	—	—	—
13	20	$9_{.017}$	$9_{.017}$	$8_{.005^+}$	$7_{.002}$
	19	$8_{.025^-}$	$8_{.025^-}$	$7_{.008}$	$6_{.003}$
	18	$7_{.026}$	$6_{.009}$	$6_{.009}$	$5_{.003}$
	17	$6_{.024}$	$6_{.024}$	$5_{.008}$	$4_{.002}$
	16	$5_{.020}$	$5_{.020}$	$4_{.007}$	$3_{.002}$
	15	$5_{.041}$	$4_{.015^+}$	$3_{.005^-}$	$3_{.005^-}$
	14	$4_{.031}$	$3_{.011}$	$2_{.003}$	$2_{.003}$
$A = 20\ B = 13$	13	$3_{.022}$	$3_{.022}$	$2_{.006}$	$1_{.001}$
	12	$3_{.041}$	$2_{.013}$	$1_{.003}$	$1_{.003}$
	11	$2_{.026}$	$1_{.007}$	$1_{.007}$	$0_{.001}$
	10	$2_{.047}$	$1_{.013}$	$0_{.002}$	$0_{.002}$
	9	$1_{.026}$	$0_{.004}$	$0_{.004}$	$0_{.004}$
	8	$1_{.047}$	$0_{.009}$	$0_{.009}$	—
	7	$0_{.018}$	$0_{.018}$	—	—
	6	$0_{.035^-}$	—	—	—
12	20	$9_{.044}$	$8_{.014}$	$7_{.004}$	$7_{.004}$
	19	$7_{.019}$	$7_{.019}$	$6_{.006}$	$5_{.002}$
	18	$6_{.018}$	$6_{.018}$	$5_{.006}$	$4_{.002}$
	17	$6_{.043}$	$5_{.016}$	$4_{.005^-}$	$4_{.005^-}$
	16	$5_{.034}$	$4_{.012}$	$3_{.003}$	$3_{.003}$
	15	$4_{.025^+}$	$3_{.008}$	$3_{.008}$	$2_{.002}$
	14	$4_{.049}$	$3_{.017}$	$2_{.005^-}$	$2_{.005^-}$
	13	$3_{.033}$	$2_{.010^-}$	$2_{.010^-}$	$1_{.002}$
	12	$2_{.020}$	$2_{.020}$	$1_{.005^-}$	$1_{.005^-}$
	11	$2_{.036}$	$1_{.009}$	$1_{.009}$	$0_{.001}$
	10	$1_{.018}$	$1_{.018}$	$0_{.003}$	$0_{.003}$
	9	$1_{.034}$	$0_{.006}$	$0_{.006}$	—
	8	$0_{.012}$	$0_{.012}$	—	—
	7	$0_{.023}$	$0_{.023}$	—	—
	6	$0_{.043}$	—	—	—
11	20	$8_{.037}$	$7_{.010^+}$	$6_{.003}$	$6_{.003}$
	19	$7_{.042}$	$6_{.013}$	$5_{.004}$	$5_{.004}$
	18	$6_{.037}$	$5_{.012}$	$4_{.003}$	$4_{.003}$
	17	$5_{.029}$	$4_{.009}$	$4_{.009}$	$3_{.002}$
	16	$4_{.021}$	$4_{.021}$	$3_{.006}$	$2_{.001}$
	15	$4_{.042}$	$3_{.014}$	$2_{.003}$	$2_{.003}$
	14	$3_{.028}$	$2_{.008}$	$2_{.008}$	$1_{.001}$

TABLE J (*continued*)

	a	0.05	0.025	0.01	0.005
				Probability	
	13	$2_{.016}$	$2_{.016}$	$1_{.003}$	$1_{.003}$
	12	$2_{.029}$	$1_{.007}$	$1_{.007}$	$0_{.001}$
	11	$1_{.014}$	$1_{.014}$	$0_{.002}$	$0_{.002}$
	10	$1_{.026}$	$0_{.004}$	$0_{.004}$	$0_{.004}$
	9	$1_{.046}$	$0_{.008}$	$0_{.008}$	—
	8	$0_{.016}$	$0_{.016}$	—	—
	7	$0_{.029}$	—	—	—
10	20	$7_{.030}$	$6_{.008}$	$6_{.008}$	$5_{.002}$
	19	$6_{.031}$	$5_{.009}$	$5_{.009}$	$4_{.002}$
	18	$5_{.026}$	$4_{.007}$	$4_{.007}$	$3_{.002}$
	17	$4_{.018}$	$4_{.018}$	$3_{.005^-}$	$3_{.005^-}$
	16	$4_{.039}$	$3_{.012}$	$2_{.003}$	$2_{.003}$
	15	$3_{.024}$	$3_{.024}$	$2_{.006}$	$1_{.001}$
	14	$3_{.045^+}$	$2_{.013}$	$1_{.003}$	$1_{.003}$
	13	$2_{.025^+}$	$1_{.006}$	$1_{.006}$	$0_{.001}$
	12	$2_{.045^-}$	$1_{.011}$	$0_{.001}$	$0_{.001}$
	11	$1_{.021}$	$1_{.021}$	$0_{.003}$	$0_{.003}$
	10	$1_{.037}$	$0_{.006}$	$0_{.006}$	—
	9	$0_{.012}$	$0_{.012}$	—	—
	8	$0_{.022}$	$0_{.022}$	—	—
	7	$0_{.038}$	—	—	—
9	20	$6_{.023}$	$6_{.023}$	$5_{.005^+}$	$4_{.001}$
	19	$5_{.022}$	$5_{.022}$	$4_{.005^+}$	$3_{.001}$
	18	$4_{.016}$	$4_{.016}$	$3_{.004}$	$3_{.004}$
	17	$4_{.037}$	$3_{.010^+}$	$2_{.002}$	$2_{.002}$
	16	$3_{.022}$	$3_{.022}$	$2_{.005^+}$	$1_{.001}$
	15	$3_{.043}$	$2_{.012}$	$1_{.002}$	$1_{.002}$
	14	$2_{.023}$	$2_{.023}$	$1_{.005^-}$	$1_{.005^-}$
	13	$2_{.041}$	$1_{.009}$	$1_{.009}$	$0_{.001}$
	12	$1_{.018}$	$1_{.018}$	$0_{.002}$	$0_{.002}$
	11	$1_{.032}$	$0_{.005^-}$	$0_{.005^-}$	$0_{.005^-}$
$A = 20\ B = 9$	10	$0_{.009}$	$0_{.009}$	$0_{.009}$	—
	9	$0_{.017}$	$0_{.017}$	—	—
	8	$0_{.029}$	—	—	—
	7	$0_{.050^-}$	—	—	—
8	20	$5_{.017}$	$5_{.017}$	$4_{.003}$	$4_{.003}$
	19	$4_{.015^-}$	$4_{.015^-}$	$3_{.003}$	$3_{.003}$
	18	$4_{.038}$	$3_{.009}$	$3_{.009}$	$2_{.002}$
	17	$3_{.022}$	$3_{.022}$	$2_{.005^-}$	$2_{.005^-}$
	16	$3_{.044}$	$2_{.011}$	$1_{.002}$	$1_{.002}$
	15	$2_{.022}$	$2_{.022}$	$1_{.004}$	$1_{.004}$
	14	$2_{.040}$	$1_{.009}$	$1_{.009}$	$0_{.001}$
	13	$1_{.016}$	$1_{.016}$	$0_{.002}$	$0_{.002}$
	12	$1_{.029}$	$0_{.004}$	$0_{.004}$	$0_{.004}$
	11	$1_{.048}$	$0_{.008}$	$0_{.008}$	—
	10	$0_{.014}$	$0_{.014}$	—	—
	9	$0_{.024}$	$0_{.024}$	—	—
	8	$0_{.041}$	—	—	—
7	20	$4_{.012}$	$4_{.012}$	$3_{.002}$	$3_{.002}$
	19	$4_{.042}$	$3_{.009}$	$3_{.009}$	$2_{.001}$
	18	$3_{.024}$	$3_{.024}$	$2_{.005^-}$	$2_{.005^-}$

TABLE J (*continued*)

	a	Probability 0.05	0.025	0.01	0.005
	17	$3_{.050^-}$	$2_{.011}$	$1_{.002}$	$1_{.002}$
	16	$2_{.023}$	$2_{.023}$	$1_{.004}$	$1_{.004}$
	15	$2_{.043}$	$1_{.009}$	$1_{.009}$	$0_{.001}$
	14	$1_{.016}$	$1_{.016}$	$0_{.002}$	$0_{.002}$
	13	$1_{.029}$	$0_{.004}$	$0_{.004}$	$0_{.004}$
	12	$1_{.048}$	$0_{.007}$	$0_{.007}$	—
	11	$0_{.013}$	$0_{.013}$	—	—
	10	$0_{.022}$	$0_{.022}$	—	—
	9	$0_{.036}$	—		
6	20	$4_{.046}$	$3_{.008}$	$3_{.008}$	$2_{.001}$
	19	$3_{.028}$	$2_{.005^-}$	$2_{.005^-}$	$2_{.005^-}$
	18	$2_{.013}$	$2_{.013}$	$1_{.002}$	$1_{.002}$
	17	$2_{.028}$	$1_{.004}$	$1_{.004}$	$1_{.004}$
	16	$1_{.010^-}$	$1_{.010^-}$	$1_{.010^-}$	$0_{.001}$
	15	$1_{.018}$	$1_{.018}$	$0_{.002}$	$0_{.002}$
	14	$1_{.032}$	$0_{.004}$	$0_{.004}$	$0_{.004}$
	13	$0_{.007}$	$0_{.007}$	$0_{.007}$	—
	12	$0_{.013}$	$0_{.013}$	—	—
	11	$0_{.022}$	$0_{.022}$	—	—
	10	$0_{.035^-}$	—	—	—
5	20	$3_{.033}$	$2_{.004}$	$2_{.004}$	$2_{.004}$
	19	$2_{.016}$	$2_{.016}$	$1_{.002}$	$1_{.002}$
	18	$2_{.038}$	$1_{.005^+}$	$1_{.005^+}$	$0_{.000}$
	17	$1_{.012}$	$1_{.012}$	$0_{.001}$	$0_{.001}$
	16	$1_{.023}$	$1_{.023}$	$0_{.002}$	$0_{.002}$
	15	$1_{.040}$	$0_{.005^-}$	$0_{.005^-}$	$0_{.005^-}$
	14	$0_{.009}$	$0_{.009}$	$0_{.009}$	—
	13	$0_{.015^-}$	$0_{.015^-}$	—	—
	12	$0_{.024}$	$0_{.024}$	—	—
	11	$0_{.038}$	—	—	—
4	20	$2_{.022}$	$2_{.022}$	$1_{.002}$	$1_{.002}$
	19	$1_{.008}$	$1_{.008}$	$1_{.008}$	$0_{.000}$
	18	$1_{.018}$	$1_{.018}$	$0_{.001}$	$0_{.001}$
	17	$1_{.035^+}$	$0_{.003}$	$0_{.003}$	$0_{.003}$
	16	$0_{.007}$	$0_{.007}$	$0_{.007}$	—
	15	$0_{.012}$	$0_{.012}$	—	—
	14	$0_{.020}$	$0_{.020}$	—	—
	13	$0_{.031}$	—	—	—
	12	$0_{.047}$	—	—	—
3	20	$1_{.012}$	$1_{.012}$	$0_{.001}$	$0_{.001}$
	19	$1_{.034}$	$0_{.002}$	$0_{.002}$	$0_{.002}$
$A = 20\ B = 3$	18	$0_{.006}$	$0_{.006}$	$0_{.006}$	—
	17	$0_{.011}$	$0_{.011}$	—	—
	16	$0_{.020}$	$0_{.020}$	—	—
	15	$0_{.032}$	—	—	—
	14	$0_{.047}$	—	—	—
2	20	$0_{.004}$	$0_{.004}$	$0_{.004}$	$0_{.004}$
	19	$0_{.013}$	$0_{.013}$	—	—
	18	$0_{.026}$	—	—	—
	17	$0_{.043}$	—	—	—
1	20	$0_{.048}$	—	—	—

TABLE K Probability Levels for the Wilcoxon Signed Rank Test

$n = 5$		$n = 8$		$n = 10$		$n = 11$		$n = 12$		$n = 13$	
T	P	T	P	T	P	T	P	T	P	T	P
[a]0	.0313	0	.0039	0	.0010	0	.0005	0	.0002	0	.0001
1	.0625	1	.0078	1	.0020	1	.0010	1	.0005	1	.0002
2	.0938	2	.0117	2	.0029	2	.0015	2	.0007	2	.0004
3	.1563	3	.0195	3	.0049	3	.0024	3	.0012	3	.0006
4	.2188	4	.0273	4	.0068	4	.0034	4	.0017	4	.0009
5	.3125	[a]5	.0391	5	.0098	5	.0049	5	.0024	5	.0012
6	.4063	6	.0547	6	.0137	6	.0068	6	.0034	6	.0017
7	.5000	7	.0742	7	.0186	7	.0093	7	.0046	7	.0023
		8	.0977	8	.0244	8	.0122	8	.0061	8	.0031
$n = 6$		9	.1250	9	.0322	9	.0161	9	.0081	9	.0040
0	.0156	10	.1563	[a]10	.0420	10	.0210	10	.0105	10	.0052
1	.0313	11	.1914	11	.0527	11	.0269	11	.0134	11	.0067
[a]2	.0469	12	.2305	12	.0654	12	.0337	12	.0171	12	.0085
3	.0781	13	.2734	13	.0801	[a]13	.0415	13	.0212	13	.0107
4	.1094	14	.3203	14	.0967	14	.0508	14	.0261	14	.0133
5	.1563	15	.3711	15	.1162	15	.0615	15	.0320	15	.0164
6	.2188	16	.4219	16	.1377	16	.0737	16	.0386	16	.0199
7	.2813	17	.4727	17	.1611	17	.0874	[a]17	.0461	17	.0239
8	.3438	18	.5273	18	.1875	18	.1030	18	.0549	18	.0287
9	.4219	$n = 9$		19	.2158	19	.1201	19	.0647	19	.0341
10	.5000	0	.0020	20	.2461	20	.1392	20	.0757	20	.0402
		1	.0039	21	.2783	21	.1602	21	.0881	[a]21	.0471
$n = 7$		2	.0059	22	.3125	22	.1826	22	.1018	22	.0549
0	.0078	3	.0098	23	.3477	23	.2065	23	.1167	23	.0636
1	.0156	4	.0137	24	.3848	24	.2324	24	.1331	24	.0732
2	.0234	5	.0195	25	.4229	25	.2598	25	.1506	25	.0839
[a]3	.0391	6	.0273	26	.4609	26	.2886	26	.1697	26	.0955
4	.0547	7	.0371	27	.5000	27	.3188	27	.1902	27	.1082
5	.0781	[a]8	.0488			28	.3501	28	.2119	28	.1219
6	.1094	9	.0645			29	.3823	29	.2349	29	.1367
7	.1484	10	.0820			30	.4155	30	.2593	30	.1527
8	.1875	11	.1016			31	.4492	31	.2847	31	.1698
9	.2344	12	.1250			32	.4829	32	.3110	32	.1879
10	.2891	13	.1504			33	.5171	33	.3386	33	.2072
11	.3438	14	.1797					34	.3667	34	.2274
12	.4063	15	.2129					35	.3955	35	.2487

[a]For given n, the smallest rank total for which the probability level is equal to or less than 0.0500.

TABLE K (*continued*)

n = 7		n = 9				n = 12		n = 13	
T	P	T	P			T	P	T	P
13	.4688	16	.2480			36	.4250	36	.2709
14	.5313	17	.2852			37	.4548	37	.2939
		18	.3262			38	.4849	38	.3177
		19	.3672			39	.5151	39	.3424
		20	.4102					40	.3677
		21	.4551					41	.3934
		22	.5000					42	.4197
								43	.4463
								44	.4730
								45	.5000

n = 14		n = 14		n = 15		n = 16		n = 17		n = 17	
T	P	T	P	T	P	T	P	T	P	T	P
0	.0001	50	.4516	47	.2444	39	.0719	25	.0064	74	.4633
2	.0002	51	.4758	48	.2622	40	.0795	26	.0075	75	.4816
3	.0003	52	.5000	49	.2807	41	.0877	27	.0087	76	.5000
4	.0004			50	.2997	42	.0964	28	.0101		
5	.0006	n = 15		51	.3193	43	.1057	29	.0116	n = 18	
6	.0009	1	.0001	52	.3394	44	.1156	30	.0133	6	.0001
7	.0012	3	.0002	53	.3599	45	.1261	31	.0153	10	.0002
8	.0015	5	.0003	54	.3808	46	.1372	32	.0174	12	.0003
9	.0020	6	.0004	55	.4020	47	.1489	33	.0198	14	.0004
10	.0026	7	.0006	56	.4235	48	.1613	34	.0224	15	.0005
11	.0034	8	.0008	57	.4452	49	.1742	35	.0253	16	.0006
12	.0043	9	.0010	58	.4670	50	.1877	36	.0284	17	.0008
13	.0054	10	.0013	59	.4890	51	.2019	37	.0319	18	.0010
14	.0067	11	.0017	60	.5110	52	.2166	38	.0357	19	.0012
15	.0083	12	.0021	n = 16		53	.2319	39	.0398	20	.0014
16	.0101	13	.0027	3	.0001	54	.2477	40	.0443	21	.0017
17	.0123	14	.0034	5	.0002	55	.2641	[a]41	.0492	22	.0020
18	.0148	15	.0042	7	.0003	56	.2809	42	.0544	23	.0024
19	.0176	16	.0051	8	.0004	57	.2983	43	.0601	24	.0028
20	.0209	17	.0062	9	.0005	58	.3161	44	.0662	25	.0033
21	.0247	18	.0075	10	.0007	59	.3343	45	.0727	26	.0038
22	.0290	19	.0090	11	.0008	60	.3529	46	.0797	27	.0045
23	.0338	20	.0108	12	.0011	61	.3718	47	.0871	28	.0052
24	.0392	21	.0128	13	.0013	62	.3910	48	.0950	29	.0060

TABLE K (continued)

n = 14		n = 15		n = 16		n = 16		n = 17		n = 18	
T	P	T	P	T	P	T	P	T	P	T	P
[a]25	.0453	22	.0151	14	.0017	63	.4104	49	.1034	30	.0069
26	.0520	23	.0177	15	.0021	64	.4301	50	.1123	31	.0080
27	.0594	24	.0206	16	.0026	65	.4500	51	.1218	32	.0091
28	.0676	25	.0240	17	.0031	66	.4699	52	.1317	33	.0104
29	.0765	26	.0277	18	.0038	67	.4900	53	.1421	34	.0118
30	.0863	27	.0319	19	.0046	68	.5100	54	.1530	35	.0134
31	.0969	28	.0365	20	.0055			55	.1645	36	.0152
32	.1083	29	.0416	21	.0065	n = 17		56	.1764	37	.0171
33	.1206	[a]30	.0473	22	.0078	4	.0001	57	.1889	38	.0192
34	.1338	31	.0535	23	.0091	8	.0002	58	.2019	39	.0216
35	.1479	32	.0603	24	.0107	9	.0003	59	.2153	40	.0241
36	.1629	33	.0677	25	.0125	11	.0004	60	.2293	41	.0269
37	.1788	34	.0757	26	.0145	12	.0005	61	.2437	42	.0300
38	.1955	35	.0844	27	.0168	13	.0007	62	.2585	43	.0333
39	.2131	36	.0938	28	.0193	14	.0008	63	.2738	44	.0368
40	.2316	37	.1039	29	.0222	15	.0010	64	.2895	45	.0407
41	.2508	38	.1147	30	.0253	16	.0013	65	.3056	46	.0449
42	.2708	39	.1262	31	.0288	17	.0016	66	.3221	[a]47	.0494
43	.2915	40	.1384	32	.0327	18	.0019	67	.3389	48	.0542
44	.3129	41	.1514	33	.0370	19	.0023	68	.3559	49	.0594
45	.3349	42	.1651	34	.0416	20	.0028	69	.3733	50	.0649
46	.3574	43	.1796	[a]35	.0467	21	.0033	70	.3910	51	.0708
47	.3804	44	.1947	36	.0523	22	.0040	70	.4088	52	.0770
48	.4039	45	.2106	37	.0583	23	.0047	72	.4268	53	.0837
49	.4276	46	.2271	38	.0649	24	.0055	73	.4450	54	.0907

n = 18		n = 19		n = 19		n = 20		n = 20		n = 21	
T	P	T	P	T	P	T	P	T	P	T	P
55	.0982	30	.0036	79	.2706	48	.0164	97	.3921	61	.0298
56	.1061	31	.0041	80	.2839	49	.0181	98	.4062	62	.0323
57	.1144	32	.0047	81	.2974	50	.0200	99	.4204	63	.0351
58	.1231	33	.0054	82	.3113	51	.0220	100	.4347	64	.0380
59	.1323	34	.0062	83	.3254	52	.0242	101	.4492	65	.0411
60	.1419	35	.0070	84	.3397	53	.0266	102	.4636	66	.0444
61	.1519	36	.0080	85	.3543	54	.0291	103	.4782	[a]67	.0479
62	.1624	37	.0090	86	.3690	55	.0319	104	.4927	68	.0516
63	.1733	38	.0102	87	.3840	56	.0348	105	.5073	69	.0555
64	.1846	39	.0115	88	.3991	57	.0379	n = 21		70	.0597
65	.1964	40	.0129	89	.4144	58	.0413	14	.0001	71	.0640
66	.2086	41	.0145	.90	.4298	59	.0448	20	.0002	72	.0686

TABLE K (continued)

n = 18		n = 19		n = 19		n = 20		n = 21		n = 21	
T	P	T	P	T	P	T	P	T	P	T	P
67	.2211	42	.0162	91	.4453	[a]60	.0487	22	.0003	73	.0735
68	.2341	43	.0180	92	.4609	61	.0527	24	.0004	74	.0786
69	.2475	44	.0201	93	.4765	62	.0570	26	.0005	75	.0839
70	.2613	45	.0223	94	.4922	63	.0615	27	.0006	76	.0895
71	.2754	46	.0247	95	.5078	64	.0664	28	.0007	77	.0953
72	.2899	47	.0273			65	.0715	29	.0008	78	.1015
73	.3047	48	.0301	n − 20		66	.0760	30	.0009	79	.1078
74	.3198	49	.0331	11	.0001	67	.0825	31	.0011	80	.1145
75	.3353	50	.0364	16	.0002	68	.0884	32	.0012	81	.1214
76	.3509	51	.0399	19	.0003	69	.0947	33	.0014	82	.1286
77	.3669	52	.0437	20	.0004	70	.1012	34	.0016	83	.1361
78	.3830	[a]53	.0478	22	.0005	71	.1081	35	.0019	84	.1439
79	.3994	54	.0521	23	.0006	72	.1153	36	.0021	85	.1519
80	.4159	55	.0567	24	.0007	73	.1227	37	.0024	86	.1602
81	.4325	56	.0616	25	.0008	74	.1305	38	.0028	87	.1688
82	.4493	57	.0668	26	.0010	75	.1387	39	.0031	88	.1777
83	.4661	58	.0723	27	.0012	76	.1471	40	.0036	89	.1869
84	.4831	59	.0782	28	.0014	77	.1559	41	.0040	90	.1963
85	.5000	60	.0844	29	.0016	78	.1650	42	.0045	91	.2060
		61	.0909	30	.0018	79	.1744	43	.0051	92	.2160
n = 19		62	.0978	31	.0021	80	.1841	44	.0057	93	.2262
9	.0001	63	.1051	32	.0024	81	.1942	45	.0063	94	.2367
13	.0002	64	.1127	33	.0028	82	.2045	46	.0071	95	.2474
15	.0003	65	.1206	34	.0032	83	.2152	47	.0079	96	.2584
17	.0004	66	.1290	35	.0036	84	.2262	48	.0088	97	.2696
18	.0005	67	.1377	36	.0042	85	.2375	49	.0097	98	.2810
19	.0006	68	.1467	37	.0047	86	.2490	50	.0108	99	.2927
20	.0007	69	.1562	38	.0053	87	.2608	51	.0119	100	.3046
21	.0008	70	.1660	39	.0060	88	.2729	52	.0132	101	.3166
22	.0010	71	.1762	40	.0068	89	.2853	53	.0145	102	.3289
23	.0012	72	.1868	41	.0077	90	.2979	54	.0160	103	.3414
24	.0014	73	.1977	42	.0086	91	.3108	55	.0175	104	.3540
25	.0017	74	.2090	43	.0096	92	.3238	56	.0192	105	.3667
26	.0020	75	.2207	44	.0107	93	.3371	57	.0210	106	.3796
27	.0023	76	.2327	45	.0120	94	.3506	58	.0230	107	.3927
28	.0027	77	.2450	46	.0133	95	.3643	59	.0251	108	.4058
29	.0031	78	.2576	47	.0148	96	.3781	60	.0273	109	.4191

TABLE K (*continued*)

n = 21		n = 22		n = 22		n = 23		n = 23		n = 24	
T	P	T	P	T	P	T	P	T	P	T	P
110	.4324	67	.0271	116	.3751	68	.0163	117	.2700	62	.0053
111	.4459	68	.0293	117	.3873	69	.0177	118	.2800	63	.0058
112	.4593	69	.0317	118	.3995	70	.0192	119	.2902	64	.0063
113	.4729	70	.0342	119	.4119	71	.0208	120	.3005	65	.0069
114	.4864	71	.0369	120	.4243	72	.0224	121	.3110	66	.0075
115	.5000	72	.0397	121	.4368	73	.0242	122	.3217	67	.0082
		73	.0427	122	.4494	74	.0261	123	.3325	68	.0089
		74	.0459	123	.4620	75	.0281	124	.3434	69	.0097
n = 22		[a]75	.0492	124	.4746	76	.0303	125	.3545	70	.0106
18	.0001	76	.0527	125	.4873	77	.0325	126	.3657	71	.0115
23	.0002	77	.0564	126	.5000	78	.0349	127	.3770	72	.0124
26	.0003	78	.0603			79	.0374	128	.3884	73	.0135
29	.0004	79	.0644	n = 23		80	.0401	129	.3999	74	.0146
30	.0005	80	.0687	21	.0001	81	.0429	130	.4115	75	.0157
32	.0006	81	.0733	28	.0002	82	.0459	131	.4231	76	.0170
33	.0007	82	.0780	31	.0003	[a]83	.0490	132	.4348	77	.0183
34	.0008	83	.0829	33	.0004	84	.0523	133	.4466	78	.0197
35	.0010	84	.0881	35	.0005	85	.0557	134	.4584	79	.0212
36	.0011	85	.0935	36	.0006	86	.0593	135	.4703	80	.0228
37	.0013	86	.0991	38	.0007	87	.0631	136	.4822	81	.0245
38	.0014	87	.1050	39	.0008	88	.0671	137	.4941	82	.0263
39	.0016	88	.1111	40	.0009	89	.0712	138	.5060	83	.0282
40	.0018	89	.1174	41	.0011	90	.0755			84	.0302
41	.0021	90	.1240	42	.0012	91	.0801	n = 24		85	.0323
42	.0023	91	.1308	43	.0014	92	.0848	25	.0001	86	.0346
43	.0026	92	.1378	44	.0015	93	.0897	32	.0002	87	.0369
44	.0030	93	.1451	45	.0017	94	.0948	36	.0003	88	.0394
45	.0033	94	.1527	46	.0019	95	.1001	38	.0004	89	.0420
46	.0037	95	.1604	47	.0022	96	.1056	40	.0005	90	.0447
47	.0042	96	.1685	48	.0024	97	.1113	42	.0006	[a]91	.0475
48	.0046	97	.1767	49	.0027	98	.1172	43	.0007	92	.0505
49	.0052	98	.1853	50	.0030	99	.1234	44	.0008	93	.0537
50	.0057	99	.1940	51	.0034	100	.1297	45	.0009	94	.0570
51	.0064	100	.2030	52	.0037	101	.1363	46	.0010	95	.0604
52	.0070	101	.2122	53	.0041	102	.1431	47	.0011	96	.0640
53	.0078	102	.2217	54	.0046	103	.1501	48	.0013	97	.0678
54	.0086	103	.2314	55	.0051	104	.1573	49	.0014	98	.0717

TABLE K (*continued*)

n = 22		n = 22		n = 23		n = 23		n = 24		n = 24	
T	P	T	P	T	P	T	P	T	P	T	P
55	.0095	104	.2413	56	.0056	105	.1647	50	.0016	99	.0758
56	.0104	105	.2514	57	.0061	106	.1723	51	.0018	100	.0800
57	.0115	106	.2618	58	.0068	107	.1802	52	.0020	101	.0844
58	.0126	107	.2723	59	.0074	108	.1883	53	.0022	102	.0890
59	.0138	108	.2830	60	.0082	109	.1965	54	.0024	103	.0938
60	.0151	109	.2940	61	.0089	110	.2050	55	.0027	104	.0987
61	.0164	110	.3051	62	.0090	111	.2137	56	.0029	105	.1038
62	.0179	111	.3164	63	.0107	112	.2226	57	.0033	106	.1091
63	.0195	112	.3278	64	.0117	113	.2317	58	.0036	107	.1146
64	.0212	113	.3394	65	.0127	114	.2410	59	.0040	108	.1203
65	.0231	114	.3512	66	.0138	115	.2505	60	.0044	109	.1261
66	.0250	115	.3631	67	.0150	116	.2601	61	.0048	110	.1322

n = 24		n = 25		n = 25		n = 25		n = 26		n = 26	
T	P	T	P	T	P	T	P	T	P	T	P
111	.1384	50	.0008	99	.0452	148	.3556	81	.0076	130	.1289
112	.1448	51	.0009	[a]100	.0479	149	.3655	82	.0082	131	.1344
113	.1515	52	.0010	101	.0507	150	.3755	83	.0088	132	.1399
114	.1583	53	.0011	102	.0537	151	.3856	84	.0095	133	.1457
115	.1653	54	.0013	103	.0567	152	.3957	85	.0102	134	.1516
116	.1724	55	.0014	104	.0600	153	.4060	86	.0110	135	.1576
117	.1798	56	.0015	105	.0633	154	.4163	87	.0118	136	.1638
118	.1874	57	.0017	106	.0668	155	.4266	88	.0127	137	.1702
119	.1951	58	.0019	107	.0705	156	.4370	89	.0136	138	.1767
120	.2031	59	.0021	108	.0742	157	.4474	90	.0146	139	.1833
121	.2112	60	.0023	109	.0782	158	.4579	91	.0156	140	.1901
122	.2195	61	.0025	110	.0822	159	.4684	92	.0167	141	.1970
123	.2279	62	.0028	111	.0865	160	.4789	93	.0179	142	.2041
124	.2366	63	.0031	112	.0909	161	.4895	94	.0191	143	.2114
125	.2454	64	.0034	113	.0954	162	.5000	95	.0204	144	.2187
126	.2544	65	.0037	114	.1001			96	.0217	145	.2262
127	.2635	66	.0040	115	.1050	n = 26		97	.0232	146	.2339
128	.2728	67	.0044	116	.1100	34	.0001	98	.0247	147	.2417
129	.2823	68	.0048	117	.1152	42	.0002	99	.0263	148	.2496
130	.2919	69	.0053	118	.1205	46	.0003	100	.0279	149	.2577
131	.3017	70	.0057	119	.1261	49	.0004	101	.0297	150	.2658
132	.3115	71	.0062	120	.1317	51	.0005	102	.0315	151	.2741
133	.3216	72	.0068	121	.1376	53	.0006	103	.0334	152	.2826
134	.3317	73	.0074	122	.1436	55	.0007	104	.0355	153	.2911

TABLE K (*continued*)

n = 24		n = 25		n = 25		n = 26		n = 26		n = 26	
T	P	T	P	T	P	T	P	T	P	T	P
135	.3420	74	.0080	123	.1498	56	.0008	105	.0376	154	.2998
136	.3524	75	.0087	124	.1562	57	.0009	106	.0398	155	.3085
137	.3629	76	.0094	125	.1627	58	.0010	107	.0421	156	.3174
138	.3735	77	.0101	126	.1694	59	.0011	108	.0455	157	.3264
139	.3841	78	.0110	127	.1763	60	.0012	109	.0470	158	.3355
140	.3949	79	.0118	128	.1833	61	.0013	[a]110	.0497	159	.3447
141	.4058	80	.0128	129	.1905	62	.0015	111	.0524	160	.3539
142	.4167	81	.0137	130	.1979	63	.0016	112	.0553	161	.3633
143	.4277	82	.0148	131	.2054	64	.0018	113	.0582	162	.3727
144	.4387	83	.0159	132	.2131	65	.0020	114	.0613	163	.3822
145	.4498	84	.0171	133	.2209	66	.0021	115	.0646	164	.3918
146	.4609	85	.0183	134	.2289	67	.0023	116	.0679	165	.4014
147	.4721	86	.0197	135	.2371	68	.0026	117	.0714	166	.4111
148	.4832	87	.0211	136	.2454	69	.0028	118	.0750	167	.4208
149	.4944	88	.0226	137	.2539	70	.0031	119	.0787	168	.4306
150	.5056	89	.0241	138	.2625	71	.0033	120	.0825	169	.4405
n = 25		90	.0258	139	.2712	72	.0036	121	.0865	170	.4503
		91	.0275	140	.2801	73	.0040	122	.0907	171	.4602
29	.0001	92	.0294	141	.2891	74	.0043	123	.0950	172	.4702
37	.0002	93	.0313	142	.2983	75	.0047	124	.0994	173	.4801
41	.0003	94	.0334	143	.3075	76	.0051	125	.1039	174	.4900
43	.0004	95	.0355	144	.3169	77	.0055	126	.1086	175	.5000
45	.0005	96	.0377	145	.3264	78	.0060	127	.1135		
47	.0006	97	.0401	146	.3360	79	.0065	128	.1185		
48	.0007	98	.0426	147	.3458	80	.0070	129	.1236		

n = 27		n = 27		n = 27		n = 28		n = 28		n = 28	
T	P	T	P	T	P	T	P	T	P	T	P
39	.0001	105	.0218	154	.2066	74	.0012	123	.0349	172	.2466
47	.0002	106	.0231	155	.2135	75	.0013	124	.0368	173	.2538
52	.0003	107	.0246	156	.2205	76	.0015	125	.0387	174	.2611
55	.0004	108	.0260	157	.2277	77	.0016	126	.0407	175	.2685
57	.0005	109	.0276	158	.2349	78	.0017	127	.0428	176	.2759
59	.0006	110	.0292	159	.2423	79	.0019	128	.0450	177	.2835
61	.0007	111	.0309	160	.2498	80	.0020	129	.0473	178	.2912
62	.0008	112	.0327	161	.2574	81	.0022	[a]130	.0496	179	.2990
64	.0009	113	.0346	162	.2652	82	.0024	131	.0521	180	.3068
65	.0010	114	.0366	163	.2730	83	.0026	132	.0546	181	.3148
66	.0011	115	.0386	164	.2810	84	.0028	133	.0573	182	.3228
67	.0012	116	.0407	165	.2890	85	.0030	134	.0600	183	.3309

TABLE K (continued)

n = 27		n = 27		n = 27		n = 28		n = 28		n = 28	
T	P	T	P	T	P	T	P	T	P	T	P
68	.0014	117	.0430	166	.2972	86	.0033	135	.0628	184	.3391
69	.0015	118	.0453	167	.3055	87	.0035	136	.0657	185	.3474
70	.0016	[a]119	.0477	168	.3138	88	.0038	137	.0688	186	.3557
71	.0018	120	.0502	169	.3223	89	.0041	138	.0719	187	.3641
72	.0019	121	.0528	170	.3308	90	.0044	139	.0751	188	.3725
73	.0021	122	.0555	171	.3395	91	.0048	140	.0785	189	.3811
74	.0023	123	.0583	172	.3482	92	.0051	141	.0819	190	.3896
75	.0025	124	.0613	173	.3570	93	.0055	142	.0855	191	.3983
76	.0027	125	.0643	174	.3659	94	.0059	143	.0891	192	.4070
77	.0030	126	.0674	175	.3748	95	.0064	144	.0929	193	.4157
78	.0032	127	.0707	176	.3838	96	.0068	145	.0968	194	.4245
79	.0035	128	.0741	177	.3929	97	.0073	146	.1008	195	.4333
80	.0038	129	.0776	178	.4020	98	.0078	147	.1049	196	.4421
81	.0041	130	.0812	179	.4112	99	.0084	148	.1091	197	.4510
82	.0044	131	.0849	180	.4204	100	.0089	149	.1135	198	.4598
83	.0048	132	.0888	181	.4297	101	.0096	150	.1180	199	.4687
84	.0052	133	.0927	182	.4390	102	.0102	151	.1225	200	4777
85	.0056	134	.0968	183	.4483	103	.0109	152	.1273	201	.4866
86	.0060	135	.1010	184	.4577	104	.0116	153	.1321	202	.4955
87	.0065	136	.1054	185	.4670	105	.0124	154	.1370	203	.5045
88	.0070	137	.1099	186	.4764	106	.0132	155	.1421		
89	.0075	138	.1145	187	.4859	107	.0140	156	.1473	n = 28	
90	.0081	139	.1193	188	.4953	108	.0149	157	.1526	50	.0001
91	.0087	140	.1242	189	.5047	109	.0159	158	.1580	59	.0002
92	.0093	141	.1292			110	.0168	159	.1636	65	.0003
93	.0100	142	.1343	n = 28		111	.0179	160	.1693	68	.0004
94	.0107	143	.1396	44	.0001	112	.0190	161	.1751	71	.0005
95	.0115	144	.1450	53	.0002	113	.0201	162	.1810	73	.0006
96	.0123	145	.1506	58	.0003	114	.0213	163	.1870	75	.0007
97	.0131	146	.1563	61	.0004	115	.0226	164	.1932	76	.0008
98	.0140	147	.1621	64	.0005	116	.0239	165	.1995	78	.0009
99	.0150	148	.1681	66	.0006	117	.0252	166	.2059	79	.0010
100	.0159	149	.1742	68	.0007	118	.0267	167	.2124	80	.0011
101	.0170	150	.1804	69	.0008	119	.0282	168	.2190	81	.0012
102	.0181	151	.1868	70	.0009	120	.0298	169	.2257	82	.0013
103	.0193	152	.1932	72	.0010	121	.0314	170	.2326	83	.0014
104	.0205	153	.1999	73	.0011	122	.0331	171	.2395	84	.0015

TABLE K (continued)

n = 29		n = 29		n = 29		n = 30		n = 30		n = 30	
T	P	T	P	T	P	T	P	T	P	T	P
85	.0016	134	.0362	183	.2340	90	.0013	139	.0275	188	.1854
86	.0018	135	.0380	184	.2406	91	.0014	140	.0288	189	.1909
87	.0019	136	.0399	185	.2473	92	.0015	141	.0303	190	.1965
88	.0021	137	.0418	186	.2541	93	.0016	142	.0318	191	.2022
89	.0022	138	.0439	187	.2611	94	.0017	143	.0333	192	.2081
90	.0024	139	.0460	188	.2681	95	.0019	144	.0349	193	.2140
91	.0026	^{a}140	.0482	189	.2752	96	.0020	145	.0366	194	.2200
92	.0028	141	.0504	190	.2824	97	.0022	146	.0384	195	.2261
93	.0030	142	.0528	191	.2896	98	.0023	147	.0402	196	.2323
94	.0032	143	.0552	192	.2970	99	.0025	148	.0420	197	.2386
95	.0035	144	.0577	193	.3044	100	.0027	149	.0440	198	.2449
96	.0037	145	.0603	194	.3120	101	.0029	150	.0460	119	.2514
97	.0040	146	.0630	195	.3196	102	.0031	^{a}151	.0481	200	.2579
98	.0043	147	.0658	196	.3272	103	.0033	152	.0502	201	.2646
99	.0046	148	.0687	197	.3350	104	.0036	153	.0524	202	.2713
100	.0049	149	.0716	198	.3428	105	.0038	154	.0547	203	.2781
101	.0053	150	.0747	199	.3507	106	.0041	155	.0571	204	.2849
102	.0057	151	.0778	200	.3586	107	.0044	156	.0595	205	.2919
103	.0061	152	.0811	201	.3666	108	.0047	157	.0621	206	.2989
104	.0065	153	.0844	202	.3747	109	.0050	158	.0647	207	.3060
105	.0069	154	.0879	203	.3828	110	.0053	159	.0674	208	.3132
106	.0074	155	.0914	204	.3909	111	.0057	160	.0701	209	.3204
107	.0079	156	.0951	205	.3991	112	.0060	161	.0730	210	.3277
108	.0084	157	.0988	206	.4074	113	.0064	162	.0759	211	.3351
109	.0089	158	.1027	207	.4157	114	.0068	163	.0790	212	.3425
110	.0095	159	.1066	208	.4240	115	.0073	164	.0821	213	.3500
111	.0101	160	.1107	209	.4324	116	.0077	165	.0853	214	.3576
112	.0108	161	.1149	210	.4408	117	.0082	166	.0886	215	.3652
113	.0115	162	.1191	211	.4492	118	.0087	167	.0920	216	.3728
114	.0122	163	.1235	212	.4576	119	.0093	168	.0955	217	.3805
115	.0129	164	.1280	213	.4661	120	.0098	169	.0990	218	.3883
116	.0137	165	.1326	214	.4745	121	.0104	170	.1027	219	.3961
117	.0145	166	.1373	215	.4830	122	.0110	171	.1065	220	.4039
118	.0154	167	.1421	216	.4915	123	.0117	172	.1103	221	.4118
119	.0163	168	.1471	217	.5000	124	.0124	173	.1143	222	.4197
120	.0173	169	.1521			125	.0131	174	.1183	223	.4276

TABLE K (continued)

n = 29		n = 29				n = 30		n = 30		n = 30	
T	P	T	P			T	P	T	P	T	P
121	.0183	170	.1572	n = 30		126	.0139	175	.1225	224	.4356
122	.0193	171	.1625	55	.0001	127	.0147	176	.1267	225	.4436
123	.0204	172	.1679	66	.0002	128	.0155	177	.1311	226	.4516
124	.0216	173	.1733	71	.0003	129	.0164	178	.1355	227	.4596
125	.0228	174	.1789	75	.0004	130	.0173	179	.1400	228	.4677
126	.0240	175	.1846	78	.0005	131	.0182	180	.1447	229	.4758
127	.0253	176	.1904	80	.0006	132	.0192	181	.1494	230	.4838
128	.0267	177	.1963	82	.0007	133	.0202	182	.1543	231	.4919
129	.0281	178	.2023	84	.0008	134	.0213	183	.1592	232	.5000
130	.0296	179	.2085	85	.0009	135	.0225	184	.1642		
131	.0311	180	.2147	87	.0010	136	.0236	185	.1694		
132	.0328	181	.2210	88	.0011	137	.0249	186	.1746		
133	.0344	182	.2274	89	.0012	138	.0261	187	.1799		

TABLE L Quantiles of the Mann – Whitney Test Statistic

n	p	m = 2	3	4	5	6	7	8	9	10	11	12	13	14	15	16	17	18	19	20
	.001	0	0	0	0	0	0	0	0	0	0	0	0	0	0	0	0	0	0	0
	.005	0	0	0	0	0	0	0	0	0	0	0	0	0	0	0	0	0	1	1
2	.01	0	0	0	0	0	0	0	0	0	0	0	1	1	1	1	1	1	2	2
	.025	0	0	0	0	0	0	1	1	1	1	2	2	2	2	2	3	3	3	3
	.05	0	0	0	1	1	1	2	2	2	2	3	3	4	4	4	4	5	5	5
	.10	0	1	1	2	2	2	3	3	4	4	5	5	5	6	6	7	7	8	8
	.001	0	0	0	0	0	0	0	0	0	0	0	0	0	0	0	1	1	1	1
	.005	0	0	0	0	0	0	0	1	1	1	2	2	2	3	3	3	3	4	4
3	.01	0	0	0	0	0	1	1	2	2	2	3	3	3	4	4	5	5	5	6
	.025	0	0	0	1	2	2	3	3	4	4	5	5	6	6	7	7	8	8	9
	.05	0	1	1	2	3	3	4	5	5	6	6	7	8	8	9	10	10	11	12
	.10	1	2	2	3	4	5	6	6	7	8	9	10	11	11	12	13	14	15	16
	.001	0	0	0	0	0	0	0	0	1	1	1	2	2	2	3	3	4	4	4
	.005	0	0	0	0	1	1	2	2	3	3	4	4	5	6	6	7	7	8	9
4	.01	0	0	0	1	2	2	3	4	4	5	6	6	7	9	8	9	10	10	11
	.025	0	0	1	2	3	4	5	5	6	7	8	9	10	11	12	12	13	14	15
	.05	0	1	2	3	4	5	6	7	8	9	10	11	12	13	15	16	17	18	19
	.10	1	2	4	5	6	7	8	10	11	12	13	14	16	17	18	19	21	22	23
	.001	0	0	0	0	0	1	2	2	3	3	4	4	5	6	6	7	8	8
	.005	0	0	0	1	2	2	3	4	5	6	7	8	8	9	10	11	12	13	14
5	.01	0	0	1	2	3	4	5	6	7	8	9	10	11	12	13	14	15	16	17
	.025	0	1	2	3	4	6	7	8	9	10	12	13	14	15	16	18	19	20	21
	.05	1	2	3	5	6	7	9	10	12	13	14	16	17	19	20	21	23	24	26
	.10	2	3	5	6	8	9	11	13	14	16	18	19	21	23	24	26	28	29	31

TABLE L (*continued*)

n	p	m = 2	3	4	5	6	7	8	9	10	11	12	13	14	15	16	17	18	19	20
	.001	0	0	0	0	0	0	2	3	4	5	5	6	7	8	9	10	11	12	13
	.005	0	0	1	2	3	4	5	6	7	8	10	11	12	13	14	16	17	18	19
6	.01	0	0	2	3	4	5	7	8	9	10	12	13	14	16	17	19	20	21	23
	.025	0	2	3	4	6	7	9	11	12	14	15	17	18	20	22	23	25	26	28
	.05	1	3	4	6	8	9	11	13	15	17	18	20	22	24	26	27	29	31	33
	.10	2	4	6	8	10	12	14	16	18	20	22	24	26	28	30	32	35	37	39
	.001	0	0	0	0	1	2	3	4	6	7	8	9	10	11	12	14	15	16	17
	.005	0	0	1	2	4	5	7	8	10	11	13	14	16	17	19	20	22	23	25
7	.01	0	1	2	4	5	7	8	10	12	13	15	17	18	20	22	24	25	27	29
	.025	0	2	4	6	7	9	11	13	15	17	19	21	23	25	27	29	31	33	35
	.05	1	3	5	7	9	12	14	16	18	20	22	25	27	29	31	34	36	38	40
	.10	2	5	7	9	12	14	17	19	22	24	27	29	32	34	37	39	42	44	47
	.001	0	0	0	1	2	3	5	6	7	9	10	12	13	15	16	18	19	21	22
	.005	0	0	2	3	5	7	8	10	12	14	16	18	19	21	23	25	27	29	31
8	.01	0	1	3	5	7	8	10	12	14	16	18	21	23	25	27	29	31	33	35
	.025	1	3	5	7	9	11	14	16	18	20	23	25	27	30	32	35	37	39	42
	.05	2	4	6	9	11	14	16	19	21	24	27	29	32	34	37	40	42	45	48
	.10	3	6	8	11	14	17	20	23	25	28	31	34	37	40	43	46	49	52	55
	.001	0	0	0	2	3	4	6	8	9	11	13	15	16	18	20	22	24	26	27
	.005	0	1	2	4	6	8	10	12	14	17	19	21	23	25	28	30	32	34	37
9	.01	0	2	4	6	8	10	12	15	17	19	22	24	27	29	32	34	37	39	41
	.025	1	3	5	8	11	13	16	18	21	24	27	29	32	35	38	40	43	46	49
	.05	2	5	7	10	13	16	19	22	25	28	31	34	37	40	43	46	49	52	55
	.10	3	6	10	13	16	19	23	26	29	32	36	39	42	46	49	53	56	59	63
	.001	0	0	1	2	4	6	7	9	11	13	15	18	20	22	24	26	28	30	33
	.005	0	1	3	5	7	10	12	14	17	19	22	25	27	30	32	35	38	40	43
10	.01	0	2	4	7	9	12	14	17	20	23	25	28	31	34	37	39	42	45	48
	.025	1	4	6	9	12	15	18	21	24	27	30	34	37	40	43	46	49	53	46
	.05	2	5	8	12	15	18	21	25	28	32	35	38	42	45	49	52	56	59	63
	.10	4	7	11	14	18	22	25	29	33	37	40	44	48	52	55	59	63	67	71

TABLE L (*continued*)

n	p	m = 2	3	4	5	6	7	8	9	10	11	12	13	14	15	16	17	18	19	20
	.001	0	0	1	3	5	7	9	11	13	16	18	21	23	25	28	30	33	35	38
	.005	0	1	3	6	8	11	14	17	19	22	25	28	31	34	37	40	43	46	49
11	.01	0	2	5	8	10	13	16	19	23	26	29	32	35	38	42	45	48	51	54
	.025	1	4	7	10	14	17	20	24	27	31	34	38	41	45	48	52	56	59	63
	.05	2	6	9	13	17	20	24	28	32	35	39	43	47	51	55	58	62	66	70
	.10	4	8	12	16	20	24	28	32	37	41	45	49	53	58	62	66	70	74	79
	.001	0	0	1	3	5	8	10	13	15	18	21	24	26	29	32	35	38	41	43
	.005	0	2	4	7	10	13	16	19	22	25	28	32	35	38	42	45	48	52	55
12	.01	0	3	6	9	12	15	18	22	25	29	32	36	39	43	47	50	54	57	61
	.025	2	5	8	12	15	19	23	27	30	34	38	42	46	50	54	58	62	66	70
	.05	3	6	10	14	18	22	27	31	35	39	43	48	52	56	61	65	69	73	78
	.10	5	9	13	18	22	27	31	36	40	45	50	54	59	64	68	73	78	82	87
	.001	0	0	2	4	6	9	12	15	18	21	24	27	30	33	36	39	43	46	49
	.005	0	2	4	8	11	14	18	21	25	28	32	35	39	43	46	50	54	58	61
13	.01	1	3	6	10	13	17	21	24	28	32	36	40	44	48	52	56	60	64	68
	.025	2	5	9	13	17	21	25	29	34	38	42	46	51	55	60	64	68	73	77
	.05	3	7	11	16	20	25	29	34	38	43	48	52	57	62	66	71	76	81	85
	.10	5	10	14	19	24	29	34	39	44	49	54	59	64	69	75	80	85	90	95
	.001	0	0	2	4	7	10	13	16	20	23	26	30	33	37	40	44	47	51	55
	.005	0	2	5	8	12	16	19	23	27	31	35	39	43	47	51	55	59	64	68
14	.01	1	3	7	11	14	18	23	27	31	35	39	44	48	52	57	61	66	70	74
	.025	2	6	10	14	18	23	27	32	37	41	46	51	56	60	65	70	75	79	84
	.05	4	8	12	17	22	27	32	37	42	47	52	57	62	67	72	78	83	88	93
	.10	5	11	16	21	26	32	37	42	48	53	59	64	70	75	81	86	92	98	103
	.001	0	0	2	5	8	11	15	18	22	25	29	33	37	41	44	48	52	56	60
	.005	0	3	6	9	13	17	21	25	30	34	38	43	47	52	56	61	65	70	74
15	.01	1	4	8	12	16	20	25	29	34	38	43	48	52	57	62	67	71	76	81
	.025	2	6	11	15	20	25	30	35	40	45	50	55	60	65	71	76	81	86	91
	.05	4	8	13	19	24	29	34	40	45	51	56	62	67	73	78	84	89	95	101
	.10	6	11	17	23	28	34	40	46	52	58	64	69	75	81	87	93	99	105	111

TABLE L (*continued*)

n	p	m = 2	3	4	5	6	7	8	9	10	11	12	13	14	15	16	17	18	19	20
	.001	0	0	3	6	9	12	16	20	24	28	32	36	40	44	49	53	57	61	66
	.005	0	3	6	10	14	19	23	28	32	37	42	46	51	56	61	66	71	75	80
16	.01	1	4	8	13	17	22	27	32	37	42	47	52	57	62	67	72	77	83	88
	.025	2	7	12	16	22	27	32	38	43	48	54	60	65	71	76	82	87	93	99
	.05	4	9	15	20	26	31	37	43	49	55	61	66	72	78	84	90	96	102	108
	.10	6	12	18	24	30	37	43	49	55	62	68	75	81	87	94	100	107	113	120
	.001	0	1	3	6	10	14	18	22	26	30	35	39	44	48	53	58	62	67	71
	.005	0	3	7	11	16	20	25	30	35	40	45	50	55	61	66	71	76	82	87
17	.01	1	5	9	14	19	24	29	34	39	45	50	56	61	67	72	78	83	89	94
	.025	3	7	12	18	23	29	35	40	46	52	58	64	70	76	82	88	94	100	106
	.05	4	10	16	21	27	34	40	46	52	58	65	71	78	84	90	97	103	110	116
	.10	7	13	19	26	32	39	46	53	59	66	73	80	86	93	100	107	114	121	128
	.001	0	1	4	7	11	15	19	24	28	33	38	43	47	52	57	62	67	72	77
	.005	0	3	7	12	17	22	27	32	38	43	48	54	59	65	71	76	82	88	93
18	.01	1	5	10	15	20	25	31	37	42	48	54	60	66	71	77	83	89	95	101
	.025	3	8	13	19	25	31	37	43	49	56	62	68	75	81	87	94	100	107	113
	.05	5	10	17	23	29	36	42	49	56	62	69	76	83	89	96	103	110	117	124
	.10	7	14	21	28	35	42	49	56	63	70	78	85	92	99	107	114	121	129	136
	.001	0	1	4	8	12	16	21	26	30	35	41	46	51	56	61	67	72	78	83
	.005	1	4	8	13	18	23	29	34	40	46	52	58	64	70	75	82	88	94	100
19	.01	2	5	10	16	21	27	33	39	45	51	57	64	70	76	83	89	95	102	108
	.025	3	8	14	20	26	33	39	46	53	59	66	73	79	86	93	100	107	114	120
	.05	5	11	18	24	31	38	45	52	59	66	73	81	88	95	102	110	117	124	131
	.10	8	15	22	29	37	44	52	59	67	74	82	90	98	105	113	121	129	136	144
	.001	0	1	4	8	13	17	22	27	33	38	43	49	55	60	66	71	77	83	89
	.005	1	4	9	14	19	25	31	37	43	49	55	61	68	74	80	87	93	100	106
20	.01	2	6	11	17	23	29	35	41	48	54	61	68	74	81	88	94	101	108	115
	.025	3	9	15	21	28	35	42	49	56	63	70	77	84	91	99	106	113	120	128
	.05	5	12	19	26	33	40	48	55	63	70	78	85	93	101	108	116	124	131	139
	.10	8	16	23	31	39	47	55	63	71	79	87	95	103	111	120	128	136	144	152

TABLE M Quantiles of the Kolmogorov Test Statistic

	One-Sided Test $p = .90$	.95	.975	.99	.995
	Two-Sided Test $p = .80$	.90	.95	.98	.99
$n = 1$	.900	.950	.975	.990	.995
2	.684	.776	.842	.900	.929
3	.565	.636	.708	.785	.829
4	.493	.565	.624	.689	.734
5	.447	.509	.563	.627	.669
6	.410	.468	.519	.577	.617
7	.381	.436	.483	.538	.576
8	.358	.410	.454	.507	.542
9	.339	.387	.430	.480	.513
10	.323	.369	.409	.457	.489
11	.308	.352	.391	.437	.468
12	.296	.338	.375	.419	.449
13	.285	.325	.361	.404	.432
14	.275	.314	.349	.390	.418
15	.266	.304	.338	.377	.404
16	.258	.295	.327	.366	.392
17	.250	.286	.318	.355	.381
18	.244	.279	.309	.346	.371
19	.237	.271	.301	.337	.361
20	.232	.265	.294	.329	.352
21	.226	.259	.287	.321	.344
22	.221	.253	.281	.314	.337
23	.216	.247	.275	.307	.330
24	.212	.242	.269	.301	.323
25	.208	.238	.264	.295	.317
26	.204	.233	.259	.290	.311
27	.200	.229	.254	.284	.305
28	.197	.225	.250	.279	.300
29	.193	.221	.246	.275	.295
30	.190	.218	.242	.270	.290
31	.187	.214	.238	.266	.285
32	.184	.211	.234	.262	.281
33	.182	.208	.231	.258	.277
34	.179	.205	.227	.254	.273
35	.177	.202	.224	.251	.269
36	.174	.199	.221	.247	.265
37	.172	.196	.218	.244	.262
38	.170	.194	.215	.241	.258
39	.168	.191	.213	.238	.255
40	.165	.189	.210	.235	.252
Approximation for $n > 40$	$\dfrac{1.07}{\sqrt{n}}$	$\dfrac{1.22}{\sqrt{n}}$	$\dfrac{1.36}{\sqrt{n}}$	$\dfrac{1.52}{\sqrt{n}}$	$\dfrac{1.63}{\sqrt{n}}$

TABLE N Critical Values of the Kruskal – Wallis Test Statistic

Sample Sizes			Critical	
n_1	n_2	n_3	Value	α
2	1	1	2.7000	.500
2	2	1	3.6000	.200
2	2	2	4.5714	.067
			3.7143	.200
3	1	1	3.2000	.300
3	2	1	4.2857	.100
			3.8571	.133
3	2	2	5.3572	.029
			4.7143	.048
			4.5000	.067
			4.4643	.105
3	3	1	5.1429	.043
			4.5714	.100
			4.0000	.129
3	3	2	6.2500	.011
			5.3611	.032
			5.1389	.061
			4.5556	.100
			4.2500	.121
3	3	3	7.2000	.004
			6.4889	.011
			5.6889	.029
			5.6000	.050
			5.0667	.086
			4.6222	.100
4	1	1	3.5714	.200
4	2	1	4.8214	.057
			4.5000	.076
			4.0179	.114
4	2	2	6.0000	.014
			5.3333	.033
			5.1250	.052
			4.4583	.100
			4.1667	.105
4	3	1	5.8333	.021
			5.2083	.050
			5.0000	.057
			4.0556	.093
			3.8889	.129

TABLE N (*continued*)

Sample Sizes			Critical	
n_1	n_2	n_3	Value	α
4	3	2	6.4444	.008
			6.3000	.011
			5.4444	.046
			5.4000	.051
			4.5111	.098
			4.4444	.102
4	3	3	6.7455	.010
			6.7091	.013
			5.7909	.046
			5.7273	.050
			4.7091	.092
			4.7000	.101
4	4	1	6.6667	.010
			6.1667	.022
			4.9667	.048
			4.8667	.054
			4.1667	.082
			4.0667	.102
4	4	2	7.0364	.006
			6.8727	.011
			5.4545	.046
			5.2364	.052
			4.5545	.098
			4.4455	.103
4	4	3	7.1439	.010
			7.1364	.011
			5.5985	.049
			5.5758	.051
			4.5455	.099
			4.4773	.102
4	4	4	7.6538	.008
			7.5385	.011
			5.6923	.049
			5.6538	.054
			4.6539	.097
			4.5001	.104
5	1	1	3.8571	.143
5	2	1	5.2500	.036
			5.0000	.048
			4.4500	.071
			4.2000	.095
			4.0500	.119

TABLE N (*continued*)

Sample Sizes			Critical Value	α
n_1	n_2	n_3		
5	2	2	6.5333	.008
			6.1333	.013
			5.1600	.034
			5.0400	.056
			4.3733	.090
			4.2933	.122
5	3	1	6.4000	.012
			4.9600	.048
			4.8711	.052
			4.0178	.095
			3.8400	.123
5	3	2	6.9091	.009
			6.8218	.010
			5.2509	.049
			5.1055	.052
			4.6509	.091
			4.4945	.101
5	3	3	7.0788	.009
			6.9818	.011
			5.6485	.049
			5.5152	.051
			4.5333	.097
			4.4121	.109
5	4	1	6.9545	.008
			6.8400	.011
			4.9855	.044
			4.8600	.056
			3.9873	.098
			3.9600	.102
5	4	2	7.2045	.009
			7.1182	.010
			5.2727	.049
			5.2682	.050
			4.5409	.098
			4.5182	.101
5	4	3	7.4449	.010
			7.3949	.011
			5.6564	.049
			5.6308	.050

TABLE N (*continued*)

Sample Sizess			Critical	
n_1	n_2	n_3	Value	α
			4.5487	.099
			4.5231	.103
5	4	4	7.7604	.009
			7.7440	.011
			5.6571	.049
			5.6176	.050
			4.6187	.100
			4.5527	.102
5	5	1	7.3091	.009
			6.8364	.011
			5.1273	.046
			4.9091	.053
			4.1091	.086
			4.0364	.105
5	5	2	7.3385	.010
			7.2692	.010
			5.3385	.047
			5.2462	.051
			4.6231	.097
			4.5077	.100
5	5	3	7.5780	.010
			7.5429	.010
			5.7055	.046
			5.6264	.051
			4.5451	.100
			4.5363	.102
5	5	4	7.8229	.010
			7.7914	.010
			5.6657	.049
			5.6429	.050
			4.5229	.099
			4.5200	.101
5	5	5	8.0000	.009
			7.9800	.010
			5.7800	.049
			5.6600	.051
			4.5600	.100
			4.5000	.102

TABLE O Exact Distribution of χ_r^2 for Tables with From 2 to 9 Sets of Three Ranks
($k = 3$; $n = 2, 3, 4, 5, 6, 7, 8, 9$; P is the probability of obtaining a value of χ_r^2 as great
as or greater than the corresponding value of χ_r^2)

χ_r^2	P	χ_r^2	P	χ_r^2	P	χ_r^2	P
n=2		n=3		n=4		n=5	
0	1.000	.000	1.000	.0	1.000	.0	1.000
1	.833	.667	.944	.5	.931	.4	.954
3	.500	2.000	.528	1.5	.653	1.2	.691
4	.167	2.667	.361	2.0	.431	1.6	.522
		4.667	1.94	3.5	.273	2.8	.367
		6.000	.028	4.5	.125	3.6	.182
				6.0	.069	4.8	.124
				6.5	.042	5.2	.093
				8.0	.0046	6.4	.039
						7.6	.024
						8.4	.0085
						10.0	.00077

χ_r^2	P	χ_r^2	P	χ_r^2	P	χ_r^2	P
n=6		n=7		n=8		n=9	
.00	1.000	.000	1.000	.00	1.000	.000	1.000
0.33	.956	.286	.964	.25	.967	.222	.971
1.00	.740	.857	.768	.75	.794	.667	.814
1.33	.570	1.143	.620	1.00	.654	.889	.865
2.33	.430	2.000	.486	1.75	.531	1.556	.569
3.00	.252	2.571	.305	2.25	.355	2.000	.398
4.00	.184	3.429	.237	3.00	.285	2.667	.328
4.33	.142	3.714	.192	3.25	.236	2.889	.278
5.33	.072	4.571	.112	4.00	.149	3.556	.187
6.33	.052	5.429	.085	4.75	.120	4.222	.154
7.00	.029	6.000	.052	5.25	.079	4.667	.107
8.33	.012	7.143	.027	6.25	.047	5.556	.069
9.00	.0081	7.714	.021	6.75	.038	6.000	.057
9.33	.0055	8.000	.016	7.00	.030	6.222	.048
10.33	.0017	8.857	.0084	7.75	.018	6.889	.031
12.00	.00013	10.286	.0036	9.00	.0099	8.000	.019
		10.571	.0027	9.25	.0080	8.222	.016
		11.143	.0012	9.75	.0048	8.667	.010
		12.286	.00032	10.75	.0024	9.556	.0060
		14.000	.000021	12.00	.0011	10.667	.0035
				12.25	.00086	10.889	.0029
				13.00	.00026	11.556	.0013
				14.25	.000061	12.667	.00066
				16.00	.0000036	13.556	.00035
						14.000	.00020
						14.222	.000097
						14.889	.000054
						16.222	.000011
						18.000	.0000006

TABLE O Exact Distribution of χ_r^2 for Tables with from 2 to 9 Sets of Three Ranks ($k = 4$; $n = 2, 3, 4$; P is the probability of obtaining a value of χ_r^2 as great as or greater than the corresponding value of χ_r^2)

χ_r^2	P	χ_r^2	P	χ_r^2	P	χ_r^2	P
.0	1.000	.2	1.000	.0	1.000	5.7	.141
.6	.958	.6	.958	.3	.992	6.0	.105
1.2	.834	1.0	.910	.6	.928	6.3	.094
1.8	.792	1.8	.727	.9	.900	6.6	.077
2.4	.625	2.2	.608	1.2	.800	6.9	.068
3.0	.542	2.6	.524	1.5	.754	7.2	.054
3.6	.458	3.4	.446	1.8	.677	7.5	.052
4.2	.375	3.8	.342	2.1	.649	7.8	.036
4.8	.208	4.2	.300	2.4	.524	8.1	.033
5.4	.167	5.0	.207	2.7	.508	8.4	.019
6.0	.042	5.4	.175	3.0	.432	8.7	.014
		5.8	.148	3.3	.389	9.3	.012
		6.6	.075	3.6	.355	9.6	.0069
		7.0	.054	3.9	.324	9.9	.0062
		7.4	.033	4.5	.242	10.2	.0027
		8.2	.017	4.8	.200	10.8	.0016
		9.0	.0017	5.1	.190	11.1	.00094
				5.4	.158	12.0	.000072

With column groupings: $n = 2$ (first pair), $n = 3$ (second pair), $n = 4$ (last two pairs).

TABLE P Critical Values of the Spearman Test Statistic. Approximate Upper-Tail Critical Values r_s^*, Where $P(r > r_s^*) \leq \alpha$, $\eta = 4(1)30$ Significance Level, α

n	.001	.005	.010	.025	.050	.100
4	—	—	—	—	.8000	.8000
5	—	—	.9000	.9000	.8000	.7000
6	—	.9429	.8857	.8286	.7714	.6000
7	.9643	.8929	.8571	.7450	.6786	.5357
8	.9286	.8571	.8095	.7143	.6190	.5000
9	.9000	.8167	.7667	.6833	.5833	.4667
10	.8667	.7818	.7333	.6364	.5515	.4424
11	.8364	.7545	.7000	.6091	.5273	.4182
12	.8182	.7273	.6713	.5804	.4965	.3986
13	.7912	.6978	.6429	.5549	.4780	.3791
14	.7670	.6747	.6220	.5341	.4593	.3626
15	.7464	.6536	.6000	.5179	.4429	.3500
16	.7265	.6324	.5824	.5000	.4265	.3382
17	.7083	.6152	.5637	.4853	.4118	.3260
18	.6904	.5975	.5480	.4716	.3994	.3148
19	.6737	.5825	.5333	.4579	.3895	.3070
20	.6586	.5684	.5203	.4451	.3789	.2977
21	.6455	.5545	.5078	.4351	.3688	.2909
22	.6318	.5426	.4963	.4241	.3597	.2829
23	.6186	.5306	.4852	.4150	.3518	.2767
24	.6070	.5200	.4748	.4061	.3435	.2704
25	.5962	.5100	.4654	.3977	.3362	.2646
26	.5856	.5002	.4564	.3894	.3299	.2588
27	.5757	.4915	.4481	.3822	.3236	.2540
28	.5660	.4828	.4401	.3749	.3175	.2490
29	.5567	.4744	.4320	.3685	.3113	.2443
30	.5479	.4665	.4251	.3620	.3059	.2400

Note: The corresponding lower-tail critical value for r_s is $-r_s^*$.

ACKNOWLEDGMENTS FOR TABLES

A. From *A Million Random Digits with 100,000 Normal Deviates* by The Rand Corporation, the Free Press, Glencoe, Ill., 1955. Reprinted by permission.

E. Reproduced from *Documenta Geigy, Scientific Tables*, Seventh Edition, 1970, courtesy of CIBA-Geigy Limited, Basel, Switzerland.

F. From A. Hald and S. A. Sinkbaek, "A Table of Percentage Points of the X^2 Distribution," *Skandinavisk Aktuarietidskrift*, *33* (1950), 168–175. Used by permission.

G. From *Biometrika Tables for Statisticians*, Third Edition, Vol. I, Bentley House, London, 1970. Reprinted by permission.

H. From *Biometrika Tables for Statisticians*, Third Edition, Vol. I, Bentley House, London, 1970. Used by permission.

J. Entries for $A = 3$, $B = 3$ through $A = 15$, $B = 2$ from Table 38 of E. S. Pearson and H. O. Hartley, *Biometrika Tables for Statisticians*, Volume 1, Third Edition, London: The Syndics of the Cambridge University Press, 1966. Entries for $A = 16$, $B = 16$ through $A = 20$, $B = 1$ from R. Latscha, "Tests of Significance in a 2×2 Contingency Table: Extension of Finney's Table," *Biometrika*, 40 (1953), 74–86; used by permission of the Biometrika Trustees.

K. From Frank Wilcoxon, S. K. Katti, and Roberta A. Wilcox, "Critical Values and Probability Levels for the Wilcoxon Rank Sum Test and the Wilcoxon Signed Rank Test," Originally prepared and distributed by Lederle Laboratories Division, American Cyanamid Company, Pearl River, New York, in cooperation with the Department of Statistics, The Florida State University, Tallahassee, Florida. Revised October 1968. Copyright 1963 by the American Cyanamid Company and the Florida State University. Reproduced by permission of S. K. Katti.

L. Adapted from L. R. Verdooren, "Extended Tables of Critical Values for Wilcoxon's Test Statistic," *Biometrika*, 50 (1963), 177–186. Used by permission of the author and E. S. Pearson on behalf of the Biometrika Trustees. The adaptation is due to W. J. Conover, *Practical Nonparametric Statistics*, Wiley, New York, 1971, 384–388.

M. From L. H. Miller, "Table of Percentage Points of Kolmogorov Statistics," *Journal of the American Statistical Association*, 51 (1956), 111–121. Reprinted by permission of the American Statistical Association. The table as reprinted here follows the format found in W. J. Conover, *Practical Nonparametric Statistics*, © 1971, by John Wiley & Sons, Inc.

N. From W. H. Kruskal and W. A. Wallis, "Use of Ranks in One-Criterion Analysis of Variance," *Journal of the American Statistical Association*, 47 (1952), 583–621; errata, ibid., 48 (9153), 907–911. Reprinted by permission of the American Statistical Association.

O. From M. Friedman, "The Use of Ranks to Avoid the Assumption of Normality Implicit in the Analysis of Variance," *Journal of the American Statistical Association*, 32 (1937), 675–701. Reprinted by permission.

P. From Gerald J. Glasser and Robert F. Winter, "Critical Values of the Coefficient of Rank Correlation for Testing the Hypothesis of Independence," *Biometrika* 48 (1961), 444–448. Used by permission. The table as reprinted here contains corrections given in W. J. Conover, *Practical Nonparametric Statistics*, © 1971, by John Wiley & Sons, Inc.

Answers to Odd-Numbered Exercises

· · · · · · · · · · · · · · ·

Chapter 2

2.3.1.

Class Interval	Frequency	Relative Frequency	Cumulative Frequency	Cumulative Relative Frequency
0– 9	102	.5025	102	.5025
10–19	52	.2562	154	.7586
20–29	25	.1232	179	.8818
30–39	12	.0591	191	.9409
40–49	7	.0345	198	.9754
50–59	3	.0148	201	.9901
60–69	0	.0000	201	.9901
70–79	2	.0098	203	1.0000
	203	1.0000		

2.3.3.

Class Interval	Frequency	Relative Frequency	Cumulative Frequency	Cumulative Relative Frequency
0–249	4	.0702	4	.0702
250–499	29	.5088	33	.5790
500–749	11	.1930	44	.7720
750–999	8	.1404	52	.9124
1000–1249	4	.0702	56	.9826
1250–1499	0	.0000	56	.9826
1500–1749	1	.0175	57	1.0000
Total	57	1.0000		

2.3.5.

Class Interval	Frequency	Relative Frequency
0–2	5	.1111
3–5	16	.3556
6–8	13	.2889
9–11	5	.1111
12–14	4	.0889
15–17	2	.0444
	45	1.0000

2.3.7.

Class Interval	Frequency	Relative Frequency
110–139	8	.0516
140–169	16	.1032
170–199	46	.2968
200–229	49	.3161
230–259	26	.1677
260–289	9	.0581
290–319	1	.0065
	155	1.0000

2.3.9.

Hospital A: Stem	Leaf	Hospital B: Stem	Leaf
17	1	12	5
18	4	13	5
19	15	14	35
20	11259	15	02445
21	233447	16	5678
22	2259	17	38
23	389	18	466
24	589	19	0059
		20	3
		21	24

2.5.1. (a) 1.8269 (b) 1.74 (c) 1.57; 1.74 (d) 1.19 (e) .09807308 (f) .31316621 (g) 17.142
2.5.3. (a) 73.52941176 (b) 72 (c) 69; 76; 84 (d) 26 (e) 76.76470588 (f) 8.761547 (g) 11.916
2.5.5. (a) 31 (b) 31.5 (c) 28; 35 (d) 12 (e) 11.78947368 (f) 3.4335803 (g) 11.076
2.7.1. $\bar{x} = 14.1059$, $s^2 = 177.071648$, $s = 13.3068$, Median = 9.451, Modal class: 0–9
2.7.3. $\bar{x} = 549.9386$, $s^2 = 89207.39348$, $s = 298.6761$, Median = 460.7069, Modal class: 250–499
2.9.5. (a) 6.53 (b) 5.85 (c) 15.1182 (d) 3.89.
2.9.7. $\bar{x} = 203.8548$, Median = 204.0918, $s^2 = 1368.4126$, $s = 36.9921$.

Review Exercises

13. $\bar{x} = 27.0476$, $s^2 = 8.347619$, $s = 2.8892$, Median $= 26$

17.

Age	Relative Frequency	Cumulative Frequency	Cumulative Relative Frequency
20–29	.101289	55	.101289
30–39	.171271	148	.272560
40–49	.208103	261	.480663
50–59	.165746	351	.646409
60–69	.156538	436	.802947
70–79	.134438	509	.937385
80–89	.053407	538	.990792
90–99	.009208	543	1.000000
Total	1.000000		

$\bar{x} = 52.4278$, $s^2 = 307.972321$, $s = 17.5491$, Median $= 51.0667$

19. Weight: $\bar{x} = 72.63$, Median $= 69.75$, $s^2 = 142.5636$, $s = 11.94$, C.V. $= 16.4395$

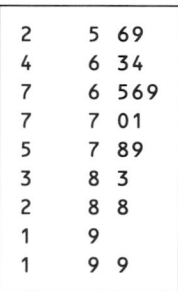

```
          2     5  69
          4     6  34
          7     6  569
          7     7  01
          5     7  89
          3     8  3
          2     8  8
          1     9
          1     9  9
```

```
                    --------------------
        -----------I        +        I-----------------------
                    --------------------
     --+---------+---------+---------+---------+---------+----Weight
      56.0      64.0      72.0      80.0      88.0      96.0
```

Height: $\bar{x} = 176.57$, Median $= 174.5$, $s^2 = 119.0281$, $s = 10.91$, C.V. $= 6.1788$

```
          2    16  14
          4    16  89
          7    17  344
          7    17  57
          5    18  034
          2    18  5
          1    19
          1    19
          1    20
          1    20  5
```

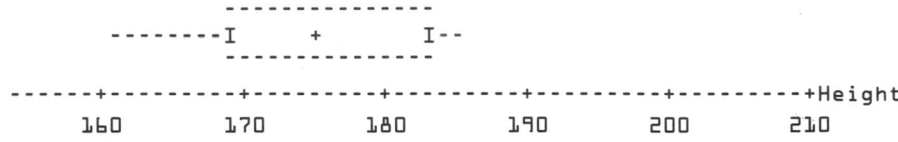

23. $\bar{x} = 3.803$, $s^2 = .243334$, $s = .493289$
25. Method 1:

$Q_1 = 22.8$, $Q_2 = 30.65$, $Q_3 = 42.40$

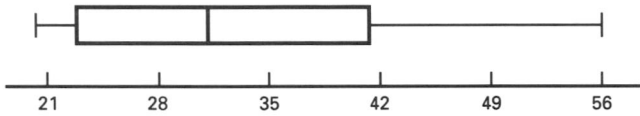

Method 2:

$Q_1 = 23.20$, $Q_2 = 28.30$, $Q_3 = 40.03$

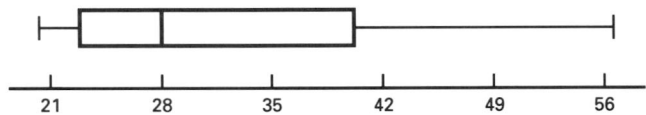

Chapter 3

3.4.1. (a) .2857 (b) marginal (d) .0559 (e) joint (f) .1043 (g) conditional (h) .5149 (i) addition rule
3.4.3. (a) clerical and able-bodied (b) clerical or able-bodied or both (c) clerical given that he/she is able-bodied (d) clerical
3.6.5. .95.
3.6.7. .301.

Review Exercises

3. (a) .1935 (b) .4752 (c) .0427 (d) .5452
7. (a) .22, .5, .055, .11, .59 (b) .3, .39, .39, .17, .07, .6
9. (a) .6, .27, .13, .25 for each area, .92, .35 (b) .01, .4, .75, .48, .08, .6
11. .006
13. .0625

Chapter 4

4.3.1. (a) .1199 (b) .9237 (c) .0763 (d) .8012
4.3.3. (a) .2219 (b) .3883 (c) .7599 (d) .8856 (e) .0012
4.3.5. 4.5, 3.15
4.3.7. (a) .001 (b) .027 (c) .972 (d) .271 (e) .972 (f) .729
4.4.1. (a) .176 (b) .384 (c) .440 (d) .427
4.4.3. (a) .105 (b) .032 (c) .007 (d) .440
4.4.5. (a) .086 (b) .946 (c) .463 (d) .664 (e) .026

4.6.1. .4236.
4.6.3. .2912
4.6.5. .0099
4.6.7. .95
4.6.9. .901
4.6.11. -2.54
4.6.13. 1.77
4.6.15. 1.32
4.7.1. (a) .6826 (b) .6915 (c) .5675
4.7.3. (a) .3446 (b) .3446 (c) .5762
4.7.5. (a) .3413 (b) .1056 (c) .0062 (d) .3830
4.7.7. (a) .0630 (b) .0166 (c) .7719

Review Exercises

15. .1719
17. (a) .0916 (b) .0905 (c) .9095 (d) .1845 (e) .2502
19. (a) .762 (b) .238 (c) .065
21. (a) .0668 (b) .6247 (c) .6826
23. (a) .0013 (b) .0668 (c) .8931
25. 57.10
27. (a) 64.75 (b) 118.45 (c) 130.15 (d) 131.8
29. 14.90
31. 10.6

Chapter 5

5.3.1. 211, 12.7279
5.3.3. (a) .1814 (b) .8016 (c) .0643
5.3.5. (a) .5 (b) .7333 (c) .9772
5.3.7. $\mu_{\bar{x}} = 5$; $\sigma_{\bar{x}}^2 = 3$
5.3.9. (a) .0853 (b) .0104 (c) .7973
5.4.1. .2578
5.4.3. .0038
5.4.5. .0139
5.5.1. .8135
5.5.3. .0217
5.5.5. (a) .1539 (b) .3409 (c) .5230
5.6.1. .008
5.6.3. .8622

Review Exercises

11. .8664
13. .0011
15. .0082
17. .7575
19. .1401
21. Normally distributed
23. .0166
25. 25, 1.4

Chapter 6

6.2.1. (a) 88, 92 (b) 87, 93 (c) 86, 94
6.2.3. (a) 7.63, 8.87 (b) 7.51, 8.99 (c) 7.28, 9.22
6.2.5. 1576.125, 1919.125
6.3.1. (a) 2.1448 (b) 2.8073 (c) 1.8946 (d) 2.0452
6.3.3. (a) 2 (b) 5.8175, 12.1825
6.3.5. (a) 66.2, 76.8 (b) 65.1, 77.9 (c) 62.7, 80.3
6.4.1. (a) .1035, 17.2964 (b) 8.1324, 29.2676 (c) -6.3316, 23.7316
6.4.3. (a) 13.7446, 22.4776 (b) 12.9085, 23.3137 (c) 11.2627, 24.9594
6.4.5. .0880, 1.0320
6.4.7. 2.1, 4.5; 1.8, 4.8; 1.3, 4.8
6.4.9. 24.7, 33.2
6.5.1. .1511, .1995
6.5.3. .035, .221
6.6.1. .0566, .2424
6.6.3. $-.0210$, .2348
6.7.1. 27, 16
6.7.3. 19
6.8.1. 683, 1068
6.8.3. 385, 289
6.9.1. .2061, .5872
6.9.3. 630, 307.86 $< \sigma^2 <$ 1,878, 027.08; 793.92 $< \sigma <$ 1,370.41
6.9.5. 1.37 $< \sigma^2 <$ 4.35; 1.17 $< \sigma <$ 2.09
6.9.7. 170.98503 $< \sigma^2 <$ 630.65006
6.10.1. .7186, 24.3392
6.10.3. .49 $< (\sigma_1^2/\sigma_2^2) <$ 2.95
6.10.5. .90 $< (\sigma_1^2/\sigma_2^2) <$ 3.52
6.10.7. 5.1263398 $< (\sigma_U^2/\sigma_N^2) <$ 60.298059

Review Exercises

13. $\bar{x} = 79.87$, $s^2 = 28.1238$, $s = 5.30$, 76.93, 82.81
15. $\hat{p} = .30$, .19, .41
17. $\hat{p}_1 = .20$, $\hat{p}_2 = .54$, .26, .42
19. $\hat{p} = .90$, .87, .93
21. $\bar{x} = 19.23$, $s^2 = 20.2268$, 16.01, 22.45
23. -12.219, -7.215
25. 7.2301, 7.5499
27. -107.3093, 429.3093
29. .2294, .3666
31. Level of confidence decreases. The interval would have no width. The level of confidence would be zero.
33. t, 1.6
35. All patients with primary atrial arrhythmias who are refractory to antiarrhythmic medications. Such patients who were available to the researchers.

Chapter 7

7.2.1. Do not reject H_0, since $-.51 > -1.28$. $p = .3085$
7.2.3. Reject H_0, since 3.5355 > 2.998. $p < .005$
7.2.5. Yes, $z = -5.73$. $p < 0.0001$
7.2.7. No, $t = -1.5$. $.05 < p < .10$

7.2.9. Yes, $z = 3.08$. $p = .0010$

7.2.11. $z = 4$, $p < .0001$

7.2.13. $t = .1271$, $p > .20$

7.2.15. $z = -4.18$. Reject H_0. $p < .0001$

7.2.17. $z = 1.67$. $p = 2(.0475) = .0950$

7.2.19. $z = -4$. $p < 0.0001$

7.3.1. Reject H_0, since $2.68 > 2.33$. $p = .0037$

7.3.3. Reject H_0, since $5.6506 > 2.0423$. $p > .01$

7.3.5. Do not reject H_0. $z = 1.40$, $p = 2(.0808) = .1616$

7.3.7. $s_p^2 = 5421.25$, $t = -6.66$. Reject H_0. $p < 2(.005) = .010$

7.3.9. $z = -3.39$ Reject H_0. $p = 2(1 - .9997) = .0006$

7.3.11. $t = -3.3567$, $p < .01$

7.4.1. Reject H_0, since $6.111 > 2.583$. $p < .005$

7.4.3. Do not reject H_0, since $2.3242 < 2.3646$. $.10 > p > .05$

7.4.5. Reject H_0, since $3.9506 > 2.9768$. $p < .01$

7.5.1. Do not reject H_0, since $1.62 < 1.645$. $p = .0526$

7.5.3. Reject H_0, since $3.17 > 1.645$. $p = .0008$

7.5.5. $z = -2.64$. $p = .0041$

7.6.1. Reject H_0, since $4.22 > 2.33$. $p < .0001$

7.6.3. Reject H_0, since $2.03 > 1.645$. $p = .0212$

7.7.1. Do not reject H_0, since $4.5187 > 3.325$. $.05 < p < .10$

7.7.3. $\chi^2 = 6.75$ Do not reject H_0. $p > .05$ (two-sided test)

7.7.5. $\chi^2 = 28.8$ Do not reject H_0. $p > .10$

7.7.7. $\chi^2 = 22.036$. $.10 > p > .05$

7.8.1. Reject H_0, since $8.7707 > 2.85$. $p < .005$

7.8.3. No, V.R. $= 1.83$, $p > .10$

7.8.5. Reject H_0. V.R. $= 4$, $.01 < p < .025$

7.8.7. V.R. $= 2.1417$, $p > .10$

7.9.1.

Alternative Value of μ	β	Value of Power Function $1 - \beta$
516	.9500	.0500
521	.8461	.1539
528	.5596	.4404
533	.3156	.6844
539	.1093	.8907
544	.0314	.9686
547	.0129	.9871

7.9.3.

Alternative Value of μ	β	Value of Power Function $1 - \beta$
4.25	.9900	.0100
4.50	.8599	.1401
4.75	.4325	.5675
5.00	.0778	.9222
5.25	.0038	.9962

7.10.1. $n = 548$; $C = 518.25$. Select a sample of size 548 and compute $\bar{x}$. If $\bar{x} \geq 518.25$, reject H_0. If $\bar{x} < 518.25$, do not reject H_0.

7.10.3. $n = 103$; $C = 4.66$. Select a sample of size 103 and compute $\bar{x}$. If $\bar{x} \geq 4.66$, reject H_0. If $\bar{x} < 4.66$, do not reject H_0.

Review Exercises

19. Reject H_0, since $2.4910 > 1.7530$. $.025 > p > .01$
21. Reject H_0, since $2.15 > 1.96$. $p = .0316$
23. $\bar{d} = .40$, $s_d^2 = .2871$, $s_d = .54$, $t = 2.869$, $.005 < p < .01$
25. $z = 1.095$, $.1379 > p > .1357$
27. $t = 3.873$, $p < .005$
29. $\bar{d} = 11.49$, $s_d^2 = 256.6790$, $s_d = 16.02$, $t = 2.485$, $.025 > p > .01$
31. Reject H_0, since $-2.286 < -1.7530$. $.01 > p > .005$

Chapter 8

8.2.1. V.R. $= 5.09$, $p = .009$.

$$HSD^* = 3.39\sqrt{18187/23} = 95.33 \, (q \text{ obtained by interpolation})$$

Since $419.9 - 305.0 = 114.9 > 95.33$, $\bar{x}_1 - \bar{x}_2$ is significant.

$$HSD^* = 3.39\sqrt{18187/15} = 118.04$$

Since $419.9 - 329.3 = 90.6 < 118.04$, $\bar{x}_1 - \bar{x}_2$ is not significant.
Since $329.3 - 305.0 = 24.3 < 118.04$, $\bar{x}_2 - \bar{x}_3$ is not significant.

8.2.3. V.R. $= 13.39$, $p = .000$.

$$HSD^* = 3.52\sqrt{27607/8} = 206.78 \, (q \text{ obtained by interpolation})$$

Since $685.9 - 617.4 = 68.5 < 206.78$, $\bar{x}_1 - \bar{x}_2$ is not significant.

$$HSD^* = 3.52\sqrt{27607/6} = 238.77$$

Since $1048.0 - 685.9 = 362.1 > 238.77$, $\bar{x}_1 - \bar{x}_3$ is significant.
Since $1048.0 - 617.4 = 430.6 > 238.77$, $\bar{x}_2 - \bar{x}_3$ is significant.

8.2.5. V.R. $= 41.19$, $p = .000$.
HSD(HSD*) $= 4.64\sqrt{.616/3} = 2.10$ for all tests. Reject H_0 for all tests except:
$\mu_1 - \mu_5, \mu_2 - \mu_3, \mu_2 - \mu_4, \mu_3 - \mu_4, \mu_5 - \mu_6$.

8.2.7. V.R. $= 61.69$, $p = .000$.

$$HSD^* = 3.36\sqrt{14/31} = 2.26$$

Since $11.839 - 8.154 = 3.685 > 1.26$, $\bar{x}_1 - \bar{x}_2$ is significant.
Since $11.839 - 2.640 = 9.199 > 2.26$, $\bar{x}_2 - \bar{x}_3$ is significant.

$$HSD^* = 3.36\sqrt{14/39} = 2.01$$

Since $8.154 - 2.640 = 5.514 > 2.01$, $\bar{x}_1 - \bar{x}_3$ is significant.

8.2.9. Total $df = 76$, Treatment $df = 3$, Within (Error) $df = 73$. $p < .005$
8.3.1. V.R. $= 21.826$, $p < .005$
8.3.3. Yes V.R. $= 30.22$, $p < .005$
8.3.5. V.R. $= 7.37$, $.025 > p > .01$

8.3.7. Total $df = 41$, Block (Dogs) $df = 5$, Treatments (Times) $df = 6$, Error $df = 30$
8.4.1. V.R. $= 2.43$, $p > .10$
8.4.3. V.R. $= 21.08$, $p < .005$
8.4.5. Total $df = 19$, Block (Subject) $df = 4$, Treatment (Time) $df = 3$, Error $df = 12$
8.5.1. WT1: V.R. (Homo) $= 18.066$, $p < .005$; V.R. (CU) $= 2.872$, $.05 < p < .10$; V.R. (Int) 1.265, $p > .10$. TDS: V.R. (Homo) $= 53.727$, $p < .005$; V.R. (CU) $= .694$, $p > .10$; V.R. (Int) $= 4.554$, $.025 < p < .05$. TDI: V.R. (Homo) $= 61.274$, $p < .005$; V.R. (CU) $= .000$, $p > .10$; V.R.(Int) $= 2.451$, $p > .10$

Review Exercises

13. V.R. $= 11.13$, $p < .005$. $q(.05) = 3.77$, obtained by interpolation. The sample mean for the control subjects is significantly different from the means of the other three categories. No other differences between sample means are significant.
15. V.R. $= .825$. Do not reject H_0. $p > .10$
17. V.R. $(A) = 6.325$, $.005 < p(A) < .01$, $p(B) < .005$, $.01 > p(AB) > .005$; V.R. $(B) = 38.856$; V.R. $(AB) = 4.970$
19. V.R. $= 14.4364$, $p < .005$
21. V.R. $= 6.32049$, $.01 > p > .005$
23. V.R. $= 3.1187$, $.05 > p > .025$. No significant differences among individual pairs of means
25. V.R. $(A) = 29.4021$, $p < .005$; V.R. $(B) = 31.4898$, $p < .005$; V.R. $(AB) = 7.11596$, $p < .005$
27. 499.5, 9, 166.5, 61.1667, 2.8889, 57.6346, $< .005$
29. (a) Completely randomized, (b) 3, (c) 30, (d) No, because $1.0438 < 3.35$
31. V.R. $= 26.06$, $p = .000$. HSD $= 2.4533$. All differences significant except $\mu_{\text{Light}} - \mu_{\text{Moderate}}$
33. V.R. $= 10.974$, $p < .005$
35. Treatment $df = 1$, Error $df = 28$, Total $df = 29$ (assuming an equal number of subjects in each group)
37. For each of the two groups established after the first observation, we have a repeated measures design. If the two groups are analyzed separately, the degrees of freedom in each group are: Subject $df = 15$, Time $df = 2$, Error $df = 14$, Total $df = 31$. It would be more appropriate to analyze the data as a factorial experiment (the two factors being intervention status and time) with repeated measures on one of the factors (time). This type of analysis is not covered in this textbook.

Chapter 9

9.3.1. (a) Direct, (b) Direct, (c) Inverse
9.3.3. $\hat{y} = -1.66 + 7.44x$
9.3.5. $\hat{y} = 2.16 + .953x$
9.3.7. $\hat{y} = 25.8 + .726x$
9.4.1. $C(4.59 \leq \beta \leq 10.29) = .95$

Predictor	Coef	Stdev	t-ratio	p
Constant	-1.6636	0.7646	-2.18	0.047
X	7.440	1.330	5.59	0.000
$s = 0.8657$	R-sq $= .691$	R-sq(adj) $= .669$		

Analysis of variance

Source	df	SS	Ms	F	p
Regression	1	23.444	23.444	31.28	0.000
Error	14	10.493	0.750		
Total	15	33.938			

9.4.3. $C(.9017 \leq \beta \leq 1.0034) = .95$

Predictor	Coef	Stdev	t-ratio	p
Constant	2.157	1.647	1.31	0.194
X	0.95257	0.02551	37.34	0.000
$s = 7.653$	R-sq $= .950$	R-sq(adj) $= .950$		

Analysis of variance

Source	df	SS	MS	F	p
Regression	1	81658	81658	1394.11	0.000
Error	73	4276	59		
Total	74	85934			

9.4.5. $C(.5588 \leq \beta \leq .8931) = .95$

Predictor	Coef	Stdev	t-ratio	p
Constant	25.770	7.494	3.44	0.001
X	0.72596	0.08287	8.76	0.000
$s = 11.10$	R-sq $= .641$	R-sq(adj) $= .633$		

Analysis of variance

Source	df	SS	MS	F	p
Regression	1	9451.1	9451.1	76.74	0.000
Error	43	5296.1	123.2		
Total	44	14747.2			

9.5.1. (a) 3.1833, 4.6490 (b) 1.9199, 5.9124
9.5.3. (a) 57.5215, 61.1015 (b) 43.8982, 74.7248
9.5.5. (a) 94.49, 102.24 (b) 75.65, 121.09
9.7.1. $r = .8019$, $t = 6.29$, $p = .000$, $C(.586 < \rho < .910) = .95$
9.7.3. Opiate: $r = .19855$, $p = .0316$, $C(.03 < \rho < .53) = .95$ Cocaine: $r = -.38423$,
　　　　$p = .0049$, $C(-.12 > \rho > -.59) = .95$
9.7.5. $r = -.8099$, $t = -12.43$, $p = .000$, $C(-.72 > \rho > -.88) = .95$

Review Exercises

17. $r = .405$, $t = 2.97$, $p < .01$

19. $\hat{y} = 0.62 + 0.0830x$

Predictor	Coef	Stdev	t-ratio	p
Constant	0.618	1.043	0.59	0.595
X	0.08301	0.01818	4.57	0.020
$s = 1.456$	R-sq $= 87.4\%$	R-sq(adj) $= 83.2\%$		

Analysis of variance

Source	df	SS	MS	F	p
Regression	1	44.176	44.176	20.84	0.020
Error	3	6.359	2.120		
Total	4	50.535			

21. $\hat{y} = 1.2714 + .8533x$, $r^2 = .6878$, $t = 5.35$

Source	SS	df	MS	V.R.
Regression	1.6498	1	1.6498	28.64
Residual	.7489	13	.0576	
Total	2.3987	14		

23. $\hat{y} = 61.8819 + .509687x$; V.R. $= 4.285$; $.10 > p > .05$; $t = 2.07$; $.10 > p > .05$. Approximate 95% confidence interval for ρ: $-.03, .79$; 110.3022; $87.7773, 132.8271$.

25. $\hat{y} = 37.4559 + .0798579x$; V.R. $= 73.957$; $p < .005$; $t = 8.6013$; $p < .01$. Approximate 95% confidence interval for ρ: $.80, .99$; $40.6150, 42.2826$.

Chapter 10

10.3.1. $\hat{y} = 7.95 - .0101x_1 - .148x_2$

10.3.3. $\hat{y} = 13.45 + 4.02x_1 + 2.81x_2$

10.3.5. $\hat{y} = -422.00 + 11.17x_1 - .63x_2$

10.4.1.

Predictor	Coef	Stdev	t-ratio	p
Constant	7.948	1.108	7.17	0.000
LOS	-0.010053	0.003453	-2.91	0.012
PAI	-0.14823	0.04883	-3.04	0.010
$s = 0.9861$	R-sq $= .610$	R-sq(adj) $= .550$		

Analysis of variance

Source	df	SS	MS	F	p
Regression	2	19.7965	9.8983	10.18	0.002
Error	13	12.6410	0.9724		
Total	15	32.4375			

10.4.3. (a) .67

(b)

Source	SS	df	MS	V.R.	p
Regression	452.56	2	226.28	7.05	$.01 < p < .025$
Residual	224.70	7	32.10		
Total	677.26	9			

(c) $t(b_1) = 3.75$; $(p < .01)$; $t(b_2) = 2.04$, $(.05 < p < .10)$

10.4.5. (a) .31

(b)

Source	SS	df	MS	V.R.	p
Regression	17,023.01	2	8,511.505	4.89	$.01 < p < .025$
Residual	38,276.99	22	1,739.86		
Total	55,300.00	24			

(c) $t(b_1) = 3.05$, $(p < .01)$; $t(b_2) = -.67$, $(p > .20)$

10.5.1. C. I.: 2.425, 3.522. P. I.: .773, 5.174

10.5.3. (a) $50.41 \pm (2.3646)(5.67)$

$$\times \sqrt{\tfrac{1}{10} + (.035757)(-1.99)^2 + (.059206)(.44)^2 + 2(.022857)(-.199)(.44)}$$

(b) Add 1 under the radical.

10.5.5. (a) $532.90 \pm 2.0739(41.71)$

$$\times \sqrt{\tfrac{1}{25} + (.007678)(-.52)^2 + (.00506)(-2.12)^2 + 2(.000002)(-.52)(-2.12)}$$

(b) Add 1 under the radical.

10.6.1. (a) Correlation Matrix

	PRISM	PSI	TISS	NUMIS	$\dot{V}02$	TUN	BCAA
PRISM	1.0000	0.9363	0.6662	0.7740	0.8319	0.8103	−0.5440
PSI	0.9363	1.0000	0.6415	0.6677	0.7190	0.7930	−0.4147
TISS	0.6662	0.6415	1.0000	0.8002	0.6084	0.8259	−0.7013
NUMIS	0.7740	0.6677	0.8002	1.0000	0.6955	0.7108	−0.6262
V02	0.8319	0.7190	0.6084	0.6955	1.0000	0.6813	−0.7806
TUN	0.8103	0.7930	0.8259	0.7108	0.6813	1.0000	−0.6603
BCAA	−0.5440	−0.4147	−0.7013	−0.6262	−0.7806	−0.6603	1.0000

(b) $R = .7681146$, $F = 3.84$, $.10 > p > .05$

(c)

```
R ( NUMIS , TUN . V02 , BCAA ) = .4226
R ( NUMIS , V02 . TUN , BCAA ) = .3036
R ( NUMIS , BCAA . TUN , V02 ) = -.0688
```

(d)

```
R ( PRISM , TUN . V02 , BCAA ) = .7490
R ( PRISM , V02 . TUN , BCAA ) = .8016
R ( PRISM , BCAA . TUN , V02 ) = .6148
```

(e)

$$
\begin{array}{l}
R\ (\ PSI\ ,\ TUN\ .\ \dot{V}O2\ ,\ BCAA\ )\ =\ .7644 \\
R\ (\ PSI\ ,\ \dot{V}O2\ .\ TUN\ ,\ BCAA\ )\ =\ .7012 \\
R\ (\ PSI\ ,\ BCAA\ .\ TUN\ ,\ \dot{V}O2\ )\ =\ .6548
\end{array}
$$

(f)

$$
\begin{array}{l}
R\ (\ TISS\ ,\ TUN\ .\ \dot{V}O2\ ,\ BCAA\ )\ =\ .6793 \\
R\ (\ TISS\ ,\ \dot{V}O2\ .\ TUN\ ,\ BCAA\ )\ =\ -.1493 \\
R\ (\ TISS\ ,\ BCAA\ .\ TUN\ ,\ \dot{V}O2\ )\ =\ -.3801
\end{array}
$$

10.6.3. (a) $R = .9517$, $F = 57.638$, $p < .005$

(b), (c) $r_{y1.2} = .9268$, $t = 8.549$, $p < .01$; $r_{y2.1} = .3785$, $t = 1.417$, $.20 > p > .10$; $r_{12.y} = -.1789$, $t = -.630$, $p > .20$

Review Exercises

7. $R = .3496\ F = .83\ (p > .10)$

9. (a) $\hat{y} = 11.43 + 1.26x_1 + 3.11x_2$

(b) $R^2 = .92$

(c)

Source	SS	df	MS	V.R.	p
Regression	1827.004659	2	913.50	69.048	< .005
Residual	158.728641	12	13.23		
	1985.7333	14			

(d) $\hat{y} = 11.43 + 1.26(10) + 3.11(5) = 39.56.$

11. $\hat{y} = -126.487 + .176285x_1 - 1.56304x_2 + 1.5745x_3 + 1.62902x_4$

(b)

Source	SS	df	MS	V.R.	p
Regression	30873.80	4	7718.440	13.655	< .005
Residual	5774.92	10	577.492		
	36648.72	14			

(c) $t_1 = 4.3967$; $t_2 = -.77684$; $t_3 = 3.53284$; $t_4 = 2.59102$

(d) $R^2_{y.1234} = .8424255$; $R_{y.1234} = .911784$

13. $\hat{y} = -.246 + .005SM1 + .00005P_{max}$

15. $r^2 = (.43)^2 = .1849$

Chapter 11

11.2.1. $\hat{y} = 2.06 + .48x_1 + .177x_2$

Less than .5: $\hat{y} = 2.06 + .48x_1$

Greater than .5: $\hat{y} = 2.237 + .48x_1$

$R - sq = .259$, $R - sq(adj) = .239$

Analysis of variance

Source	df	SS	MS	F	p
Regression	2	48.708	24.354	13.43	0.000
Error	77	139.609	1.813		
Total	79	188.317			

Since $p = .596$ for $t = .53$, conclude that the difference between outputs between the two methods may not have any effect on the ability to predict Td from a knowledge of TEB.

11.2.3. $\hat{y} = 29.9 + 11.7x_1 + 6.37x_2$.

Female: $\hat{y} = 36.27 + 11.7x_1$.

Male: $\hat{y} = 29.9 + 11.7x_1$.

$R - sq = .215$, $R - sq(adj) = .084$

Analysis of variance

Source	df	SS	MS	F	p
Regression	2	282.49	141.25	1.65	0.234
Error	12	1030.22	85.85		
Total	14	1312.72			

Since $p = .209$ for $t = 1.33$, conclude that gender may have no effect on the relationship between mexiletine and theophylline metabolism.

11.3.1. Summary of Stepwise Procedure for Dependent Variable COUNT

Step	Variable Entered	Removed	Number In	Partial R^2	Model R^2	F	Prob > F
1	NETWGT		1	0.1586	0.1586	5.4649	0.0265
2	NOTBIG2		2	0.1234	0.2820	4.8138	0.0367
3	MAXDOSE		3	0.0351	0.3171	1.3867	0.2492
4		NETWGT	2	0.0335	0.2836	1.3230	0.2601
5	NOTBIG		3	0.0519	0.3355	2.1089	0.1580
6		NOTBIG	2	0.0519	0.2836	2.1089	0.1580

11.3.3.

```
STEPWISE REGRESSION OF    GEW   ON   7 PREDICTORS, WITH N.=    28
    STEP                    1               2               3
CONSTANT               4.8213          5.5770          0.6937

BMPR2                   0.307           0.391           0.401
T-RATIO                 2.96            4.19            4.89

SX                                     -1.02           -0.88
T-RATIO                                -3.18           -3.07

GG                                                      1.51
T-RATIO                                                 2.88

S                       0.886           0.762           0.671
R-SQ                   25.16           46.72           60.40
```

11.4.1. Partial SAS printout:

Variable	DF	Parameter Estimate	Odds Ratio
INTERCPT	1	-2.9957	
GOODNUT	1	3.2677	26.250

Review Exercises

15. $\hat{y} = 1.87 + 6.3772x_1 + 1.9251x_2$

Coefficient	Standard Error	t
1.867	.3182	5.87
6.3772	.3972	16.06
1.9251	.3387	5.68
$R^2 = .942$		

Source	SS	df	MS	VR
Regression	284.6529	2	142.3265	202.36954
Residual	17.5813	25	.7033	
	302.2342	27		

17. $\hat{y} = -1.1361 + .07648x_1 + .7433x_2 - .8239x_3 - .02772x_1x_2 + .03204x_1x_3$

Coefficient	Standard Deviation	t	p^a
-1.1361	.4904	-2.32	$.05 > p > .02$
.07648	.01523	5.02	$< .01$
.7433	.6388	1.16	$> .20$
$-.8239$	.6298	-1.31	$.20 > p > .10$
$-.02772$	.02039	-1.36	$.20 > p > .10$
.03204	.01974	1.62	$.20 > p > .10$

[a]Approximate. Obtained by using 35 df.

$R^2 = .834$

Source	SS	df	MS	VR
Regression	3.03754	5	.60751	34.04325
Residual	.60646	34	.01784	
	3.64400	39		

$$x_2 = \begin{cases} 1 \text{ if } A \\ 0 \text{ if otherwise} \end{cases} \qquad x_3 = \begin{cases} 1 \text{ if } B \\ 0 \text{ if otherwise} \end{cases}$$

For A: $\hat{y} = (-1.1361 + .7433) + (.07648 - .02772)x_1 = -.3928 + .04875x_1$
For B: $\hat{y} = (-1.1361 - .8239) + (.07648 + .03204)x_1 = -1.96 + .10852x_1$
For C: $\hat{y} = -1.1361 + .07648x_1$
19. $\hat{y} = 2.016 - .308x_1 - .104x_2 + .00765x_3 - .00723x_4$

Chapter 12

12.3.1. $X^2 = 2.072 \, p > .005$
12.3.3. $X^2 = 3.417 \, p > .10$
12.3.5. $X^2 = 2.21 \, p > .10$
12.4.1. $X^2 = 28.553$, $p < .005$ Combining last two rows: $X^2 = 26.113$, $p < .005$
12.4.3. $X^2 = 14.881$, $p < .005$
12.4.5. $X^2 = 42.579$, $p < .005$

12.5.1. $X^2 = 8.575$, $.10 > p > .05$

12.5.3. $X^2 = 9.821$, $p < .005$

12.5.5. $X^2 = 82.373$ with 2 d.f. Reject H_0. $p < .005$

12.6.1. Since $b = 6 > 4$ (for $A = 19$, $B = 14$, $a = 13$), $p < 2(.027) = .054$. Do not reject H_0.

12.6.3. Since $b = 4 < 8$ (for $A = 13$, $B = 12$, $a = 13$), $p = .039$. Reject H_0 and conclude that chance of death is higher among those who hemmorage.

12.7.1. $\widehat{RR} = 1.1361$, $X_2 = .95321$. 95% C. I. for RR: .88, 1.45. Since the interval contains 1, conclude that RR may be 1.

12.7.3. $\widehat{OR} = 2.2286$, $X^2 = 3.25858$, $p > .05$. 95% C. I. for OR: .90, 11.75.

12.7.5. $\chi^2_{MH} = 5.2722$, $.025 > p > .01$. $OR = 3.12$

Review Exercises

15. $X^2 = 7.004$, $.01 > p > .005$

17. $X^2 = 2.40516$, $p > .10$

19. $X^2 = 5.1675$, $p > .10$

21. $X^2 = 67.8015$ $p < .005$

23. $X^2 = 7.2577$ $.05 > p > .025$

25. Independence

27. Homogeneity

29. Since $b = 4 > 1$ (for $A = 8$, $B = 5$, $a = 7$), $p > 2(.032) = .064$

31. $X^2 = 3.893$, $p > .10$

Chapter 13

13.3.1. $P = .3036$, $p = .3036$

13.3.3. $P(x \leq 2 | 13, .5) = .0112$. Since $.0112 < .05$, reject H_0. $p = .0112$

13.4.1. $T_+ = 48.5$. $.1613 < p < .174$

13.4.3. Let $d_i = A_i - B_i$. H_0: $\mu_d \leq 0$, H_A: $\mu_d > 0$. $T_+ = 55$, Test statistic $= T_- = 0$. $p = .0010$. Reject H_0.

13.5.1. $X^2 = 16.13$, $p < .005$.

13.6.1. $S = 177.5$, $T = 111.5$. $w_{1-.001} = 121 - 16 = 105$. Since $111.5 > 105$, reject H_0 at the .002 level.

13.6.3. $S = 65.5$, $T = 10.5$, $.005 < p < .01$

13.7.1. $D = .3241$, $p < .01$

13.7.3. $D = .1319$, $p > .20$

13.8.1. $H = 13.12$ (adjusted for ties), $p < .005$

13.8.3. $H = 15.06$ (adjusted for ties), $p < .005$

13.8.5. $H = 23.28$ (adjusted for ties), $p < .005$

13.8.7. $H = 19.55$, $p < .005$

13.9.1. $\chi^2_r = 8.67$, $p = .01$

13.9.3. $\chi^2_r = 25.42$, $p < .005$

13.10.1. $r_s = -0.07$, $p > .20$

13.10.3. $r_s = -.534$, $.005 > p > .001$

13.10.5. $r_s = -.610$, $.01 > p > .005$

13.10.7. $r_s = .6979$

$.002 < p < .010$

13.11.1. $\hat{\beta} = 1.429$

$\hat{\alpha}_{1,M} = -176.685$

$\hat{\alpha}_{2,M} = -176.63$

Review Exercises

7. $P(X \leq 1 \mid 10, .5) = 1 - .9893 = .0107$, $p = .09127$
9. $\chi_r^2 = 16.2$, $p < .005$
11. $D = .1587$, $p > .20$
13. $r_s = .6397$, $p < .005$

Chapter 14

14.2.1. (a) 10.4 (b) 10.1, 11.0 (c) 16.1 (d) 21.5 (e) 16.9 (f) 47.6 (g) 15.2, 27.3
14.3.1. (a) 97.0, 165.4, 125.0, 62.4, 5.8, 3.5
      (b) 2413 (c) 405, 1312, 1937, 2249, 2378, 2413
      (d) 76.5

INDEX